Coronary Restenosis

FUNDAMENTAL AND CLINICAL CARDIOLOGY

1. *Drug Treatment of Hyperlipidemia*, edited by Basil M. Rifkind
2. *Cardiotonic Drugs: A Clinical Review, Second Edition, Revised and Expanded*, edited by Carl V. Leier
3. *Complications of Coronary Angioplasty*, edited by Alexander J. R. Black, H. Vernon Anderson, and Stephen G. Ellis
4. *Unstable Angina*, edited by John D. Rutherford
5. *Beta-Blockers and Cardiac Arrhythmias*, edited by Prakash C. Deedwania
6. *Exercise and the Heart in Health and Disease*, edited by Roy J. Shephard and Henry S. Miller, Jr.
7. *Cardiopulmonary Physiology in Critical Care*, edited by Steven M. Scharf
8. *Atherosclerotic Cardiovascular Disease, Hemostasis, and Endothelial Function*, edited by Robert Boyer Francis, Jr.
9. *Coronary Heart Disease Prevention*, edited by Frank G. Yanowitz
10. *Thrombolysis and Adjunctive Therapy for Acute Myocardial Infarction*, edited by Eric R. Bates
11. *Stunned Myocardium: Properties, Mechanisms, and Clinical Manifestations*, edited by Robert A. Kloner and Karin Przyklenk
12. *Prevention of Venous Thromboembolism*, edited by Samuel Z. Goldhaber
13. *Silent Myocardial Ischemia and Infarction: Third Edition*, Peter F. Cohn
14. *Congestive Cardiac Failure: Pathophysiology and Treatment*, edited by David B. Barnett, Hubert Pouleur, and Gary S. Francis

15. *Heart Failure: Basic Science and Clinical Aspects*, edited by Judith K. Gwathmey, G. Maurice Briggs, and Paul D. Allen
16. *Coronary Thrombolysis in Perspective: Principles Underlying Conjunctive and Adjunctive Therapy*, edited by Burton E. Sobel and Désiré Collen
17. *Cardiovascular Disease in the Elderly Patient*, edited by Donald D. Tresch and Wilbert S. Aronow
18. *Systemic Cardiac Embolism*, edited by Michael D. Ezekowitz
19. *Low-Molecular-Weight Heparins in Prophylaxis and Therapy of Thromboembolic Diseases*, edited by Henri Bounameaux
20. *Valvular Heart Disease*, edited by Muayed Al Zaibag and Carlos M. G. Duran
21. *Implantable Cardioverter-Defibrillators: A Comprehensive Textbook*, edited by N. A. Mark Estes III, Antonis S. Manolis, and Paul J. Wang
22. *Individualized Therapy of Hypertension*, edited by Norman M. Kaplan and C. Venkata S. Ram
23. *Atlas of Coronary Balloon Angioplasty*, Bernhard Meier and Vivek K. Mehan
24. *Lowering Cholesterol in High-Risk Individuals and Populations*, edited by Basil M. Rifkind
25. *Interventional Cardiology: New Techniques and Strategies for Diagnosis and Treatment*, edited by Christopher J. White and Stephen R. Ramee
26. *Molecular Genetics and Gene Therapy of Cardiovascular Diseases*, edited by Stephen C. Mockrin
27. *The Pericardium: A Comprehensive Textbook*, David H. Spodick
28. *Coronary Restenosis: From Genetics to Therapeutics*, edited by Giora Z. Feuerstein

ADDITIONAL VOLUMES IN PREPARATION

The Endothelium in Clinical Practice: Source and Target of Novel Therapies, edited by Gabor M. Rubanyi and Victor J. Dzau

Molecular Biology of Cardiovascular Disease, edited by Andrew R. Marks and Mark B. Taubman

Coronary Restenosis

From Genetics to Therapeutics

edited by

Giora Z. Feuerstein
SmithKline Beecham Pharmaceuticals
King of Prussia, Pennsylvania

Marcel Dekker, Inc. New York•Basel•Hong Kong

Library of Congress Cataloging-in-Publication Data

Coronary restenosis: from genetics to therapeutics / edited by Giora
Z. Feuerstein.
p. cm.— (Fundamental and clinical cardiology ; 28)
Includes index.
ISBN 0-8247-9767-1 (hardcover : alk. paper)
1. Coronary artery stenosis—Pathophysiology. 2. Transluminal angioplasty—Complications. 3. Coronary artery stenosis—Molecular aspects. I. Feuerstein, Giora Z. II. Series. III. Series: Fundamental and clinical cardiology ; v. 28. [DNLM: 1. Coronary Disease—physiopathology. 2. Coronary Disease-therapy. 3. Coronary Thrombosis—physiopathology. 4. Recurrence. W1 FU538TD v.28 1997 / WG 300 C8262 1997]
RC685.C58C6926 1997
616.1'23—dc20
DNLM/DLC
for Library of Congress 96-43176
CIP

The publisher offers discounts on this book when ordered in bulk quantities. For more information, write to Special Sales/Professional Marketing at the address below.

This book is printed on acid-free paper.

Marcel Dekker, Inc.
270 Madison Avenue, New York, New York 10016

Current printing (last digit):
10 9 8 7 6 5 4 3 2 1

PRINTED IN THE UNITED STATES OF AMERICA

To my wife, Nili, my son, Ron, and my daughter, Sheira, for their faithful support of my work.

Series Introduction

Marcel Dekker, Inc., has focused on the development of various sets of beautifully produced books in different branches of medicine. These series have facilitated the integration of rapidly advancing information for both the clinical specialist and the researcher.

My goal as editor of the Fundamental and Clinical Cardiology series is to assemble the talents of world-renowned authorities to discuss virtually every area of cardiovascular medicine. In the current monograph, *Coronary Restenosis: From Genetics to Therapeutics*, Dr. Giora Z. Feuerstein has edited a much needed and timely book. Future contributions to this series will include books on molecular biology, interventional cardiology, and clinical management of such problems as coronary artery disease and ventricular arrhythmias.

Samuel Z. Goldhaber

Preface

Modern medicine is a discipline founded on the premise that humans can alleviate their suffering from diseases by interventions that alter the cause and course of the disease. Over the past two millennia, humans developed diverse ways to interfere with diseases by using physical, chemical, mental, and, most recently, genetic means aimed at improving the quality and duration of life. However, in the course of proactive interventions in disease processes, undesired consequences are often produced while attempting to gain benefits. This experience led ancient medical practitioners to caution, "primum non nocera," a warning to the medical profession to avoid harm prior to considering intervention.

In today's medicine, new interventions are required to establish a clinically acceptable "therapeutic index"—meaning that benefits clearly must surpass any liabilities or harmful consequences to the patient. This philosophy also underwrites the charters of modern regulatory agencies, which seek "safety and efficacy" as the basis for drug or device approval for medical use.

With this in mind, *Coronary Restenosis: From Genetics to Therapeutics* reflects the reality of modern interventional cardiology—mitigating the consequences of an old disease, atherosclerosis, while at the same time eliciting a new pathology, restenosis. The need to relieve obstructions to blood flow in essential blood vessels such as the coronary arteries has led to novel and powerful interventions that produce rapid relief from life-threatening events such as abrupt vessel obstruction. PTCA, stents, and other interventions have proven to be of great benefit to patients in danger of death from myocardial infarction. In particular, the use of PTCA and stents is currently a common practice in many medical centers, with success rates of over 96%, and minimal hospitalization time, morbidity, and mortality. The only real "shadow" cast over this modern success in conquering coronary (and other vessel) obstruction and heart attacks is the phenomenon of restenosis, or, simply, reocclusion of vessels that have been successfully opened by direct mechanical intervention.

Restenosis is a new disease, one of many that medicine has encountered en route to introducing physical (e.g., radiation) or chemical (drugs) agents for therapeutic use. Restenosis, however, was not a predicted liability (unlike consequences to chemotherapy or radiation), because the pathology underlying restenosis differs substantially from the pathology of the disease leading to the obstruction of the blood vessel in the first place, namely, atherosclerosis and thrombosis. Restenosis is a significant medical problem because it occurs in a large proportion of patients (30–50%) undergoing PTCA or stent placement, may result in morbidity and mortality, and adds significant burden on medical costs.

Why does restenosis occur? A definitive answer to this question has not yet been delivered, but significant strides have been made in understanding major components in the evolution of restenosis. This book is designed to provide the reader with a state-of-the-art review of five aspects of the problem. First, it highlights the key conceptual underpinnings of research on restenosis, with emphasis on the mechanisms of "neointima formation" (a key event in restenosis) and elaborates on the phenomenon of vascular remodeling, a fundamental process that shapes the overall capacity of blood vessels to respond to physiological and pathological conditions. In this respect, the authors must be commended for a clear and succinct review of the molecular and cellular events that shape the vessel wall in response to injuries introduced by mechanical interventions (PTCA, stents).

Second, this book provides the readers with an updated and comprehensive review of the pharmacology of restenosis. This area is of particular importance since no drug has received regulatory agency approval for treatment of restenosis, in spite of enormous basic research, animal experimentation, and costly clinical trials. Better understanding of the role of animal models in pharmacological studies of restenosis is necessary, and careful analyses of the benefits and limitations of animal models of restenosis are essential for effective progression of pharmacological agents into clinical practice.

Third, the role of thrombosis in restenosis is of great interest and importance, since blood cells and blood-borne factors play a key role in initiation and propagation of many of the processes in neointima formation and vascular remodeling in response to injury. Several chapters address the issue of thrombosis in restenosis, where the role of platelets and coagulation factors is reviewed, and strategies for interventions in various aspects of the coagulation cascade and platelet aggregation are evaluated. The importance of thrombosis in acute occlusion of vessels subjected to intervention has recently been demonstrated by clinical trials with ReoPro (an antibody that blocks the platelet fibrinogen receptor, GPIIb/IIIa), which have shown significant efficacy in reducing morbidity and mortality in patients undergoing PTCA (EPIC trial). However, it is still unclear whether ReoPro (or other antithrombotic agents) is capable of combating the restenosis process per se.

Fourth, this book aims to carefully document all key issues concerning clinical trials in restenosis. In particular, patient selection, protocol design, and surrogate and clinical end points are reviewed carefully vis-á-vis the numerous trials conducted so far. In addition, the book provides insights into unmet clinical needs that should drive development of improved PTCA and stent technologies as well as targets for adjunct medical treatment and better interventions.

Finally, this book addresses the potential of gene therapy in restenosis. Gene (or DNA) therapy is an emerging concept and technology, in which extensive research is being conducted for cardiovascular disease. In fact, two protocols are currently being pursued where human genes are deployed for improved vascularization (e.g., VEGF gene transfer for enhanced vascularization), which hopefully will help pave the way for future gene therapy. A simple and straightforward description of the technologies available for gene therapy is laid out, the pros and cons of various delivery systems are explained, and examples of success (proof of hypothesis) in in vivo animal models are provided. While this form of restenosis therapy may not be available for some time, it is important for researchers and clinicians to become familiar with this technology.

The objectives of this book are presented in a consecutive format, by experts in each particular field. The material was selected for a diverse audience, and obviously was not designed to provide an exhaustive review of all published reports; rather, emphasis has been placed on conceptual frameworks underscoring research trends, analysis of main issues and directions in both preclinical and clinical investigations, and setting the stage for future opportunities in both intervention technology, pharmacology, and genomic medicine.

We hope that this unique and stimulating approach to the problem of restenosis will help basic scientists to readily identify research directions and novel targets for therapeutics and help clinicians to better design and execute productive clinical trials. This book will also be useful for graduate students in various biology disciplines as well as physicians-in-training who seek rapid introduction to the multiple dimensions of this new medical condition—restenosis.

Giora Z. Feuerstein

Contents

Contributors

Karen M. Anderson, Ph.D. Associate Senior Investigator, Department of Cardiovascular Pharmacology, SmithKline Beecham Pharmaceuticals, King of Prussia, Pennsylvania

H. Vernon Anderson, M.D. Associate Professor of Medicine, Cardiology Division, University of Texas Health Science Center, Houston, Texas

Juan J. Badimon, Ph.D. Associate Professor of Medicine, The Cardiovascular Institute, Mount Sinai Medical Center, New York, New York

Lina Badimon The Cardiovascular Institute, Mount Sinai Medical Center, New York, New York

Michelle P. Bendeck, Ph.D. Assistant Professor of Medicine and Pathology, St. Michael's Hospital and University of Toronto, Toronto, Ontario, Canada

Mary E. Brawner Department of Gene Expression Sciences, SmithKline Beecham Pharmaceuticals, King of Prussia, Pennsylvania

Peter Carmeliet Adjunct Director and Associate Professor, Center for Transgene Technology and Gene Therapy, Flanders Interuniversity Institute for Biotechnology, Leuven, Belgium

James H. Chesebro The Cardiovascular Institute, Mount Sinai Medical Center, New York, New York

Désiré Collen Flanders Interuniversity Institute for Biotechnology, Leuven, Belgium

Stephen A. Douglas, B.Sc., M. Phil., Ph.D. Department of Cardiovascular Pharmacology, SmithKline Beecham Pharmaceuticals, King of Prussia, Pennsylvania

David Eccleston, M.B.B.S. Cleveland Clinic Foundation, Cleveland, Ohio

Giora Z. Feuerstein, M.D. Department of Cardiovascular Pharmacology, SmithKline Beecham Pharmaceuticals, King of Prussia, Pennsylvania

Valentin Fuster The Cardiovascular Institute, Mount Sinai Medical Center, New York, New York

Richard Gallo, M.D., F.R.C.P.(C). Research Associate, The Cardiovascular Institute, Mount Sinai Medical Center, New York, New York

David P. Hajjar Cornell University Medical College, New York, New York

Richard Hayes The Cardiovascular Institute, Mount Sinai Medical Center, New York, New York

Osamu Hori Columbia University College of Physicians and Surgeons, New York, New York

William R. Huckle, Ph.D. Senior Research Biochemist, Merck Research Laboratories, West Point, Pennsylvania

Bernard E. Ilson, M.D., A.A.C.P. Director, Clinical Research, SmithKline Beecham Pharmaceuticals, and Assistant Clinical Professor of Medicine, University of Pennsylvania, Philadelphia, Pennsylvania

Robert K. Jackson, D.V.M. SmithKline Beecham Pharmaceuticals, King of Prussia, Pennsylvania

Robert G. Johnson, Jr., M.D., Ph.D. Director, Department of Pharmacology, Merck Research Laboratories, West Point, Pennsylvania

Diane K. Jorkasky, M.D., F.A.C.P. Vice President, Clinical Pharmacology, SmithKline Beecham Pharmaceuticals and Associate Clinical Professor of Medicine, University of Pennsylvania, Philadelphia, Pennsylvania

Robert J. Kaner Cornell University Medical College, New York, New York

Arvinder S. Kurbaan, M.B., M.R.C.P. Department of Invasive Cardiology, Royal Brompton Hospital and National Heart and Lung Institute, London, England

Calvert Louden, Ph.D. SmithKline Beecham Pharmaceuticals, King of Prussia, Pennsylvania

Andrew J. Nichols Department of Advanced Technologies in Genetics, SmithKline Beecham Pharmaceuticals, King of Prussia, Pennsylvania

Andrew C. Nicholson, D.V.M., Ph.D. Department of Pathology, Cornell University Medical College, New York, New York

Eliot H. Ohlstein SmithKline Beecham Pharmaceuticals, King of Prussia, Pennsylvania

Michael A. Reidy, Ph.D. Professor, Department of Pathology, University of Washington, Seattle, Washington

Robert R. Ruffolo, Jr., Ph.D. Vice President, Pharmacological Sciences, SmithKline Beecham Pharmaceuticals, King of Prussia, Pennsylvania

Ann Marie Schmidt Columbia University College of Physicians and Surgeons, New York, New York

Robert S. Schwartz, M.D. Professor, Department of Medicine, Mayo Clinic and Mayo Foundation, Rochester, Minnesota

Stephen M. Schwartz, M.D., Ph.D. Professor, Department of Pathology, University of Washington, Seattle, Washington

U. Sigwart Director, Department of Invasive Cardiology, Royal Brompton Hospital and National Heart and Lung Institute, London, England

Jeffrey M. Stadel, Ph.D. Associate Director, Department of Cardiovascular Pharmacology, SmithKline Beecham Pharmaceuticals, King of Prussia, Pennsylvania

David Stern Professor, Department of Physiology, Columbia University College of Physicians and Surgeons, New York, New York

Eric J. Topol, M.D. Chairman and Professor, Department of Cardiology, Cleveland Clinic Foundation, Cleveland, Ohio

XinKang Wang Associate Senior Investigator, Department of Cardiovascular Pharmacology, SmithKline Beecham Pharmaceuticals, King of Prussia, Pennsylvania

Robert N. Willette, Ph.D. Senior Investigator, Department of Cardiovascular Pharmacology, SmithKline Beecham Pharmaceuticals, King of Prussia, Pennsylvania

Shi Du Yan Columbia University College of Physicians and Surgeons, New York, New York

Tian-Li Yue, Ph.D. Senior Investigator, Department of Cardiovascular Pharmacology, SmithKline Beecham Pharmaceuticals, King of Prussia, Pennsylvania

Coronary Restenosis

1

Restenosis: Basic Research and Clinical Perspective

Giora Z. Feuerstein
SmithKline Beecham Pharmaceuticals, King of Prussia, Pennsylvania

Almost 20 years ago practicing cardiologists were introduced to a revolutionary technology for treatment of coronary artery disease—percutaneous transluminal coronary angioplasty (PTCA) (1). Prior to the "PTCA era," coronary artery bypass graft (CABG) surgery and palliative medical therapy were the primary medical practices for angina pectoris (a symptom emanating from high stenosis of coronary vessels), which offered no remedy for the arterial disease itself. The introduction of PTCA has dramatically reduced the morbidity and mortality from coronary artery disease (CAD) as the practice spread from a few highly specialized centers in the late 1970s to numerous cardiology clinics performing an estimated million procedures worldwide.

PTCA (and its stent variants) is a highly successful procedure, having reached in many centers a success rate of over 90%. The major acute risk of the procedure—abrupt occlusion of the vessel by thrombosis and/or recoil—has been aggressively dealt with by antithrombotic agents (aspirin, heparin, ticlopidine, and GPIIb/IIIa antagonists such as ReoPro) and vasodilators. However, shortly after the introduction of PTCA, it became clear that even in the hands of the most skillful interventionalists practicing in the best "high-throughput" facilities, repeated interventions had to be offered within 6–12 months of the original procedure. The need for late repeated interventions was recognized as a consequence of the formation of a new layer of intimal tissue (marked by cellularity and abundance of matrix)—the "neointima" formation—and/or failure of "remodeling" processes that result in vessel enlargement and increase in lumen size.

Restenosis is commonly referred to as the process where a stenotic coronary artery, which regained significant patency following mechanical intervention, reverts to its former state of insufficient lumen diameter (practically $\geq$ 50% loss of the gain by PTCA, stent, or atherectomy). Coronary restenosis is an iatrogenic disease, i.e., it is initiated by the very procedure aimed to increase coronary patency to provide critical blood flow to the heart. This process is believed to be a fundamental response to injury elicited within the manipulated blood vessel wall.

The importance of restenosis is apparent by its consequences: significant patient morbidity and medical costs. Of the estimated 500,000 coronary interventions (PTCA/stents) conducted in the United States in 1995, 30–50% of the patients experienced relapse of their primary disease within 6–12 months following the intervention, to the extent that repeated interventions had to be offered. At an estimated total cost of about $10,000 per procedure ($5,000–$15,000) and a minimum of 30% rate of secondary (repeated) intervention per year, the estimated annual medical cost of restenosis exceeds $1.5 billion.

Furthermore, morbidity and mortality of secondary procedures are higher than the primary ones, and often CABG becomes the procedure of choice, marked by significant additional costs and patient morbidity. Taken together, this entirely unexpected phenomenon of restenosis has had a major impact on the overall management of atherosclerotic CAD and the long-term success of PTCA, stents, and atherectomies.

It is, therefore, no surprise that restenosis became a target of intense basic and clinical research to explore its underlying mechanisms, clarify the risk factors to develop restenosis, and, most important, contemplate strategies to prevent restenosis by improved device technology and pharmacological/medical treatments. In this book, the key areas in restenosis research conducted over the past 10 years will be highlighted and analyzed.

Two major schools of thought emerged that point toward two very different pathomechanisms in restenosis. The first one emphasizes the growth of new intimal tissue (neointima formation), which infringes on the vessel lumen and ultimately results in reocclusion of the artery. The second research hypothesis points toward a vascular remodeling phenomenon—the process of enlargement of the injured vessel that prevents occlusion (in spite of neointima formation)—as the important event in securing critical

Table 1 Comparative Effects on Restenosis (Animal vs. Human Models)

Drug	Rat	Rabbit	Pig	Baboon	Human[a]
Carvedilol	+		-		-
Cilazapril	+	+	-	-	-
Enoxaparin		+	E		-
Lovastatin	+	+			-
Prostacyclin		+			-
Hirudin		E	+		-
N-3FAs				+	-
Angiopeptin		+	+		E

-, No significant effect; +, effective; E, equivocal.
[a]Randomized placebo-control double-blind trial (phase III).

lumen volume. Thus, failure of appropriate remodeling may also contribute to reocclusion.

Nevertheless, it is clear that the injury to the arterial wall induced by PTCA, stents, or other interventions elicits numerous biochemical, molecular, and cellular reactions in the blood vessel wall, including gene expression, metabolic and synthetic processes, cell proliferation, migration and activation, apoptosis, thrombosis, inflammation, coagulation, and immune responses. All these events are under intense investigation and seem to contribute in varying degrees to the overall complex phenomenon of neointima formation, vascular remodeling, and ultimately restenosis.

Significant strides toward understanding the events leading to restenosis have been made over the past 5 years. Basic research efforts have yielded a plethora of opportunities, some of which have already been tested in clinical trials in patients undergoing PTCA. Interestingly, in spite of highly encouraging preclinical data that lay out strong rationale for the potential therapeutic value of many drugs, no clear benefits have been demonstrated in any of the clinical studies conducted to date. Moreover, this reality is highlighted by the marked contrast between the failure to demonstrate the capacity to block restenosis in patients by adjunct medical therapy versus the demonstrated efficacy of the same agents to inhibit restenosis in certain animal models. As shown in Table 1, the lack of demonstrable reduction in restenosis in clinical studies by any drug so far makes it impossible to qualify standard animal models that are used to study the phenomenon of restenosis. These issues are dealt with specifically in several chapters of this book.

While the search for therapeutic agents for restenosis continues (no such agent has been identified as yet), the intensive work on restenosis has already greatly affected two areas of technology: gene therapy and device development. The latter draws from the early success that stent technology has demonstrated in clinical trials to the extent that stents are now the most rapidly growing intervention for treatment of coronary stenosis. Innovative stent technology aimed to minimize vessel injury coupled to sophisticated applications methods that allow for local delivery of pharmacological agents aimed to suppress restenosis are being explored. Equally exciting are the advances in gene therapy that stem from early explorations of the genomic driving force of the restenosis phenomenon, which is marked by robust expression of genes that normally have little or no expression in cellular components of blood vessels. In particular, genes expressing growth factors, cytokines, cell-cycle regulators, transcription and signal-transduction factors (in particular kinases and phosphatases), adhesion molecules and matrix proteins are being explored. The importance of upregulation of new genes in restenosis is exemplified by remarkable research in animal models of restenosis using antisense technology and genetic models (transgenic or gene "knock-out" models) illustrating substantial capacity to tame the process of restenosis by selective suppression of specific genes and their products. These recent discoveries are already being examined in pilot clinical trials aimed to manipulate the restenosis phenomenon using recombinant DNA technology. Thus, attempts to modulate restenosis by transgenes (or recombinant DNA) have emerged at the forefront of cardiovascular gene therapy and will be addressed specifically in this book.

Finally, the scope of issues and themes under investigation by basic and clinical scientists engaged in restenosis research are too broad to be systematically dealt with in this book. Rather than producing an exhaustive compilation of information, we focus on concepts, issues, and research directions that complement and extend recent publications (1–3). In particular, issues concerning vascular remodeling, the hemostatic systems (coagulation, fibrinolysis, and thrombosis), analysis of pharmacological strategies, and clinical issues are the main topics selected for in-depth review. It is also clear that this highly dynamic field is subject to rapid developments, at both the basic research and clinical levels, which hopefully will culminate in successful therapeutic remedies for restenosis.

REFERENCES

1. Gruentzig, A. Transluminal dilatation of coronary artery stenosis. Lancet 1978; 1:263.
2. Schwartz RS. Coronary Restenosis. Blackwell Scientific Publication. Series on Interventional Cardiology, 1993.
3. Schwartz SM, deBois D, OBrien RM. The intima: soil for atherosclerosis and restenosis. Circ Res 1995; 77:445—465.

2

Arterial Remodeling in Disease

Stephen M. Schwartz
University of Washington, Seattle, Washington

I. INTRODUCTION

The cells of the arterial wall comprise a living tissue with complex, biochemical functions. Most attention has been paid to the endothelium. Antithrombotic, anticoagulant, and hemostatic functions and even the permeability functions of the arterial lining depend upon specific structural proteins, receptors, endocrine factors, and enzymes synthesized by the endothelial cell. Smooth muscle cells not only provide a motor to control vessel wall tone, they secrete proteins important to vessel wall structure and synthesize molecules that may control their own growth. Smooth muscle hypertrophy and hyperplasia are central to current concepts of the morphological changes underlying the major diseases involving obstruction of the vascular lumen: atherosclerotic vascular disease and hypertension (1,2). In contrast to the endothelium, much less is known about the molecules that control smooth muscle function. We do know, however, that rearrangement of the layers of arterial smooth muscle by migration or proliferation plays a key role in the ontogeny of vascular disease. This chapter will consider how these rearrangements, often called "remodeling," occur.

II. CELLS OF THE VESSEL WALL

A modern view of vascular pathology must begin by reviewing how endothelial and smooth muscle cells come together to form blood vessels (3). This two-cell composition means that blood vessels have a simpler structure than most other organs. Much of the pathology of blood vessels can be understood by analyzing the function and dysfunction of these two cells.

III. EMBRYONIC DEVELOPMENT OF BLOOD VESSELS

The earliest vascular primordia in the embryo are isolated cells that display endothelial and primitive hematopoietic immunological markers (4). The precursors of endothelium coalesce to form "blood islands" lined with recognizable endothelium. Some of these endothelial sacs also contain primitive blood cells. The islands extend by processes forming hollow tubes and fuse to form a network. The network eventually becomes connected with the heart to form the primitive circulation (5–7).

Investment by smooth muscle cells is a secondary event. The endothelial tubes become surrounded by locally derived, irregularly shaped mesenchymal cells that include the precursors of smooth muscle cells and adventitial fibroblasts (8–11). By the fourth fetal month in humans, the three coats of the arterial wall become clearly evident. Cell layers delimited by elastic lamellae become more identifiable in large arteries, and the cells take on a more characteristic structural appearance (12). At parturition, most arteries appear to have developed their adult number of layers of smooth muscle (13). After this stage, the number of layers in the wall does not increase, and the medial thickening is due to the production of connective tissue, increase in cell number, or increase in cell mass (14,15). Expression of the full phenotype of smooth muscle cells, that is, of cells with all of the characteristic contractile proteins, is not seen until the third trimester (16).

The best evidence indicates that endothelial cells signal differentiation of smooth muscle cells from the surrounding embryonic milieu. This hypothesis is supported by studies of isolated and cultured vessel wall cells. Studies from this laboratory attempted to explore the ability of adult bovine endothelial cells to induce changes in the developing chick embryo. These bovine endothelial cells elicited a marked angiogenic response in the chicken system. Bovine fibroblasts and smooth muscle cells were not similarly angiogenic (17). Endothelial cells have also been shown to produce fibroblast growth factor (FGF), a peptide that is angiogenic (18), as well as being mitogenic for smooth muscle cells, and platelet-derived growth factor (PDGF), a peptide that is chemotactic for smooth muscle cells (19–24). Perhaps one of these peptides is responsible for the recruitment of smooth muscle cells. More direct evidence for endothelial induction of a smooth muscle count comes from a recent study of vascular embryology. Using quail chick hybrids, Ekblom et al. (25) showed that smooth muscle cells of the kidney vasculature are derived locally, while the endothelium is derived entirely from endothelial cells in the primitive vessels that vascularize the renal precursor.

The identity of smooth muscle cells remains somewhat confusing. While we generally assume that the smooth muscle cell has a well-defined phenotype, the most characteristic markers of this phenotype are lost when these cells are placed in culture. This is especially true of markers typically expressed late in development, such as myosin or calponin (26–34). Moreover, the marker most commonly cited, smooth muscle α-actin, is certainly not restricted to smooth muscle cells, as smooth muscle α-actin has also been described in bone marrow, hepatocytes, and also in neurons (35–37). Recently, however, evidence has been found for markers that may be shared by all muscle lineages. One of these, a troponinlike molecule called SM-22α, appears to be restricted to smooth muscle in adult animals as demonstrated recently using a promoter construct (34).

IV. LAYERS OF THE ARTERIAL WALL

Atherosclerotic occlusion mainly represents the pathology of the tunica intima of larger muscular arteries. The major cell type between the endothelium and the internal elastic lamina (IEL) is an intimal smooth muscle cell. Other resident cells of the intima include lymphocytes, macrophages, and other inflammatory cells derived from the blood (38–40). Even in large vessels, very little tunica intima is seen at birth; however, the intima thickens as we age (41–43).

Hypertension affects all layers of the vessel, but the most important functional changes are due to pathology of the tunica media, the layer responsible for regulating blood flow. The narrow lumen of these vessels produces an increased resistance, reducing blood pressure to levels appropriate for exchange across the thin-walled capillaries where exchange occurs. Thus, these vessels serve to reduce pressure to maintain systemic capillary levels while increasing systemic pressure by regulation of total peripheral resistance. Pathological change in the ratio of wall thickness to size of the lumen is central to elevation of blood pressure in hypertension (44).

In both hypertension and atherosclerosis, the critical issue is lumen size. This is obvious in hypertension, since peripheral resistance is the product of a decreased lumen size. What may be less apparent is that lumen size is dependent on structural changes in the vessel wall as well as on active vasoconstriction (45). These structural changes in hypertensive microvasculature are called "remodeling," that is, adaptive restructuring of the vessel wall, which also occurs in larger arteries with atherosclerosis. As the intimal plaque increases in mass, the remainder of vessel wall dilates to accommodate the demand for flow (46). The mechanisms underlying remodeling are unknown, although studies by Langille and colleagues (47–50), as well as by Mulvany (45), suggest that endothelial-mediated signaling allows the vessel to respond to changes in flow while the thickness of the vessel wall adjusts to normalize wall tension. Interestingly, the cellular processes responsible for remodeling are also unclear; replication may play a minor role, while rearrangement of vessel wall components and programmed cell death could play critical roles (51).

V. CONTROL OF SMOOTH MUSCLE PROLIFERATION

At least three mechanisms have been proposed for the control of smooth muscle proliferation: control by growth factors released from blood cells, control by inhibitors derived from the vessel wall, or control by growth stimulants produced by the cells of the vessel wall themselves.

Until recently, the predominant hypothesis of proliferation suggested that cell growth was initiated by actions of growth factors derived from platelets or leukocytes. The factor usually discussed was PDGF (1,52). The idea that a platelet factor controlled smooth muscle replication grew out of the observation that smooth muscle cells would not replicate in serum prepared without platelet release (52). This led to the suggestion that PDGF was required for smooth muscle replication. This hypothesis was supported by the observation by Stemerman and others that denudation of arteries by a balloon embolectomy catheter produces intimal proliferation. Immediately after balloon catheterization, the denuded surface shows a prominent platelet carpet (53,54). Antiplatelet serum inhibits the smooth muscle proliferative response (55).

It is important to point out that mitogenic substances other than PDGF may also be present at sites of vascular wall injury (56–58). As already noted, FGF may be released from many cells as these cells are lysed (20). Perhaps most relevant to atherosclerosis, the most obvious stimulus may be a growth factor derived from macrophages. Since these cells accumulate in the intima soon after commencement of a high-fat diet (59–61), monocytes could be critical to smooth muscle proliferation. In vitro, monocytes or macrophages produce several mitogens (62–64).

The most significant growth factors for vascular response to injury may be synthesized by the vessel wall cells themselves. Cultured endothelial cells secrete soluble polypeptide mitogens that can stimulate smooth muscle replication. Part of this activity is due to a material that competes with the PDGF receptor and is neutralized by the PDGF antibody (65). The identity of the non-PDGF mitogen remains unknown (66,67). Although FGF is synthesized by endothelial cells, the protein either is not secreted or remains bound to the extracellular matrix (20,68). The PDGF gene is expressed at high levels by cultured endothelial cells, and expression of the PDGF gene is seen in endothelium in vivo (69). At least in culture, production of PDGF by endothelium appears to be controlled by several factors, including the state of differentiation, exposure to thrombin, or exposure to lipoproteins (19,21,70). We do not know whether levels of PDGF protein production can be altered in vivo. We do know, however, that endothelial cells in atherosclerotic plaques can synthesize message for PDGF-B chain. Barrett and Benditt (71) used Northern hybridization of human carotid artery plaques to detect message in patterns of atherosclerotic plaques. They found mRNA for von Willebrand factor (an endothelial protein), fms (a leukocyte marker), smooth muscle actin, and both PDGF genes. Correlations between the concentrations of these messages suggested that macrophages were the major source of PDGF B-chain, but left open the possibility that endothelium could be involved. Wilcox and collaborators (72) used in situ hybridization on the same tissue and found a high level of B-chain localization, and some A-chain, over small vessels penetrating the plaques. The large masses of macrophages were negative, suggesting that Barrett's Northern blot hybridizations may have been detecting fms in macrophage associated with these small vessels and suggesting that plaque endothelium is the major source of PDGF B-chain message. As noted below, however, plaque smooth muscle cells may also be an important source of these mRNAs. Libby and coworkers extended these studies by cell culture, showing that plaque smooth muscle cells synthesize PDGF-A (73). Ross and colleagues (74) used a monoclonal antibody and came to a somewhat different conclusion. Their data suggested that monocytes were the major source of PDGF-B. They did not study PDGF-A, so the data are not inconsistent with the earlier reports of Wilcox et al. (72) and Libby et al. (73). The prevalence of protein in macrophages and RNA in endothelial cells could mean that there is a difference in translation, storage, or even that macrophages take up PDGF produced by other cells.

Perhaps more surprising is recent evidence that smooth muscle cells themselves may be able to stimulate their own growth by synthesis of FGF, PDGF, and insulin growth factor-1 (IGF-1). Clemmons and colleagues (75) have found that PDGF is able to stimulate smooth muscle cells to produce

IGF-1. This is particularly interesting because of evidence cited above that IGF-1 is a cofactor required by smooth muscle cells for completion of the cell cycle following stimulation with PDGF (76–79). The role of IGF-1 in growth responses of the vessel wall is unexplored. The discovery that cultured smooth muscle cells from fetal rats spontaneously produce PDGF-like material grew out of the observation that growth of smooth muscle cells derived from newborn rat aortas cannot be arrested by putting cells in PDGF-deficient serum (80). The culture medium from these fetal cells stimulates 3T3 cell and smooth muscle cell replication. The mitogen responsible for this activity is inactivated by anti-PDGF antibody and the conditioned medium competes for the PDGF receptor. Thus, it appears likely that fetal smooth muscle cells, at least in one species, can make this important mitogen (80). There is also evidence that adult smooth muscle cells can be induced to produce similar material. As already noted, PDGF is secreted by human smooth muscle cells cultured from plaques (73). Primary cultures of smooth muscle from aorta express A chain message and synthesize a PDGF-like protein, and the A-chain can also be detected in fresh aortic tissue (81,82). With passage, however, cultured rat arterial smooth muscle cells produce low or absent levels of PDGF-like material unless those cells are derived from balloon-injured vessels; these cells produced levels similar to those seen in cultured cells from the immature aorta (83). It is important to point out that since the observations of protein production can only be made on cells placed in culture, there is no direct evidence for comparable levels of production in vivo. Nonetheless, the appearance of activity in cells derived from the balloon-injured vessel and from the human plaque implies that some dramatic change has occurred in the capabilities of the smooth muscle cells making up the injured vessel wall. An intriguing possibility is that this change could be responsible for both the commitment to replication and the maintenance of replication during the days and weeks after injury (84). As with observations of endothelial cell-derived mitogens, interpretation of these observations depends on whether the results reflect some property in vivo. As already noted, Wilcox and colleagues began to address this question using in situ hybridization. These studies have shown localization of PDGF message in two cells within human carotid lesions. One cell type, already noted, is the endothelial lining of the capillaries found inside plaques. The other cell type is the intimal mesenchymal cell, presumably a dedifferentiated smooth muscle cell (72). These results are somewhat surprising, given the high level of PDGF production by macrophages in vitro (52). It will be important to ask whether protein, as well as message, is being produced in the plaques.

In vivo studies of the response to angioplasty may be most relevant to human disease. At least in the rat, several growth factors seem to play a role in the changes occurring after balloon injury. Critical molecules include angiotensin, PDGF, FGF, and transforming growth factor-β (TGF-β). The balloon injury model begins with complete destruction of the endothelium as well as extensive death of medial smooth muscle cells (85). The first response to balloon injury, called "first wave," consists of medial smooth muscle cell proliferation and begins about 24 h after the injury. In elegant studies, Reidy and colleagues have shown that this wave of replication can be completely accounted for by release of basic FGF (bFGF) from dying smooth muscle cells (86, 87). Among other candidate molecules, studies with infused PDGF, as well as studies with anti-PDGF antibodies, have shown that this molecule does not play a significant role as a mitogen (88,89). In addition, other molecules may be active, as more limited data suggest that α-adrenergic antagonists and angiotensin II (AII) can block medical replication (90–92).

Thus, FGF and, perhaps, AII, appear to be critical to mitogenic responses in the rat model of arterial response to injury. However, while we know that these molecules are critical to the initiation of growth, much less is known about how growth continues. Once smooth muscle cells arrive in the intima, they may replicate for weeks to months (93). This replication is called the "third wave." As of the time of writing this review, no specific molecular antagonist has been shown to inhibit this replication. Even antibodies to bFGF, which are so effective in inhibiting the first wave, are impotent against third-wave replication (87). Therefore, although we cannot say that any specific molecule has definitively been identified as a third-wave mitogen, a few potential candidates appear to be present in the intima. For example, PDGF-A chain is overexpressed in the intima but will not stimulate replication if infused, nor do antibodies of PDGF suppress third-wave replication (88,94,95). Other growth control molecules that appear to be overexpressed in the rat neointima include the AII receptor and TGF-β (96,97). IGF-1 is also overexpressed following injury; however, it is overexpressed in the media (98). While we cannot identify the critical molecules that sustain elevated replication in the third wave, we do know that the neointima can be stimulated to show a further increase of replication by infusion of other molecules. This increased responsiveness to mitogens can be called a "fourth wave," and involves at least TGF-β, bFGF, or AII as agonists (86, 90, 96). Again, PDGF does not appear to be mitogenic (88).

The role of the angiotensin system in neointimal formation is of particular relevance because of the failure of extensive clinical trials using angiotensin-converting enzyme (ACE) inhibitors to prevent restenosis (99). With all the evidence from studies in the rat, why did the clinical studies fail? One explanation may lie in a misunderstanding of the pharmacology of converting enzyme inhibitors. Existing studies with ACE inhibitors are inconclusive in part because higher drug doses are needed to achieve significant suppression of intimal thickening (3–30 mg/kg/day) than to obtain a maximal (20%) reduction of blood pressure in the same strain of normotensive rats (3 mg/kg/day) (100). This difference in dosage requirements may reflect the higher doses necessary to achieve inhibition of vascular tissue ACE or to effectively block degradation of bradykinin at the site of injury (101). The latter is of special interest because of evidence that bradykinin elevation as a result of inhibition of the normal catabolism by converting enzyme may act as an endogenous inhibitor of neointimal formation (102). Finally, recent studies have identified a second enzyme able to produce active, AII, chymase. Chymase is present in plaque and could be an important factor in the local production of angiotensin (103,104). The best studied model for in vivo replication, neointimal formation, is the response of the rat carotid artery to balloon angioplasty (54,85,105). It is important to realize that this model is much simpler than the same response in larger, more complex human arteries that already exhibit disease. First, the rat carotid artery has only rare intimal cells (106). Even normal arteries in larger animals have a preexisting intima (107,108). Second, unlike the response of arteries in larger animals, including rabbits, swine, and nonhuman primates, the response of rat arteries to most injuries involves platelets, but there is no deposition of fibrillar fibrin or adherence of leukocytes (109–118). The simplicity of the rat model has made it possible to develop methods for detailed kinetic analyses of the processes leading to neointimal formation and to define four waves of response to injury with the molecules responsible for each of these waves (55, 119–123).

Stimulation of proliferation may not be the whole story. There is also evidence that the vessel wall normally contains inhibitors of smooth muscle proliferation. The best studied of these are proteoglycans belonging to the heparan class. Clowes et al. discovered that exogenous heparin could inhibit proliferation in response to removal of the endothelium (84,122,124). This effect may have mimicked the actions of materials present in the normal vessel wall and identified as crude extracts by previous studies. Nam et al. (125) showed that an aqueous extract of pig aorta injected intraperitoneally into 8-week-old living swine, in quantities as low as 500 g of protein, drastically reduced the rate of entry of arterial smooth muscle cells into mitosis, with no demonstrable effect on epidermal mitosis. Eisenstein et al. (126) reported two classes of molecules derived from bovine aortic extracts that are able to inhibit cell growth. One class, comprised of structural polyanions, including heparans and proteoglycans, inhibited the growth of both smooth muscle and endothelial cells. Alcohol precipitates from aqueous extracts of the pig intima plus media were fractionated to produce both stimulators and inhibitors of synthetic state smooth muscle in culture (127).

The most obvious question is the source of synthesis of such inhibitors. Possible cellular sources are suggested by studies showing that cultured vessel wall cells, including both endothelium and smooth muscle, can synthesize heparan sulfates capable of inhibiting smooth muscle growth (128–131). Smooth muscle cells themselves can synthesize a growth inhibitor for their own growth. Fritze et al. (130), continuing the work of Castellot, have shown that smooth muscle cells also make a growth-inhibitory heparan sulfate. This material is most prominent in quiescent cultures. By analogy to smooth muscle cells in vivo, the quiescent, untraumatized wall may be refractory to stimulation by PDGF (130). It is conceivable that heparan sulfate released from quiescent endothelial cells could inhibit smooth muscle cell proliferation as the region becomes covered with endothelium. Maintenance of the normal wall in a quiescent state could reflect heparan sulfate synthesis by both endothelial cells and smooth muscle cells.

The role of endogenous heparan sulfates in controlling cell proliferation after an arterial wound provides an alternative to the usual hypothesis that growth requires stimulation by release of a mitogen into the injured wall. One could imagine that balloon denudation results in a release of enzymes that digest the extracellular matrix, removing its inhibitory effect and thereby allowing the cells to replicate. Platelets contain a heparan sulfate—degrading endoglycosidase that could act in this way (132–134). Incubation of endothelial cells with a crude platelet enzyme preparation or with a partially purified preparation of heparan sulfate—degrading endoglycosidase from the same source causes a marked release of cell surface heparan sulfate, which appears in the incubation medium as oligosaccharides. Castellot et al. (135) proposed that following endothelial denudation of injury, platelets are deposited on the subendothelium releasing heparitinase, platelet factor 4, and PDGF. The heparitinase cleaves heparinlike substances on the endothelium and smooth muscle into fragments that diffuse away, with additional inactivation of the substance by platelet factor 4 (136). Thus, it is possible that balloon injury allows growth by initiating breakdown of heparan sulfate.

The hypothesis that growth is initiated by platelet-released factors at the site of denuding injury does not easily explain the continuation of proliferation lasting weeks after a balloon injury, while platelet release lasts only hours to days (119,137). Several possibilities exist. The possibility has just been discussed that growth may depend on loss of inhibitors; nothing is known about how long a time would be required to restore endogenous inhibitory factors. Somewhat anecdotal evidence supports the possibility that mitogens might be released from cells within the plaque. Gajdusek and Schwartz reported that dead, cultured smooth muscle cells release a cytoplasmic mitogen distinct from PDGF (138). More recent reports suggest that this material is FGF (20), a suggestion that seems consistent with evidence in vivo that FGF is a critical mitogen following angioplasty. Interestingly, Imai et al. (139) found a high correlation of evidence of cell death and stimulation of smooth muscle proliferation in fat-fed swine. They attributed this correlation to the extent of oxidation in cholesterol preparations used to feed the animals. Thus, cell death and platelet release in the plaque may be synergistic in the release of mitogens and hydrolysis of heparinlike molecules. FGF is very sticky (140,141) and could remain active in the wall for many days. Vlodavsky and colleagues have suggested that FGF in vivo may be stored in a bound form localized in the extracellular matrix (68,142). Smith et al. (143) found that residual PDGF on the culture dish could maintain smooth muscle cell growth for days even in the presence of medium containing no PDGF. FGF, possibly released from dying cells, is also very sticky and might persist in areas of cell death for very long periods of time. The sticky properties of growth factors may explain the claims of Savion et al. (144) that cells can grow on "extracellular matrices" prepared by detergent solubilization of cell cultures grown in the presence of growth factors.

Finally, while we have emphasized replication, formation of an intima also requires the migration of smooth muscle cells across the internal elastic lamina. Smooth muscle cells are readily observed on the luminal side of the internal elastic lamina 4 days after injury (85). The duration of the second wave is not known. Several molecules can contribute to smooth muscle migration, including PDGF, TFG-β, bFGF, and AII. The relative contributions of these different molecules are not known, nor do we know whether other molecules are involved (87,92,96). The migration effect of PDGF is noteworthy, given the indication from in vitro studies that this molecule is a mitogen, despite the apparent lack of mitogenicity in vivo (88). Again, the effects of ACE inhibitors are of special interest because of the widespread clinical use of these drugs and their failure in clinical trials to suppress restenosis. Again, we lack dose-response data. Such data could be vital, because, as discussed above, the effects of ACE inhibitors may result from the ability of these drugs to elevate bradykinin levels by preventing its degradation rather than the expected effect of these agents on lowering levels of AII. ACE inhibitors are not specific of the conversion of AI to AII (102,145–147). Depending on dose, these drugs inhibit degradation of bradykinin, and there is evidence from studies involving bradykinin antagonists that elevation of bradykinin can explain part of the effect of ACE inhibitors on neointimal formation (102; deBlois and Schwartz, unpublished data). Relative dose controlling migration vs. proliferation is not known.

In summary, the emerging picture of growth control in arterial smooth muscle is a complex balance of stimuli and inhibitors of migration and replication. This concept has recently become even more complex with the renewed recognition that cell death also plays a role in intimal formation and turnover (148).

VI. MONOCLONALITY AND ORIGINS OF THE ATHEROSCLEROTIC LESION IN THE INTIMA

As previously discussed, the cells of the tunica intima of arteries include smooth muscle cells and blood-derived white blood cells. This population is the soil in which smooth muscle cells proliferate to form the characteristic morphology of atherosclerosis.

Two different lesions have been proposed as the initial lesion of atherosclerosis (149,150). The simplest is a local accumulation of fat in the vessel wall, resulting in a lesion sometimes referred to as a fatty spot or fatty streak. Alternatively, atherosclerosis may begin with focal accumulations of intimal smooth muscle cells called intimal cell masses.

Fatty streaks can be seen both in young humans and in experimental animals fed high-fat diets. Originally it was thought that the major fatty cell of the lesion was the macrophage. Interest in the macrophage decreased with the discovery in the early 1970s that many fat-filled cells were modified smooth muscle cells (149,151,152). A balanced view today suggests that those cells with the greatest amount of lipid are indeed macrophages; however, smooth muscle cells may also contain fat. Fat-filled macrophages and fat-filled smooth muscle cells are together called "foam cells."

There is reason to believe that the fatty spot is not the initial lesion. Children who die accidentally at a young age will usually show large numbers of fatty spots in many parts of their arterial tree. The distribution of fatty infiltration in children, however, is somewhat unlike the distribution of more characteristic atherosclerotic lesions in adults. For example, fatty infiltration is common in the thoracic aorta, while atherosclerosis in adults is typical in the abdominal aorta. Nonetheless, many people believe that fatty infiltration represents the initial lesion of atherosclerosis with other factors controlling the distribution of the final, more clinically significant lesions (150,153).

The alternative candidate for the initial lesion is the "intimal cell mass" (Fig. 1) (3,154). The intimal cell mass consists of accumulations of smooth muscle cells and associated connective tissue. Intimal cell masses near arterial branch sites are called "cushions." Intimal cell masses may be found in other locations within the intima (154,155). Studies of fat-fed swine, as well as autopsy studies of human tissue, suggest that these focal

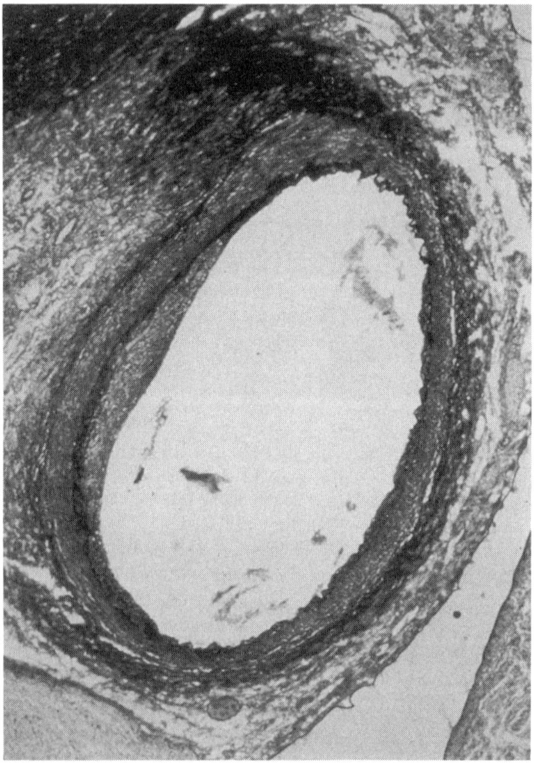

Figure 1 Intimal mass. Small masses like this can be found in a 6-month-old human left or anterior descending artery. These masses may be the progenitors of plaques.

accumulations of smooth muscle cells may have a predilection to the development of atherosclerotic lesions (41,153,154,156).

The presence of intimal cell masses in normal young people suggests that the initial stages of lesion development may occur early in the human life span. Accumulation of smooth muscle cells in the intima, however, is a normal part of the aging process. Arteries from older people show diffuse intimal thickening. Since this is part of the aging process and since it occurs diffusely throughout large arteries, many investigators would like to distinguish "normal" intimal thickening from the focal pathological events leading to atherosclerosis (150).

Despite these reservations, there is compelling evidence that smooth muscle proliferation is an essential part of atherosclerosis and intrinsic to its earliest phases. Morphological studies of fat-fed animals as well as later studies using tritiated thymidine autoradiography demonstrate that smooth muscle proliferation is a major part of the response of animals to fat-feeding (52,157). Moreover, careful cell kinetic studies imply that the proliferative lesion in fat-fed pigs also begins in a preexisting intimal cell mass (154).

While similar isotopic labeling studies have not been done in humans, advanced atherosclerotic lesions have been labeled in vitro with [^{3}H]thymidine using tissue excised into organ culture. These studies suggest that smooth muscle replication at this stage of lesion development is, if anything, quite low (158,159). These data are supported by more recent studies using cell cycle-specific markers to identify replicating cells in atherosclerotic plaques (Fig. 2) (160—164).

Despite these low values from cell kinetic studies, evidence for proliferation in the early stages of human atherosclerotic lesions comes from a surprising direction. Many tumors can be shown to be the result of monoclonal proliferations because the presence of genetic markers specific for only a small number of the cells in the tissue of origin can be used to detect clonal growths. For example, we know that the leiomyoma of the uterus is monoclonal. This conclusion depends upon the fact that a large proportion of African American women are heterozygotic for glucose-6-phosphate dehydrogenase (G6PD). The gene for G6PD is located on the X chromosome. Each female cell turns off one or the other X chromosome early during differentiation. In a heterozygotic individual, each tissue consists of a mosaic of cells, some expressing one allele and others the other allele of G6PD. The mixture of alleles in a cell mass, when compared with the random mixture in the underlying tissue, is a measure of the clonality of proliferation. Benditt utilized this fact to study the origins of human atherosclerotic lesions. He observed that a large proportion of atherosclerotic plaques of vessels in African American females were monoclonal. The individual lesions showed a high preponderance of one or the other allele, well beyond the chance distribution that might be expected from a random selection of large numbers of cells from underlying tissue (165).

Lee and Thomas and their collaborators have offered a different interpretation of monoclonality (154–169). This group has attempted to reconcile the data in humans with their own experimental work in animal models. Extensive cell kinetic analysis of fat-fed swine has been interpreted as showing that smooth muscle proliferation occurs by repetitive waves of replication and cell death. On the basis of a mathematical model, they argued that monoclonality might arise by a repeated resampling of a proliferative population in which several clones have become expanded. While this model might appear attractive mathematically, it is important to point

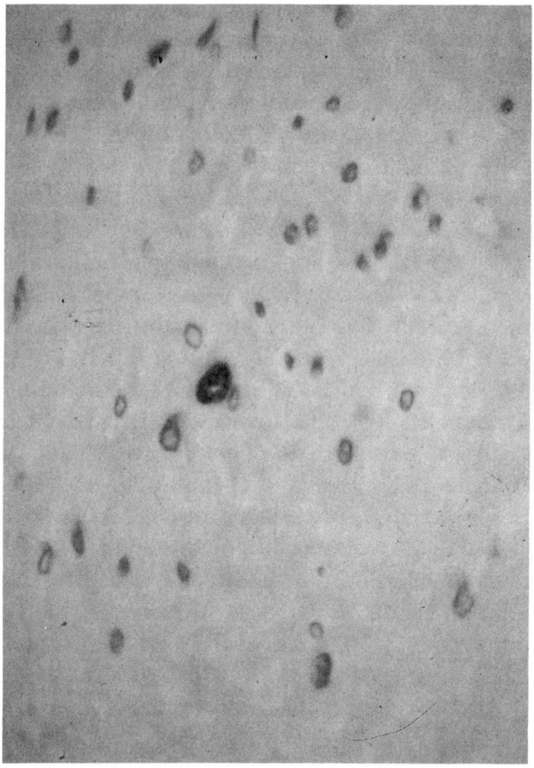

Figure 2 Replicating cells in atherosclerotic plaques. Although human DNA cannot usually be labeled with thymidine derivatives, we can detect replicating cells with antibodies directed at proteins associated with replicating cells of nucleic acid probes, via in situ hybridization, for cell cycle-specific RNAs. This figure shows a rare replicating cell, stained for proliferating cell nucleus antigen, in an atherosclerotic plaque.

out that the group has been unsuccessful in producing monoclonal lesions in fat-fed animals. This experiment was performed in hybrid hares bred between two species differing in the G6PD allotype. The failure to demonstrate monoclonality in the animal model must be seen as a serious reservation in our interpretation of smooth muscle cell proliferation in animal model systems (170–172).

Benditt used monoclonal data as evidence that atherosclerotic lesions are benign neoplasms. Benditt's hypothesis has much to recommend it. By definition, a benign neoplasm is a focal overgrowth of a single cell type.

Benign neoplasms do not metastasize or invade. Thus, a nodule of smooth muscle cells growing in the uterus is called a "leiomyoma." This may seem like semantics, but it is worth noting that if the plaque is comprised of a focal proliferation of smooth muscle cells, then the atherosclerotic plaque is, *by definition,* a benign neoplasm of smooth muscle cells.

The equation of plaques with leiomyomas leads to intriguing questions. For example, Benditt has proposed that the risk associated with smoking might be due to the accumulation of mutagens from cigarette smoke (165). Interestingly, he observed that polycyclic aromatic hydrocarbons distribute in lipoproteins and that human vascular smooth muscle cells respond to chemical mutagens as, of course, might have been expected (173). An additional avenue stimulated by the observation of monoclonality has been the search for possible oncogenic viruses. The Fabricants and their collaborators have reported that the incidence of fatty lesions in chickens is greatly increased by infection with Marek's disease virus (174,175). This is a virus of the herpes group. In collaboration with McDougall, Benditt and Barrett showed that herpesvirus genomes could be detected in atherosclerotic plaques by in situ hybridization (176). This observation has been confirmed by Gyorkey et al. (177). In addition, Melnik et al. reported the presence of cytomegalovirus antigen within human arterial smooth muscle cells and high levels of antibody in the serum of patients undergoing vascular surgery to treat atherosclerosis (178,179).

Benditt's neoplasm hypothesis needs to be considered in the context of current concepts of the control of normal and neoplastic growth. The last decade has seen the identification of a number of proteins, initially identified as mRNA species or as genomic DNA sequences specific for neoplasia. These mammalian genomic species were identified by their presence in transforming retroviruses. The discovery that these were originally derived from mammalian genomic sequences has turned out to be a very powerful tool in understanding the normal replication of the cell. Alterations in the activity of the protein products of these genes, including structural alterations in the protein so as to increase or decrease their activity, as well as alterations in the gene so as to increase or decrease the amount of protein synthesis, may cause severe imbalances that control cell replication and an overproliferation of cells (180). Penn et al. (181) used DNA transfection to demonstrate that there are transforming sequences in human atherosclerotic tissue. This assay depends on the shearing of cellular DNA and the insertion of that DNA into target assay cells, usually the NIH 3T3 cell line. When this is done, there is always a small frequency of transformation (182). An increased frequency of transformation may be seen either when the source DNA contains genomic species that are altered in some way so as to stimulate cell proliferation or when the source DNA is inserted into the recipient cells in such a way as to cause overexpression. Penn et al. (181) found an increased frequency of positive transformants. It is difficult to determine what this means. The sequence responsible for transformation is not known. Even if the sequence were known, the possibility exists that this sequence is a normal cellular gene, somehow made more available for transfection by the content of the plaque. Even that result, however, would illustrate an important point: by elucidating a smooth muscle–derived transforming gene, we might learn more about normal mechanisms of smooth muscle growth control.

In summary, the monoclonal part of the "monoclonal hypothesis" is probably a fact. It is difficult or impossible to see how monoclonality could arise in response, for example, to a diffuse injury. Clonal origin must be among the earliest events in ontogeny of the atherosclerotic plaque. It is important, however, to put this discussion of plaque origins in perspective. First, very few doublings would be required to convert the mass of the normal intima into the mass of an occlusive lesion. Such doublings might occur at rare intervals, intervals too rare to detect by the random samplings we now have. These doublings might even occur in bursts, consistent with angiographic studies that demonstrate rapid growth, or at least loss of lumen, at sites that are initially relatively normal (183). Finally, we also need to consider proliferation of cells other than smooth muscle cells. A recent study from this laboratory shows focal levels of endothelial replication as high as 10% (164). This may be evidence that angiogenesis is a very active and chronic process adding to plaque mass. Finally, while most studies have focused attention on the smooth muscle cell, Gordon et al. found more impressive evidence for macrophage replication than for smooth muscle replication (162). Thus, even if plaques originate as a clonal growth, in the long term, other processes may be more important for determining the mass of the plaque.

VII. DOES PLAQUE REPLICATION NARROW THE LUMEN?

It is not obvious that the result of intimal hyperplasia would be a narrowed lumen. Glagov et al. found that human vessels can undergo massive accumulations of atherosclerotic mass without lumen narrowing (46). The vessel wall compensates for the new mass by dilating to permit a normal level of blood flow until an adaptational limit is exceeded. This limit appears to occur when approximately 40% or more of the area bounded by the internal elastic lamina is occupied by intimal mass. The compensatory dilation is a structural change in the vessel wall and is usually called "remodeling." Decreased lumen size probably does not occur until Glagov's limit is exceeded and may depend on pharmacological mechanisms associated with the neointima or the plaque that cause a failure of normal remodeling events.

Remodeling is a normal response that allows the vessel to maintain normal levels of blood flow and wall stress and can be seen in small muscular arteries as well as in large elastic arteries (44,49). Branching patterns of conduit vessels seem to be genetically determined (184). Thus, the only way arteries can respond to a demand for an increase or decrease in blood flow is by changing vessel caliber. These changes rely on rearrangement of existing vessel wall components rather than synthesis of new mass or cell replication (45). Until recently, the concept of vessel wall remodeling as a part of the response to injury had been largely ignored in animal models of arterial injury and repair. The extent of remodeling versus loss of lumen due to intimal formation is illustrated by an important experiment. When Jamal and colleagues studied the balloon-injured rabbit carotid artery, they found no narrowing of the lumen despite a 100% increase in wall thickness (49). The same study, however, showed a significant (14%) narrowing in response to an experimental restriction of flow in the vicinity of the thyroid artery where endothelium had regenerated. This effect of the endothelium in an injured vessel is consistent with observations that structural adaptation to changes in flow requires an endothelium (49). Since reendothelialization generally correlates with a diminution of intimal thickening, these data may even imply a negative correlation of intimal mass with luminal narrowing (185). The role of the endothelium in controlling lumen size may be especially important given the often neglected fact that plaques have a prominent microcirculation comprised of capillaries arising from the adventitia (186–188). The role of these small vessels in regulating structural change, or, for that matter, contractile properties of the atherosclerotic vessel, remains unexplored. As shown in Figure 3, endothelium may play a similar role in vascular remodeling after angioplasty.

If the correlation of intimal (or plaque) mass with lumen caliber is not a simple one, how do we account for angiographic changes seen after aggressive lipid-lowering therapy (189–191)? The actual degree of improvement of stenosis diameter in these studies is small (e.g., 0.7–5.3%, or an increase of 0.003 to 0.117 mm in minimum absolute diameter). To put these results in perspective, one should note that 6 months after percutaneous coronary angioplasty, there is an average improvement of 16% diameter stenosis units and a 0.47 mm increase in minimum absolute diameter (192). It is critical to realize that angiographic studies provide no insight into the mechanisms that may account for loss of lumen caliber. Thus, it is possible that apparent changes in mass reflect changes in adherent thrombotic material or state of vasospasm rather than in the extent of lumen narrowing due to accumulation of lipid and necrotic material in the atherosclerotic intima (193).

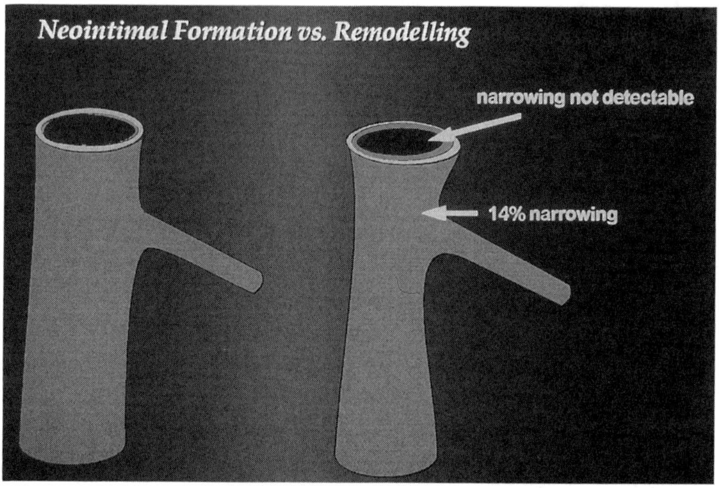

Figure 3 Remodeling vs. intimal hyperplasia. When Langille and coworkers injured rabbit carotid arteries, they found a twofold increase in intimal mass. This, however, was not sufficient to narrow the lumen. In contrast, with reduced flow, the reendothelialization portion of the vessel produced a 14% narrowing.

These angiographic regression studies showed only a modest change in lumen caliber compared to the beneficial change in clinical events (189, 191). This raises the intriguing possibility that lipid-lowering therapies may improve clinical outcome by stabilizing the lesion rather than by altering the lumen. Davies and others have suggested that the formation of fissures in plaques is the critical step leading to vascular occlusion (194–196). They propose that fissuring results from a combination of biochemical events that weaken the fibrous cap over lesions and may include the expression of certain proteases (197). Another group has added to this concept by proposing that accumulation of tumor necrosis factor-α may lead to necrotic changes that result in plaque rupture (40). While Arbustini and colleagues were unable to find a clear correlation of fissuring with acute ischemic heart disease and Davies et al. found a high incidence of fissuring in atherosclerotic "control" arteries of patients dying of noncoronary events, the control patients may have had undetected myocardial infarctions and these fissures may simply represent sequelae of advanced atherosclerosis (40, 195, 198). Davies' hypothesis would imply that we may be able to develop diagnostic tests, based on plaque composition as assessed by magnetic resonance imaging, intravascular ultrasound, or even gene expression patterns in atherectomy specimens, that might indicate lesion prognosis or the effectiveness of drugs targeted at stabilizing the lesion.

VIII. DOES REPLICATION OCCUR IN RESTENOSIS?

Restenosis seems like a simple problem; when 30% or more of angioplasties fail, most investigators assume that this is the result of neointimal formation by hyperplasia, as discussed above. This point of view is supported by morphological studies that show proliferative smooth muscle cells in restenotic tissue. "Proliferation," as used here, however, is only a term describing a morphological change. Until recently, no one had asked whether the cells that make up restenotic tissue were actually replicating by objective criteria.

As discussed above, we have used immunocytochemical labeling for the proliferating cell nuclear antigen (PCNA) to determine the proliferative profile of atherosclerotic lesions and found only very low levels of smooth muscle replication. We have used the same method to study 100 restenotic coronary atherectomy specimens (163). To our surprise, the vast majority of the restenotic specimens (74%) showed no evidence of PCNA labeling. Moreover, in those specimens with proliferation, only a modest number of PCNA-positive cells were present per slide (typically < 50 cells per slide). PCNA labeling was detected over a wide time interval after the initial procedure (e.g., one day to 390 days) with no obvious proliferative peak. There were no differences in the proliferative profiles of restenotic specimens collected in the first 3 months, 4–6 months, 7–9 months, or > 9 months after the initial interventional procedure (Spearman rank correlation coefficient = 0.081, $p = 0.43$). Furthermore, only 12 of 30 specimens obtained within 60 days of the initial coronary interventional procedure had one or more PCNA-positive nucleus per slide (including nine specimens collected within 6 days of the initial procedure, only three of which had immunolabeling of 1, 7, and 20 cells per slide). In support of these findings, a recent preliminary study using in vitro bromodeoxyuridine labeling also found low levels of proliferation in restenotic atherectomy specimens (199). Similarly, Strauss et al. found no PCNA-positive cells in atherectomy specimens from seven restenotic stented coronary artery lesions (200).

These results and those of Strauss et al. (200) contrast with a recent report by Pickering et al. (201). In the latter study, both primary and restenotic coronary and peripheral arterial specimens had surprisingly high percentages of cells that were considered PCNA-positive (e.g., mean ± SD: 15.2 ± 13.6% and 20.6 ± 18.2% by immunocytochemistry and in situ hybridization, respectively). However, only 4 of the 19 restenotic atherectomy specimens were obtained from coronary artery lesions, and none were obtained within one month of the initial interventional procedure (e.g., 1.6, 5.2, 6.1, and 7.9 months). Overall, the labeling indices reported by Pickering et al. seem exceptionally high (e.g., as high as 59% of cells being PCNA-positive) and resemble those of malignant neoplasms (202). It is important, however, to realize that PCNA is not a direct measure of replication. Thus, the detection of differences in the frequency of PCNA-positive cells in the Pickering study should raise concerns that differences between primary and restenotic tissue in Pickering's study could reflect changes specific to peripheral arterial lesions, a tissue not included in our study.

These data return us to the discussion above of remodeling. We cannot assume that an increase in intimal mass after angioplasty would narrow a vessel. Further, animal studies may be misleading and we must reconsider the relevance of animal models to the human problem. Almost all animal studies, particularly those done in the rat, measure a decrease in lumen size from the initially normal situation. This can rightly be called "stenosis." In contrast, the clinical problem is defined by the extent of dilatation that is lost after an atherosclerotic vessel has been dilated to achieve what the interventional cardiologist believes is an optimal diameter. The loss of this optimal diameter, rather than the preexisting vessel caliber, is rightly called "restenosis" (e.g., a popular clinical definition of restenosis is > 50% loss of initial luminal diameter gain). By current angiographic criteria, even a return of the human vessel to its predilation diameter would be defined as restenosis, despite no change in intimal mass. To the best of our knowledge, angiographic studies in humans do not show that angioplasty produces stenoses similar to those seen in animal models. Of course, this would be difficult to demonstrate angiographically, as the initial lesion usually already has a critical stenosis. Furthermore, animal models, perhaps by design, require that all manipulated arteries show narrowing, i.e., stenosis. There is no animal model in which 50% (or any significant percentage) of manipulated arteries remain dilated beyond their initial, unmanipulated caliber; yet this 50% rate (or higher) is the success rate seen when atherosclerotic human arteries are dilated with an angioplasty balloon. Perhaps, with more than 50% of human arteries remaining free of restenosis months after angioplasty, we may want to ask whether we have a sufficient animal model that allows us to explain why angioplasty is ever successful in the first place.

Finally, as noted in the discussion of the atherosclerotic lesion, it is difficult to imagine that replication does not occur sometime during the formation of these lesions as well. It is important to remember that only very few doublings, occurring episodically after angioplasty, would be enough to produce a large intimal mass by geometric progression. Detecting such a transient and rare event may be too difficult for current methods.

IV. MORPHOLOGICAL PATHOLOGY OF HYPERTENSION

While remodeling is a relatively new idea in understanding atherosclerosis, it is quite old in the study of hypertension. Whatever the mechanism of initiation of blood pressure, most studies agree that the maintenance of blood pressure depends upon fixed structural changes sometimes called chronic autoregulation (44,203). Folkow (44) has suggested that these changes may themselves be important for the maintenance of elevated blood pressure. An understanding of the mechanisms involved in modeling or remodeling of blood vessels may very well be important to our understanding of the pathological consequences of this disease.

The possible significance of this smooth muscle pathology depends upon understanding the central role played by "peripheral resistance" in control of blood pressure. The vasculature comprises a simple circuit, not unlike a high school science laboratory demonstration in which a transformer, some large wires, some resistances, and capacitors are connected together. The resistors in the vascular circuit are the small arteries and arterioles. If the resistance is too high, no flow occurs. If resistance is too low, the circuit overheats and small wires, the capillaries, will melt down. Vascular resistance is controlled either by restriction of lumen size, called arterial narrowing, or by a decrease in the number of vessels called rarefaction. In the former case, narrowing can be the result of increased wall thickness or active contraction. Most studies, however, show that increased wall thickness is a common feature of chronic hypertension regardless of the mechanism initiating elevation of pressure (13,204,205). Morphometric studies have further shown that this increase includes all components of the vessel wall, that is, smooth muscle cell mass and connective tissue are both elevated (206,207). Since the cell's own mass and the surrounding connective tissue are both synthesized by smooth muscle cells, hypertension is characterized by a fundamental, morphological smooth muscle lesion. We will examine the evidence for an increased vascular mass and discuss possible mechanisms underlying that increase.

It is important to realize that an increase in vascular smooth muscle mass occurs in resistance vessels in a wide variety of forms of hypertension, including forms in which we know the increase in mass is not itself the primary etiology. Forms of hypertension due to changes in blood volume may effectively increase resistance due to increased flow of blood through the microvascular bed. For example, Cowley and colleagues induced hypertension in dogs by resection of two thirds of the renal mass followed by infusion of salt and water (203,208). The initial response was an elevated cardiac output and blood volume. Peripheral resistance actually decreased.

By 48 h, however, cardiac output and blood volume were within normal limits and maintenance of pressure elevation was due to increase peripheral resistance (203). While Cowley used this experiment to illustrate the central role of volume even when no elevation of volume is measurable, it is also apparent that the elevation of pressure depended upon restriction of the lumen of the resistance vessels.

The lumen may be restricted either by active contraction of the vessel wall or by increase in the structural mass of the vessel wall or both. The rapid drop in blood pressure, when hypertensive animals or humans are treated with smooth muscle relaxants, implies that active constriction is very important. Folkow (44), however, has pointed out that it is important to think of the increased mass not only in terms of its passive role in obstructing the vessel lumen, but as amplifying the artery's response to extrinsic vasoactive stimuli. He has suggested that some component of elevation of blood pressure in humans and animals with hypertension must be attributed to a structural change.

If there are structural changes, we might expect to be able to measure a morphological change in wall mass. Such changes have been analyzed by careful morphometric analysis of the vessel wall. It is important to point out that very small changes in radius should produce a massive increase in resistance. Since resistance is inversely proportional to the fourth power of the radius, a change of only 5% in the radius of a 100-mm resistance vessel would be expected to produce a 20% increase in blood pressure (44). Against this background, it is likely that morphological changes will only be detectable when there is significant elevation of pressure. Some authors have found surprising evidence for an increase in vascular mass prior to changes in blood pressure (209,210).

The changes in wall mass seen in morphometric studies are subtle quantitative changes that are only believable when carefully analyzed on a population basis. It is not surprising, therefore, that most pathologists find that the morphology of hypertensive vascular thickening is not diagnostic of hypertension. Other changes have been purported to be more diagnostic. Diffuse intimal thickening of elastic arteries and large muscular arteries, hyaline change, and reduplication of the internal elastic lamina in resistance arteries or arterioles are a normal part of the aging process. These changes are called benign arteriosclerosis and are said to appear at an accelerated rate in individuals with hypertensive atherosclerosis of large arteries and are also "accelerated" in individuals with chronic hypertension.

As shown in Figures 4 and 5, severe elevations of blood pressure, e.g., malignant hypertension, produce more dramatic changes at the microvascular level. The retinal vessels of hypertensive individuals are sufficiently abnormal to allow the diagnosis of hypertension on the basis of

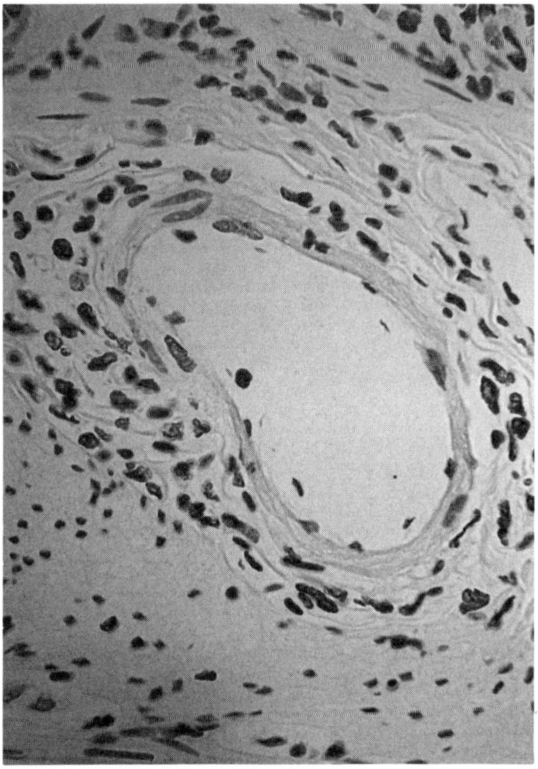

Figure 4 Onion skinning. Infusion of high doses of angiotensin-II produces two sorts of injury. In small, 50 μ vessels, there is severe dilation followed by macrophage infiltration and replication. The second injury is shown in Figure 3.

ophthalmoscopy alone. Arteries show segmental constriction and dilation; the arterioles are unable to resist the change in pressure, resulting in aneurysmal formation, hemorrhage, and scarring. These changes are typical of the pathology of other resistance vessels with severe rapid elevation of blood pressure, typically to diastolic blood pressures above 110 mmHg. Smooth muscle cells in the vessel wall in dilated segments undergo necrosis, endothelial integrity is lost, and there are great increases in vascular permeability (211,212). Studies of animals undergoing a rapid severe elevation of pressure show that the period of acute injury is reflected by endothelial denudation in the dilated segments followed by exudation of plasma proteins and deposition of platelets (213,214). In humans or animals the result is necrosis, deposition of fibrin, and entry of plasma proteins into the vessel

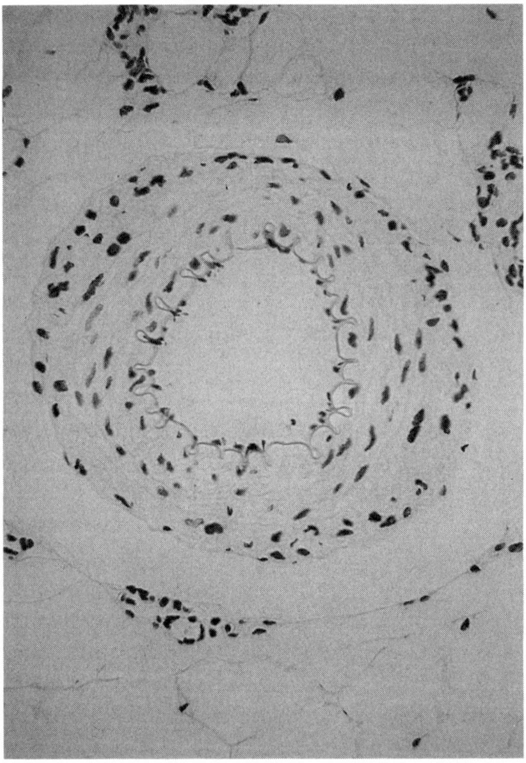

Figure 5 Resistance vessel hyperplasia. Large arteries, the 100–200 μ resistance vessels, undergo hyperplasia. This produces a thickened wall.

wall. This combination has been called "fibrinoid necrosis." This breakdown of vascular integrity is followed by smooth muscle proliferation, with a dramatic increase in the numbers of layers of smooth muscle cells seen in hypertensive vessels, sometimes called "onion skinning."

X. MECHANISM OF SMOOTH MUSCLE REPLICATION IN MALIGNANT HYPERTENSION

The proliferation of smooth muscle cells at sites of endothelial denudation and vascular dilation in small resistance vessels subjected to severe elevations in pressure is not surprising given our knowledge of the response of larger arteries to mechanical denudation described in the discussion of atherosclerosis (211–214). It is reasonable to suppose that smooth muscle proliferation at these sites is the result of release of mitogens from platelets and necrotic vessel wall cells at the site of injury.

The key observations began in the 1970s with autoradiographic studies by Crane and Dutta (215) and later by Bevan (216) showing that smooth muscle replication was markedly increased in response to acute elevation of blood pressure. Using a coarctation model, Bevan demonstrated that DNA synthesis occurs in response to hypertension. Although the microvascular data were not quantitative, she showed a rough correlation of replication in small resistance vessels with the replication observed in large vessels. The latter showed an increase within 3 days of onset of hypertension with a gradual decrease over the following days and weeks (216).

The presence of endothelial denudation in small arterioles has been shown in several animal models for high blood pressure (211–214). Furthermore, this microvascular change is specifically associated with focal areas of extreme dilation with high levels of permeability to plasma solutes (211,212,214) and endothelial denudation with thrombosis (211,212,213). Indirect evidence supports the proposition that a platelet-dependent mechanism may be operative. Crane and Dutta (215) published an interesting autoradiographic study showing a diffusion gradient of replication at sites of hypertensive injury. Replication was prominent in the endothelium and smooth muscle cells of small renal arteries. Low levels were seen in the adjacent fibroblasts, and still lower but significant levels of replication were seen in adjacent epithelium of the collecting tubules. As they propose, these data suggest a role for a diffusible factor released at the site of injury (215). The hypertensive microvessel may well be the best candidate for a vascular wall undergoing a proliferative response following release of platelet factors.

XI. MECHANISM OF SMOOTH MUSCLE REPLICATION IN MODERATE HYPERTENSION

The mechanism eliciting smooth muscle replication in resistance vessels during moderate elevations in pressure may be less obvious. As just discussed, endothelial denudation is a prominent feature of acute hypertension induced by a variety of vasoactive agents. Thus, it is reasonable to attempt to explain smooth muscle replication in small arteries of Goldblatt hypertensive animals by the response to injury mechanism. As far as we know, however, mild hypertension, even the chronic elevation of pressure seen in a hypertensive rat, does not cause endothelial denudation. Even severe hypertension does not cause denudation in large arteries. There is also evidence that changes a vessel wall mass occur in coarctation hypertension, even in protected vessels. This suggests the presence of a humoral trophic factor that might also affect DNA synthesis (217).

Unlike the acute changes in pressure seen in hypertensive models studied by Bevan (216) and by Crane and Dutta (215), the spontaneously hypertensive rat (SHR) shows only a slow increase in pressure. There are no reports of endothelial denudation or platelet deposition in either the microvessels or the large vessels of this rat strain. Before discarding denudation as an important component of hypertensive smooth muscle proliferation, it is interesting to note that Lee and colleagues found evidence of apparently necrotic endothelial cells in the microvasculature of the salt-fed Dahl hypertensive rat, another animal model in which the rise in blood pressure is relatively small (218). It is certainly possible that microvascular injury occurs episodically in the SHR. Nonetheless, it would be dangerous to conclude from the presence of hyperplasia in the microvasculature of chronically hypertensive animals that the mechanism of increase in smooth muscle cells is the same as that occurring in malignant hypertension or in the response of large vessels to the balloon catheter.

The sympathetic nervous system is an attractive alternative candidate for regulation of smooth muscle growth. Motor neurons can exert a trophic influence on skeletal muscle (219). Similarly, sympathetic nerves exert a trophic influence on the structure and function of smooth muscle. Bevan and Tsuru (220) found that sympathectomy inhibited the increase in DNA mass of the developing rabbit ear artery. Similarly, extracts of sympathetic ganglia were shown to maintain cultured smooth muscle cells in a differentiated state (221). Finally, Rorive et al. (222), among others, found that the ability of antihypertensive drugs to inhibit smooth muscle DNA replication depended on the presence or absence of effects on the sympathetic nervous system. We do know that hypertension increases the DNA content as well as the mass of large vessels.

XII. SMOOTH MUSCLE MASS VERSUS SMOOTH MUSCLE CELL NUMBER

Until this point, smooth muscle proliferation and wall thickening have been discussed as if they were a single entity. By definition this need not be true—organ mass can increase by increasing cell number, hyperplasia by increasing cell mass, and hypertrophy or both may occur at the same time. For example, Owens and Schwartz (223,224) measured cell size in smooth muscle cells extracted from the aortas of SHR or Goldblatt hypertensive rats. They found that individual cells of the hypertensive animals were bigger and the increase in cell size was adequate to account for the increase in wall mass. However, when the DNA content of the isolated cells was corrected for cell number, there was more DNA than there should have been given the normal mammalian content of DNA per cell. A combination of image analysis and flow cytometric techniques were used to demonstrate that this increase in DNA was due to an increase in smooth muscle ploidy. In other words, there were no more smooth muscle cells, however, there was more DNA. This work has been confirmed by others (225,226). Polyploid cells account for most of the increased mass of the hypertensive rate vessel (223,227). Thus it appears, at least in large vessels of the rat, that DNA synthesis is important to the increase in mass.

Two reservations need to be expressed about these observations. First the data have only been obtained from studies in the rat. We have recently obtained limited data from humans (131). In a study of about 200 autopsies, at the University of Washington, we were able to examine ploidy in the aortas of seven hypertensive and seven control patients. Our postmortem diagnosis of hypertension was based upon patient history and confirmed by the presence of a hypertrophied heart in these individuals. Clinical data, however, were very limited. No evidence was found in this study of an increase in ploidy and mean ploidy levels between the hypertensives and the controls. However, a startling correlation was found between the frequency of elevated ploidy and the age of patients in the hypertensive, but not the control, population. This at least suggests that we may be seeing a progressive change whose magnitude was limited by the use of antihypertensive therapy in this small number of patients.

The second reservation has to do with vessel size. While large vessels may be affected by hypertension, the possibility of an increase in total cell number is more important for microvessels. Obviously, the microvascular resistance vessels provide the major source of peripheral resistance and therefore are the site of most interest in hypertension. As already noted, resistance vessels in humans and all other animals with hypertension show an increase in total mass. The available data suggest that these vessels show a true hyperplasia, that is, an increase in the number of diploid cells (228–230). These studies, however, only estimated the number of cells by counting profiles in sections. Data in a two-dimensional image of a complex structure are insufficient to permit anything more than a rough estimate of the number of cells from the number of profiles that can be seen in a single plane of section. Several attempts have been made to circumvent this problem.

Five different approaches have been used to estimate the number of cells in vessel walls. Todd et al. (231) used three-dimensional reconstruction techniques to derive a model of all the smooth muscle cells located in the vessel wall. This arduous technique provided important and detailed data on the structure of the vessel wall and, at least in theory, could be used to count the number of cells in microvessels. The problem obviously would be the limited number vessels that could be studied in this way. As yet, Todd's method has not been applied to the problem of hypertensive small vessels. A more limited sampling approach has been employed by Thomas and colleagues to estimate the numbers of cells in the aortas of athero-sclerotic swine. These investigators used serial sections to estimate the length of different cells (169). They argued that differences in cell length were inversely proportional to differences in frequency of representation of cells in section. Estimates of cell length could be used to derive correction factors that could be applied to data gained in section. This relatively simple approach has not been applied to microvessels, perhaps because of concerns that changes in the size or shape of cells in different conditions would invalidate the approximation. A third technique grows out of the work on cell ploidy. If one knows the ploidy of cells in a vessel, it is possible to calculate the number of cells directly from the biochemical measurement of total DNA. The limitation of applying this method to microvessels is the difficulty in getting pure samples of microvascular smooth muscle cell free of endothelial cells and adventitial cells. A fourth approach has been applied to hypertensive vessels by Lee and his colleagues. These workers used the relationship of cell surface to cell volume as a means of estimating the probability of an increase in numbers of profiles of smooth muscle cells representing an increase in cell number or an increase in mass. They argued that increased numbers of objects, without a change in size or shape, should not change the ratio of surface area to volume. An increase in cell size should appear as a decrease in the surface/volume relationship. This method has been applied to the microvasculature, and the authors have interpreted their data as supporting an increase in cell number in the hypertensive microvasculature (207). The fifth and most practical approach has come from the work of Mulvany et al. (232) on a technique called the "dissector." The dissector depends upon the assumption that the numbers of bottoms of nuclei seen in successive serial sections is proportional to the total number of cells.

Mulvany used the dissector to study mesenteric arteries of SHR. These arteries contained an increased number of cells, consistent with the semi-quantitative conclusions by others. The dissector, like most morphometric approaches, is arduous, and only small numbers of vessels were studied. This has led to some surprising findings. Mulvany, studying both animal and human microvessels, was unable to find a change in either cell number or total wall mass of hypertensive vessel walls. However, since physiological studies tell us that these vessel walls must be thickened to account for the contractile properties of the hypertensive wall, Mulvany concludes that the primary wall change must be a *rearrangement* or remodeling of the existing vessel wall mass, rather than an accretion of new mass (233,234).

Unfortunately, we have very little data on the mechanism underlying remodeling. Obviously, few clues can come from studies of smooth muscle replication after injury, and the distinction between hyperploid replication and true proliferation may not be critical to the most important implication of a proliferative response to hypertension. Nonetheless, maintenance of high blood pressure implies either chronic stimulation by a stimulus exogenous to the vessel wall or a chronic change in the responsiveness of the vessel wall.

On the other hand, the dissector is not necessarily conclusive. The method is arduous and might allow changes in cell number at a level that is biologically significant. One might imagine some sort of initial stimulus, an as yet undefined injury, that results in a chronic change we recognize as high blood pressure and is associated with an increase in cell number. This sort of "memory" might occur at many levels, ranging from resetting of renal or central physiological mechanisms, positive feedback regulation of electrolyte levels, or direct changes in the effector system—the smooth muscles themselves. Change in DNA content of the vessel wall is a special alternative. If one imagines that the microvasculature replicates in response to episodes of acute hypertension, then the wall would retain an increased DNA content as a "memory" of the earlier event. In turn, this increased DNA could alter the ability of the vascular system to regulate synthesis and degradation of the contractile protein mass of arterial smooth muscle cells, possibly producing a fixed increase in peripheral vessel wall mass. Such a mechanism might account for the well-established increase in structural resistance of the peripheral vasculature in humans and animals with hypertension (44,235).

Treatment studies may be important in the concept of a memory of vascular mass. The reversal of mass changes in SHR resistance vessels was accomplished by proportional reductions in cellular and extracellular material (236). Is there a change in cell number with treatment? Warshaw et al. (236) showed that the number of profiles of smooth muscle cells in vessel cross sections were reduced by 12% in treated SHR. As discussed previously, this measure can only give a rough estimate of cell number. Carlier and Rorive (237) have shown that early treatment of renal hypertension of unclipping can reverse DNA content changes, but that after 3 weeks of hypertension, these DNA changes were permanent. DNA synthesis, elevated in renal and genetic hypertensions, is decreased with treatment in both of these models (222,238,239). It would be interesting to see if models of hypertension with different degrees of DNA change would react differently to subsequent episodes of hypertension. Freis et al. (240) have found that treatment of spontaneous hypertension can effectively reduce pressure, but when treatment is released, pressure rapidly rises to pretreatment levels and then proceeds to rise at the same rate as untreated controls. Limas et al. (241) studied effects of treatment release on aortic medial wall thickening in SHR and found that treatment prevented further wall thickening, but release resulted in a return to hypertensive levels after 20 weeks. This further suggests an internally coded memory of the appropriate response to hypertension, and indeed a programmed response may be resumed at the same stage present in this memory. Changes in ploidy of vascular smooth muscle are not reversed in SHR by treatment (242) or in DOCA hypertension by a low-salt diet (243). These results, as well as those of Carlier and Rorive (237,244), imply that DNA change could well be involved as irreversible events (memory) resulting from hypertension and resulting in structural hypertrophy.

Whether increases in arterial DNA are important in maintenance of elevated peripheral resistance depends on as yet unanswered questions:

1. Is the dissector sensitive enough to detect small changes in vessel wall cell number?
2. How does an increase in the number of cells or the amount of DNA per cell or total DNA per vessel length affect the steady-state mass of the vessel wall?
3 If DNA content changes, how does an increase in DNA affect the response of the vessel wall to trophic stimuli from nerves or circulating factors?
4. How does an increased amount of DNA affect the response to subsequent hypertensive episodes?

XIII. RELATIONSHIP OF MASS CHANGES TO REPLICATION

The most obvious reason for being interested in this increase in DNA is the possibility that our available knowledge of the control of DNA synthesis might provide insights into the control of vascular mass in resistance vessels. The fact that most known changes in vascular mass are associated with increases in DNA content leads one to think that the two cellular changes may somehow be related.

Relatively little is known about the factors controlling vessel wall mass. Two recent experiments, however, seem particularly relevant. The first, reported by Langille et al., (245), studied the adaptation of the common carotid to deceased flow. This was accomplished by ligating the external carotid artery. Within 48 h, the remaining carotid artery underwent active contraction, decreasing the effective lumen size. Within 2 weeks this was followed by remodeling, so that now the vessel had an increased wall thickness and a decreased lumen diameter (245,246). These changes that occurred in a large vessel are strikingly similar to changes described by Joshua et al. (247) in the cremasteric circulation of rats with 1-kidney, 1-clip hypertension. Initially, they found an active constriction of the precapillary arterioles. By 2 weeks this was converted to a structural change in the larger vessels, restricting flow in a fashion no longer relaxable with papaverine. With time, the "structural" component spread to smaller vessels. Joshua and colleagues suggested that the structural changes in the larger vessels were in local response adapted to protecting the smaller vessels from damage by elevated pressure (247). It is tempting to equate these hyperplastic changes to Cowley's findings of increased peripheral resistance due to autoregulation after a few days of high-volume hypertension due to excess salt intake (203).

Langille's experiment also provides possible clues as to the mechanisms controlling vascular mass independent of replication. Endothelial denudation of the common carotoid prevented both the active contraction and the later remodeling change. Two known functions of the endothelium may be relevant. First, the endothelium is the source of endothelial-derived relaxing factor (248–250). Whether endothelial-derived relaxing factor somehow interacts with the underlying wall to maintain normal tone is not known, although it is obviously difficult to see how the presence of a source of a relaxing factor would encourage vasoconstriction. Second, and easier to consider, is the discovery, reviewed above, that endothelial cells are a potent source of polypeptide mitogens, including PDGF. While these peptide hormones have traditionally been thought of as growth factors, they have also been shown to be vasoactive (251,252). It is possible that endothelial-derived PDGF, released in response to some flow-dependent stimulus, causes both an initial constriction response and a later trophic remodeling response.

Another possible clue comes from reports of the effects of various therapeutic regimes in cardiovascular mass. If there is a relationship between blood pressure and cardiovascular mass, then reversal or prevention of hypertension should prevent or reverse structural changes seen in hypertensive animals. A substantial literature shows that antihypertensive agents can reverse or prevent cardiovascular hypertrophy. However, the efficacy of pharmacological treatment is not universal and depends in part upon the model and duration of hypertension, the form and duration of reversal, and the type of structural change of interest. For example, when blood pressures were controlled by captopril, aortic hypertrophy was prevented in

SHR (253) but the DNA synthesis associated with renal hypertension was not (222). Reserpine, however, was effective in preventing DNA synthesis in renal hypertension (222). There is evidence that the reversal of SHR hypertension requires extended treatment (253,254), whereas in early stages of renal hypertension, treatment effects are relatively rapid (254). Established renal hypertension is more difficult to reverse than developing renal hypertension (244,254). A number of reports show that cardiac hypertrophy induced by hypertension can be prevented by captopril, but not by hydralazine, although both treatments achieve normotension (253,255). Hydralazine has an effect on the ratio of aortic weight to length after prolonged treatment, but not in mesenteric vessels (253).

It is intriguing to consider the possibility that the link is control of vascular mass by the sympathetic nervous system. Probably the best evidence from treatment studies is the differential effects of vasodilators, which may reduce blood pressure but not affect cardiovascular mass, or sympathetic agents, calcium channel blockers, and angiotensin antagonists, which do prevent or reduce cardiovascular hypertrophy.

Hydralazine prevents hypertension, but also stimulates sympathetic output, while captopril reduces sympathetic stimulation by reducing AII levels (253,255). The effects of sympathetic agents are more direct, such as reserpine, which rapidly depletes catecholamines, providing a clearer view of the possible mechanism of sympathetic control over mass. It has already been noted that Bevan found that unilateral sympathectomy of the ears of developing rabbits decreased growth in ear artery DNA content. Wall-to-lumen ratio of Wistar-Kyoto mesenteric vessels has also been reduced by sympathectomy (256). Sympathectomy can prevent hypertrophy (257,258) in hypertensive vessels, but it appears that the completeness and maintenance of sympathectomy are important issues in how effective this treatment is (256,259).

An alternative hypothesis has been proposed by Loeb et al. (210,239), who found that calcium channel blockers were effective in preventing hypertension-induced aortic DNA synthesis. They have argued that similar effects by captopril and hydralazine were also calcium-mediated. This was further supported by ouabain treatment of normal animals that also stimulated DNA synthesis. The separation of hypertension from DNA synthesis and the lack of control over possible sympathetic stimulation by ouabain makes these results difficult to interpret. The effectiveness of calcium channel blockers in reducing or preventing hypertrophy is also somewhat unpredictable, but this is an interesting hypothesis which deserves further study.

In summary, the stimuli controlling smooth muscle replication in hypertension remain unknown. Growth factors released by platelets may play an important role in microvascular changes in malignant hypertension, but platelet-released factors are not likely to by involved in large vessels or in any vessel affected by milder and more chronic forms of high blood pressure. Wall tension and sympathetic activity are intriguing alternatives that need more exploration.

The thesis of this chapter begins with a very simple idea—that vascular structure, that is, lumen size and wall thickness, is a critical target for understanding the pathology of atherosclerosis and hypertension. In the former case, we have seen how lesions are primarily a problem of intimal mass. The factors contributing to this mass include smooth muscle growth, but this may be an early event, perhaps preceding the characteristic lipid accumulation and inflammation seen as lesion progress. It is even possible that the smooth muscle replication ascribed to the response to injury is reparative, strengthening otherwise fragile advanced lesions.

This intimal smooth muscle proliferation may only play an early role in lesion formation. Perhaps more important to the clinical outcome of the lesion may be the role of medial smooth muscle cells in accommodating the vessel to change as the lesion grows. In a sense, occlusive atherosclerotic arterial disease may be best characterized as a failure of this mechanism of accommodation.

Remodeling also appears to be a critical process during the response to clinical injury, that is, restenosis after angioplasty. To the best of our knowledge, this is a healing process, restoring the vessel to its preexisting narrowed caliber rather than narrowing the vessel beyond its already pathological state. Nonetheless, the mechanisms of this specialized form of wound healing need to be studied. We have no idea, for example, how restenosis after injury relates to physiological remodeling seen when blood flow is changed.

Finally, the best clues to understanding remodeling may come from studies of the change in wall properties seen in the hypertensive microvasculature. We have tried to review this literature; however, the picture needs a lot of clarification. The best available data implicate the endothelium as the transducer of changes in flow. The candidates for secondary messengers mediating structural changes include nitric oxide, ET-1, and PDGF, but no definitive experiments have tested these molecular hypotheses. Even less is known about the pharmacological mediators controlling wall mass.

REFERENCES

1. Ross R. The pathogenesis of atherosclerosis—a perspective for the 1990's. Nature 1993; 362:801–809.
2. Schwartz SM, Heimark RL, Majesky MW. Developmental mechanisms underlying pathology of arteries. Physiol Rev 1990; 70:1177–1209.

3. Schwartz SM, Campbell GR, Campbell JH. Replication of smooth muscle cells in vascular disease. Circ Res 1986; 58:427–444.
4. Pardanaud L, Altmann C, Kitos P, Dieterlen-Lievre F, Buck CA. Vasculogenesis in the early quail blastodisc as studied with a monoclonal antibody recognizing endothelial cells. Development 1987; 100:339–349.
5. Le Douarin NM. Cell migrations in embryos. Cell 1984; 38:353–360.
6. Peault BM, Thiery JP, Le Douarin NM. A surface marker for the hemopoietic and endothelial cell lineages in the quail species defined by a monoclonal antibody. Proc Natl Acad Sci USA 1983; 80:2976–2980.
7. Noden DM. Origins and assembly of avian embryonic blood vessels. Ann NY Acad Sci 1990; 588:236–249.
8. Manasek FJ. The ultrastructure of embryonic myocardial blood vessels. Devel Biol 1971; 26:42–54.
9. De Simone-Santoro I, Renda T. Recherches ultrastructurales, histochimiques et histoenzymologiques sur la paroi aortique pendant sa morphogenese chez l'embryon de poulet. Annal Histochim 1971; 16:171–181.
10. Blatt HJ. Über die Entwicklung der Coronararterien bei der Ratte—licht- und elektronenmikroskopische Untersuchungen. Z Anat Entwicklungsgesch 1973; 142:53–64.
11. Gonzalez-Crussi F. Vasculogenesis in the chick embryo. An ultrastructural study. Am J Anat 1971; 130:441–460.
12. Karrer HE. An electron microscope study of the aorta in young and aging mice. J Ultrastruct Res 1961; 5:1–27.
13. Wolinsky H, Glagov S. A lamellar unit of aortic medial structure and function in mammals. Circ Res 1967; 20:99–101.
14. Looker T, Berry CL. The growth and development of the rat aorta. II. Changes in nucleic acid and scleroprotein content. J Anat 1972; 113:17–34.
15. Olivetti G, Anversa P, Melissori M, Loud AV. Morphometric study of early postnatal development of the thoracic aorta in the rat. Circ Res 1980; 47:417–424.
16. Bochaton-Piallat ML, Gabbiani F, Ropraz P, Gabbiani G. Cultured aortic smooth muscle cells from newborn and adult rats show distinct cytoskeletal features. Differentiation 1992; 49:175–185.
17. Harris-Hooker SA, Gajdusek CM, Wight TN, Schwartz SM. Neovascular responses induced by cultured aortic endothelial cells. J Cell Physiol 1983; 114:302–310.
18. Montesano R, Vassalli JD, Baird A, Guillemin R, Orci L. Basic fibroblast growth factor induces angiogenesis in vitro. Proc Natl Acad Sci USA 1986; 83:7297–7301.
19. Gajdusek CM, Carbon S, Ross R, Nawroth P, Stern D. Activation of coagulation releases endothelial cell mitogens. J Cell Biol 1986; 103:419–428.
20. Schweigerer L, Neufeld G, Friedman J, Abraham JA, Fiddes JC, Gospodarowicz D. Capillary endothelial cells express basic fibroblast growth factor, a mitogen that promotes their own growth. Nature 1987; 325:257–259.
21. Fox PL, DiCorleto PE. Modified low density lipoproteins suppress production

of a platelet-derived growth factor-like protein by cultured endothelial cells. Proc Natl Acad Sci USA 1986; 83:4774–4778.
22. Abraham JA, Whang JL, Tumolo A, Mergia A, Friedman J, Gospodarowicz D, Fiddes JC. Human fibroblast growth factor: nucleotide sequence and genomic organization. EMBO J 1986; 5:2523–2528.
23. Tong BD, Levine SE, Jaye M, Ricca G, Drohan W, Maciag T, Deuel TF. Isolation and sequencing of a cDNA clone homologous to the v-sis oncogene from human endothelial cells. Mol Cell Biol 1986; 6:3018–3022.
24. Burgess WH, Mehlman T, Marshak DR, Fraser BA, Maciag T. Structural evidence that endothelial cell growth factor-β is the precursor of both endothelial cell growth factor-α and acidic fibroblast growth factor. Proc Natl Acad Sci USA 1986; 83:7216–7220.
25. Ekblom P, Sariola H, Karkinen-Jaaskelainen M. Saxen L. The origin of the glomerular endothelium. Cell Differ 1982; 11:35–39.
26. Kuro-o M, Nagai R, Nakahara K, Katoh H, Tsai RC, Tsuchimochi H, Yazaki Y, Ohkubo A, Takaku F. cDNA cloning of a myosin heavy chain isoform in embryonic smooth muscle and its expression during vascular development and in arteriosclerosis. J Biol Chem 1991; 266:3768–3773.
27. Thyberg J, Blomgren K. Phenotype modulation in primary cultures of rat aortic smooth muscle cells. Effects of drugs that interfere with the functions of the vascular system and the cytoskeleton. Virchows Arch B Cell Pathol Incl Molec Pathol 1990; 59:1–10.
28. Okamato E, Imataka K, Fujii J, Juro-o M, Nakahara K, Nishimura H, Yazaki Y, Nagai R. Heterogeneity in smooth muscle cell population accumulating in the neointimas and the media of poststenotic dilatation of the rabbit carotid artery. Biochem Biophys Res Commun 1992; 185:459–464.
29. Shirinsky VP, Birukov KG, Koteliansky VE, Glukhova MA, Spanidis E, Rogers JD, Campbell JH, Campbell GR. Density-related expression of caldesmon and vinculin in cultured rabbit aortic smooth muscle cells. Exp Cell Res 1991; 194:186–189.
30. Desmouliere A, Gabbiani G. The cytoskeleton of arterial smooth muscle cells during human and experimental atheromatosis. Kidney Int. 1992; 37(suppl):S87–S89.
31. Glukhova MA, Frid MG, Koteliansky VE. Phenotypic changes of human aortic smooth muscle cells during development and in the adult vessel. Am J Physiol 1991; 261(4 suppl):78–80.
32. Zanellato AM, Borrione AC, Tonello M, Scannapieco G, Pauletto P, Sartore S. Myosin isoform expression and smooth muscle cell heterogeneity in normal and atherosclerotic rabbit aorta. Arteriosclerosis 1990; 10:996–1009.
33. Kim HS, Aikawa M, Kimura K, Kuro-o M, Nakahara K, Suzuki T, Katoh H, Okamoto E, Yazaki Y, Nagai R. Ductus arteriosus. Advanced differentiation of smooth muscle cells demonstrated by myosin heavy chain isoform expression in rabbits. Circulation 1993; 88(4 Pt 1):1804–1810.
34. Solway J, Seltzer J, Samaha FF, Kim S, Alger LE, Niu Q, Morrisey EE, Ip

HS, Parmacek MS. Structure and expression of a smooth muscle cell-specific gene, SM22-α. J Biol Chem 1995; 270:13460–13469.
35. Rockey DC, Boyles JK, Gabbiani G, Friedman SL. Rat hepatic lipocytes expression smooth muscle actin upon activation in vivo and in culture. J Submicrosc Cytol Pathol 1992; 24:193–203.
36. Sugimoto T, Ueyama H, Hosoi H, Inazawa J, Kato T, Kemshead JT, Reynolds CP, Gown Am, Mine H, Sawada T. α-smooth muscle actin and desmin expressions in human neuroblastoma cell lines. Int J Cancer 1991; 48:277–283.
37. Peled A, Zipori D, Abramsky O, Ovadia H, Shezen E. Expression of α-smooth muscle actin in murine bone marrow stromal cells. Blood 1991; 78:304–309.
38. Jonasson L, Holm J, Skalli O, Bondjers G, Hansson GK. Regional accumulations of T cells, macrophages, and smooth muscle cells in the human atherosclerotic plaque. Arteriosclerosis 1986; 6:131–138.
39. Gown AM, Tsukada T, Ross R. Human atherosclerosis. II. Immunocytochemical analysis of the cellular composition of human atherosclerotic lesions. Am J Pathol 1986; 125:191–207.
40. Arbustini E, Grasso M, Diegoli M, Pucci A, Bramerio M, Ardissino D, Angoli L, de Servi S, Bramucci E, Mussini A. Coronary atherosclerotic plaques with and without thrombus in ischemic heart syndromes: a morphologic, immunohistochemical, and biochemical study. Am J Cardiol 1991; 68:36B–50B.
41. Velican D, Velican C. Intimal thickening in developing coronary arteries and its relevance to atherosclerotic involvement. Atherosclerosis 1976; 23:345–355.
42. Stary HC, Strong JP. the fine structure of non-atherosclerotic intimal thickening of developing and of regressing atherosclerotic lesions at the bifurcation of the left coronary artery. Adv Exp Med Biol 1976; 67:89–108.
43. Sims FH, Gavin JB, Vanderwee MA. The intima of human coronary arteries. Am Heart J 1989; 118:32–38.
44. Folkow B. Physiological aspects of primary hypertension. Physiol Rev 1982; 62:347–504.
45. Mulvany MJ. Determinants of vascular structure. J Cardiovasc Pharmacol 1992; 19(suppl 5):S1–S6.
46. Glagov S, Weisenberg E, Zarins CK, Stankunavicius R, Kolettis GJ. Compensatory enlargement of human atherosclerotic coronary arteries. N Engl J Med 1987; 316:1371–1375.
47. Langille BL. Remodeling of developing and mature arteries: endothelium, smooth muscle, and matrix. J Cardiovasc Pharmacol 1993; 21(suppl 1): S11–S17.
48. Langille BL, Adamson SL. Thoracic aortic pressure-flow relationships and vascular impedance in fetal sheep. Am J Physiol 1992; 263(3 Pt 2):H824–H832.
49. Jamal A, Bendeck M, Langille BL. Structural changes and recovery of function after arterial injury. Arterioscler Thromb 1992; 12:307–317.

50. Bendeck MP, Langille BL. Rapid accumulation of elastin and collagen in the aortas of sheep in the immediate perinatal period. Circ Res 1991; 69:1165–1169.
51. Cho A, Courtman DW, Langille BL. Apoptosis (programmed cell death) in arteries of the neonatal lamb. Circ Res 1995; 76:168–175.
52. Ross R. The pathogenesis of atherosclerosis—an update. N Engl J Med 1986; 314:488–500.
53. Stemerman MB, Ross R. Fibrous plaque formation in primate, an electron microscope study. J Exp Med 1972; 136:769–789.
54. Schwartz SM, Stemerman MB, Benditt EP. The aortic intima. II. Repair of the aortic lining after mechanical denudation. Am J Pathol 1975; 81:15–42.
55. Friedman RJ, Stemerman MB, Wenz B, Moore S, Gauldie J, Gent M, Tiell ML, Spaet TH. The effect of thrombocytopenia on experimental atherosclerotic lesion formation in rabbits. Smooth muscle cell proliferation and re-endothelialization. J Clin Invest 1977; 60:1191–1201.
56. Oka Y, Orth DN. Human plasma epidermal growth factor/β-urogastrone is associated with blood platelets. J Clin Invest 1983; 72:249–259.
57. Assoian RK, Grotendorst GR, Miller DM, Sporn MB. Cellular transformation by coordinated action of three peptide growth factors from human platelets. Nature 1984; 309:804–806.
58. Tucker RF, Shipley GD, Moses HL, Holley RW. Growth inhibitor from BSC-1 cells closely related to platelet type-β transforming growth factor. Science 1984; 226:705–707.
59. Gerrity RG. The role of the monocyte in atherogenesis. I. Transition of bloodborne monocytes into foam cells in fatty lesions. Am J Pathol 1981; 103:181–190.
60. Faggiotto A, Ross R. Studies of hypercholesterolemia in the nonhuman primate. II. Fatty streak conversion to fibrous plaque. Arteriosclerosis 1984; 4:341–356.
61. Faggiotto A, Ross R, Harker L. Studies of hypercholesterolemia in the nonhuman primate. I. Changes that lead to fatty streak formation. Arteriosclerosis 1984; 4:323–340.
62. Leibovich SJ, Ross R. A macrophage-dependent factor that stimulates the proliferation of fibroblasts in vitro. Am J Pathol 1976; 84:501–513.
63. Curwen KD, Gimbrone MA Jr, Handin RI. In vitro studies of thromboresistance. The role of prostacyclin (PGI_2) in platelet adhesion to cultured normal and virally transformed human vascular endothelial cells. Lab Invest 1980; 42:366–374.
64. Shimokado K, Raines EW, Ross R. Activated macrophages secrete a PDGF-like molecule (abstract). J Cell Biochem 1985; (suppl)9A:137.
65. DiCorleto PE, Bowen-Pope DF. Cultured endothelial cells produce a platelet-derived growth factor-like protein. Proc Natl Acad Sci USA 1983; 80:1919–1923.
66. DiCorleto PE. Cultured endothelial cells produce multiple growth factors for connective tissue cells. Exp Cell Res 1984; 153:167–172.

67. Gajdusek CM. Release of endothelial cell-derived growth factor (ECDGF) by heparin. J Cell Physiol 1984; 121:13–21.
68. Vlodavsky I, Folkman J, Sullivan R, Fridman R, Ishai-Michaeli R, Sasse J, Klagsbrun M. Endothelial cell-derived basic fibroblast growth factor: Synthesis and deposition into subendothelial extracellular matrix. Proc Natl Acad Sci USA 1987; 84:2292–2296.
69. Barrett TB, Sampson P, Owens GK, Schwartz SM, Benditt EP, Polyploid nuclei in human artery wall smooth muscle cells. Proc Natl Acad Sci USA 1983; 80:882–885.
70. Jaye M, Maciag T. Modulation of the sis gene transcript during endothelial cell differentiation in vitro. Science 1985; 228:882–884.
71. Barrett TB, Benditt EP. Platelet-derived growth factor gene expression in human atherosclerotic plaques and normal artery wall. Proc Natl Acad Sci USA 1988; 85:2810–2814.
72. Wilcox JN, Smith KM, Williams LT, Schwartz SM, Gordon D. Platelet-derived growth factor mRNA detection in human atherosclerotic plaques by in situ hybridization. J Clin Invest 1988; 82:1134–1143.
73. Libby P, Warner SJ, Salmon RN, Birinyi LK. Production of platelet-derived growth factor-like mitogen by smooth muscle cells from human atheroma. N Engl J Med 1988; 318:1493–1498.
74. Ross R, Raines EW, Bowen-Pope DF. The biology of platelet-derived growth factor. Cell 1986; 46:155–169.
75. Clemmons DR, Underwood LE, Chatelain PG, Van Wyk JJ. Liberation of immunoreactive somatomedin-C from its binding proteins by proteolytic enzymes and heparin. J Clin Endocrinol Metabol 1983; 56:384.
76. O'Keefe EJ, Pledger WJ. A model of cell cycle control: sequential events regulated by growth factors. Mol Cell Endocrinol 1983; 31:167–186.
77. Singh JP, Chaikin MA, Pledger WJ, Scher CD, Stiles CD. Persistence of the mitogenic response to platelet-derived growth factor (competence) does not reflect a long-term interaction between the growth factor and the target cell. J Cell Biol 1983; 96:1497–1502.
78. Clemmons DR. Interaction of circulating cell-derived and plasma growth factors in stimulating cultured smooth muscle cell replication. J Cell Physiol 1984; 121:425–430.
79. Russell WE, Van Wyk JJ, Pledger WJ. Inhibition of the mitogenic effects of plasma by a monoclonal antibody to somatomedin C. Proc Natl Acad Sci USA 1984; 81:2389–2392.
80. Seifert RA, Schwartz SM, Bowen-Pope DF. Developmentally regulated production of platelet-derived growth factor-like molecules. Nature 1984; 311:669–671.
81. Nilsson J, Sjolund M, Palmberg L, Thyberg J, Heldin CH. Arterial smooth muscle cells in primary culture produce a platelet-derived growth factor-like protein. Proc Natl Acad Sci USA 1985; 82:4418–4422.
82. Majesky MW, Benditt EP, Schwartz SM. Expression and developmental control of platelet-derived growth factor A-chain and B-chain/sis genes in rat aortic smooth muscle cells. Proc Natl Acad Sci USA 1988; 85:1524–1528.

83. Walker LN, Bowen-Pope DF, Reidy MA. Secretion of platelet-derived growth factor (PDGF)-like activity by arterial smooth muscle cells is induced as a response to injury. J Cell Biol 1984; 99:416a.
84. Clowes AW, Clowes MM. Kinetics of cellular proliferation after arterial injury. IV. Heparin inhibits rat smooth muscle mitogenesis and migration. Circ Res 1986; 58:839–845.
85. Clowes Aw, Clowes MM, Reidy MA. Kinetics of cellular proliferation after arterial injury. I. Smooth muscle growth in the absence of endothelium. Lab Invest 1983; 49:327–333.
86. Lindner V, Reidy MA. Proliferation of smooth muscle cells after vascular injury is inhibited by an antibody against basic fibroblast growth factor. Proc Natl Acad Sci USA 1991; 88:3739–3743.
87. Olson NE, Chao S, Lindner V, Reidy MA. Intimal smooth muscle cell proliferation after balloon catheter injury. The role of basic fibroblast growth factor. Am J Pathol 1992; 140:1017–1023.
88. Jawien A, Bowen-Pope DF, Lindner V, Schwartz SM, Clowes AW. Platelet-derived growth factor promotes smooth muscle migration and intimal thickening in a rat model of balloon of balloon angioplasty. J Clin Invest 1992; 89:507–511.
89. Ferns GAA, Raines EW, Sprugel KH, Motani AS, Reidy MA, Ross, R. Inhibition of neointimal smooth muscle accumulation after angioplasty by an antibody to PDGF. Science 1991; 253:1129–1132.
90. Daemen MJAP, Lombardi DM, Bosman FT, Schwartz SM. Angiotensin II induces smooth muscle cell proliferation in the normal and injured arterial wall. Circ Res 1991; 68:450–456.
91. Van Kleef EM, Smits JFM, DeMey JGR, Cleutjens JPM, Lombardi DM, Schwartz SM, Daemen MJAP. α-1-Adrenoreceptor blockade reduces the angiotensin II-induced vascular smooth muscle cell DNA synthesis in the rat thoracic aorta and carotid artery. Circ Res 1992; 70:1122–1127.
92. Prescott M, Webb R, Reidy MA. ACE inhibitors vs. AII, AT1 receptor antagonist: effects on smooth muscle cell migration and proliferation after balloon catheter injury. Am J Pathol 1991; 139;1291–1302.
93. Clowes AW, Clowes MM, Reidy MA. Kinetics of cellular proliferation after arterial injury. III. Endothelial and smooth muscle growth in chronically denuded vessels. Lab Invest 1986; 54:295–303.
94. Majesky MW, Reidy MA, Bowen-Pope DF, Wilcox JN, Schwartz SM. Platelet-derived growth factor (PDGF) ligand and receptor gene expression during repair of arterial injury. J Cell Biol 1990; 111:2149–2158.
95. Jackson CL. Raines EW, Ross R, Reidy MA. Role of endogenous platelet-derived growth factor in arterial smooth muscle cell migration after balloon catheter injury. Arterioscler Thromb 1993; 13:1218–1226.
96. Majesky MW, Lindner V, Twardzik DR, Schwartz SM, Reidy MA. Production of transforming growth factor β1 during repair of arterial injury. J Clin Invest 1991; 88:904–910.
97. Viswanathan M, Stromberg C, Seltzer A, Saavedra JM. Balloon angioplasty

enhances the expression of angiotensin II AT1 receptors in neointima of rat aorta. J Clin Invest 1992; 90:1707–1712.
98. Cercek B, Fishbein MC, Forrester JS, Helfant RH, Fagin JA. Induction of insulin-like growth factor 1 messenger RNA in rat aorta after balloon denudation. Circ Res 1990; 66:1755–1760.
99. MERCATOR Study Group. Does the new angiotensin-converting enzyme inhibitor cilazapril prevent restenosis after percutaneous transluminal coronary angioplasty? Circulation 1992; 86:100–110.
100. Powell JS, Muller RKM, Rouge M, Kuhn H, Hefti F, Baumgartner HR. the proliferative response to vascular injury is suppressed by angiotensin-converting enzyme inhibition. J Cardiovasc Pharmacol 1990; 16(suppl 4):S42–S49.
101. Rakugi H, Dzau VJ, Pratt RE. Importance of tissue angiotensin-converting enzyme (ACE) in neointimal hyperplasia. Circulation 1992; 86(suppl I):I–169.
102. Farhy RD, Carretero OA, Ho KL, Scicli AG. Role of kinins and nitric oxide in the effects of angiotensin-converting enzyme inhibitors on neointima formation. Circ Res 1993; 72:1202–1210.
103. Kaartinen M, Penttila A, Kovanen PT. Mast cells of two types differing in neutral protease composition in the human aortic intima. Demonstration of tryptase- and tryptase/chymase-containing mast cells in normal intimas, fatty streaks, and the shoulder region of atheromas. Arterioscler Thromb 1994; 14:966–972.
104. Urata H, Kinoshita A, Misono KS, Bumpus FM, Husain A. Identification of a highly specific chymase as the major angiotensin II-forming enzyme in the human heart. J Biol Chem 1990; 265:22348–22357.
105. Baumgartner HR. Eine neue Methode zur Erzeugung der Thromben durch gezielte Überdehnung der Gefasswantd. Z Ges Exp Med 1963; 137:227–234.
106. Salisbury BG, Hajjar DP, Minick CR. Altered glycosaminoglycan metabolism in injured arterial wall. Exp Molec Pathol 1985; 42:306–319.
107. Vesselinovitch D. Animal models and the study of atherosclerosis. Arch Pathol Lab Med 1988; 112:1011–1017.
108. Anderson PG. Animal models and morphometric techniques in studies of the vascular response to injury. Cardiovasc Pathol 192; 1:263–278.
109. Schwartz SM, Haudenschild CC, Eddy EM. Endothelial regeneration. I. Quantitative analysis of initial stages of endothelial regeneration in rat aortic intima. Lab Invest 1978; 38:568–580.
110. Bjorkerud S. Reaction of the aortic wall of the rabbit after superficial, longitudinal, mechanical trauma. Virchows Arch 1969; 347:197–210.
111. Reidy MA, Yoshida K, Harker LA, Schwartz SM. Vascular injury: quantification of experimental focal endothelial denudation in rats using indium-111-labeled platelets. Arteriosclerosis 1986; 6:305–311.
112. Richardson M, Hatton MWC, Buchanan MR, Moore S. Wound healing in the media of the normolipemic rabbit carotid artery injured by air drying or by balloon catheter de-endothelialization. Am J Pathol 1990; 137:1453–1465.

113. Reddick RL, Read MS, Brinkhous KM, Bellinger D, Nichols T, Griggs TR. Coronary atherosclerosis in the pig. Induced plaque injury and platelet response. Arteriosclerosis 1990; 10:541–550.
114. Weidinger FF, McLenachan JM, Cybulsky MI, Fallon JT, Hollenberg NK, Cooke JP, Ganz P. Hypercholesterolemia enhances macrophage recruitment and dysfunction of regenerated endothelium after balloon injury of the rabbit iliac artery. Circulation 1991; 84:755–767.
115. Scott RF, Imai H, Makita T, Thomas WA, Keiner JM. Lining cell and intimal smooth muscle cell response and Evans blue staining in abdominal aortae of young swine after denudation by balloon catheter. Exp Molec Pathol 1980; 33:185–202.
116. Stadius ML, Rowan R, Fleischhauer JF, Kernoff R, Billingham M, Gown AM. Time course and cellular characteristics of the iliac artery response to acute balloon injury. An angiographic, morphometric, and immunocytochemical analysis in the cholesterol-fed New Zealand white rabbit. Arterioscler Thromb 1992; 12:1267–1273.
117. Groves HM, Kinlough-Rathbone RL, Richardson M. Platelet interaction with damaged rabbit aorta. Lab Invest 1979; 40:194–206.
118. Nichols TC, Bellinger DA, Reddick RL, Read MS, Koch GG. Brinkhous KM, Griggs TR. Role of von Willebrand factor in arterial thrombosis. Studies in normal and von Willebrand disease pigs. Circulation 1991; 83(6 suppl):IV56–IV64.
119. Clowes AW, Schwartz SM. Significance of quiescent smooth muscle migration in the injured rat carotid artery. Circ Res 1985; 56:139–145.
120. Schwartz SM, Reidy MA, Clowes A. Kinetics of atherosclerosis, a stem cell model. Ann NY Acad Sci 1985; 454:292–304.
121. Miano JM, Vlasic N, Tota RR, Stemerman MB. Smooth muscle cell immediate-early gene and growth factor actin follows vascular injury. A putative in vivo mechanism for autocrine growth. Arterioscler Thromb 1993; 13:211–219.
122. Majesky MW, Schwartz SM, Clowes MM, Clowes AW. Heparin regulates smooth muscle S phase entry in the injured rat carotid artery. Circ Res 1987; 61:296–300.
123. Hanke H, Strohschneider T, Oberhoff M, Betz E, Karsch KR. Time course of smooth muscle cell proliferation in the intima and media of arteries following experimental angioplasty. Circ Res 1990; 67:651–659.
124. Clowes AW, Karnovsky MJ. Suppression by heparin of smooth muscle cell proliferation in injured arteries. Nature 1977; 265:625–626.
125. Nam SC, Florentin RA, Janakidevi K, Lee KT, Reiner J, Thomas WA. Population dynamics of arterial smooth muscle cells. III. Inhibition by aortic tissue extracts of proliferative response to intimal injury in hypercholesterolemic swine. Exp Mol Pathol 1974; 21:259.
126. Eisenstein R, Harper E, Kuettner KE, Schumacher B, Matijevitch B. Growth regulators in connective tissue. II. Evidence for the presence of several growth inhibitors in aortic extracts. Paroi Arterielle 1979; 5:163–169.

127. Chamley-Campbell JH, Campbell GR, Ross R. Phenotype-dependent response of cultured aortic smooth muscle to serum mitogens. J Cell Biol 1981; 89:379–383.
128. Castellot JJ Jr, Addonizio ML, Rosenberg R, Karnovsky MJ. Cultured endothelial cells produce a heparin-like inhibitor of smooth muscle cell growth. J Cell Biol 1981; 90:372–379.
129. Campbell GR, Campbell JH. Smooth muscle phenotypic changes in arterial wall homeostasis: implications for the pathogenesis of atherosclerosis. Exp Mol Path 1985; 42:139–162.
130. Fritze LMS, Reilly CF, Rosenberg RD. An antiproliferative heparan sulfate species produced by postconfluent smooth muscle cells. J Cell Biol 1985; 100:1041–1049.
131. Reilly DF, Gordon D, Schwartz SM. Determination and comparison of the aortic polyploid smooth muscle content of human hypertensive subjects and normotensive controls. Acta Physiol Scand 1988; 133(suppl 571):181–188.
132. Wasteson A, Glimelius B, Busch C, Westermark B, Heldin C-H, Norling B. Effect of a platelet endoglycosidase on cell surface associated heparan sulphate of human cultured endothelial and glial cells. Thrombosis Res 1977; 11:309–321.
133. Wasteson A, Hook M, Westermark B. Demonstration of a platelet enzyme, degrading heparan sulphate. FEBS Lett 1976; 64:218–221.
134. Oosta GM, Favreau LV, Beeler DL, Rosenberg RD. Purification and properties of human platelet heparitinase. J Biol Chem 1982; 257:11249–11255.
135. Castellot JJ Jr, Favreau LV, Karnovsky MJ, Rosenberg RD. Inhibition of vascular smooth muscle cell growth by endothelial cell-derived heparin. Possible role of a platelet endoglycosidase. J Biol Chem 1982; 257:11256–11260.
136. Handin RI, Cohen JH. Purification and binding properties of human platelet factor four. J Biol Chem 1976; 251:4273–4282.
137. Reidy MA, Chao SS, Kirkman TR, Clowes AW. Endothelial regeneration. VI. Chronic nondenuding injury in baboon vascular grafts. Am J Pathol 1986; 123:432–439.
138. Gajdusek CM, Schwartz SM. Comparison of intracellular and extracellular mitogen activity. J Cell Physiol 1984; 121:316–322.
139. Imai H, Werthessen NT, Taylor CB, Lee KT. Angiotoxicity and arteriosclerosis due to contaminants of USP-grade cholesterol. Arch Pathol Lab Med 1976; 100:565–572.
140. Vlodavsky I, Fridman R, Sullivan R, Sasse J, Klagsbrun M. Aortic endothelial cells synthesize basic fibroblast growth factor which remains cell associated and platelet-derived growth factor-like protein which is secreted. J Cell Physiol 1987; 131:402–408.
141. Baird A, Ling N. Fibroblast growth factors are present in the extracellular matrix produced by endothelial cells in vitro: implications for a role of heparinase-like enzymes in the neovascular response. Biochem Biophys Res Commun 1987; 142:428–435.
142. Bar-Ner M, Eldor A, Wasserman L, Matzner Y, Cohen IR, Fuks Z,

Vlodavsky I. Inhibition of heparanase-mediated degradation of extracellular matrix heparan sulfate by non-anticoagulant heparin species. Blood 1987; 70:551–557.
143. Smith JC, Singh JP, Lilliquist JS, Goon DS, Stiles CD. Growth factors adherent to cell substrate are mitogenically active in situ. Nature 1982; 296:154–156.
144. Savion N, Vlodavsky I, Greenburg G, Gospodarowicz D. Synthesis and distribution of cytoskeletal elements in endothelial cells as a function of cell growth and organization. J Cell Physiol 1982; 110:129–141.
145. Kauffman RF, Bean JS, Zimmerman KM, Brown RF, Steinberg MI. Losartan, a nonpeptide AII receptor antagonist, inhibits neointima formation following balloon injury to rat carotid arteries. Life Sci 1991; 49: PL223–PL228.
146. Dzau VJ. Gibbons GH, Pratt RE. Molecular mechanisms of vascular renin-angiotensin system in myointimal hyperplasia. Hypertension 1991; 18(4 suppl):II100–II105.
147. Bunning P, Holmquist B, Riordan JF. Substrate specificity and kinetic characteristics of angiotensin-converting enzyme. Biochem 1983; 22:103–110.
148. Schwartz SM, Bennett MR. Death by any other name. Am J Pathol 1995; 147:229–234.
149. Haust MD, More RH, Movat HZ. The role of smooth muscle cells in the fibrogenesis of arteriosclerosis. Am J Pathol 1960; 37:377–389.
150. McGill HC Jr. Persistent problems in the pathogenesis of atherosclerosis. Arteriosclerosis 1984; 4:443–451.
151. Geer JC. Fine structure of human aortic intimal thickening fatty streaks. Lab Invest 1965; 14:1764–1783.
152. Parker F, Odland GF. A correlative histochemical, biochemical and electron microscopic study of experimental atherosclerosis in the rabbit aorta with special reference to the myointimal cell. Am J Pathol 1966; 48:197–239.
153. Wissler RW, McCallister HA Jr, Vesselinovitch D. A histopathologic study of the fatty streak in aortas and coronary arteries of young American military personnel. Am J Pathol 1975; 78:64a.
154. Thomas WA, Lee KT, Kim DN. Cell population kinetics in atherogenesis. Cell births and losses in intimal cell mass-derived lesions in the abdominal aorta of swine. Ann NY Acad Sci 1985; 454:305–315.
155. Velican C, Velican D. Differences in the pattern of atherosclerotic involvement between non-branched regions and adjacent branching points of human coronary arteries. Atherosclerosis 1985; 54:333–342.
156. Velican C, Velican D. The precursors of coronary atherosclerotic plaques in subjects up to 40 years old. Atherosclerosis 1980; 37:33–46.
157. Stary HC, McMillan GC. Kinetics of cellular proliferation in experimental atherosclerosis. Arch Path 1970; 89:173–183.
158. Spagnoli LG, Villaschi S, Neri L, Palmieri G, Taurino M, Faraglia V, Fiorani P. Autoradiographic studies of the smooth muscle cells in human arteries. Paroi Arterielle 1981; 7;107–112.

159. Villaschi S, Spagnoli LG. Autoradiographic and ultrastructural studies on the human fibro-atheromatous plaque. Atherosclerosis 1983; 48:95–100.
160. Katsuda S. Coltrera MD, Ross R, Gown AM. Human atherosclerosis IV. Immunocytochemical analysis of cell activation and proliferation in lesions of young adults. Am J Pathol 1993; 142:1787–1793.
161. Rekhter M, Nicholls S, Ferguson M, Gordon D. Cell proliferation in human arteriovenous fistulas used for hemodialysis. Arterioscler Thromb 1993; 13:609–617.
162. Gordon D, Reidy MA, Benditt EP, Schwartz SM. Cell proliferation in human coronary arteries. Proc Natl Acad Sci USA 1990; 87:4600–4604.
163. O'Brien ER, Alpers CE, Stewart DK, Ferguson M, Tran N, Gordon D, Benditt EP, Hinohara T, Simpson JB, Schwartz SM. Proliferation in primary and restenotic coronary atherectomy tissue: Implications for antiproliferative therapy. Circ Res 1993; 73:223–231.
164. O'Brien ER, Garvin MR, Dev R, Stewart DK, Hinohara T, Simpson JB, Schwartz SM. Angiogenesis in human coronary atherosclerotic plaques. Am J Pathol 1994; 145:883–894.
165. Benditt EP, Gown Am. Atheroma: the artery wall and the environment. Int Rev Exp Path 1980; 21:55–118.
166. Lee KT, Thomas WA, Florentin RA, Reiner JM, Lee WM. Evidence for a polyclonal origin and proliferative heterogeneity of atherosclerotic lesions induced by dietary cholesterol in swine. Ann NY Sci 1976; 275:336–347.
167. Thomas WA, Florentin RA, Reiner JM, Lee WM, Lee KT. Alterations in population dynamics of arterial smooth muscle cell during atherogenesis. IV. Evidence for a polyclonal origin of hypercholesterolemia diet-induced atherosclerotic lesions in young swine. Exp Mol Pathol 1976; 24:244–260.
168. Thomas WA, Reiner JM, Janakidevi K, Florentin RA, Lee KT. Population dynamics of arterial cells during atherogenesis. X. Study of monotypism in atherosclerotic lesions of black women heterozygous for glucose-6-phosphate dehydrogenase (G6PD). Exp Mol Pathol 1979; 31:367–386.
169. Thomas, WA, Reiner JM, Florentin RA, Scott RF. Population dynamics of arterial cells during atherogenesis. VIII. Separation of the roles of injury and growth stimulation in early aortic atherogenesis in swine originating in preexisting intimal smooth muscle cell masses. Exp Mol Pathol 1979; 31:124–144.
170. Lee KT, Janakidevi K, Kroms M, Schmee J, Thomas WA. Mosaicism in female hybrid hares heterozygous for glucose-6-phosphate dehydrogenase. VII. Evidence for selective advantage of one phenotype over the other in ditypic samples from aortas of hares fed cholesterol oxidation products. Exp Mol Pathol 1985; 42:71–77.
171. Pearson TA, Dillman JM, Heptinstall RH. Clonal mapping of the human aorta. Relationship of monoclonal characteristics, lesion thickness, and age in normal intima and atherosclerotic lesions. Am J Pathol 1987; 126:33–39.
172. Pearson TA, Dillman J, Malmros H, Sternby N, Heptinstall RH. Cholesterol-induced atherosclerosis. Clonal characteristics of arterial lesions in the hybrid hare. Arteriosclerosis 1983; 3:574.

173. Bond JA, Kocan RM, Benditt EP, Juchau MR. Metabolism of benzo-[a]pyrene and 7, 12-dimethylbenz[a]anthracene in cultured human fetal aortic smooth muscle cells. Life Sci 1979; 25:425–430.
174. Minick CR, Fabricant CG, Fabricant J, Litrenta MM. Atheroarteriosclerosis induced by infection with a herpesvirus. Am J Pathol 1979; 96:673–706.
175. Fabricant CG, Fabricant J, Minick CR, Litrenta MM. Herpesvirus-induced atherosclerosis in chickens. Fed Proc 1983; 42:2476–2479.
176. Benditt EP, Barrett T, McDougall JK. Viruses in the etiology of atherosclerosis. Proc Natl Acad Sci USA 1983; 80:6386–6389.
177. Gyorkey F, Melnick JL, Guinn GA, Gyorkey P, DeBakey ME. Herpesviridae in the endothelial and smooth muscle cells of the proximal aorta in arteriosclerotic patients. Exp Mol Pathol 1984; 40:328–339.
178. Melnick JL, Petrie BL, Dreesman GR, Burek J, McCollum CH, DeBakey ME. Cytomegalovirus antigen within human arterial smooth muscle cells. Lancet 1983; 2:644–647.
179. Adam E, Melnick JL, Probstfield JL, Petrie BL, Burek J, Bailey KR, McCollum CH, DeBakey ME. High levels of cytomegalovirus antibody in patients requiring vascular surgery for atherosclerosis. Lancet 1987; 2:291–193.
180. Stiles CD. The biological role of oncogenes—insights from platelet-derived growth factor. Cancer Res 1985; 45:5215–5218.
181. Penn A, Garte SJ, Warren L, Nesta D, Mindich B. Transforming gene in human atherosclerotic plaque DNA. Proc Natl Acad Sci USA 1986; 83: 7951–7955.
182. Weinberg RA. The action of oncogenes in the cytoplasm and nucleus. Science 1985; 230:770–776.
183. Waters D, Higginson L, Gladstone P, Kimball B, LeMay M, Boccuzzi SJ, Lesperance J. Effects of monotherapy with an HMG-CoA reductase inhibitor on the progression of coronary atherosclerosis as assessed by serial quantitative arteriography. Circulation 1994; 89:959–968.
184. Dilley RJ, Schwartz SM. Vascular remodeling in the growth hormone transgenic mouse. Circ Res 1989; 65:1233–1240.
185. Haudenschild CC, Schwartz SM. Endothelial regeneration. II. Restitution of endothelial continuity. Lab Invest 1979; 41:407–418.
186. Koester W. Endarteritis and arteritis. Berl Klin Wochenschr 1876; 13:454–455.
187. Geiringer E. Intimal vascularization and atherosclerosis. J Pathol Bacteriol 1951; 63:201–211.
188. Barger AC, Beeuwkes R, Lainey LL, Silverman KJ. Vasa vasorum and neovascularization of human coronary arteries. N Engl J Med 1984; 310:175–177.
189. Brown BG, Albers JJ, Fisher LD, Schaefer SM, Lin JT, Kaplan CK, Zhao XQ, Bisson BD, Fitzpatrick VF, Dodge HT. Regression of coronary artery disease as a result of intensive lipid-lowering therapy in men with high levels of apolipoprotein B. N Engl J Med 1990; 323:1289–1298.
190. Blankenhorn DH, Nessim SA, Johnson RL, Sanmarco RE, Azen SP, Cachin-Hamphill L. Beneficial effects of colestipol niacin therapy on coro-

nary atherosclerosis and coronary venous bypass grafts. JAMA 1987; 257: 3233–3240.
191. Watts GF, Lewis B, Brunt JN, Lewis ES, Coltart DJ, Smith LD, Mann JI, Swan AV. Effects on coronary artery disease of lipid-lowering diet, or diet plus cholestyramine, in the St. Thomas' Atherosclerosis Regression Study (STARS). Lancet 1992; 339:563–569.
192. Gould KL. Quantitative analysis of coronary artery restenosis after coronary angioplasty—Has the rose lost its bloom? J Am Coll Cardiol 1992; 19:946–947.
193. Kragel AH, Reddy SG, Wittes JT, Roberts WC. Morphometric analysis of the composition of atherosclerotic plaques in the four major epicardial coronary arteries in acute myocardial infarction and in sudden coronary death. Circulation 1989; 80:1747–1765.
194. Constantinides P. Plaque fissures in human coronary thrombosis. J Atheroscler Res 1966; 6:1–17.
195. Davies MJ, Thomas AC. Plaque fissuring—the cause of acute myocardial infarction, sudden ischemic death, and crescendo angina. Br Heart J 1985; 53:363–373.
196. Falk E. Morphologic features of unstable atherothrombotic plaques underlying acute coronary syndromes. Am J Cardiol 1989; 63:114E–120E.
197. Henney AM, Wakeley PR, Davies MJ, Foster K, Hembry R, Murphy G, Humphries S. Localization of stromelysin gene expression in atherosclerotic plaques by in situ hybridization. Proc Natl Acad Sci USA 1991; 88:8154–8158.
198. Davies MJ. Anatomic features in victims of sudden coronary death. Coronary artery pathology. Circulation 1992; 85(1 suppl):I19–I24.
199. Leclerc G, Kearney M, Schneider D, Rosenfield K, Losordo DW, Isner JM. Assessment of cell kinetics in human restenotic lesions by in vitro bromodeoxyuridine labeling of excised atherectomy specimens (abstract). Clin Res 1993; 41:343A.
200. Strauss BH, Umans VA, vanSuylen RJ, Defeyter PJ, Marco J, Robertson GC, Renkin J, Heyndrickx G, Vuzevski VD, Bosman FT. Directional atherectomy for treatment of restenosis within coronary stents: clinical, angiographic and histological results. J Am Coll Cardio 1992; 20:1465–1473.
201. Pickering JG, Weir L, Jekanowski J, Kearney MA, Isner JM. Proliferative activity in peripheral and coronary atherosclerotic plaque among patients undergoing percutaneous revascularization. J Clin Invest 1993; 91:1469–1480.
202. Garcia RL, Coltrera MD, Gown AM. Analysis of proliferative grade using anti-PCNA/cycin monoclonal antibodies in fixed, embedded tissues: Comparison with flow cytometric analysis. Am J Pathol 1989; 134:733–739.
203. Cowley AW. The concept of autoregulation of total blood flow and its role in hpertension. In: Laragh JH, ed. Topics in Hypertension. New York: Yorke Medical Books, 1980:184–200.
204. Mulvany MJ, Hansen PK, Aalkjaer C. Direct evidence that the greater contractility of resistance vessels in spontaneously hypertensive rats is associated

with a narrowed lumen, a thickened media, and an increased number of smooth muscle cell layers. Circ Res 1978,43.854–863.
205. Aalkjaer C, Heagerty AM, Mulvany MJ. In vitro characteristics of vessels from patients with essential hypertension. J Clin Hypertens 1987; 3:317–322.
206. Pang SC, Scott TM. Stereological analysis of the tunica media of the aorta and renal artery during the development of hypertension in the spontaneously hypertensive rat. J Anat 1981; 133:513–526.
207. Lee RM, Forrest JB, Garfield RE, Daniel EE. Ultrastructural changes in mesenteric arteries from spontaneously hypertensive rats. A morphometric study. Blood Vessels 1983; 20:72–91.
208. Cowley AW, Guyton AC. Baroreceptor reflex effects on transient and steady-state hemodynamics of salt-loading hypertension in dogs. Circ Res 1975; 36:536.
209. Lee RMKW. Vascular changes at the prehypertensive phase in the mesenteric arteries from spontaneously hypertensive rats. Blood Vessels 1985; 22:105–126.
210. Loeb AL, Mandel G, Straw JA, Bean BL. Increased aortic DNA synthesis precedes renal hypertension in rats. An obligatory step? Hypertension 1986; 8;754–761.
211. Goldby FS, Beilin LJ. Relationship between arterial pressure and the permeability of arterioles to carbon particles in acute hypertension in the rat. Cardiovasc Res 1972; 6:384–390.
212. Goldby FS, Beilin LJ. How an acute rise in arterial pressure damages arterioles. Cardiovasc Res 1972; 6:569–584.
213. Reidy MA. Schwartz SM. A technique to investigate surface morphology and endothelial cell replication of small arteries. A study in acute angiotensin-induced hypertensive rats. Microvasc Res 1982; 24:158–167.
214. Giese J. Renin, angiotensin and hypertensive vascular damage: A review. Am J Med 1973; 55:315–331.
215. Crane WAJ, Dutta LP. The utilisation of tritiated thymidine for deoxyribonucleic acid synthesis by the lesions of experimental hypertension in rats. J Path Bact 1963; 86:83–97.
216. Bevan RD. An autoradiographic and pathological study of cellular proliferation in rabbit arteries correlated with an increase in arterial pressure. Blood Vessels 1976; 13:100–128.
217. Plunkett WC, Overbeck HW. Increased arteriolar wall-to-lumen ratio in a normotensive vascular bed in coarctation hypertension. Am J Physiol 1985; 249:H859–H866.
218. Lee RM, Triggle CR. Morphometric study of mesenteric arteries from genetically hypertensive Dahl Strain rats. Blood Vessels 1986; 23:199–224.
219. Gutmann E. Neutrophic relations. Ann Rev Physiol 1976; 38:177–216.
220. Bevan RD, Tsuru H. Long-term denervation of vascular smooth muscle causes not only functional but structural damage. Blood Vessels 1979; 16:109–112.
221. Chamley-Campbell JH, Campbell GR. Development of smooth muscle and

autonomic nerves in culture. In: Burnstock G, O'Brien R, Vrbova G, eds. Somatic and Autonomic Nerve-Muscle Interactions. Amsterdam: Elsevier, 1983:35–56.
222. Rorive GL, Carlier PJ, Foidart JM. Hyperplasia of rat arteries smooth muscle cells associated with development and reversal of renal hypertension. Clin Sci 1980; 59:335–338.
223. Owens GK, Schwartz SM. Alterations in vascular smooth muscle mass in the spontaneously hypertensive rat. Role in cellular hypertrophy, hyperploidy, and hyperplasia. Circ Res 1982; 51:280–289.
224. Owens GK, Schwartz SM. Vascular smooth muscle cell hypertrophy and hyperploidy in the Goldblatt hypertensive rat. Circ Res 1983; 53:491–501.
225. Leitschuh M, Chobanian AV. Inhibition of nuclear polyploidy by propranolol in aortic smooth muscle cells of hypertensive rats. Hypertension 1987; 9:III-106-III-109.
226. Lichtenstein AH, Brecher P, Chobanian AV. Effects of deoxycorticosterone-salt hypertension on cell ploidy in the rat aorta. Hypertension 1986; 8:II-50;II;54.
227. Goldberg ID, Rosen EM, Shapiro HM, Zoller LC, Myrick K, Levenson SE, Christenson L. Isolation and culture of a tetraploid subpopulation of smooth muscle cells from the normal rat aorta. Science 1984; 226:559–561.
228. Halpern W, Warshaw DM, Mulvany MJ. Mechanical and morphological properties of arterial resistance vessels in young and old spontaneously hypertensive rats. Circ. Res 1979; 45:250–259.
229. Mulvany MJ. Blood pressure regulation and characteristics of small arteries in hypertension. Acta Med Scand 1982; 670(suppl):21–28.
230. Mulvany MJ. Determinants of vascular hemodynamic characteristics. Hypertension 1984; 6:III-13-III-18.
231. Todd ME, Laye CG, Osborne DN. The dimensional characteristics of smooth muscle in rat blood vessels. A computer-assisted analysis. Circ Res 1983; 53:319–331.
232. Mulvany MJ, Baandrup U, Gundersen HJG. Evidence for hyperplasia in mesenteric resistance vessels of spontaneously hypertensive rats using a three-dimensional disector. Circ Res 1985; 57:794–800.
233. Mulvany MJ. Resistance vessel structure in hypertension: Growth or remodeling? J Cardiovasc Pharmacol 1993; 22(suppl 5):S44–S47.
234. Falloon BJ, Bund SJ, Tulip JR, Heagerty AM. In vitro perfusion studies of resistance artery function in genetic hypertension. Hypertension 1993; 22: 486–495.
235. Folkow B. Brief historical background and clinical implications of early structural changes. Hypertension 1984; 6:II-1-III-3.
236. Warshaw DM, Root PT, Halpern W. Effects of antihypertensive drug therapy on the morphology and mechanics of resistance arteries from spontaneously hypertensive rats. Blood Vessels 1980; 17:257–270.
237. Carlier PG, Rorive GL. Pathogenesis and reversibility of the aortic changes in experimental hypertension. J Cardiovasc Pharmacol 1985; 7:S46–S51.

238. Owens GK. Influence of blood pressure on development of aortic medial smooth muscle hypertrophy in spontaneously hypertensive rats. Hypertension 1987; 9:178–187.
239. Loeb AL, Bean BL. Antihypertensive drugs inhibit hypertension-associated aortic DNA synthesis in the rat. Hypertension 1986; 8:1135–1142.
240. Freis ED, Ragan D, Pillsbury H, Mathews M. Alteration of the course of hypertension in the spontaneously hypertensive rat. Circ Res 1972; 31:1–7.
241. Limas C, Westrum B, Limas CJ. Effect of antihypertensive therapy on the vascular changes of spontaneously hypertensive rats. Am J Pathol 1983; 111:380–393.
242. Owens GK. Differential effects of antihypertensive drug therapy on vascular smooth muscle cell hypertrophy, hyperploidy, and hyperplasia in the spontaneously hypertensive rat. Circ Res 1985; 56:525–536.
243. Chobanian AV, Lichtenstein AH, Schwartz JH, Hanspal J, Brecher P. Effects of deoxycorticosterone/salt hypertension on cell ploidy in rat aortic smooth muscle cells. Circulation 1987; 75:I-102–I-106.
244. Carlier PG, Rorive GL. Evolution at aortic hyperplasia after reversal of renovascular hypertension in the rat. Arch Int Physiol Biochim 1983; 91:205–213.
245. Langille BL, Reidy MA, Kline RL. Injury and repair of endothelium at sites of flow disturbances near abdominal aortic coarctations in rabbits. Arteriosclerosis 1986; 6:146–154.
246. Langille BL, O'Donnell F. Reductions in arterial diameter produced by chronic decreases in blood flow are endothelium-dependent. Science 1986; 231:405–407.
247. Joshua IG, Wiegman DL, Harris PD, Miller FN. Progressive microvascular alterations with the development of renovascular hypertension. Hypertension 1984;6:61–67.
248. Radomski MW, Palmer RMJ, Moncada S. Comparative pharmacology of endothelium-derived relaxing factor, nitric oxide and prostacyclin in platelets. Br J Pharm 1987; 92:181–187.
249. Cocks TM, Angus JA, Campbell JH, Campbell GR. Release and properties of endothelium-derived relaxing factor (EDRF) from endothelial cells in culture. J Cell Physiol 1985; 123:310–320.
250. Vanhoutte PM. Could the absence or malfunction of vascular endothelium precipitate the occurrence of vasospasm? J Mol Cell Cardiol 1986; 18: 67–89.
252. Berk, BC, Alexander RW, Brock TA, Gimbrone MA Jr, Webb RC. Vasoconstriction: a new activity for platelet-derived growth factor. Science 1986; 232:87–90.
252. Berk BC, Brock TA, Gimbrne MA Jr, Alexander RW. Early agonist-mediated ionic events in cultured vascular smooth muscle cells. Calcium mobilization is associated with intracellular acidification. J Biol Chem 1987; 262:5065–5072.
253. Freslon JJ, Giudicelli JF. Compared myocardial and vascular effects of

captropil and dihydralazine during hypertension development in spontaneously hypertensive rats. Br J Pharmacol 1983; 80:533–543.
254. Lundgren Y. Adaptive changes of cardiovascular design in spontaneous and renal hypertension. Hemodynamic studies in rats. Acta Physiol Scand Suppl 1974; 408:1–62
255. Limas C, Westrum B, Limas CJ. Comparative effects of hydralazine and captopril on the cardiovascular changes in spontaneously hyperactive rats. Am J Pathol 1984; 117:360–371.
256. Nyborg NCB, Mulvany MJ. Lack of effect of antihypertensive treatment with felodiprine on cardiovascular structure of young spontaneously hypertensive rats. Cardiovasc Res 1985; 19:528–536.
257. Sadoshima S, Fujii K, Yao H, Ibayashi S, Fujishima M. Effect of chronic sympathetic denervation on cerebrovascular hypertrophy during the development of hypertension in rats. Brain Res 1986; 379:205–209.
258. Hart MN, Heistad DD, Brody MJ. Effect of chronic hypertension and sympathetic denervation on wall/lumen ratio of cerebral vessels. Hypertension 1980; 2:419–423.
259. Lee RMKW, Smeda JS. Primary versus secondary structural changes of the blood vessels in hypertension. Can J Physiol Pharmacol 1985; 63:392–401.

3

The Development of Arterial Lesions: A Process Controlled by Multiple Factors

Michael A. Reidy
University of Washington, Seattle, Washington

Michelle P. Bendeck
St. Michael's Hospital and University of Toronto, Toronto, Ontario, Canada

The identification of factors controlling the proliferation of arterial smooth muscle cells (SMCs) has been a much-pursued aim in vascular biology. While significant advances have been made, this goal still has not been attained. In 1967, Ross and colleagues put forward the theory that platelet-derived growth factor (PDGF) was the critical growth factor for SMC replication and that one of the early events in atherosclerosis was endothelial cell loss and platelet adhesion. Platelet α-granules are rich in PDGF, and thus SMC proliferation and intimal lesion development were hypothesized to occur at sites of arterial denudation.

Many studies demonstrated that PDGF was indeed a potent SMC mitogen in vitro, but the reaction to injury hypothesis as first described could not explain the events that take place in arteries. Very early in our work, we repeatedly showed that deliberate removal of endothelium, which was always accompanied by platelet adherence, did not necessarily lead to intimal lesion development. In these studies, arterial endothelial cells were denuded with fine nylon wire. While no SMC replication was detected and no intimal lesions formed, we did note that these wounds rapidly reendothelialized. In subsequent studies, we observed that as the width of the denuded zone was made larger, small increases in SMC replication were observed although no intimal lesions developed. This led us to hypothesize that smooth muscle growth was directly controlled by the presence of the endothelium, and that the main reason these arterial injuries did not initiate intimal lesion growth was because of the relatively rapid regrowth of endothelium suppressing SMC proliferation. Indeed, several groups had shown that heparan sulfate made by endothelial cells suppresses SMC growth. Once the injury was sufficiently extensive to delay endothelial cell regrowth, such as balloon catheter injury, then intimal lesions were commonly observed. At that time, we were unable to discern why these results were different from other denuding injuries, but they clearly showed that platelet interaction with the denuded artery was not critical for lesion growth. These results suggested that factors other than PDGF may be important for SMC proliferation.

I. MEDIAL CELL REPLICATION

Since the early studies mentioned above, many laboratories have adopted the balloon catheter as the standard technique for experimentally injuring arteries (6–8). This model yields uniform results in most laboratories and has an additional feature in that it closely resembles the process of angioplasty, which is performed on thousands of patients each year. Thus, we hope that information gained from these studies will have direct beneficial relevance to the disease process in humans. It should be noted, however, that in this laboratory, the balloon catheter injury is used to try to understand the process of SMC proliferation. While data gained in this manner may be relevant to humans, the lesions that develop in injured rat arteries are in some ways dissimilar to those in humans.

We have divided the response of an artery to balloon catheter injury into various stages or "waves." These stages are based upon the temporal sequence of events that take place in the artery after a widespread denuding injury and corresponds to the involvement of different stimuli (9). Within 24 h of balloon catheter injury to rat arteries, medial SMCs begin to replicate (Fig. 1a), and by day 4 these cells can be seen to have migrated into the intima (Fig. 1b). We have referred to these events as the first and second waves of the SMC response. Once SMCs have reached the intima, they undergo a sustained period of replication, which we call the third wave (11).

The first-wave response by SMCs has perhaps received the most attention in recent years. Results from a number of studies over the past several years have allowed us to draw some firm conclusions as to factors that control this process. After balloon injury, medial SMC replication can be detected within the first 24 h after injury and reaches its peak between 48 and 72 h after injury. An important issue was to identify

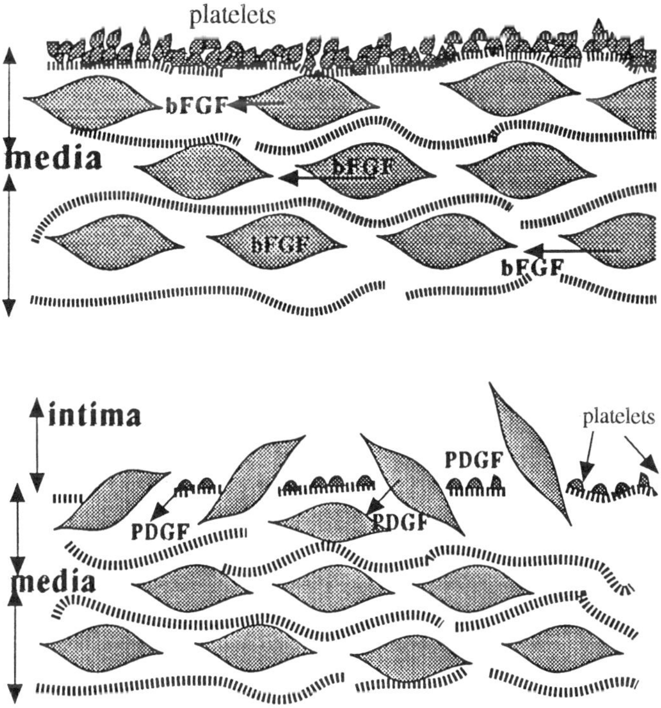

Figure 1 SMC are induced to migrate to the intimal surface within 4 days after balloon catheter injury. PDGF, which is released from the platelets and is synthesized by the SMC, has been shown to be important for this process.

the factor(s) that controlled this process. One key result came from a study in which rats were made thrombocytopenic and then subjected to balloon catheter injury (12). We observed that the absence of platelets, and presumable platelet factors, made no difference in the rate of SMC replication. In fact, SMC proliferation in the arteries of thrombocytopenic animals was identical to that observed in control animals. More recently, the role of PDGF in SMC replication has been addressed more directly by either administering recombinant PDGF to animals or by blocking PDGF with a neutralizing antibody. Neither of these treatments had any effect on the medial SMC replication in these balloon catheter-injured rat arteries (13,14).

We now believe that basic fibroblast growth factor (bFGF) is critical for stimulating the first wave of SMC replication and that its release is related to the degree of injury inflicted on the arterial wall cells. One key fact that influenced our selection of bFGF was that this protein has no signal sequence (15) and therefore is not secreted in the normal manner. This fact had led several investigators to suggest that cell injury is a mechanism by which bFGF is released (16). Thus, cell injury caused by use of the balloon catheter may be responsible for release of bFGF from the injured SMCs and therefore for the increase in cell replication. Consistent with these data is the observation that when arteries are subjected to a denuding injury that does not traumatize the arterial SMCs, only a small increase in replication occurs (10). Thus, the degree of arterial injury and release of bFGF from injured cells may be the molecular trigger for the rapid stimulation of arterial SMCs following a mechanical injury. This would also explain the results referred to above in which small zones of endothelium were removed with nylon wire and no SMC replication was observed (1,3).

One important consideration in the above theory is whether arterial SMCs synthesize bFGF. SMC have been shown to express bFGF in vitro (17) but no data were available for these cells in vivo. Northern blots of normal rat arteries showed the SMCs express bFGF and, interestingly, that a decrease in expression was observed after injury (18). Immunolocalization studies also revealed that bFGF was readily detected in the cells of normal uninjured arteries; following injury, this pattern of cellular staining was lost. This observation was confirmed by immunoblots, which also showed a fall in bFGF protein levels after injury. That the quiescent normal artery was rich in bFGF was something of a puzzle, since it might be expected that presence of the mitogen would be associated with an increase in cell division. However, SMC replication in these arteries is on the order of approximately 0.04%. One explanation as to why bFGF in the artery does not initiate replication is that the mitogen is located in a cellular compartment where it is inaccessible to the high-affinity receptors. Presumably, after injury there must be a shift in the distribution of bFGF, which is associated with entry into the cell cycle. Our immunocytochemical data show that bFGF is localized to the SMCs, and several reports have indicated that bFGF is frequently localized to the nuclei of quiescent cells. Immunocytochemistry also showed a dramatic loss of bFGF from the medial cells following injury. We therefore believe that balloon catheter injury causes damage to the SMCs, allowing bFGF to be released into the extracellular pool, and therefore is able to stimulate cell replication via the high-affinity receptors.

Thus, arterial SMCs do synthesize bFGF, but we next needed to establish that bFGF is indeed mitogenic for these cells in vivo. Accordingly, rat arteries were subjected to balloon catheter or gentle injury and bFGF was directly infused into the arterial circulation (19). This caused a dramatic increase in SMC replication, and daily infusion of bFGF led to a striking increase in intimal lesion size. In fact, the highest rates of SMC replication thus far observed in rat arteries were achieved by the addition of bFGF. We therefore concluded that in vivo bFGF is a potent mitogen for arterial SMCs. To validate that bFGF was indeed the critical mitogen for SMC replication in injured arteries, we made an antibody to bFGF to block its mitogenic action and infused it into animals immediately prior to balloon catheter injury. A single injection of this antibody (10 g/rat) caused a highly significant reduction in SMC replication (13% to 1.5%) when measured 24–48 h after balloon catheter injury (20). We believe this result strongly supports our hypothesis that bFGF is the critical mitogen involved in the stimulation of arterial medial SMCs after mechanical injury (first wave). Interestingly, this single injection of bFGF antibody did not block the growth of intimal lesions seen after 7 days, which would suggest that other pathways, independent of medial replication, are important for the growth of arterial lesions.

II. SMOOTH MUSCLE CELL MIGRATION

As with many other small animals, there are no intimal SMCs in the arteries of rats. Consequently, SMCs must migrate from the media into the intima for intimal lesions to develop. Little attention has been paid to the process of SMC migration in arterial lesion development. We first became aware of migration as a separate and differentially controlled process in studies using thrombocytopenic rats. After balloon catheter injury in platelet-deprived rats, we noted no change in intimal or medial SMC replication, but there was a marked suppression of lesion growth (12). We therefore concluded that platelet factors and possibly PDGF were important for the migration of cells into the intima. Administering PDGF antibody to rats subjected to balloon injury had no effect on cell replication, but markedly suppressed the size of the intimal lesion (14). These results suggested that PDGF played a significant role in promoting SMC migration, but not SMC replication. A similar conclusion was reached in a study in which PDGF was given to rats whose arteries had been injured with a balloon catheter (13). Chronic infusion of PDGF did not change the replication of either intimal or medial SMCs, but did significantly increase the size of the intimal lesions. Taken together, the results from the above studies strongly support the idea that PDGF stimulates SMC migration into the intima, but does not stimulate cell replication. Further, these studies emphasize that cell migration is a critical component for the growth of an intimal lesion.

Migration of SMCs presumable requires degradation of matrix surrounding the cells, so we examined expression of matrix-degrading proteases by injured arteries. Proteases such as plasmin and matrix metalloproteinases (MMPs) facilitate cell movement in situations such as tumor invasion and metastasis (21,22). After balloon catheter injury, rat arteries express increased amounts of uPA and tPA, and a marked increase in plasmin activity was detected between 3 and 10 days after injury (23). This time sequence of PA activity is interesting because SMCs are found in the intima starting 4 days after injury, therefore approximately correlating with SMC migration into the intima. In an attempt to link the presence of plasminogen activator/plasmin with SMC migration, we infused rats with transexamic acid, which binds to the lysine-binding site of plasminogen and plasmin, thus inhibiting vessel wall plasmin production (24,25). In these studies, we noted a significant reduction in the rate of SMC migration in ballooned arteries in the absence of a change in cell replication. We believe that these data support the concept that plasmin is important for the migration of SMCs into the intima, probably by degrading various matrix components of the arterial wall or by activating other proteases, such as collagenase.

In other studies, we investigated the role of growth factors on SMC protease expression. An antibody against PDGF inhibited the increase in plasmin activity seen after balloon catheter injury (23). This suggests that chemoattractants such as PDGF are able to induce expression of these proteases and may well explain how PDGF is able to promote SMC migration. bFGF is also linked to cell migration; administration of bFGF to rats with injured arteries stimulated the movement of SMCs into the intima and, as with PDGF, antibodies of bFGF were able to block this process (26). The FGF antibody, however, blocked cell migration, but did not reduce plasmin activity in these injured arteries. This suggests that other proteases may be important for the migration of SMCs.

MMPs are another family of enzymes that have the ability to degrade a variety of matrix molecules; they are expressed during normal and pathological tissue remodeling (27–31). We have characterized MMP expression in the rat carotid after two forms of arterial injury, using gelatin zymograms, Northern blots, and in situ hybridization (32). In normal, uninjured arteries, two prominent bands of gelatinolytic activity were present on zymograms (MW 70 and 62 kDa), representing latent and active MMP-2 (Fig. 2). An additional band of gelatinolytic activity (MW 88 kDa), corresponding to MMP-9, was induced within 1 day after balloon catheter injury, and this activity was present until 6 days after injury (Fig. 2). We were also able to detect an increased expression of rat MMP-9 by Northern blot and in situ hybridization. The early induction of this enzymatic activity preceded the appearance of smooth muscle cells in the intima (4 days after injury), and thus may have served to facilitate migration of cells within the media. MMP-9 activity and mRNA were not present in the vessel at 2 weeks after injury, a time when intimal smooth muscle cells were actively

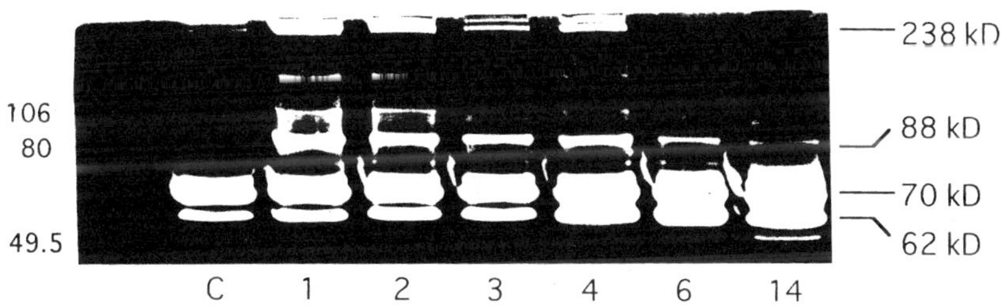

Figure 2 Time course of gelatinolytic activity in rat carotid arteries after balloon catheter injury. Arteries were taken from control animals (C) and 1,2,3,4,6, and 14 days after injury.

replicating. Thus, there was no correlation between MMP-9 activity and intimal smooth muscle cell replication. Furthermore, the administration of an MMP inhibitor, the peptide hydroxamic acid GM 6001, dramatically inhibited the migration of medial smooth muscle cells into the intima (Fig. 3) with no effect on SMC replication in media or intima (Fig. 4). These data suggest a strong link between gelatinases and SMC migration.

One final aspect relating to cell migration is whether the process of cell movement from the media into the intima is necessary for lesion growth in arteries that already possess intimal SMCs. One possible consequence of

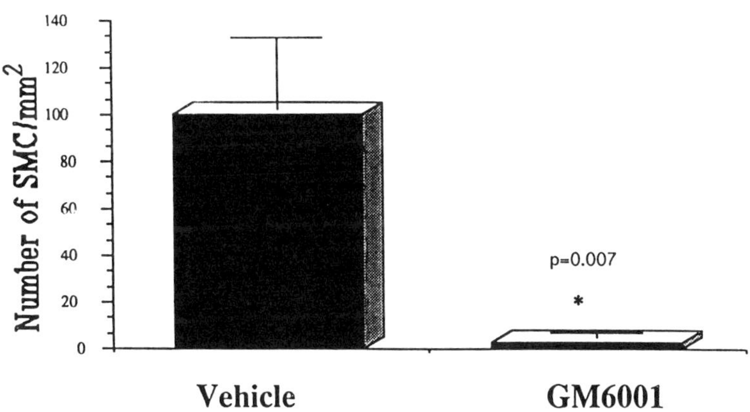

Figure 3 SMC migration onto the intimal surface 4 days after balloon injury of rat carotid artery. The MMP (GM6001) inhibitor was given daily for the experimental period.

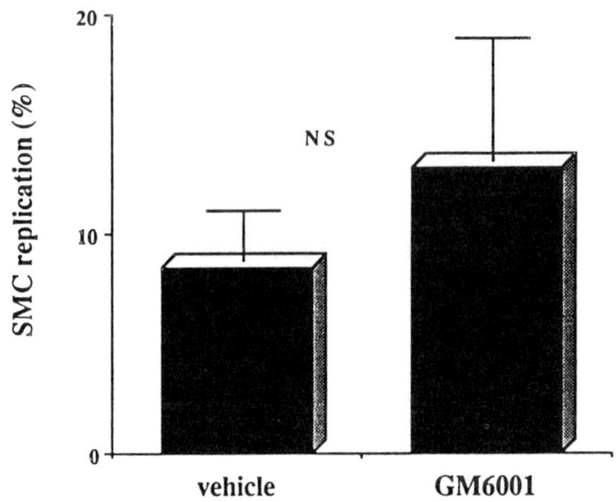

Figure 4 Medial SMC replication 4 days after balloon catheter injury. The MMP (GM6001) inhibitor was given daily for the experimental period.

injury to such arteries is that intimal lesion growth is due solely to replication of the existing intimal cells. Currently there are no reliable markers for cell migration. We can only detect cell migration by quantitating the number of SMCs in the intima when cells first begin to move. In the ballooned rat carotid, we detect the first intimal SMCs on the third day after injury, and we quantitate migration by counting the intimal cells within 24 h, at 4 days after injury. Beyond that time, any change in intimal cell number could be attributed to both intimal replication and cell migration. In arteries with existing intimal SMCs, counting the number of intimal cells would not be a valid technique to measure cell migration. This is problematic in humans, since we are currently unable to assess whether SMC migration plays a role in human lesion development. Clearly, much more work will be required before these questions are answered.

III. INTIMAL SMOOTH MUSCLE CELL REPLICATION

The highest rates of SMC replication in an injured artery are found in the intima, not the media, and this intimal replication, unlike that of the media, is sustained for several weeks. Relatively little is known about the control of intimal SMC replication, in part because the experiments on intimal cell replication have failed to discern a clear pathway as to their growth control. We have examined the role of bFGF on intimal SMCs, since one possibility was the FGF, synthesized by intimal SMCs, was responsible for this continued replication. Northern blot analysis showed no upregulation of bFGF mRNA by intimal SMCs; in fact, a decrease was observed (18). Further examination of Western blots of rat arteries showed a decrease in bFGF protein after injury. We have also tried to inhibit intimal SMC replication with our bFGF antibody, and although it was able to block medial SMC replication, no reduction in intimal SMC replication was achieved. These data suggest that perhaps bFGF has little to do with intimal replication. In a recent study, however, bFGF expression was observed in intimal lesions using a new *en face* technique (34). Of interest was the bFGF expression was high at early times after injury and almost undetectable at later times (6 weeks after injury). This association of bFGF expression and cell replication is intriguing and could suggest that bFGF is important for the proliferation of intimal SMCs. Unlike the case of a recently balloon-injured artery, we have no data of widespread cell death at these late times, and so the mechanism for bFGF release is unclear. One possibility is that blood flow over these SMC leads to nonlethal trauma and may precipitate release of bFGF (35–37). This has been found to occur with endothelial cells (38). In our studies, the SMCs that express bFGF line the luminal surface of the artery and so are in contact with flowing blood. A working hypothesis, therefore, is that bFGF can be released from these cells via nonlethal trauma and so stimulate surrounding SMCs.

Other studies examining the role of known growth factors on intimal SMC replication focused on whether these cells respond to PDGF. Data from Jawien et al. (13) showed that administration of PDGF to animals did not initiate intimal SMC replication. Infusion of PDGF antibodies, when delivered at a sufficient concentration to block SMC migration, likewise had no effect on intimal SMC replication (14). Taken together, these data suggest that PDGF is not an important mitogen for intimal SMCs. One interesting fact in these studies is that when PDGF was given to animals with quiescent intimal lesions, a small but significant increase in intimal SMC replication was detected (13). The actual replication rate was increased to approximately 2%, which is far less than we have observed after the addition of bFGF. It should be remembered, however, that the replication rate of normal uninjured arteries is approximately 0.04%, and therefore this represents a significant increase above normal replication rates. Further, a SMC replication rate of 2% per day over several months would result in an approximate doubling of SMCs in a rat carotid artery, which could have a marked impact on the pathology of the artery.

If PDGF does play a role in intimal cell proliferation, then we need to identify the source of this mitogen. In animal studies, platelet adhesion to the denuded artery is complete within the first 24 h. Once SMCs form a luminal surface (approximately 4 days), almost no adherent platelets are present (39). Therefore, if PDGF were to play any role in the chronic replication of SMCs, the source would not be from platelets. The obvious source would be the SMCs themselves. Several years ago, we showed that intimal SMCs grown in culture were able to synthesize PDGF B-chain; in contrast, no expression was observed in medial SMCs (40). The role of PDGF as an endogenously synthesized mitogen has received renewed interest with the recent finding that intimal SMCs of rat arterial lesions do express PDGF B-chain (41). These data were obtained using an *en face* approach to in situ hybridization, a technique that appears to be more sensitive than convention in situ hybridization on histological cross sections (34). Approximately 10% of intimal SMCs were found to express PDGF-B chain, and these cells were scattered throughout the lesion. This finding could suggest an autocrine or paracrine pathway for the stimulation of intimal cells, since intimal SMCs express the PDGF-β-receptor. Thus, endogenous synthesis of PDGF by SMCs may be responsible for the small but chronic increase in intimal replication. Recently published studies show that after angioplasty, the replication rate of cells in human lesions rarely exceeds more that 1–2%. Such low rates of replication are often dismissed as having little significance, but it should be remembered that a low rate of replication for several months would lead to a significant increase in lesion size. It would be interesting to see if PDGF B-chain was expressed in these lesions. This pathway is only speculative, since the current data from animal studies show that PDGF plays a role in migration but not SMC replication.

In summary, we can now divide the response of an artery to balloon catheter injury into three or more distinct stages. The first wave is medial SMC replication, which is primarily controlled by bFGF. Within 3–4 days after injury, cells begin to migrate to the intima (the second wave), and this appears to be controlled by the expression of several proteases. Blocking antibodies to both PDGF and bFGF inhibit the migration of SMCs. Finally, the third wave of response to balloon injury is the replication of intimal SMCs. Intimal SMCs respond weakly to bFGF and almost not at all to PDGF. However, the recent data showing that a selected population of intimal SMCs expresses both bFGF and PDGF is suggestive that these mitogens may play a role in intimal SMC replication.

REFERENCES

1. Reidy MA, Schwartz SM. Endothelial regeneration. III. Time course of intimal changes after small defined injury to rat aortic endothelium. Lab Invest 1981; 44:301–308.
2. Reidy MA, Silver M. Endothelial regeneration. VII. Lack of intimal proliferation after defined injury to rat aorta. Am J Pathol 1985; 118:173–177.

3. Tada T, Reidy MA. Endothelial regeneration. IX. Arterial injury followed by rapid endothelial repair induces smooth-muscle-cell proliferation but not intimal thickening. Am J Pathol 1987; 129:429–433.
4. Clowes AW, Karnovsky MJ. Suppression by heparin of smooth muscle cell proliferation in injured arteries. Nature 1977; 265:625–626.
5. Castellot JJ, Jr., Wright TC, Karnovsky MJ. Regulation of vascular smooth muscle cell growth by heparin and heparan sulfates. Sem Thromb Hemost 1987; 13:489–503.
6. Baumgartner H-R, Studer A. Folgen des Gefass kalheterismus am normo- und hypercholesterinaemischen Kaninchen. Pathol Microbiol 1966; 29:393.
7. Stemerman M, Ross R. Experimental arteriosclerosis. I. Fibrous plaque formation in primates, an electron microscope study. J Exp Med 1972; 136:769–789.
8. Clowes AW, Reidy MA, Clowes MM. Kinetics of cellular proliferation after arterial injury. I. Smooth muscle growth in the absence of endothelium. Lab Invest 1983; 49:327–333.
9. Reidy MA, Jackson J, Lindner V. Neointimal proliferation: Control of vascular smooth muscle growth. Vasc Med Rev 1992; 3:156–167.
10. Fingerle J, Au YP, Clowes AW, Reidy MA. Intimal lesion formation in rat carotid arteries after endothelial denudation in absence of medial injury. Arteriosclerosis 1990; 10:1082–1087.
11. Clowes AW, Clowes MM, Reidy MA. Kinetics of cellular proliferation after arterial injury. III. Endothelial and smooth muscle growth in chronically denuded vessels. Lab Invest 1986; 54:295–303.
12. Fingerle J, Johnson R, Clowes AW, Majesky MW, Reidy MA. Role of platelets in smooth muscle cell proliferation and migration after vascular injury in rat carotid artery. Proc Natl Acad Sci USA 1989; 86:8412–8416.
13. Jawien AD, Bowen-Pope DF, Lindner V, Schwartz SM, Clowes AW. Platelet-derived growth factor promotes smooth muscle migration and intimal thickening in a rat model of balloon angioplasty. J Clin Invest 1992; 89:507–511.
14. Ferns GAA, Raines EW, Sprugel KH, Motani AS, Reidy MA, Ross R. Inhibition of neointimal smooth muscle accumulation after angioplasty by an antibody to PDGF. Science 1991; 253:1129–1132.
15. Abraham JA, Mergia A, Whang JL, Tumolo A, Friedman J, Hjerrild KA, Gospodarowicz D, Fiddes JC. Nucleotide sequence of a bovine clone encoding the angiogenic protein, basic fibroblast growth factor. Science 1986; 233:545–548.
16. Klagsbrun M, Edelman ER. Biological and biochemical properties of fibroblast growth factors. Implications for the pathogenesis of atherosclerosis. Arteriosclerosis 1989;9:269–278.
17. Winkles JA, Friesel R, Burgess WH, Howk R, Mehlman T, Weinstein R, Maciag T. Human vascular smooth muscle cells both express and respond to heparin-binding growth factor I (endothelial cell growth factor). Proc Natl Acad Sci USA 1987; 84:7124–7128.
18. Olson NE, Chao S, Lindner V, Reidy MA. Intimal smooth muscle cell prolif-

eration after balloon catheter injury: The role of basic fibroblast growth factor. Am J Pathol 1992; 140:1017–1023.
19. Lindner V, Lappi DA, Baird A, Majack RA, Reidy MA. Role of basic fibroblast growth factor in vascular lesion formation. Circ Res 1991; 68: 106–113.
20. Lindner V, Reidy MA. Proliferation of smooth muscle cells after vascular injury is inhibited by an antibody against basic fibroblast growth factor. Proc Natl Acad Sci USA 1991; 88:3739–3743.
21. Laiho M, Keski-Oja J. Growth factors in the regulation of pericellular proteolysis: A review. Cancer Res 1989; 49:2533–2553.
22. Dano K, Andreasen PA, Grondahl-Hansen J, Kristensen P, Nielsen LS, Skriver L. Plasminogen activators, tissue degradation and cancer. Adv Cancer Res 1985; 44:139–266.
23. Jackson CL, Raines E, Ross R, Reidy MA. Role of endogenous platelet-derived growth factor in arterial smooth muscle cell migration after balloon catheter injury. Arteriosclerosis 1993; 13:1218–1226.
24. Verstraete M. Clinical application of inhibitors of fibrinolysis. Drugs 1985; 29:236–261.
25. Takada A, Takada Y. Inhibition by transexamic acid of the conversion of single-chain tissue plasminogen activator to its two chain form by plasmin: the presence on tissue plasminogen activator of a site to bind with lysine binding sites of plasmin. Thromb Res 1989; 55:717–725.
26. Jackson CL, Reidy MA. Basic fibroblast growth factor: Its role in the control of smooth muscle cell migration. Am J Pathol 1992; 143:1024–1031.
27. Matrisian LM. The matrix-degrading metalloproteinases. BioEssays 1992; 14:455–463.
28. Sreenath T, Matrisian LM, Stetler-Stevenson W, Gattoni-Celli S, Pozzatti RO. Expression of matrix metalloproteinase genes in transformed rat cell lines of high and low metastatic potential. Cancer Res 1992; 52:4942–4947.
29. Unemori EN, Bouhana KS, Werb Z. Vectorial secretion of extracellular matrix proteins, matrix-degrading proteinases, and tissue inhibitor of metalloproteinases by endothelial cells. J Biol Chem 1990; 265:445–451.
30. Alexander CM, Werb Z. Targeted disruption of the tissue inhibitor of metalloproteinases gene increases the invasive behavior of primitive mesenchymal cells derived from embryonic stem cells *in vitro*. J Cell Biol 1992; 118:727–739.
31. Werb Z. Textbook of Rheumatology. 2d ed. Philadelphia: W. B. Saunders, 1989:300–321.
32. Bendeck MP, Zempo N, Clowes AW, Galardy RE, Reidy MA. Smooth muscle cell migration and matrix metalloproteinase expression after arterial injury in the rat. Circ Res 1994; 75:539–545.
33. Grobelny D, Poncz L, Galardy RE. Inhibition of human skin fibroblast collagenase, thermolysin, and Pseudomonas aeruginosa elastase by peptide hydroxamic acids. Biochemistry 1992; 31:7152–7154.
34. Lindner V, Reidy MA. Expression of basic fibroblast growth factor and its

receptor by smooth muscle cells and endothelium in injured rat arteries: an *en face* study. Circ Res 1993; 73:589–595.

35. McNeil PL, Ito S. Molecular traffic through plasma membrane disruptions of cells *in vivo*. J Cell Sci 1990; 96:549–556.
36. McNeil PL, Muthukrishnan L, Warder E, D'Amore PA. Growth factors are released by mechanically wounded endothelial cells. J Cell Biol 1989; 109: 811–922.
37. Muthukrishnan L, Warder E, McNeil PL. Basic fibroblast growth factor is efficiently released from a cytolsolic storage site through plasma membrane disruptions of endothelial cells. J Cell Physiol 1991; 148:1–16.
38. Yu QC, McNeil PL. Transient disruptions of aortic endothelial cell plasma membranes. Am J Pathol 1992; 141:1349–1360.
39. Reidy MA, Chao SS, Kirkman TR, Clowes AW. Endothelial regeneration: chronic nondenuding injury in baboon vascular grafts. Am J Pathol 1986; 123:432–439.
40. Walker LN, Bowen-Pope DF, Ross R, Reidy MA. Production of platelet-derived growth factor-like molecules by cultured arterial smooth muscle cells accompanies proliferation after arterial injury. Proc Natl Acad Sci USA 1986; 83:7311–7315.

4

Vascular Smooth Muscle Cell Migration, Integrin Adhesion Receptors, and Neointima Formation in Restenosis

Tian-Li Yue, XinKang Wang, Jeffrey M. Stadel, and Giora Z. Feuerstein
SmithKline Beecham Pharmaceuticals, King of Prussia, Pennsylvania

I. VASCULAR SMOOTH MUSCLE CELL MIGRATION IN NEOINTIMAL FORMATION

Research on arterial remodeling following localized mechanical damage of the arterial lumen has rapidly increased in the past decade, owing to the increase in intervention procedures, such as percutaneous transluminal coronary angioplasty (PTCA), endarterectomy, and coronary artery bypass grafting (CABG) (1). While PTCAs (or stents) are highly successful procedures at the onset, disappointing results due to restenosis (30–50%) have been noted in the long term (6–12 months) (2). The mechanism of restenosis following PTCA of human atherosclerotic vessel is complex and poorly understood (3,4). To date only limited information has been obtained from humans concerning the time course of changes in vessel wall architecture that leads to restenosis (5). Knowledge of the sequence of events has mainly come from studies of experimental animals, in particular, the rat carotid artery balloon catheter injury model, which is the most extensively studied animal model for pharmacological studies of neointima formation (4,6).

A three-wave model has been introduced to explain the major events in vascular remodeling following balloon injury (Fig. 1). The first wave occurs during the first few days and consists of an increase in the replication rate of

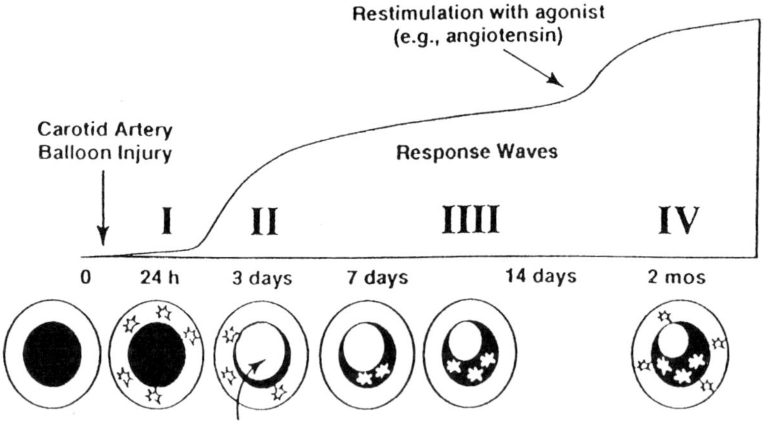

Figure 1 Balloon injury to the rat carotid artery produces medial smooth muscle cell (SMC) proliferation (first wave), followed by migration of SMC across the internal elastic lamina and formation of neointima (second wave), and then intimal SMC replication that lasts a few weeks (third wave). (From Ref. 4.)

medial vascular smooth muscle cells (SMCs) at the injury site. SMCs start synthesizing DNA within 24 h after arterial injury. This repair response does not directly contribute to the accumulation of cells in the intima, but it is possible that this first wave is necessary to provide cells that ultimately form the intimal lesion. During the second wave, SMCs cross the internal elastic lamina and form a neointima by 4–5 days after injury. The migration wave is followed by the third wave, in which smooth muscle cell replication proceeds at a lower rate that lasts weeks or months. During this period, a significant extracellular matrix production is also observed.

SMC migration following balloon injury was first demonstrated a decade ago (7) and further confirmed by electron microscopic inspection of the intimal surface. The peak of SMC migration from the media to the intima was observed at day 4–5 after balloon injury of the rat carotid artery (8,9). The importance of cellular migration in neointimal formation following angioplasty was highlighted in a study by Ross and colleagues (10). Administration of neutralizing antibodies directed against the SMC chemotactic agent, PDGF, inhibited the migration of smooth muscle cells from the media to the intima and significantly reduced the balloon injury–induced neointima formation. In contrast, there was no difference in [^{3}H]thymidine incorporation in the intima or the media of the artery after administration of either anti-PDGF or nonimmune IgG, suggesting the PDGF mediates its action principally by stimulating chemotactic migration of the SMC into the media. The data clearly demonstrate that SMC migration is essential to the development of neointimal thickening following balloon injury.

The mechanisms relating to SMC migration are not well understood. SMC movement presumably requires degradation of the basement membrane and extracellular matrix surrounding the cells. It has recently been reported that balloon injury in rat induced an 88 kDa gelatinase, and administration of a metalloproteinase inhibitor after balloon injury reduced SMC migration into the intima (9). Furthermore, cell attachment, spreading, and cytoskeleton changes are also requisite for cell migration (11,12). Firm attachment of the cell to the matrix is determined by the number of contacts localized within focal adhesions, and the connection to the cellular cytoskeleton provides the tension/traction necessary for cell motility (Fig. 2) (13). Cell migration is probably initiated by the specific recognition of extracellular matrix proteins by a family of cell surface adhesion receptors known as integrins (14,15), a large family of cell surface adhesion receptors composed of two noncovalently associated chains: the α and β chains (Fig. 3) (16). Each subunit contains a single transmembrane domain that separates a large ectodomain from its cytoplasmic tail, which in most cases is shorter than 50 amino acids. Upon ligand recognition, integrins typically cluster at the site of cell-substrate interface leading to polymerization of the actin cytoskeleton (17). In this context, they form a bridge between the extracellular and intracellular environments and affect cellular behavior by transmitting extracellular signals to the intracellular compartment, lead to gross changes in cellular morphology orchestrated by the actin cytoskeleton that facilitate cell migration. An increasing body of evidence has indicated that integrin $\alpha_v\beta_3$ is an important adhesion molecule for the mediation of vascular SMC migration. The purpose of this chapter is to provide a brief overview about the roles of $\alpha_v\beta_3$ integrin and its ligands, osteopontin and vitronectin, in neointima formation following vascular injury. The data suggest that integrin $\alpha_v\beta_3$ may be a new target for suppression of neointimal formation following angioplasty, by suppression of osteopontin or other $\alpha_v\beta_3$ ligand–induced SMC migration (18).

II. INTEGRIN $\alpha_v\beta_3$, OSTEOPONTIN, AND SMC MIGRATION

A. Integrin $\alpha_v\beta_3$ in Vascular SMCs

Integrin $\alpha_v\beta_3$ displays a broad tissue distribution and is expressed in a variety of cell types (19); however, the expression and regulation of this

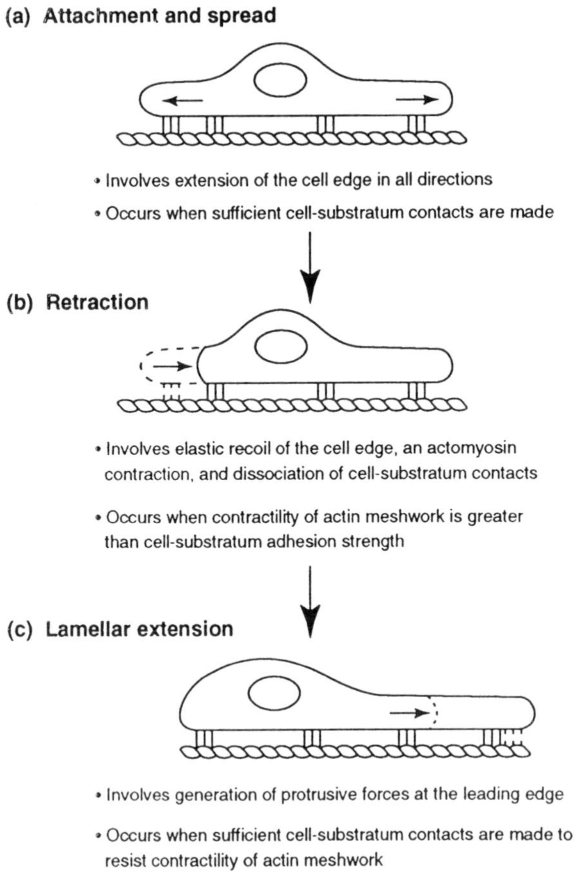

Figure 2 A schematic model of cell movement. (From Ref. 13.)

integrin in vascular SMCs are not well characterized (20). The presence of $\alpha_v\beta_3$ integrin on the human SMC surface has been detected with indirect immunofluorescence staining (21), mRNA analysis by Northern hybridization (22), and immunoprecipitation techniques (22,23). The constitutive expression of $\alpha_v\beta_3$ integrin in human aortic SMCs is quite low (22). Liaw et al. compared $\alpha_v\beta_3$ levels in adult and newborn infant aortic SMCs using flow cytometry techniques further verified by radioimmunoprecipitation of surface-labeled proteins (23). An interesting finding in the above study was that $\alpha_v\beta_3$ levels were lower in adult human SMCs compared to newborn infant SMCs; however, it is not clear how many samples from adult humans and infants were tested. Janat et al. reported that expression of

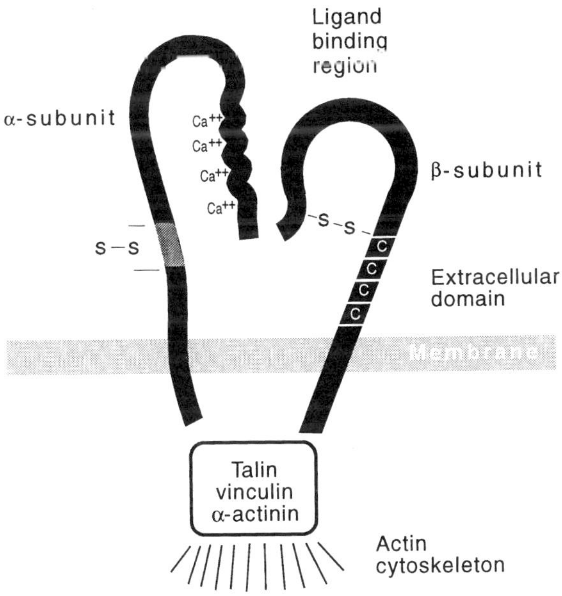

Figure 3 Schematic structure of $\alpha_v\beta_3$ integrin. (From Ref. 16.)

the $\alpha_v\beta_3$ integrin complex in rabbit aortic SMC was induced by TGF-β and PDGF, although TGF-β appeared to be the more potent inducer (20). The β_3 subunit mRNA was undetectable in quiescent cells and enhanced by both growth factors, while the α_v subunit mRNA did not change in the presence of growth factors. The results suggest that appearance of the $\alpha_v\beta_3$ integrin after growth factor stimulation was due to increased expression of the β_3 subunit mRNA. However, a recent study reported that both β_3 and α_v subunit could be upregulated by TGF-β_1 and thrombin (22). Upregulation of $\alpha_v\beta_3$ by TGF-β_1 was also observed in other cell lines such as human and mouse fibroblasts (24) and by retinoic acid in human melanoma cells (25). A recent study has demonstrated that $\alpha_v\beta_3$ is present both in the normal artery and in sites of SMC accumulation and angiogenesis in atherosclerotic plaques (26). It has been demonstrated that the NPXY structural motif within the β_3 subunit, comprising residues 744–747, is essential for cell migratory responses mediated by integrin $\alpha_v\beta_3$ in vitro and in vivo (27).

The ligands known to bind to $\alpha_v\beta_3$ integrin include vitronectin, fibrinogen, thrombospondin, von Willebrand factor, collagens, laminin, and fibronectin. The role of β_3 integrin in SMC adhesion and migration has been studied using lamb ductus arteriosus SMCs. The results indicate that SMC migration over surfaces coated with extracellular matrix proteins such as vitronectin, fibronectin, and laminin depended to a large extent on the $\alpha_v\beta_3$ receptor. In contrast, SMC adhesion to these matrix proteins depended exclusively on β_1 integrin (28). Recently, osteopontin, a matrix protein found in human atherosclerosis, has been found to possess an RGD motif through which it binds to $\alpha_v\beta_3$ integrin and thereby induces SMC migration.

B. Osteopontin: A Matrix Protein Associated with SMC Migration

Osteopontin (OPN), an Arg-Gly-Asp (RGD)–containing acidic phosphoglycoprotein, is an extracellular matrix protein first identified as a major sialylated protein in bone and subsequently found in a variety of tissues, such as kidney, placenta, and brain (29). Recent studies have found that OPN mRNA is expressed in rat aorta and carotid arteries, and markedly elevated following balloon angioplasty, suggesting a previously unappreciated role for this molecule in vascular biology and pathophysiology (30). More recently, studies have demonstrated that OPN is elevated during neointima formation in rat arteries as well as in human atherosclerotic vessels (31–35).

In vitro analysis of OPN expression in vascular SMCs has demonstrated that addition of 10% FCS-supplemented medium to subconfluent quiescent SMCs led to a strong and time-dependent induction of OPN mRNA expression and that OPN expression was associated with cell proliferation (36). Further studies on the regulation of OPN expression in cultured SMCs in our laboratory have demonstrated that PDGF is the major growth factor that upregulates OPN expression (Fig. 4), and that TGF-β_1, bFGF, and EGF showed much less effect on OPN expression compared to PDGF (Fig. 5).

Our studies and the data reported by Liaw et al. (37) have demonstrated that OPN is a powerful inducer of SMC migration. OPN enhances rat aortic SMC migration in a time-and concentration-dependent manner with an EC_{50} value of about 50–100 nM (Fig. 6A) (37,38). OPN was more effective than many other agents reported to induce SMC migration (38). Checkerboard analysis indicated that OPN-induced rat SMC migration is chemotactic in nature. OPN also promotes VSMC adhesion and spreading (37). However, OPN neither enhances SMC proliferation nor potentiates the mitogenic effect of PDGF (38).

OPN-induced rat aortic SMC migration can be blocked by the monoclonal antibody, F_{11}, which recognizes the rat integrin β_3 (Fig. 6B) (38). This

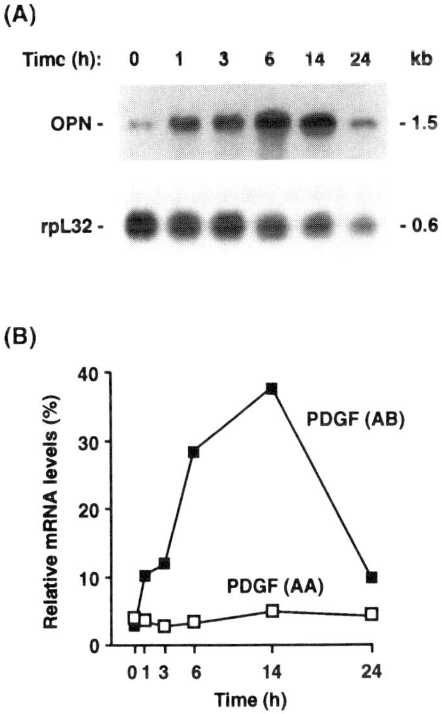

Figure 4 Northern analysis of expression of OPN mRNA in rat aortic smooth muscle cells (RASMC) induced by PDGF. (A) A representative Northern blot. (B) Quantitative OPN mRNA data in PDGF-stimulated RASMCs after normalizing with rpL32, a housekeeping gene.

was also demonstrated in human aortic SMCs in which OPN-induced cell migration was inhibited by the monoclonal antihuman $\alpha_v\beta_3$ antibody, LM609. Integrin $\alpha_v\beta_3$ are also involved in OPN-induced SMC adhesion but not in cell migration, indicating that the adhesive and migratory effects of OPN are mediated via distinct cell surface integrins (37).

While most investigations thus far have focused on the smooth muscle effects of OPN, recent observations indicate the OPN modulates the functions of endothelial cells and macrophages, suggesting that these cell types might also be targets for OPN during vascular remodeling (39–41). Since the important role played by macrophages and endothelial cells in atherosclerosis and restenosis is well recognized, the effect of OPN on these cells is of considerable interest.

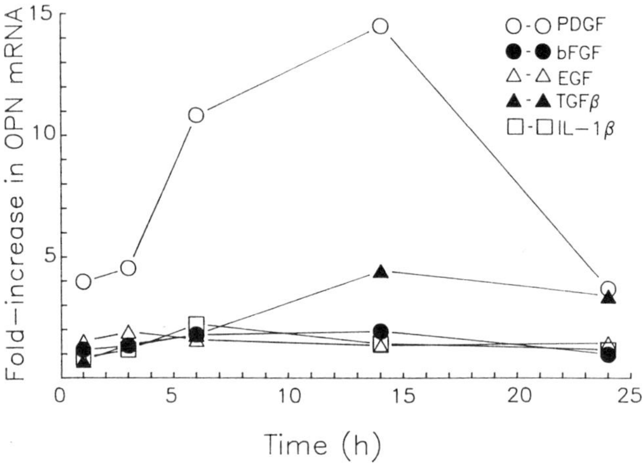

Figure 5 Effects of different growth factor/cytokines on OPN mRNA expression in cultured RASMC. The serum-deprived RASMC were challenged with 1 nM of PDGF, bFGF, EGF, and IL-1β or 5 ng/ml TGF-β_1 for 1,3,6,14, and 24 h. Total cellular RNA was isolated and analyzed using Northern hybridization. The relative intensity of OPN was determined using PhosphorImage analysis and plotted graphically after normalization with rpL32.

III. BLOCKING $\alpha_v\beta_3$ INTEGRIN RECEPTOR INHIBITS VASCULAR SMOOTH MUSCLE CELL MIGRATION *IN VITRO* AND PREVENTS NEOINTIMA FORMATION *IN VIVO*

A. In Vitro Studies

Blocking $\alpha_v\beta_3$ integrin with the RGD peptide analog, SK&F107260 (42) inhibited vitronectin-induced rat aortic SMC migration in a dose-dependent manner (Fig. 7A). Similar results were also observed when echistatin, a snake venom peptide with potent nonselective Arg-Gly-Asp antagonist activity, was used on vitronectin-induced rat and human VSMC migration (Fig. 7B). As mentioned previously, F_{11}, a monoclonal antibody specifically directed toward the rat β_3 integrin subunit, blocked OPN-induced rat aortic SMC migration. This antibody has no effect on fibronectin-induced RASMC migration, which can be inhibited by anti–integrin β_1 antibody. It was also reported recently that $\alpha_v\beta_3$-mediated human aortic SMC migration can be blocked by anti-$\alpha_v\beta_3$ antiserum (22).

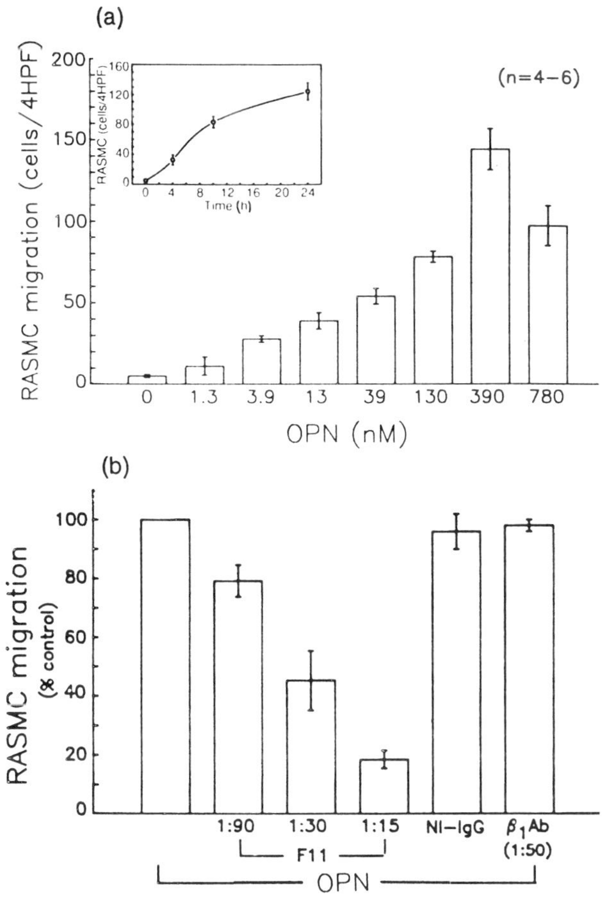

Figure 6 (a) Concentration dependency of OPN-induced rat aortic smooth muscle cell (RASMC) migration. The inset is the time course of OPN-induced RASMC migration. (b) Inhibition of OPN-induced RASMC migration by a specific antirat β_3 integrin antibodies, F_{11}. (From Ref. 38.)

B. In Vivo Studies

A cyclic RGD peptide antagonist to the $\alpha_v\beta_3$ integrin, GpenGRGDSPCA, has recently been tested in a rabbit balloon angioplasty model. The peptide was administered locally to rabbit carotid artery after balloon angioplasty, and the animals were sacrificed 2 weeks after balloon injury. The neointimal area and the ratio of intima to media were determined. Both

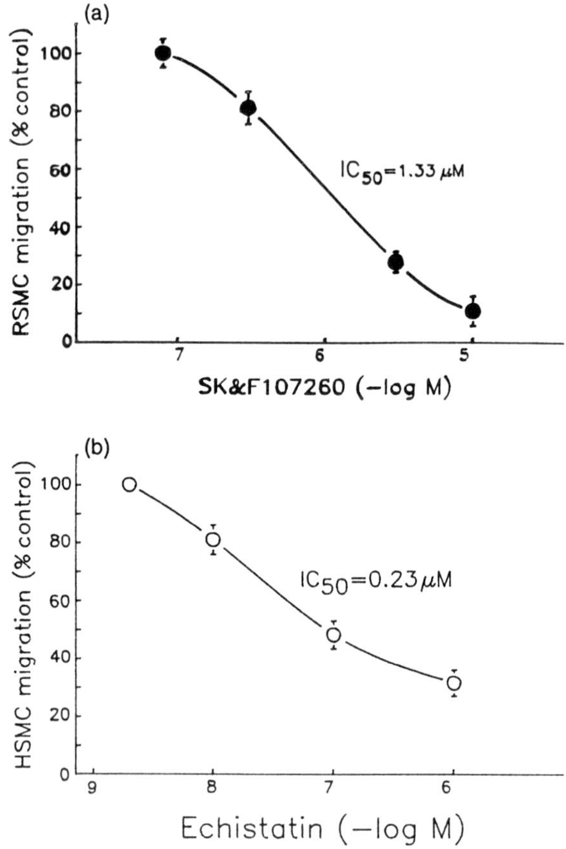

Figure 7 Inhibition of vitronectin-induced vascular smooth muscle cell migration by SK&F107260 (a) and echistatin (b).

neointima area and intima/media ratio showed a significant reduction with GpenGRGDSPCA administration (Fig. 8) (43).

The effect of SK&F107260 on neointima formation in rat carotid artery following balloon angioplasty has recently been studied in our laboratory. The peptide (SK&F107260) was delivered by osmotic minipumps at 16 mg/rat/day, and the animals were sacrificed 2 weeks after balloon injury. The results showed that the neointima cross-sectional area and the ratio of the neointima versus the media were significantly reduced by 39% and 32% respectively, in the SK&F107260-treated group versus the vehicle-treated group (Fig. 9). Furthermore, a cyclic RGD-containing peptide, G4120, which binds to both $\alpha_v\beta_3$ and $\alpha_{IIb}\beta_3$, has recently been tested in a hamster

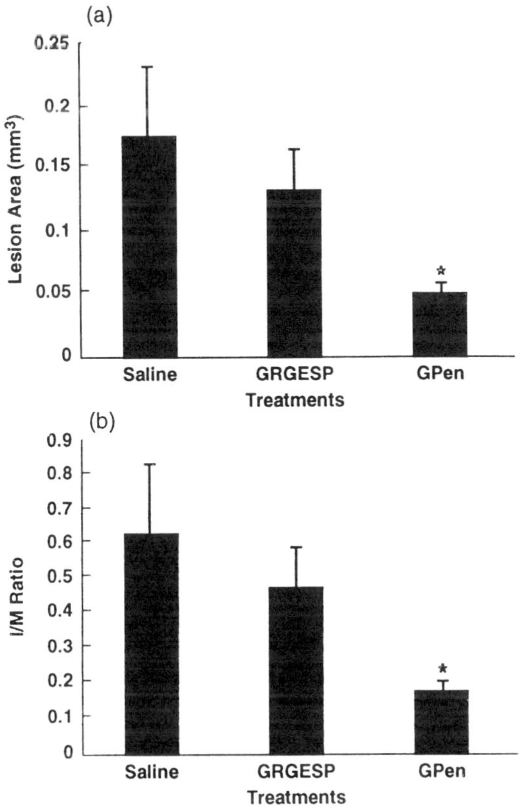

Figure 8 Inhibition of neointimal hyperplasia in a rabbit carotid artery balloon angioplasty model by a peptide $\alpha_v\beta_3$ antagonist GpenGRGDSPCA. (a) $p < 0.05$ vs. vehicle-treated group or (b) $p < 0.01$ vs. vehicle-treated group. (From Ref. 43.)

balloon angioplasty model (44). G4120 was administered by a continuous intravenous infusion using an implanted osmotic minipump. The infusion was started either 1 hour before or 30 min after balloon injury and continued for 3, 7, or 14 days. The ratio between the neointima area and the total area within the internal elastic lamina was determined. The result showed that the peptide inhibited neointima formation at the dose of 100 μg/kg/h. Since the peptide is a dual β_3 antagonist, the effect might be due both to blocking SMC $\alpha_v\beta_3$ as well as platelet $\alpha_{IIb}\beta_3$ (44).

A clinical study of monoclonal anti-β_3 integrin antibody, c7E3 Fab, significantly reduced symptoms of restenosis in angioplasty patients (45). Although the contribution of each component, $\alpha_v\beta_3$ and $\alpha_{IIb}\beta_3$, to the

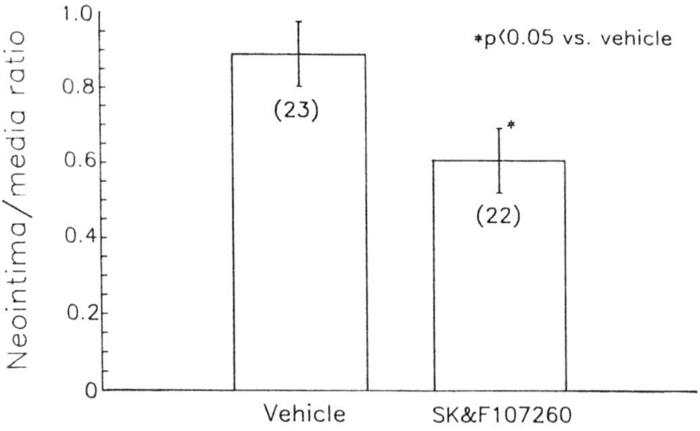

Figure 9 Inhibition of neointimal formation in rat carotid artery angioplasty model by SK&F107260. SK&F107260 (16 mg/rat/day) was delivered by osmotic minipumps (Alzet) embedded in abdominal cavity. Animals were sacrificed 14 days after balloon injury.

protective effect of the antibody is not known, inhibition of $\alpha_v\beta_3$ may have contributed to the reduction in clinical restenosis by c7E3 Fab (46). A clear advantage of a specific $\alpha_v\beta_3$ inhibitor is the absence of the risk of bleeding that was observed in patients under treatment with c7E3 Fab.

IV. SUMMARY

Vascular SMC migration is believed to play a critical role in neointima formation following angioplasty. Osteopontin and some other extracellular matrix proteins potently promote vascular SMC migration via integrin $\alpha_v\beta_3$. In vitro studies have demonstrated that blocking $\alpha_v\beta_3$ integrin inhibits SMC migration in response to certain ligands such as osteopontin and vitronectin. In vivo animal models of restenosis have suggested that RGD-containing peptides with marked selectivity against $\alpha_v\beta_3$ or both $\alpha_v\beta_3$ and $\alpha_{IIb}\beta_3$ reduced neointima formation following balloon angioplasty. Moreover, clinical data with the monoclonal anti-β_3 antibody, c7E3, significantly reduced the number of ischemic events and death in patients after coronary angioplasty. Taken together, the data suggest that development of specific $\alpha_v\beta_3$ antagonists or dual antagonists against both $\alpha_v\beta_3$ and $\alpha_{IIb}\beta_3$ may have therapeutic utility in limiting restenosis following balloon angioplasty or other vascular interventions.

REFERENCES

1. Gibbons GH, Dzau VJ. The emerging concept of vascular remodeling. N Engl J Med 1994; 330:1431–1438.
2. Bobir A, Campbell JH. Vascular derived growth factors: cell biology, pathology, and pharmacology. Pharmacol Rev 1993; 45:2–42.
3. Ross R. Cell biology of atherosclerosis. Annu Rev Physiol 1995; 57: 791–804.
4. O'Brien ER, Schwartz SM. Update on the biology and clinical study of restenosis. Trends Cardiovasc Med 1994; 4:169–178.
5. Nobuyoshi M, Kimura T, Nosaka. Restenosis after successful percutaneous transluminal coronary angioplasty: serial angiographic follow-up 229 patients. J Am Coll Cardiol 1988; 12:616–623.
6. Struijker-Boudier HA, Smits JFM, De Mey JGR. Pharmacology of cardiac and vascular remodeling. Ann Rev Pharmacol 1995; 35:509–539.
7. Clowes AW, Schwartz SN. Significance of quiescent smooth muscle migration in the injured rat carotid artery. Circ Res 1985; 56:139–145.
8. Jackson CL, Raines EW, Ross R, Reidy MA. Role of endogenous platelet-derived growth factor in arterial smooth muscle cell migration after balloon catheter injury. Arterioscler Thromb 1993; 13:1218–1226.
9. Bendeck MP, Zempo N, Clowes AW, Galardy RE, Reidy MA. Smooth muscle cell migration and matrix metalloproteinase expression after arterial injury in the rat. Circ Res 1994; 75:539–545.
10. Ferns GAA, Raines EW, Sprugel KH, Motani AS, Reidy MA, Ross R. Inhibition of neointimal smooth muscle accumulation after angioplasty by an antibody of PDGF. Science 1991; 253:1129–1132.
11. Hynes RO, Lander AD. Contact and adhesive specificities in the associations, migrations, and targeting of cells and axons. Cell 1992; 68:303–322.
12. Pollard TD, Goldman RD. Cytoplasm and cell motility. Curr Opin Cell Biol 1992; 4:1–3.
13. Lee J, Ishihara A. Jakabson K. How do cells move along surfaces? Trends Cell Biol 1993, 3:366–370.
14. Ruoslahti E. Integrins. J Clin Invest 1991; 87:1–5.
15. Hynes RO. Integrins: versatility, modulation, and signalling in cell adhesion. Cell 1992; 69:11–25.
16. Albeld SM, Buck CA. Integrins and other cell adhesion molecules. FASEB J 1990; 4:2868–2880.
17. Burridge K, Fath K, Kelly T, Nuckolls G, Turner C. Focal Adhesion: transmembrane junctions between the extracellular matrix and the cytoskeleton. Annu Rev Cell Biol 1988; 4:487–525.
18. Matsuno H, Stasen JM, Vermylen J, Deckmyn H. Inhibition of integrin function by a cyclic RGD-containing peptide prevents neointima formation. Circulation 1994; 90:2203–2206.
19. Cheresh DA. Structural and biologic properties of integrin-mediated cell adhesion. Lab Immunol 1992; 12:217–236.
20. Janat MF, Argraves WS, Liau G. Regulation of vascular smooth muscle cell

integrin expression by transforming growth factor b1 and by platelet-derived growth factor-BB. J Cell Physiol 1992; 151:588–595.
21. Choi ET, Engel L, Callow AD, Sun S, Trachtenberg J, Santoro S, Ryan US. Inhibition of neointimal hyperplasia by blocking $\alpha_v\beta_3$ integrin with a small peptide antagonist GpenGRGDSPCA. J Vasc Surg 1994; 19:125–134.
22. Brown SL, Lundgren CH, Nordt T, Fujii S. Stimulation of migration of human aortic smooth muscle cells by vitronection: implications for atherosclerosis. Cardiovasc Res 1994; 28:1815–1820.
23. Liaw L, Skinner MP, Raines EW, Ross R, Cheresh DA, Schwartz SM. The adhesive and migratory effects of osteopontin are mediated via distinct cell surface integrins. J Clin Invest 1995; 95:713–724.
24. Ignotz RA, Heino J, Massague J. Regulation of cell adhesion receptors by transforming growth factor-b. J Biol Chem 1989; 264:389–392.
25. Santos CLS, Giorgi RR, Frochtengarten F, Elias MCQB, Chammas R, Brentani RR. Regulation of vitronectin receptor expression by retinoic acid on human melanoma cells. Int J Clin Res 1994; 24:148–153.
26. Hoshiga M, Alpers CE, Smith LL, Giachelli CM, Schwartz SM. $\alpha v\beta 3$ integrin expression in normal and atherosclerotic artery. Circ Res 1994; 77:1129–1135.
27. Filardo EJ, Brooks PC, Deming SL, Damsky C, Cheresh DA. Requirement of the NPXY motif in the integrin β_3 subunit cytoplasmic tail for melanoma cell migration in vitro and in vivo. J Cell Biol 1995; 130:441–450.
28. Clyman RI, Mauray F, Kramer RH. b_1 and b_3 integrins have different roles in the adhesion and migration of vascular smooth muscle cells on extracellular matrix. Exp Cell Biol 1992; 200:272–284.
29. Butler WT. The nature and significance of osteopontin. Connect Tissue Res 1989; 23:123–136.
30. Giachelli C, Bae N, Lombardi D, Majesky M, Schwartz S. Molecular cloning and characterization of 2B7, a rat mRNA which distinguishes smooth muscle cell phenotypes in vitro and is identical to osteopontin (secreted phosphoprotein I, 2aR). Biochem Biophys Res Commun 1991; 177:867–873.
31. Giachelli C, Bae N, Almeida M, Denhardt DT, Alpers CE, Schwartz SM. Osteopontin is elevated during neointima formation in rat arteries and is a noval component of human atherosclerotic plaques. J Clin Invest 1993; 92:1686–1696.
32. Ikeda T, Shirasawa T, Esaki Y, Yoshiki S, Hirokawa K. Osteopontin mRNA is expressed by smooth muscle-deprived foam cells in human atherosclerotic lesions of the aorta. J Clin Invest 1993; 92:2814–2820.
33. Hirota S, Imakita M, Kohri K. Expression of osteopontin messenger RNA by macrophages in atherosclerotic plaques. Am J Pathol 1993; 143:1003–1008.
34. Shanahan CM, Cary NR, Metcalfe JC, Weissberg PL. High expression of genes for calcification-regulating proteins in human atherosclerotic plaques. J Clin Invest 1994; 93:2393–2402.
35. O'Brien ER, Garvin MR, Stewart DK. Osteopontin is synthesized by macrophage, smooth muscle and endothelial cells in primary and restenotic

human coronary atherosclerotic plaques. Arterioscler Thromb 1994; 14: 1648–1656.
36. Gadeau A-P, Campan M, Millet D, Candresse T, Desgranges C. Osteopontin overexpression is associated with arterial smooth muscle cell proliferation in vitro. Arterioscler Thromb 1993; 13:120–125.
37. Liaw L, Almeida M, Hart CE, Schwartz SM, Giachalli CM. Osteopontin promotes vascular cell adhesion and spreading and is chemotactic for smooth muscle cells in vitro. Circ Res 1994; 74:214–224.
38. Yue TL, McKenna PJ, Ohlstein EH, Farach-Carson MC, Butier WT, Johanson K, McDevitt P, Feuerstein GZ, Stadel JM. Osteopontin-stimulated vascular smooth muscle cell migration is mediated by β integrin. Exp Cell Res 1994; 214:459–464.
39. Murry CE, Giachelli CM, Schwartz SM, Vracko R. Macrophages express osteopontin during repair of myocardial necrosis. Am J Pathol 1994; 145: 1450–1462.
40. O'Brien ER, Garvin MR, Stewart DK, Hinohara T, Simpson JB, Schwartz SM, Giachelli CM. Osteopontin is synthesized by macrophage, smooth muscle, and endothelial cells in primary and restenotic human coronary atherosclerotic plaques. Arterioscler Thromb 1994; 14:1648–1656.
41. Giachelli CM, Schwartz SM, Liaw L. Molecular and cellular biology of osteopontin. Trends Cardiovasc Med 1994; 5:88–95.
42. Samanen J, Ali FE, Romoff T, Calvo R, Sorensos E, Vasko J, Berry D, Bennett D, Strohsacker M, Powers DJS, Nichols A. Development of a small RGD-peptide fibrinogen receptor antagonist with potent antiaggregatory activity in vitro. J Med Chem 1991; 34:3114–3125.
43. Choi ET, Engel L, Callow AD, Sun S, Trachtenberg J, Santoro S, Ryan US. Inhibition of neointimal hyperplasia by blocking $\alpha_v\beta_3$ integrin with a small peptide antagonist GpenGRGDSPCA. J Vasc Surg 1994; 19:125–34.
44. Matsuno H, Stassen JM, Vermylen J, Deckmyn H. Inhibition of integrin function by a cyclic RGD-containing peptide prevents neointima formation. Circulation 1994; 90:2203–2206.
45. EPIC investigators: Use of a monoclonal antibody directed against the platelet glycoprotein llb/llla receptor in high-risk coronary angioplasty. N Engl J Med 1994; 330:956–961.
46. Lefkovits J, Plow EF, Topol EJ. Platelet glycoprotein llb/llla receptors in cardiovascular medicine. N Engl J Med 1995; 332:1553–1559.

5

Advanced Glycation End Products Interacting with Their Cellular Receptor Induce Oxidant Stress: Implications for the Pathogenesis of Vascular Disease in Aging and Diabetes

Ann Marie Schmidt, Osamu Hori, Shi Du Yan, and David Stern
Columbia University College of Physicians and Surgeons, New York, New York

I. INTRODUCTION

Proteins or lipids exposed to aldose sugars undergo nonenzymatic glycation and oxidation (1–7). The initial, reversibly formed products of these interactions are the Schiff bases/Amadori products, the best known of which is hemoglobin A_{1c}, used clinically as a measure of diabetic glycemia control over a period of weeks. In the presence of persistent glycation, further complex molecular rearrangements may occur; the ultimate products of these irreversible reactions are known as advanced glycation end products, or AGEs. AGEs, a heterogeneous group of structures, are composed of yellow-brown pigments and are characterized by their fluorescence and their ability to form cross-links and to result in the generation of reactive oxygen intermediates (7–9). AGEs accumulate in the plasma and the vessel wall during the process of normal aging, but to an accelerated degree in patients with diabetes, proportional to the extent and duration of hyperglycemia, and are believed to be contributory factors in the pathogenesis of vascular disease associated with these two states (1,2,4).

AGEs are further characterized by their ability to recognize a class of receptors on cellular surfaces (11–14). The AGE-receptor interaction appears critical in the delivery of oxidant stress to the cells, a process likely contributory to ongoing vascular damage and ultimately the development of vascular disease.

II. CHARACTERIZATION OF CELLULAR RECEPTORS FOR AGEs

A. Identification of AGE-Binding Polypeptides

Our initial characterization of cellular receptors for AGEs began with extract of bovine lung, a material rich in endothelial cells, selected as a starting material since this particular cell type demonstrated dose-dependent, saturable binding of ^{125}I-AGE albumin, a prototypic ligand prepared in vitro by incubating albumin with glucose or other aldose sugars, with dissociation constants in the range of 50–200 nM (12,15,16). Further, as the binding of ligand to cultured endothelial cells was destroyed in the presence of trypsin or detergent (12), it was concluded that the cellular binding sites were likely composed, at least in part, of polypeptide(s). We thus undertook the isolation of these cellular binding proteins by subjecting bovine lung detergent extract to sequential chromatography on hydroxylapatite, followed by FPLC Mono S and gel filtration. By this process, we identified two polypeptides based on their ability to bind AGEs. The first, a newly identified member of the immunoglobulin superfamily of cell surface molecules, is known as RAGE, or the receptor for AGE. The other is a lactoferrinlike polypeptide based on amino-terminal sequence analysis and shared immunoreactivity with purified antibodies to lactoferrin, an iron-binding protein (12,13,17). This chapter will focus on the former molecule, RAGE.

B. RAGE: Molecular Cloning Studies

Molecular cloning studies revealed a significantly shared homology (>90%) among the bovine, human, murine, and rat counterparts of RAGE. The putative hydropathy plot (Fig. 1) reveals that the molecule is composed of an extracellular domain composed of three putative immunoglobulinlike domains: one "V"-type domain followed by two "C"-type domains. This portion of the molecule shares its greatest homology to the neural cell adhesion molecule. Following this extracellular domain is a hydrophobic putative transmembrane-spanning domain followed by a short highly charged cytosolic tail, which bears homology to CD20, a marker of B-cell activation (13). Upon transfection of the cDNA for RAGE into 293 cells, the cells acquire the ability to bind AGEs, which is blocked by anti-RAGE IgG (Fig. 2), suggesting that RAGE, a membrane-spanning polypeptide, is likely to be a cellular binding site for AGEs (13).

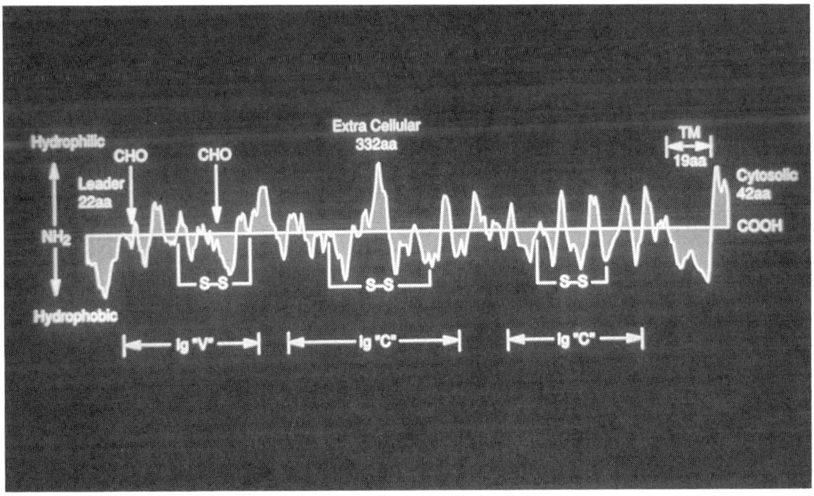

Figure 1 Hydrophilicity plot of bovine RAGE. The hydropathy plot of bovine RAGE generated from the Hopp and Woods program of intelligenetics. NH_2, amino terminus; COOH, carboxyl terminus; CHO, N-linked glycosylation sites; TM, transmembrane spanning domain; S-S, disulfide-linked cysteine residues; IgG and IgC, immunoglobulinlike variable and constant domains, respectively.

C. Histological Survey of the Cellular Distribution of RAGE

Using monospecific antibody to RAGE, the presence of RAGE has been identified in a number of diverse cell types (18). RAGE expression has been demonstrated in the endothelium and vascular smooth muscle, as well as in mononuclear phagocytes (in all cases both in cultured cells and tissue sections from organs). The identification of RAGE in these cell types places it in a unique position to be critically important in the development of vasculopathy mediated by AGEs, affecting a number of physiological systems. Further, RAGE is present in other cell types (mesangial cells), as well as in a certain population of central nervous system neurons (18). In addition to the indications for a role of RAGE in potentially mediating diabetic complications observed in the kidney and nervous system, these data further suggest that RAGE may have important functions via interaction with alternative ligands in other physiological/pathophysiological settings. For example, experiments with cultured rat embryonic neurons have suggested a role for RAGE in mediating neurite outgrowth on specific matrices (unpublished observations).

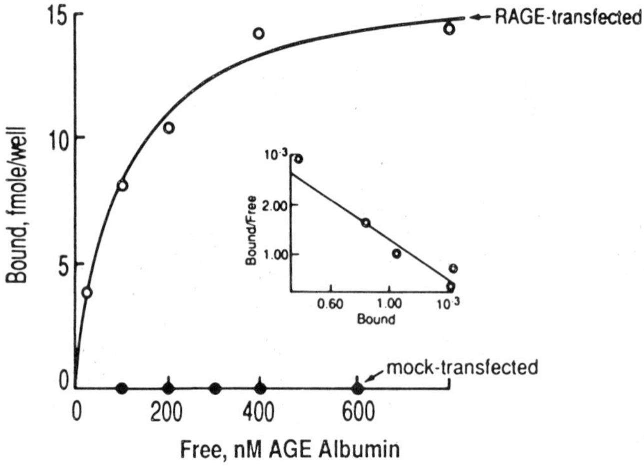

Figure 2 Binding of ^{125}I-AGE albumin by transfected 293 cells. A radioligand binding assay was performed on 293 cells transfected with the cDNA for RAGE (open circles) or mock-transfected 293 control cells (closed circles) by adding the indicated concentrations of ^{125}I-AGE albumin alone or in the presence of unlabeled AGE albumin (at a 20-fold molar excess). After an incubation period of 2 h, the cultures were washed and cell-bound radioactivity eluted with minimal essential medium containing Triton X-100 (1%). Each point is the mean of quadruplicate determinations, and the inset shows Scatchard analysis of the same data. Parameters of binding are $K_D = 100 \pm 20$ nM (value ± standard error) and $n = 17 \pm 1$ fmol/well.

III. ROLE OF AGE-RAGE INTERACTION IN THE DEVELOPMENT OF CELLULAR OXIDANT STRESS

Numerous previous studies have strongly linked glycation and oxidation and have demonstrated that AGEs can result in the generation of reactive oxygen intermediates (8,9). We hypothesized that AGEs interacting with their cellular receptor, RAGE, might result in the generation of an oxidant stress imparted to the vasculature. In this context, one may postulate that this interaction might therefore be responsible for a range of alterations in the normal homeostatic mechanisms of the cell (2). Our previous studies have demonstrated that incubation of AGE albumin prepared in vitro, AGEs immunoisolated from the plasma of diabetic patients (19), AGE-β_2-microglobulin [a glycated form of the plasma protein accumulates in patients with renal failure and likely plays a role in the development of hemodialysis-associated arthritis (20,21)], or diabetic red blood cells (22,23) results in the generation of oxidant stress to cultured endothelium as demonstrated by the generation of thiobarbituric acid–reactive substances, induction of mRNA for heme oxygenase-1, and activation of the transcription factor NF-kB (19) [the latter two observations have been linked to the presence of oxidant stress was demonstrated by the studies of others (24,25)]. Each of these AGE-induced phenomena indicative of cellular oxidant stress was inhibited in the presence of antioxidants placed in the culture medium or in the presence of blocking antibodies to RAGE (19).

The critical test of our hypothesis that AGE-RAGE interaction imparted an oxidant stress to the cell with consequent changes in cellular properties was whether these observations could be extended to the in vivo setting. In this context, infusion of AGE mouse albumin into normal mice resulted in the generation of oxidant stress as demonstrated by the presence of malondialdehyde-specific epitopes in the vascular wall (Fig. 3A). In contrast, infusion of nonglycated native albumin did not result in immunoreactivity for malondialdehyde epitopes within the vasculature (Fig. 3B). Furthermore, immunoreactivity was not found in the presence of nonimmune IgG, in place of antimalondialdehyde IgG (Fig. 3C). Further evidence of AGE-induced oxidant stress in vivo was manifested by RAGE-mediated generation of thiobarbituric acid–reactive substances in a range of organs, as well as by the induction of mRNA for heme oxygenase-1 and the activation of NF-kB in the livers of AGE-treated animals (Fig. 4). After infusion of AGE albumin into normal mice, the livers were removed and nuclear extracts prepared. Electrophoretic mobility shift assay with ^{32}P-labeled probe for consensus sequence of NF-kb revealed the presence of DNA-binding activity in the presence of AGEs (Fig. 4, lanes 2 and 6). In contrast, no significant increase in DNA-binding activity was noted after infusion of native albumin (Fig. 4, lane 1). The specificity of this DNA-binding activity in the presence of AGEs is indicated by complete competition in the presence of excess unlabeled NF-kB probe compared with lack of inhibition in the presence of an irrelevant probe, Spl (Fig. 4, lanes 7 and 8, respectively). The central role of RAGE in mediating the effects of AGEs was demonstrated by inhibition of the activation of NF-kB in the presence of anti-RAGE IgG (Fig. 4, lane 3). In contrast, nonimmune IgG was without effect (data not shown). That these results are due to the generation of AGE-RAGE–mediated oxidant stress is demonstrated by the inhibition of AGE-induced activation of NF-kB in the presence of the antioxidant probucol (Fig. 4, lane 4).

These data suggest that the interaction of AGEs with their cellular receptor results in the generation of an oxidant stress both in vitro and in vivo. The important significance of activation of NF-kB in the development

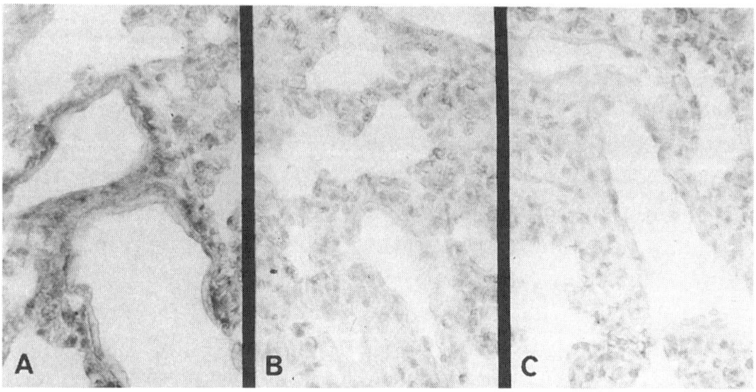

Figure 3 Immunohistological demonstration of malondialdehyde epitopes in the vasculature of rats after infusion of AGE rat serum albumin. Rats were infused with either AGE rat serum albumin (1 mg/animal; A) or native rat serum albumin (1 mg/animal; B). After 60 min, rats were humanely sacrificed and tissues processed for the detection of malondialdehyde epitopes by indirect immunoalkaline phosphatase. In panel C, sections from an animal infused with AGE albumin were reacted with nonimmune IgG and then processed as in A and B. (Magnification ×400.)

of vascular lesions has been suggested by the work of others suggesting a critical link in the activation of this transcription factor with the ultimate transcriptional regulation of cytokines, long believed to play a critical role in the development of atherogenesis (26). In addition, the activation of NF-kB has been linked to the transcriptional regulation of cellular adherence molecules, also believed to play a role in the development of vascular disease (26).

IV. AGE-RAGE INTERACTION RESULTS IN THE ENHANCED EXPRESSION OF VASCULAR CELL ADHESION MOLECULE-1 IN ENDOTHELIAL CELLS BOTH IN VITRO AND IN VIVO

An important component of the development of vascular pathology is the expression of inducible adherence molecules, which render the vasculature a selective target for the attraction of circulating mononuclear cells. Previous work by others has demonstrated that VCAM-1 is likely to be especially important in this process since its enhanced expression has been observed in the vasculature in experimental hypercholesterolemia-induced atherosclerosis (27,28) and in the vasculature of alloxan-treated diabetic rabbits (29). Furthermore, enhanced vascular VCAM-1 expression has

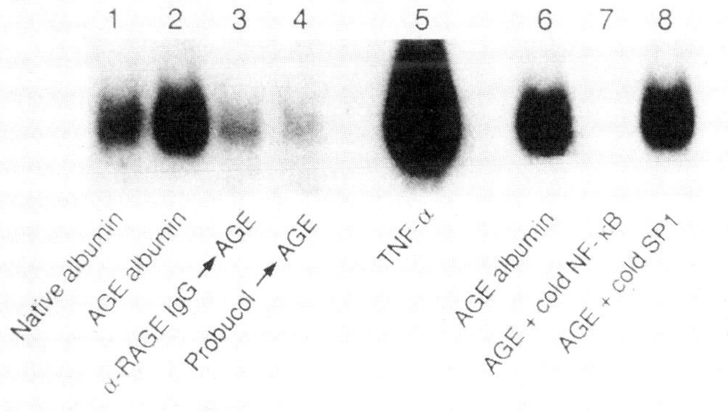

Figure 4 AGE-induced cellular oxidant stress: activation of NF-kB in vivo. Mice were infused with either AGE albumin, native albumin, or tumor necrosis factor alpha. Livers were then harvested and nuclear extracts prepared. Where indicated, mice were pretreated with either anti-RAGE IgG or probucol, as noted in the figure. The binding of nuclear proteins to the NF-kB site was demonstrated using electrophoretic gel shift mobility assay. All lanes contain the labeled probe, and other additions are as indicated below the numbered lane.

been demonstrated in human atherosclerotic lesions (30). Since previous work by others has demonstrated that the transcriptional regulation of VCAM-1 is, at least in part, due to the role of redox-sensitive pathways (31), we postulated that AGE-RAGE–induced oxidant stress might also result in enhanced expression of VCAM-1 within the vasculature.

Incubation of cultured human endothelial cells with AGE albumin or AGEs immunoisolated from the plasma of diabetic patients results in time-dependent enhanced adhesivity of Molt-4 cells (mononuclear cells that bear the counterligand for VCAM-1, VLA-4), a process inhibited in the presence of anti-VCAM $F(ab')_2$ as well as by antioxidants, anti-RAGE $F(ab')_2$, and soluble RAGE (sRAGE, the extracellular two thirds of the molecule) (32). Consistent with these data, AGEs result in increased expression of VCAM-1 antigen as measured by ELISA in cultured human endothelial cells, a process also inhibited by antioxidants and RAGE blockade. That this increase in VCAM-1 antigen and functional activity was due to increased transcription of VCAM-1 mRNA was demonstrated both by Northern blot and nuclear run-on experiments (32), processes dependent on generation of oxidant stress and RAGE.

Since NF-kB binding sites in the promoter of the VCAM-1 gene have been implicated in the regulation of VCAM-1 expression in response to certain cytokines such as tumor necrosis factor alpha (TNF-2), mediated at least in part by an oxidant-sensitive mechanism (31–33), we postulated that AGE-induced cellular oxidant stress might result in enhanced VCAM-1 expression, at least in part by the activation of NF-kB. Indeed, exposure of endothelial cells to AGE albumin resulted in activation of NF-kB binding to specific DNA sequences in the promoter of the VCAM-1 gene by electrophoretic mobility shift assay (Fig. 5, lanes 3, 6, and 10). In contrast, native albumin had no effect (Fig. 5, lane 2). This AGE-induced DNA-binding activity was sequence-specific since its appearance was blocked in the presence of excess unlabeled NF-kB probe, but not in the presence of excess unlabeled mutationally inactivated NF-kB probe (Fig. 5, lanes 4 and 5, respectively). DNA binding was dependent on the p50 and p65 proteins of the NF-kB proteins in the nucleus as indicated by the distinct retardation patterns of AGE-induced gel shift bands in the presence of anti-p65 IgG, anti-p50 IgG, or both anti-p65 and anti-p50 IgG together (Fig. 5, lanes 7, 8, and 9, respectively). The importance of AGE-RAGE interaction in the activation of NF-kB was demonstrated by dose-dependent inhibition in the presence of anti-RAGE IgG (Fig. 5, lanes 11 and 12) but not in the presence of nonimmune IgG (Fig. 5, lane 13). Furthermore, the role of oxidant stress in this process is demonstrated by inhibition of AGE-induced activation of NF-kB by N-acetylcysteine (Fig. 5, lane 14). These data indicate that AGE–endothelial RAGE interaction activates nuclear-binding activity for the VCAM-1 NF-kB site, likely via an oxidant-sensitive mechanism.

Consistent with these in vitro data, infusion of AGE albumin into normal mice resulted in increased expression of VCAM-1 in the vasculature (Fig. 6B). In contrast, native albumin was without effect (Fig. 6A).

We further found that exposure of cultured endothelial cells to AGEs resulted not only in increased expression of cell-associated VCAM-1 antigen, but also in increased soluble VCAM-1 (sVCAM-1) as measured in culture supernatants by ELISA (32). We postulated that since this material did not appear to antagonize the binding of Molt-4 cells to TNF-2–treated endothelial cells in pilot studies, that perhaps sVCAM-1 might be a marker of vascular dysfunction as manifested by enhanced expression of cellular VCAM-1. In this context, we found that in an unselected group of diabetic individuals (the only exclusion was evidence of renal insufficiency; defined as serum creatinine > 1.2 mg/dl), higher levels of sVCAM-1 were found in their plasma compared to nondiabetic individuals (1,115 ng/ml vs. 632 ng/ml, $p < 0.001$, respectively) and that this increase parallelled increased levels of AGE-immunoreactive material in the plasma of the diabetic patients versus that in the normal controls (244 ng/ml AGE albumin equivalents vs. 157 ng/ml AGE albumin equivalents, $P < 0.001$, respectively). Further examination of diabetic patients revealed that patients with mi-

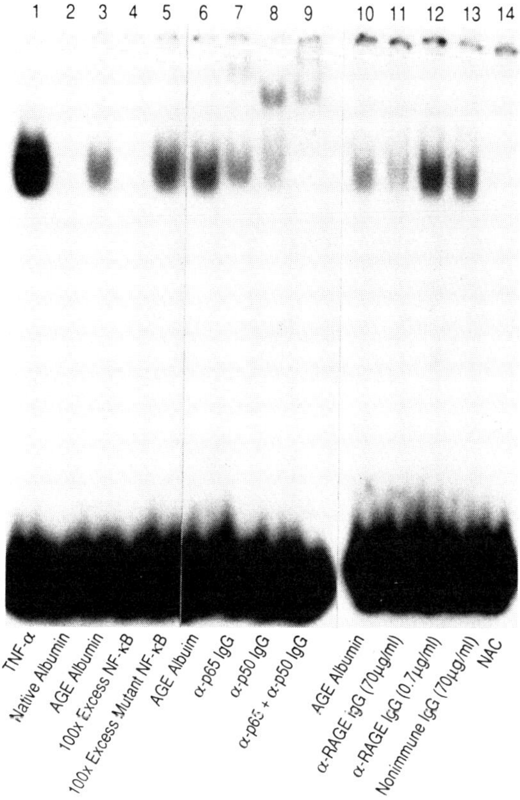

Figure 5 AGE albumin–mediated induction of endothelial VCAM-1: activation of NF-kB via binding of endothelial nuclear proteins to the NF-kB binding site in the VCAM-1 promoter. All lanes in this electrophoretic gel shift mobility assay contain the labeled probe. Endothelial cells were treated with AGE albumin, native albumin, or tumor necrosis factor alpha. Cells were then harvested and nuclear extracts prepared. Where indicated, cells were pretreated with anti-RAGE IgG (70 μg/ml or 0.7 μg/ml), nonimmune IgG, or N-acetylcysteine as noted in the figure. Other additions, including competition studies and supershift experiments, are indicated below each numbered lane.

croalbuminuria, considered a likely marker of diffuse vascular dysfunction in diabetes, had significantly higher levels of sVCAM-1 compared with diabetic patients with normoalbuminuria (757 ng/ml vs. 505 ng/ml, $p < 0.05$). We hypothesize that while the significance of elevated sVCAM-1 in this context is not clear, it is possible that at least sVCAM-1 may serve as a marker of the extent of vascular perturbation in diabetes. Of course, while

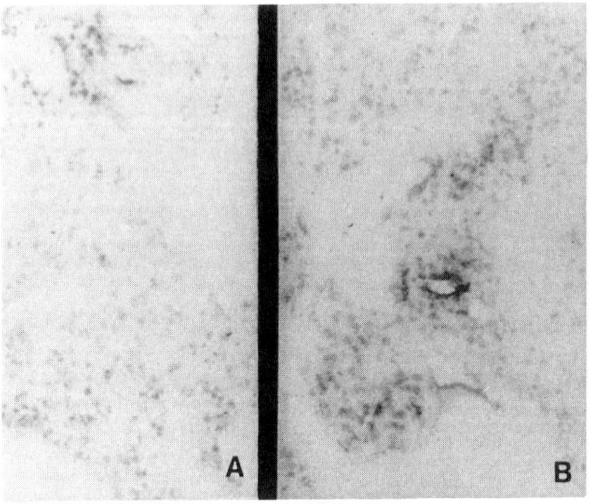

Figure 6 AGE albumin infusion into mice induces vascular expression of VCAM-1. Mice were infused with either native albumin (500 μg/ml; A) or AGE albumin (500 μg/ml;B). After 6 h, lung was harvested and immunohistochemistry performed with antimurine VCAM-1 antibody.

endothelial expression of VCAM-1 may occur in response to diverse stimuli, such as cytokines (34), as well as by oxidant stress, which results directly from hyperglycemia itself (35), it is nevertheless possible that serial measurement of sVCAM-1 levels might be of benefit not only in identifying the extent of vascular dysfunction in patients with diabetes, but also in monitoring the effectiveness of therapeutic interventions.

V. CONCLUSION

Irreversibly glycated proteins accumulate in the presence of elevated levels of plasma glucose as well as on long-lived molecules present within the vascular wall. These characteristics prime AGEs to be contributory in the pathogenesis of vascular disease both during the normal aging process and especially in diabetes. AGEs, via interaction with their cellular receptor, RAGE, a newly identified member of the immunoglobulin superfamily of cell surface molecules, impart an enhanced oxidant stress to vascular cells, both in vitro and in vivo (Fig. 7). One of the critical consequences of this ligand-receptor interaction is activation of the transcription factor NF-kB,

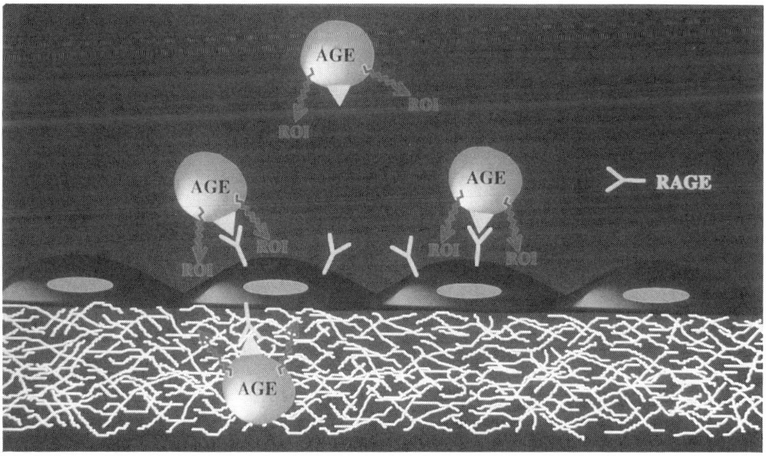

Figure 7 AGEs induce cellular oxidant stress via interaction with RAGE. AGEs, whether circulating as irreversibly modified plasma proteins or on the surface of diabetic red blood cells, or those immobilized on long-loved vascular wall proteins, interact with cellular RAGE. One of the consequences of this ligand-receptor interaction is the delivery of an oxidant stress to the vasculature. The central hypothesis of this work is that AGE-RAGE–induced oxidant stress sets into motion a series of events likely to result in ongoing chronic vascular dysfunction, characteristic of the alterations in homeostasis observed in aging and especially in diabetes.

a process linked to the transcriptional regulation of cytokines and cellular adherence molecules, such as VCAM-1, factors likely to be critical in the development of vascular pathology. Central to this oxidant-sensitive AGE-induced activation of NF-kB and enhanced expression of endothelial VCAM-1 is inhibition in the presence of RAGE blockade, either by anti-RAGE IgG or sRAGE. It is likely that the inhibitory effect of sRAGE and anti-RAGE IgG derive, at least in part, from their ability to delay the interaction of vascular AGEs with the vessel wall (36). Taken together, we conclude that these data suggest a future receptor-directed therapeutic target in the treatment of vascular dysfunction observed in both diabetes and aging.

REFERENCES

1. Ruderman N, Williamson J, Brownlee M. Glucose and diabetic vascular disease. FASEB J 1992; 6:2905–2914.
2. Baynes J. Role of oxidative stress in development of complications in diabetes. Diabetes 1991; 40:405–412

3. Sell D, Monnier V. Structure elucidation of a senescence cross-link from human extracellular matrix: implication of pentoses in the aging process. J Biol Chem 1989; 264:21597–21602.
4. Brownlee M, Cerami A, Vlassara H. Advanced glycosylation end products in tissue and the biochemical basis of diabetic complications. N Engl J Med 1988; 318:1315–1320.
5. Bucala R, Makita Z, Koschinsky T, Cerami A, Vlassara H. Lipid advanced glycosylation: pathway for lipid oxidation in vivo. Proc Natl Acad Sci USA 1993; 90:6434–6438.
6. Hicks M, Delbridge L, Yue D, Reeve R. Catalysis of lipid peroxidation by glucose and glycosylated proteins. Biochem Biophys Res Commun 1988; 151:649-655.
7. Hunt J, Smith C, Wolff S. Autooxidative glycosylation and possible involvement of peroxides and free radicals in LDL modification by glucose. Diabetes 1990; 30:1420–1424.
8. Mullarkey C, Edelstein D, Brownlee M. Free radical generation by early glycation products: a mechanism for accelerated atherogenesis in diabetes. Biochem Biophys Res Commun 1990; 173:932–939.
9. Sakurai T, Tsuchiya S. Superoxide production from nonenzymatically glycated protein. FEBS Lett 1988; 236:406–410.
10. Klein R, Klein B, Moss S, Davis M, DeMets DL. Glycosylated haemoglobin predicts the incidence and progression of diabetic retinopathy. JAMA 1989; 260:2864–2868.
11. Yang Z, Makita J, Horii y, Brunelle S. Cerami A, Sehajpal P, Suthanthiran M, Vlassara H. Two novel rat liver membrane proteins that bind advanced glycosylation end products: relationship to macrophage receptor for glucose-modified proteins. J Exp Med 1991; 174:515–524.
12. Schmidt AM, Vianna M, Gerlach M, Brett J, Ryan J, Kao J, Esposito C. Hegarty H, Hurley W, Clauss M, Wang F, Pan YC, Tsang T, Stern D. Isolation and characterization of binding proteins for advanced glycation endproducts for lung tissue which are present on the endothelial cell surface. J Biol Chem 1992; 267:14987–14997.
13. Neeper M, Schmidt AM, Brett J, Yan SD, Wang F, Pan YC, Elliston K, Stern D, Shaw A. Cloning and expression of RAGE: a cell surface receptor for advanced glycation end products of proteins. J Biol Chem 1992; 267: 14998–15004.
14. El-Khoury J, Thomas CA, Loike J, Cao L, Silverstein SC. Macrophages adhere to glucose-modified basement membrane collagen IV via their scavenger receptors. J Biol Chem 1994; 269:10197–10200.
15. Esposito C, Gerlach H, Brett J, Stern D, Vlassara H. Endothelial receptor-mediated binding of glucose-modified albumin is associated with increased monolayer permeability and modulation of cell surface coagulant properties. J Exp Med 1989; 170:1387–1407.
16. Schmidt AM, Yan SD, Brett J, Mora R, Nowygrod R, Stern D. Regulation of human mononuclear phagocyte migration by cell surface-binding pro-

teins for advanced glycation end products in vivo. J Clin Invest 1993; 92:2155–2168.
17. Schmidt AM, Mora R, Cao R, Yan SD, Brett J, Ramakrishnan R, Tsang TC, Simionescu M, Stern D. The endothelial cell binding site for advanced glycation end products consists of a complex: an integral membrane protein and a lactoferrin-like polypeptide. J Biol Chem 1994; 269:9882–9888.
18. Brett J, Schmidt AM, Yan SD, Zou YS, Weidman E, Pinsky D, Nowygrod R, Neeper M, Przysiecki C, Shaw A, Migheli A, Stern D. Survey of the distribution of an newly characterized receptor for advanced glycation end products in tissues. Am J Pathol 1993; 143:1699–1712.
19. Yan SD, Schmidt AM, Anderson GM, Zhang J, Brett J, Zou YS, Pinsky D, Stern D. Enhanced cellular oxidant stress by the interaction of advanced glycation end products with their receptors/binding proteins. J Biol Chem 1994; 269:9889–9897.
20. Miyata T, Inagi R, Iida Y, Sato M, Yamada N, Oda O, Maeda K, Seo H. Involvement of β_2-microglobulin modified with advanced glycation end products in the pathogenesis of hemodialysis-associated amyloidosis. J Clin Invest 1994; 93:521–528
21. Schmidt AM, Yan SD, Hori O, Stern D, Miyata T. The monocyte interaction site of glucose-modified β_2-microglobulin is the receptor for advanced glycation endproducts. Circulation 1994; 90(part 2) abstract #1251.
22. Wautier JL, Paton C, Wautier MP, Pintigny D, Abadie E, Passa P, Caen J. Increased adhesion of erythrocytes to endothelial cells in diabetes mellitus and its relation to vascular complications. N Engl J Med 1981; 305:237–242
23. Wautier JL, Wautier MP, Schmidt AM, Anderson GM, Hori O, Zoukourian C, Capron L, Chappey O, Yan SD, Brett J, Guillausseau PJ, Stern D. Advanced glycation end products (AGEs) on the surface of diabetic red cells bind to the vessel wall via a specific receptor inducing oxidant stress in the vasculature: a link between surface-associated AGEs and diabetic complications. Proc Natl Acad Sci USA 1994; 91:7742–7746.
24. Keyse S, Applegate L, Tromvoukis Y, Tyrell R. Oxidant stress leads to transcriptional activation of the human heme oxygenase gene in cultured skin fibroblasts. Mol Cell Biol 1990; 10:4967–4969.
25. Schreck R, Rieber P, Baeuerle P. Reactive oxygen intermediates as apparently widely used messengers in the activation of the NF-kB transcription factor and HIV-1. EMBO J 1991; 10:2247–2258.
26. Collins T. Endothelial nuclear factor kB and the initiation of the atherosclerotic lesion. Lab Invest 1993; 68:499–508.
27. Cybulsky M, Gimbrone M. Endothelial expression of a mononuclear leukocyte adhesion molecule during atherogenesis. Science 1991; 251:788–791.
28. Li H, Cybulsky M, Gimbrone M. Libby. An atherogenic diet rapidly induces VCAM-1, a cytokine-regulatable mononuclear leukocyte adhesion molecule, in rabbit aortic endothelium. Arterioscler Thromb 1993; 13:197–204.
29. Richardson M, Hadcock S, DeReske M, Cybulsky M. Increased expression in vivo of VCAM-1 and E-selectin by the aortic endothelium of normo-

lipemic and hyperlipemic diabetic rabbits. Arterioscler Thromb 1994; 14: 760–769.
30. O'Brien KD, Allen MD, McDonald TO, Chait A, Harlan JM, Fishbein J, McCarty J, Ferguson M, Hudkins K, Benjamin CD, Lobb R, Alpers CE. Vascular cell adhesion molecule-1 is expressed in human coronary atherosclerotic plaques. Implications for the mode of progression of advanced coronary atherosclerosis. J Clin Invest 1993; 92:945–951.
31. Marui N, Offermann M, Swerlick R, Kunsch C. Raosen C, Ahmad M, Alexander R, Medford R. VCAM-1 gene transcription and expression are regulated through an oxidant-sensitive mechanism in human vascular endothelial cells. J Clin Invest 1993; 92:1866–1874.
32. Schmidt AM, Hori O, Chen JX, Li JF, Crandall J, Zhang J, Cao R, yan SD, Brett J, Stern D. Advanced glycation endproducts interacting with their endothelial receptor induce expression of vascular cell adhesion molecule-1 (VCAM-1) in cultured human endothelial cells and in mice: a potential mechanism for the accelerated vasculopathy of diabetes. J Clin Invest. In press.
33. Neish A, Williams A, Palmer H, Whitley M. Collins T. Functional analysis of the human VCAM-1 promoter. J Exp Med 1992; 176:1583–1593.
34. Iademarco M, McQuillan J, Dean D. VCAM-1: contrasting transcriptional control mechanisms in muscle and endothelium. PNAS USA 1993; 90:3943–3947.
35. Pober J, Cotran R. Cytokines and endothelial cell biology. Physiol Rev 1990; 70:427–451.
36. Schmidt AM, Hasu M, Popov D, Zhang JH, Chen J, Yan SD, Brett J, Cao R, Kuwabara K, Costache G, Simionescu N, Simionescu M, Stern D. Receptor for advanced glycation end products (AGEs) has a central role in vessel wall interactions and gene activation in response to circulating AGE proteins. PNAS USA 1994; 91:8807–8811.

6

Transforming Growth Factor-β in Restenosis

Karen M. Anderson, Mary E. Brawner, and Andrew J. Nichols
SmithKline Beecham Pharmaceuticals, King of Prussia, Pennsylvania

I. INTRODUCTION

Following an acute injury, a complex set of cellular and molecular interactions are initiated at the site of injury to stimulate tissue repair. The reparative process frequently results in normal healing and restoration of function, but under certain (yet largely unpredictable) circumstances it will proceed to a fibroproliferative scar/lesion and subsequent related pathology (1). Progression of the normal intimal fibroproliferative response to restenosis following interventional revasularization in some patients likely involves dysregulated, excessive, or persistent action of mediator(s) involved in the normal wound-healing response. Transforming growth factor-β (TGF-β) is a multifunctional cytokine which is upregulated in response to tissue injury. TGF-β influences both migration and proliferation of vascular cells and plays a unique role in regulation of extracellular matrix deposition. Significant evidence now exists that establishes TGF-β as an important factor in vascular remodeling associated with restenosis. This chapter will review the cellular and molecular biology of TGF-β and its receptors, the vascular effects of TGF-β, the role of TGF-β in wound healing and tissue repair, and the evidence that implicates TGF-β in restenosis. The multifunctional nature of TGF-β makes inhibition of this cytokine an attractive therapeutic target for prevention of restenosis. Data from a limited number of studies that examined the effect of inhibiting TGF-β activity in fibroproliferative disorders, including restenosis, will also be discussed.

II. THE TGF-βs

A. The Superfamily of TGF-β–Related Peptides

TGF-β is a 25 kDa homodimeric protein. Three structurally related mammalian isoforms—TGF-β_1, TGF-β_2, and TGF-β_3—have been identified and cloned (2–4). The amino acid sequences of the mature forms of these peptides share 70–75% identity (5). Together with a number of more distantly related peptides, including the activins, inhibins, bone morphogenetic proteins, growth differentiation factors, and Müllerian inhibiting substance, the TGF-βs comprise a superfamily of multifunctional proteins involved in tissue development, differentiation, and repair (5–9). The TGF-βs themselves influence a wide range of processes associated with cellular proliferation and differentiation. By regulating angiogenesis, cellular migration, cellular proliferation, and extracellular matrix turnover, TGF-β plays a critical role in inflammation and wound repair. TGF-α, an additional but structurally distinct transforming growth factor, is a homolog of epidermal growth factor (EGF) that binds to the EGF receptors. TGF-α is not a member of the superfamily of TGF-β–related peptides and will not be discussed further in this chapter.

B. TGF-β Expression

The TGF-βs are expressed by virtually all cells and tissues. Although there are reports that certain cell types including fibroblasts and vascular smooth muscle cells express all three TGF-β isoforms when maintained in continual culture (4,10–12), important recent data provide examples of both cell-specific (13–17) and tissue-specific (17–20) patterns of isoform expression and evidence for different temporal patterns of expression by cells or tissues that co-express two or all three TGF-βs (12,21–27). Differential expression of TGF-β isoforms in vivo has been well documented, particularly during embryogenesis (21–27), and differential regulation by a variety of stimuli has been described in vitro, mainly in cultured cells (28–33). The TGF-βs regulate their own expression in a complex manner, as indicated by evidence that TGF-β_2 upregulates expression of all three isoforms, while TGF-β_1 upregulates its own expression but downregulates TGF-β_2 and TGF-β_3 expression (112). The genes encoding TGF-β_1, TGF-β_2, and TGF-β_3 are located on different chromosomes (34–36). Molecular cloning and characterization of the promoter regions of these three genes reveals little sequence similarity and, thus, provides a molecular basis for involvement of various signal transduction molecules and sequence-specific transcription factors in differential transcriptional activation of the three genes (37–47). Recent data indicating differential patterns of posttranscriptional regulation of the three TGF-β isoforms (12,48) adds further complexity to mechanisms by which the TGF-β system is regulated.

C. Regulation of TGF-β Activity

Each mature TGF-β molecule is composed of two identical 112-amino-acid subunits, which represent the carboxyl termini of two identical 390-amino-acid prepropeptides (Fig. 1). Following removal of a short signal peptide from the prepropeptide, endoproteolytic processing releases the mature TGF-β from the precursor. The enzymes involved in this intracellular processing step are not well understood. Dubois and colleagues (49) recently demonstrated that human furin, a member of a newly identified six-member family of calcium-dependent serine proteases called SPCs (subtilisinlike pro-protein convertases), efficiently and accurately processes the TGF-β_1 propeptide both in vitro and in vivo. In addition, they provided evidence that TGF-β_1 significantly increases furin expression in NIH-3T3 cells and synovial cells, suggesting that TGF-β_1 upregulates expression of its own converting enzyme. These observations together with ubiquitous expression of both furin and TGF-β_1, colocalization of their intracellular localization, and the presence of an optimum furin consensus cleavage motif in the pro-TGF-β_1 amino acid sequence led these investigators to conclude that furin is a physiologically relevant human TGF-β_1 convertase. PACE4, another member of the SPC family, may also serve as a TGF-β–converting enzyme (49).

The mature processed TGF-β secreted by most cells is not able to bind to its signaling receptors and, therefore, is biologically inactive (50). This is due to noncovalent association of the aminoterminal portion of the processed dimeric precursor protein (at this point referred to as the latency associated peptide, LAP) with the mature TGF-β homodimer (5,7,50,51) (Fig. 1). In some cells, including platelets, the LAP is further associated by disulfide bonds with a second protein, the latent TGF-β binding protein (LTBP), although this protein is not necessary to confer latency on TGF-β (51). The mechanisms responsible for activating the latent secreted form of TGF-β in vivo are not well understood. Release of the biologically active TGF-β dimer has been demonstrated in vitro by a variety of means including acidosis, glycosidases, or proteolytic digestion by cathepsin D or plasmin (52–57). The tissue enzyme transglutaminase, which cross-links latent TGF-β to cell surfaces or matrix molecules, may also be required for activation of latent TGF-β (58). Potential relevance of these data to in vivo

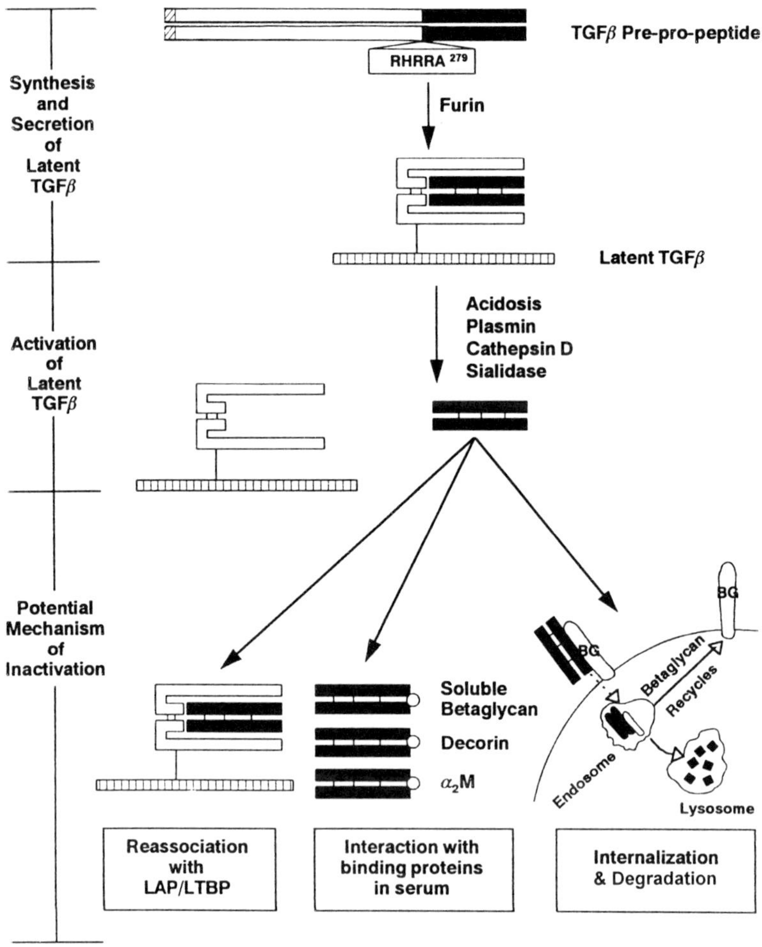

Figure 1 Mechanisms of TGF-β processing. Schematic representation of the processes involved in synthesis and secretion of latent TGF-β, proteolytic processing of the mature peptide from the prepropeptide, and mechanisms of activation/inactivation of the peptide. Refer to text for details.

situations is indicated by the presence of local acidic microenvironments in injured tissues (7,9,59), secretion of sialidase by activated macrophages (60), and activities of cell surface plasmin and cathepsin D (54,55). The TGF-β_1 propeptide contains mannose-6-phosphate, through which it can bind to the cation-independent mannose-6-phosphate/IGF-II receptor. Binding of latent TGF-β_1 to the IGF-II receptor on both endothelial cells and vascular smooth muscle cells may be necessary for its subsequent activation (61–63). In addition, latent TGF-β is able to bind to the nonsignaling (type III, betaglycan) TGF-β receptor (9). It is possible that binding (i.e., capturing) the inactive TGF-β by these receptors or other TGF-β binding proteins serves to concentrate TGF-β at the cell surface for subsequent proteolytic activation by cell surface proteases.

Once activated, TGF-β is capable of binding to its specific signaling cell surface receptors to initiate its various biological responses (see below). Potential mechanisms by which TGF-β is subsequently inactivated (Fig. 1) include reassociation with the latency-associated peptide, binding to circulating TGF-β binding proteins such as soluble betaglycan, decorin, or α_2-macroglobulin, and internalization of the TGF-β–surface receptor complex (8,64–66).

III. TGF-β RECEPTORS

A. Multiple TGF-β Receptor Subtypes

The cellular action of TGF-β is mediated through binding to cell surface receptors. Affinity labeling and cross-linking of iodinated TGF-β_1 to cell surface proteins has revealed multiple TGF-β binding proteins and led to the identification of three distinct high-affinity (picomolar) TGF-β receptors named type I, type II, and type III according to their relative mobility in nondenaturing gels (6,8,67,68). Within the last 4 years, all three TGF-β receptor subtypes have been cloned (69–74), thus facilitating studies to advance our understanding of the mechanisms through which TGF-β elicits its diverse biological effects. The type III receptor is an 853-amino-acid cell surface proteoglycan with a large extracellular domain containing both heparan sulfate and chondroitan sulfate glycosaminoglycan side chains (72–75); it has been renamed betaglycan. The type I and type II receptors are single membrane-spanning serine/threonine kinase receptors (69–71). The type I receptor is also referred to as the ALK5 receptor, as it was once one of six cloned orphan serine/threonine kinase receptors originally named *a*ctivin-*l*ike *k*inase receptors 1–6, but since identified as functional type I receptors for various members of the superfamily of TGF-β-related peptides (6,69,76–78).

B. TGF-β Receptor Distribution

Examination of TGF-β receptor expression by chemical cross-linking of radiolabeled TGF-β to a variety of normal (i.e., nontransformed) cell lines indicates broad (but not ubiquitous) expression of the type III receptor and ubiquitous expression of both the type I and type II receptors (79–81).

Northern analysis of TGF-β receptor mRNA expression patterns in a limited panel of normal human tissues also suggests that the receptors are ubiquitously expressed, but that there are differences in the levels of expression of the three receptors among the tissues examined (69,71,72). Extensive examination of TGF-β receptor expression by reverse transcriptase-polymerase chain reaction analysis of 30 normal adult porcine tissues indicates that all three TGF-β receptors are indeed universally expressed (K. M. Anderson, M.D. Kelly, A. J. Nichols, unpublished). Changes in the pattern of TGF-β receptor expression have been noted both in vitro in response to various culture conditions (81–92) and in vivo during development (93,94). Whether the expression of TGF-β receptors—including the ratio of the three subtypes—is altered in disease is a significant issue, which must be addressed if we are to understand the role of the TGF-β system in fibroproliferative disorders such as restenosis and atherosclerosis. Of potential importance to the vascular function of TGF-β is the observation that endothelial cells do not express betaglycan (type III) receptor. They do, however, express endoglin, a large cell surface proteoglycan that, like betaglycan, is capable of binding the TGF-βs (95).

C. Mechanisms of TGF-β Receptor Activation and Intracellular Signaling

Molecular cloning of the type III TGF-β receptor (72–74) revealed a short cytoplasmic domain, which has a high content of serine and threonine residues, but which does not have any known signaling motif. TGF-βs bind to the core protein of this cell surface proteoglycan. All three isoforms bind with equivalent affinity, but the function of the receptor subsequent to TGF-β binding is not clear (5). Betaglycan is the most abundantly expressed TGF-β receptor and, relative to the type I and type II receptors, it has a lower affinity for the TGF-βs. Thus, it has been proposed that betaglycan may serve as a high-density, lower-affinity receptor which binds TGF-β to locally increase the peptide concentration on the cell surface, thereby enhancing activation of the peptide and binding to the type I and type II receptors (5,8). Evidence in support of this model includes increased binding and activation of type II receptors in cells transfected with complementary DNA for the type III receptor (73,96). However, data showing a paradoxical increase in type I receptor binding with concomitant decreased binding to type III and type II receptors (90) suggest that this may not be a universal model.

The mechanisms of activation of the type I and type II receptors have been studied predominantly by expression of the receptors (native, mutated, or truncated) in various cell lines (naive, transformed, or chemically mutated). Based on these studies, two general models have evolved for mechanisms of TGF-β binding and activation of intracellular signaling cascades (97–100). As shown in Figure 2 (left), the fundamental premise of the first (Massagué) model is that both type I and type II receptor subtypes are absolutely required to elicit biological responses to TGF-β and that the type I and type II receptors form a functional heterodimer subsequent to TGF-β binding, but that *all* signaling occurs through the type I receptor. According to this model, the type II receptor is a constitutively active kinase whose activity is not increased by ligand binding; the type I receptor is unable to bind TGF-β free in solution (i.e., extracellular), but the type II receptor is capable of binding free TGF-β. It is proposed that TGF-β binds first to the type III receptor to either concentrate or activate the TGF-β for subsequent binding to the type II receptor. TGF-β binding to the type II receptor induces recruitment of the type I receptor, which is then capable of binding TGF-β to form a stable heterotrimeric complex with the type II receptor and bound TGF-β. Upon formation of this complex, the type II receptor phosphorylates the type I receptor at multiple cytoplasmic serine and threonine residues (97,98). The type I receptor does not phosphorylate itself or the type II receptor. The substrates for the type I receptor serine/threonine kinase–mediated phosphorylation are not known, and, therefore, subsequent intracellular signaling mechanisms have not been characterized. However, the model suggests that the type I receptor kinase activity is required for signal propagation and that all signal transduction results from type I receptor phosphorylation activity. Again, the recent evidence that bone morphogenetic protein 2 induces simultaneous increased binding to the type I receptor and decreased binding to the type II and III receptors (90) suggest that this model may not be universally correct. According to data from studies using the yeast two-hybrid system and double immunoprecipitation analyses (99), Derynck et al. propose (Fig. 2, right) that direct interaction of the cytoplasmic domains of the type I and type II receptors occurs even in the absence of TGF-β. These interactions lead to the formation of type I–type II heterodimers, type I homodimers, and type II homodimers. TGF-β binding is proposed to stabilize these complexes. The type II homodimer binds TGF-β and may mediate TGF-β responses. It is not clear whether the type I homodimer is capable of binding TGF-β. In agreement with the Massague model, the Derynck model proposes that the major signaling events result from binding of TGF-β to the type I–type II heterodimer. Derynck et al. provide evidence that transphosphorylation occurs between both receptor subtypes, but acknowledge that the predominant result of TGF-β binding to the complex is type II receptor–mediated phosphorylation of the type I receptor. The seminal difference between the two models is that Derynck et al. propose that both receptors are capable of mediating functional re-

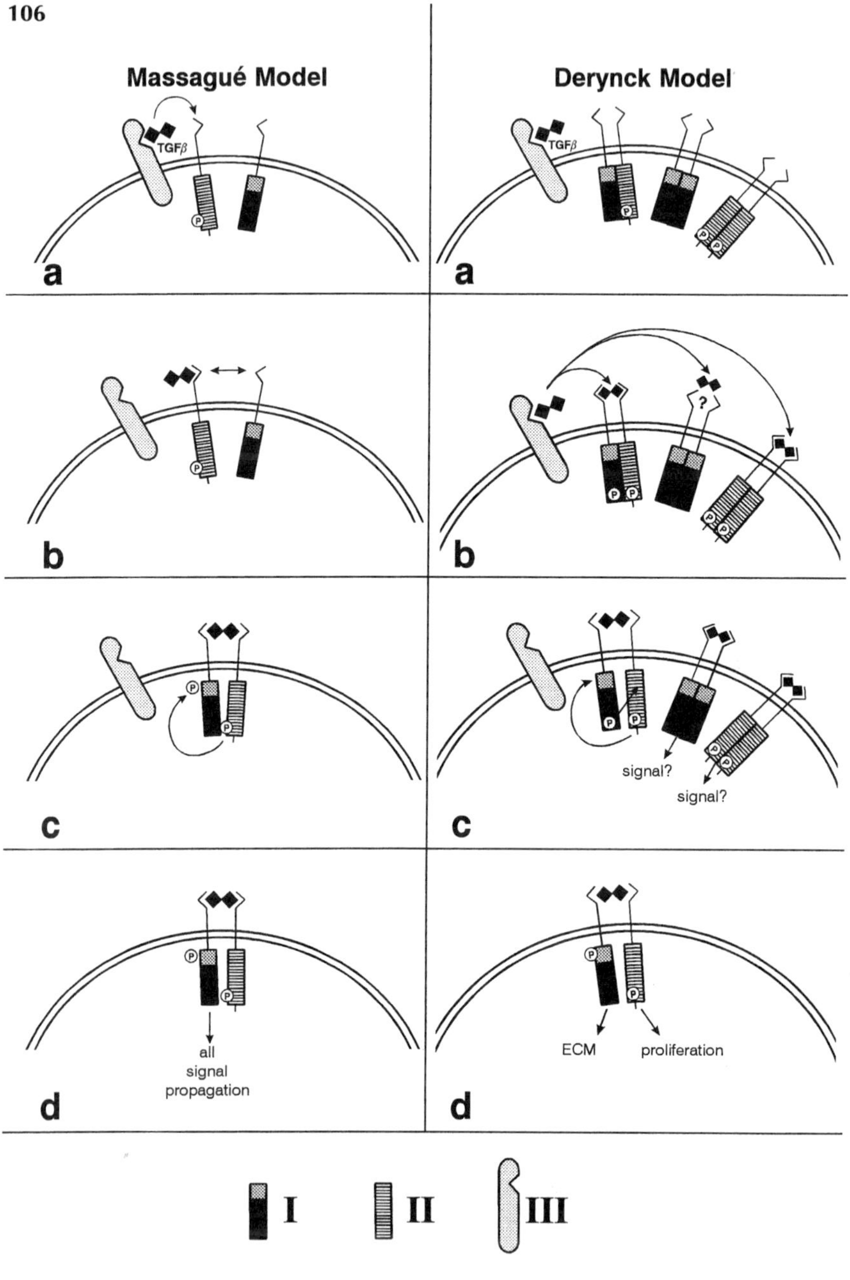

Figure 2 Proposed models of TGF-β receptor activation and signaling. TGF-β binding and activation of receptors: Massagué model (left panel) proposes that the type III receptor binds TGF-β first and transfers TGF-β to the type II receptor,

sponses and, importantly, that they mediate distinct responses to TGF-β (100). Specifically, it is proposed that the type I receptor mediates the effects of TGF-β on extracellular matrix turnover, while the type II receptors are responsible for the effect of TGF-β on cellular proliferation. There are functional data from independent laboratories to support this model (90,101,102) and identification of the retinoblastoma gene product as a selective substrate in the type II receptor pathway (100). However, dissection of the intracellular pathways involved in TGF-β–mediated responses and determination of whether one of these models—or both—represents actual physiological mechanisms through which TGF-β elicits biological responses awaits further research.

IV. BIOLOGICAL ACTIVITIES OF TGF-β

A. Overview

The biological effects mediated by TGF-β are numerous and diverse. In addition to influencing cellular differentiation, proliferation, adhesion, migration, and extracellular matrix deposition, TGF-β modulates inflammatory and immune responses, as well as carbohydrate and protein metabolism (5–9). Modulation of a particular biological response by TGF-β may itself actually represent the culmination of the interaction of a number of specific TGF-β–mediated effects. For example, TGF-β produces extracellular matrix accumulation by concomitant potent stimulation of extracellular matrix protein synthesis and inhibition of degradation of matrix proteins—two processes that themselves result from multiple biochemical effects of TGF-β to regulate numerous enzymes. Related to its multifunctional nature, alterations in TGF-β activity have been implicated in a broad range of pathologies including a host of neoplastic diseases and nearly all fibrotic disorders. A review of the extensive body of literature detailing the various biological activities of TGF-β on its multitude of effectors is well beyond the scope of this chapter and will not be attempted.

---

which then recruits the type I receptor into a stable heterotrimeric complex. Derynk et al. (99) propose (right panel) that preexisting type I–type II receptor heterodimers, type I receptor homodimers, and type II receptor homodimers are stabilized by TGF-β binding. Signaling: Massagué proposes that all TGF-β responses are signaled exclusively by type I receptor–mediated phosphorylation events. Derynk et al. propose that the type I and type II receptor subtypes mediate distinct cellular responses. Refer to text for further details.

Rather, because of the implications for restenosis, this chapter will review the vascular effects of TGF-β and the effects of TGF-β as a mediator of wound healing and tissue repair.

B. Vascular Responses to TGF-β

1. Effects of TGF-β on Endothelial and Vascular Smooth Muscle Cells In Vitro

Understanding the biology of TGF-β has been confounded largely because of two issues. First, initial observations in several in vitro assays suggested that the biological activity of the three isoforms is similar (103). Based on this observation, it became somewhat conventional to refer to the results obtained by addition of any isoform as a generic response to TGF-β. However, there are now reports in the literature describing different potencies and distinct biological effects of the TGF-βs (103–111). The initial assumption that the TGF-βs are biologically equivalent and insufficient detail regarding the isoform(s) used in particular studies makes interpretation and comparison of data difficult and contributes to potentially misleading conclusions about TGF-β activity. Strict attention must now be given to the isoforms used in particular studies, and one must be cautious in drawing general conclusions about TGF-β activity based on responses to a given isoform. The second issue clouding our understanding of the biology of TGF-β is that the results obtained upon addition of TGF-β to a particular cell type in culture vary depending on experimental conditions of cell density, growth substrate, media components, TGF-β concentration, and incubation interval. As summarized in Table 1, TGF-β_1 reportedly stimulates (112–117), inhibits (104, 118, 119), or has no effect (120–123) on proliferation of vascular smooth muscle cells in vitro. Similarly, TGF-β_1 reportedly stimulates (105,124–126), inhibits (104,126–132), or has no effect (104) on proliferation of endothelial cells in culture. TGF-β_1 stimulates (110,133) or has no effect (104) on migration of cultured vascular smooth muscle cells. In contrast, it inhibits endothelial cell migration (104, 127, 128, 134). TGF-β_1 potently and consistently stimulates synthesis of extracellular matrix proteins from both cell types (123,134–141) and has been shown to increase synthesis of plasminogen activator inhibitor in both cells (142,143). In addition, TGF-β_1 upregulates integrin receptor expression in these cells (110,133,144). The relevance of these in vitro vascular responses to in vivo biology is largely unknown. The variable nature of the vascular responses to TGF-β makes it particularly difficult to draw inferences about potential relevance to in vivo physiology and pathophysiology.

Table 1 Vascular Effects of TGF-β In Vitro

Cell type	Proliferation	Migration	ECM deposition	Integrin receptors
VSM	+−NE	+NE	+++	++
Endothelial cells	+−NE	−	+++	++

2. *Effects of TGF-β on Endothelial and Vascular Smooth Muscle Cells In Vivo*

Emerging in vivo data are beginning to clarify our understanding of the vascular effects of TGF-β (Table 2). Recent demonstrations of a neointimal fibroproliferative response to infusion of recombinant TGF-β_1 into rats (145) or genetic transfer of the gene encoding TGF-β_1 into porcine arteries (146) and attenuation of the injury-induced hyperplastic response by antibodies to TGF-β_1 (147) convincingly establish that TGF-β_1 stimulates vascular smooth muscle cell migration and proliferation in vivo. The effect of TGF-β_1 to induce small vessel endothelial cell migration and proliferation in vivo is fundamental to TGF-β–induced angiogenesis (148–150). In contrast, large vessel endothelial cell migration and proliferation are inhibited by TGF-β_1 (128). In agreement with the in vitro data, TGF-β potently increases in vivo extracellular matrix production (145–147) and integrin receptor expression (108).

C. TGF-β in Wound Healing and Tissue Repair

Numerous studies predominantly using wound healing following linear skin incisions as a model—but which share important parallels to the process of repair in other soft tissues—have firmly established that release of cytokines in response to tissue damage is the central event in initializing repair. Among the cytokines released, TGF-β plays the most critical role (151–153). TGF-β_1 protein has been detected as early as 5 min after injury to human skin (154). Platelets represent the most concentrated source of TGF-β (155) and, although porcine platelets contain approximately 20% TGF-β_2 (156), human platelets contain exclusively TGF-β_1 (13). Thus, degranulation of aggregated human platelets at an injury site releases TGF-β_1 into the surrounding tissue (112). At femtomolar concentrations, activated TGF-β_1 attracts monocytes, neutrophils, and fibroblasts to the locus of injury (157–159). Autocrine and/or paracrine induction of TGF-β synthesis increases local TGF-β concentrations further. In response to higher (picomolar) local concentrations, fibroblasts proliferate and synthesize extracellular matrix proteins, and the monocytes secrete other growth factors (IL-1, FGF, TNF-α), which act in concert with PDGF to further stimulate cellular proliferation.

Table 2 Vascular Effects of TGF-β In Vivo

Cell type	Proliferation	Migration	ECM deposition	Integrin receptors
VSM	+	+	+++	++
Endothelial cells	+−	+−	+++	++

The extracellular matrix molecules (collagens, fibronectin, proteoglycans) secreted by fibroblasts and resident cells begin to accumulate due to the simultaneous action of TGF-β to block matrix degradation by directly decreasing the synthesis of matrix proteases (collagenase, stromelysin, plasminogen activator) and increasing the inhibitors of these proteins (plasminogen activator inhibitor-1 and tissue inhibitors of metalloproteinases) (5,7,151). In addition, TGF-β increases the expression of integrin receptors on the surface of target cells thereby strengthening cell-matrix interactions and influencing cell adhesion and migration (160,161). An important component of the healing effect of TGF-β is its action to stimulate angiogenesis, an effect that has been demonstrated in vivo (148,149) and that may be due to the direct effects of TGF-β on endothelial cell migration and proliferation (124,132) or indirect effects through the activation and release of other growth factors such as PDGF and vascular endothelial growth factor (VEGF) (162,163). The overall process of wound healing is generally categorized into three somewhat overlapping stages, each with its unique molecular and cellular interactions (151): (a) the initial inflammatory stage; (b) formation of granulation tissue composed of numerous mesenchymal (fibroblast and myofibroblasts) and nonmesenchymal (monocytes, macrophages) cells and neovasculature enmeshed within a loosely assembled matrix of collagen, fibronectin, and proteoglycans; and (c) a final phase predominantly characterized by continuous biosynthesis and remodeling of the extracellular matrix. As reviewed herein, TGF-β plays a critical role in each of these phases and, in fact, is unique among growth factors in that regard.

V. ROLE OF TGF-β IN RESTENOSIS

In 1990, approximately 300,000 patients underwent percutaneous transluminal coronary angioplasty (PTCA) in the United States alone, and it was estimated that nearly 500,000 patients would undergo PTCA in the United States in 1995 (164). At present, the immediate success rate of PTCA is reported to be approximately 95% (164,165). However, the restenosis rate after PTCA still ranges from 30 to 50% within one year (165), suggesting that, of the estimated 500,000 PTCAs performed in 1995,

142,000–238,000 patients will develop restenosis. The expectations that new technologies would reduce the incidence of restenosis have not yet been fulfilled (164): the frequency of restenosis among patients after excimer laser angioplasty, directional coronary atherectomy, and rotational atherectomy is reportedly 50, 50, and 54%, respectively. Clearly, restenosis represents a significant challenge in interventional cardiology.

Vascular smooth muscle proliferation and extracellular matrix accumulation represent the fundamental mechanisms for formation of a restenotic lesion following intimal injury. The fibroproliferative tissue typical of human restenosis is characterized by foci of hypercellularity in which cells with phenotypic characteristics of proliferative vascular smooth muscle cells are associated with an abundant, loose, proteoglycan-rich extracellular matrix (166). The ballooned rat carotid artery model has been used extensively to study mechanisms responsible for injury-induced intimal hyperplasia and its associated restenosis. Detailed characterization of this model (167,168) has established that the inflated balloon catheter physically removes the endothelium and approximately 25% of the medial vascular smooth muscle cells. The remaining medial vascular smooth muscle cells start proliferating 1 day after injury. Migrating medial smooth muscle cells start to form a neointima after 4 days, and these cells continue to proliferate in the intima for approximately 2 weeks. Thereafter, the vascular smooth muscle cell proliferative rate returns to its low basal level, but the intima is further thickened by substantial progressive accumulation of extracellular matrix proteins including elastin, collagens, and proteoglycans. In fact, it is estimated that, at 3 months after injury, the extracellular matrix comprises ≥80% of the lesion. The substantial in vitro data that established that TGF-β_1 is a potent stimulator of extracellular matrix production and a potential stimulator for vascular smooth muscle migration and proliferation, together with the evidence of involvement of TGF-β in tissue repair, begged the hypothesis that TGF-β could be directly involved in restenosis after vascular injury.

Madri et al. (128) first published immunohistochemical data showing TGF-β_1 in the intima and media of chronically deendothelialized regions of ballooned rat carotid arteries, thereby suggesting a role for TGF-β in restenosis. Several subsequent studies (145,147,169,170) using the balloon-injured rat carotid artery and porcine iliac artery models have confirmed that TGF-β_1 expression is elevated following arterial injury. Northern analysis or semiquantitative reverse transcriptase-polymerase chain reaction analysis demonstrated that TGF-β_1 mRNA increased within 2 h (169) or 6 h (145) of balloon injury, reached maximum (five- to sevenfold increase over control) by 24 h (145), and remained at, or near, maximum levels of expression over the duration of the 2-week (145,147,169) or 6-week (170) studies. No (128,146) or little (145) TGF-β_1 expression was detected in control vessels. Immunohistochemical staining and in situ hybridization showing localization of the TGF-β_1 protein within the vascular smooth muscle cells (145), and demonstration that in vivo cyclohexamide infusion attenuated the balloon injury–induced increase in TGF-β_1 expression (169) indicate that injury induces TGF-β_1 expression de novo. In all these studies, elevated TGF-β_1 expression was correlated with evidence of increased extracellular matrix proteins including collagens I and II (128,145,146,170), fibronectin (128,145,147,170), elastin (170), and proteoglycans (146,147), suggesting a causal relationship between increased TGF-β_1 and developing fibroproliferative lesions. More definitive evidence for a causal role of TGF-β_1 in restenosis include: (a) transfection of the gene encoding TGF-β_1 into the vascular smooth muscle cells of a normal porcine iliac artery resulted in intimal and medial hyperplasia with increased deposition of extracellular matrix proteins (146) and (b) administration of neutralizing anti-TGF-β_1 antibodies significantly reduced the size of the intimal lesions that developed after balloon injury of the rat carotid artery (147). It is important to note that in vivo TGF-β_1 has greater stimulatory effect on extracellular matrix production than on vascular smooth muscle cell proliferation (145,147). This is in contrast to other growth factors such as PDGF-BB, which are highly mitogenic but have little effect on extracellular matrix metabolism (146). Thus, in vivo, as in vitro, TGF-β_1 appears unique among growth factors in its influence on extracellular matrix accumulation. It is unlikely that TGF-β_2 and TGF-β_3 are involved in development of restenotic lesions. Northern analysis indicates that little or no TGF-β_2 or TGF-β_3 is expressed in control rat carotid arteries and that neither isoform is upregulated in response to injury (145).

Recent examination of human restenotic lesions obtained by directional atherectomy also implicate TGF-β_1 in restenosis (171–173). In situ hybridization revealed significantly (≈fivefold) and persistently increased TGF-β_1 expression relative to controls in studies of 5 samples (173), 28 samples (172), and 62 samples (171). Increased TGF-β_1 expression occurred in all specimens regardless of the length of time between the original balloon angioplasty procedure and the atherectomy [1 h to 25 months (172,173)], and was independent of the vessel source (coronary artery, peripheral artery, saphenous bypass graft). Immunohistochemical analysis confirmed that vascular smooth muscle cells were the source of the TGF-β_1 and that the staining was primarily intracellular (172). In general, the level of TGF-β_1 expression was not correlated with the number of balloon angioplasty events to which the vessel had been exposed (171), and restenotic lesions expressed more TGF-β_1 than primary atherosclerotic lesions, which, in turn, expressed more TGF-β_1 than control arteries (171). TGF-β_1 expression did not correlate with known risk factors for coronary artery disease such as age, sex, smoking, systemic hypertension, diabetes, and total serum cholesterol (171). Consistent with the animal data, TGF-β_2 and TGF-β_3 are likely not involved with the restenotic process as their mRNAs could not be detected by in situ hybridization (172). Together with the animal data, these data from atherectomy samples of human restenotic lesions clearly implicate TGF-β in the vascular response to injury and restenosis consequent to the resultant fibroproliferative lesion.

Elevated TGF-β_1 expression and corresponding fibroblast proliferation and matrix accumulation has been noted in the adventitia of balloon-injured arteries (173). In addition, TGF-β–mediated inhibition of nitric oxide production has been documented (174). Adventitial matrix accumulation and associated scar contraction and decreased release of nitric oxide in a restenosing vessel would both contribute to a reduced ability of the vessel to remodel appropriately in response to the developing lesion (175), and therefore represent additional possible mechanisms of TGF-β–mediated restenosis.

VI. THERAPEUTIC POTENTIAL OF TGF-β ANTAGONISM FOR PREVENTION OF RESTENOSIS

Shortly after the introduction of PTCA to clinical practice in 1977 (176), it became evident that restenosis represents a clear limitation to the success of this procedure. Nearly two decades of intensive basic and clinical research has failed to identify a successful pharmacological means for management/prevention of human restenosis. It has been proposed that the failure to identify an effective therapeutic agent in the clinic may be related to design of the clinical trials including such issues as dose of compound, time of administration, and statistical power of the experiments (177). An additional possibility is that the clinical interventions to date have been aimed at the wrong target. Previous therapeutic approaches for prevention of restenosis have included inhibition of thrombosis, inflammation, coronary vasospasm, and lipid metabolism. However, the major focus of most studies of restenosis has been on prevention of vascular smooth muscle proliferation to reduce lesion size and, therefore, clinical restenosis (165,177). Despite the fact that the extracellular matrix deposited in a restenotic lesion accounts for greater than 80% of the lesion volume, little if any attention has been paid to inhibiting matrix accumulation to prevent restenosis.

The multifunctional nature of TGF-β together with the fact that TGF-β is the most potent inducer of extracellular matrix accumulation (178) makes inhibition of this cytokine an attractive therapeutic target for prevention of restenosis. The complexity of the TGF-β system provides a number of targets for therapeutic intervention: processing of the mature peptide from the prepropeptide, activation of the inactive TGF-β homodimer, interaction of TGF-β with its receptors, and mechanisms of inactivation of the peptide all represent potential steps for inhibition of TGF-β activity (Fig. 1). Injection of soluble decorin, a small proteoglycan that binds TGF-β, successfully inhibited excessive matrix accumulation in nephritic rats (179). Neutralizing antibodies to TGF-β reduced matrix accumulation and subsequent fibrosis in the kidney (180), synovium (181), lung (182), central nervous system (183), and skin (111,184) without adverse effects on normal healing. Interestingly, it has recently been demonstrated that administration of low concentrations of TGF-β_3 or combined inhibition of TGF-β_1 and TGF-β_2 were equally effective in reducing scar formation in skin (111). We have reviewed above the data from the rat carotid artery model of PTCA, which indicates that neutralizing antibody to TGF-β_1 significantly attenuated the size of the injury-induced lesion (147). Taken together, these data clearly indicate that there exists real therapeutic potential in taking the approach of TGF-β antagonism for prevention of restenosis.

REFERENCES

1. Bitterman PB, Henke CA. Fibroproliferative disorders. Chest 1991; 99(3): 81S–84S
2. Derynck R, Jarrett JA, Chen EY, Eaton DH, Bell JR, Assoian RK, Roberts AB, Sporn MB, Goeddel DV. Human transforming growth factor-beta cDNA sequence and expression in normal and transformed cells. Nature 1985; 316:701-705.
3. Madisen L, Webb NR, Rose TM, Marquardt H, Ikeda T, Twardzik D., Seyedin S, Purchio AF. Transforming growth factor-β2: cDNA cloning and sequence analysis. DNA 1988; 7:1–8
4. Derynck R, Lindquist PB, Lee A, Wen D, Tamm J, Graycar JL, Rhee L, Mason AJ, Miller DA, Coffey RJ, Moses HL, Chen EY. A new type of transforming growth factor-β, TGf-β3. EMBO J 1988; 7:3737–3743.
5. Roberts AB, Sporn MB. The transforming growth factor-βs. In: Sporn MB, Roberts AB, eds. Peptide Growth Factors and Their Receptors. New York: Springer-Verlag, 1991:419–472.
6. Kingsley DM. The TGF-β superfamily: new members, new receptors, and new genetic tests of function in different organisms. Genes Dev 1944; 8:133–146.
7. Barnard JA, Lyons RM, Moses HL. The cell biology of transforming growth factor β. Biochim Biophys Acta 1990; 79–87.
8. Attisano L, Wrana JL, Lopez-Casillas F, Massagué J. TGF-β receptors and actions. Biochim Biophys Acta 1994; 71–80.

9. Pimentel E. Transforming growth factors. In: Pimentel E., ed., Handbook of Growth Factors. Vol. II: Peptide Growth Factors. Boca Raton, FL: CRC Press, 1994; 263–323.
10. Lawerence DA, Pirchner R, Kryceve-Martinerie C, Jullien P. Normal embryo fibroblasts release transforming growth factors in a latent form. J Cell Physiol 1984; 121:184–188.
11. Bobik A, Campbell JH. Vascular derived growth factors: cell biology, pathophsiology and pharmacology. Pharmacol Rev 1993; 45(1):1–42.
12. Bascom CC, Wofshohl JR, Coffey RJ, Jr., Madisen L, Webb NR, Purchio AR, Derynck R, Moses HL. Complex regulation of transforming growth factor B1, B2, and B3 mRNA expression in mouse fibroblasts and keratinocytes by transforming growth factors B1 and B2. Mol Cell Biol 1989; 9(12):5508–5515.
13. Assoian RK, Komoriya A, Meyers CA, Miller DM, Sporn MB. Transforming growth factor-beta in human platelets: identification of a major storage site, purification and characterization. J Biol Chem 1983; 258:7155–7160.
14. Danielpour D, Dart LL, Flanders KC, Roberts AB, Sporn MB. Immunodetection and quantitation of the two forms of transforming growth factor-beta (TGF-beta 1 and TGF-beta 2) secreted by cells in culture. J Cell Physiol 1989; 138:79–86.
15. Flanders KC, Cissel DS, Roberts AB Sporn MB, Unsicker K. Immunohistochemical localization of transforming growth factors-βs in the nervous system of the mouse embryo. J Cell Biochem 1990; 14F(S):88.
16. Heine UI, Munoz EF, Flanders KC, Ellingsworth LR, Lam HYP, Thompson NL, Roberts AB, Sporn MB. Role of transforming growth factor-β in the development of the mouse embryo. J Cell Biol 1987; 105:2861–2876.
17. Thompson NL, Flanders KC, Smith M, Ellingsworth LR, Roberts AB, Sporn MB. Expression of transforming growth factor-β1 in specific cells and tissues of adult and neonatal mice. J Cell Biol 1989; 108:661-669.
18. Miller DA, Lee A, Pelton RW, Chen EY, Moses HL, Derynck R. Murine transforming growth factor-β2 cDNA sequence and expression in adult tissues and embryos. Mol Endocrinol 1989; 3:1108–1114.
19. Jampel HD, Roche NS, Stark WJ, Roberts AB. Transforming growth factor beta in human aqueous humor. Curr Eye Res 1990; 9:963–969.
20. Connor TB, Roberts AB, Sporn MB, Danielpour D, Dart LL, Michels RG, deBustros S, Enger C, Kato H, Lansing M, Hayashi H, Glaser BM. Correlation of fibrosis and transforming growth factor-beta type 2 levels in the eye. J Clin Invest 1989; 83:1661–1662.
21. Gatherer D, ten Dijke P, Baird DT, Akhurst RJ. Expression of TGFB isoforms during first trimester human embryogenesis. Development 1990; 109:445–460.
22. Fitzpatrick DR, Denhez F, Kondaiah P, Akhurst RJ. Differential expression of TGF-beta isoforms in murine palatogenesis. Development 1990; 109: 585–596.
23. Millan FA, Denhez F, Kondaiah P, Ankhurst RJ. Embryonic gene expression

patterns of TGFβ1, β2 and β3 suggest different developmental functions in vivo. Development 1991; 111:131–144.
24. Schmid P, Cox D, Bilbe G, Maier R, McMaster GK. Differential expression of TGFβ1, β2 and β3 genes during mouse embryogenesis. Development 1991; 111:117–130.
25. Pelton RW, Dickinson ME, Moses HL, Hogan BLM. In situ hybridization analysis of TGFβ3 RNA expression during mouse development: comparative studies with TGFβ1 and TGFβ2. Development 1990; 110:609–620.
26. Pelton RW, Saxena B, Jones M, Moses HL, Gold LI. Immunohistochemical localization of TGFβ1, TGFβ2 and TGFβ3 in the mouse embryo: expression patterns suggest multiple roles during embryonic development. J Cell Biol 1991; 115:1091–1105.
27. Pelton RW, Hogan BLM, Miller DA Moses HL. Differential expression of genes encoding TGFs β1, β2 and β3 during murine palate development. Dev Biol 1990; 141:456–460.
28. Escherick JS, DiCunto F, Flanders KC, Missero C, Dotto GP. Transforming growth factor beta 1 induction is associated with transforming growth factors beta 2 and beta 3 down-modulation in 12–0-tetradecanoylphorbol-13-acetate-induced skin hyperplasia. Cancer Res 1993; 53(22):5517–5522.
29. Danielpour D, Kim KY, Winukur TS, Sporn MB. Differential regulation of TGFβ1 and TGFβ2 expression by retinoic acid and epidermal growth factor in NRK and A549 cells. J Cell Biochem 1990; 14C (suppl):292.
30. Coletta AA, Wakefield LM, Howell FV, van Roozendaal KEP, Danielpour D, Ebbs SR, Sporn MB, Baum M. Anti-oestrogens induce the secretion of active transforming growth factor-B from human fibroblasts. B J Cancer 1990; 62:405-409.
31. Glick AB, Flanders KC, Danielpour D, Yuspa SH, Sporn MB. Retinoic acid induces transforming growth factor-β2 in cultured keratinocytes and mouse epidermis. Cell Regul 1989; 1:87–97.
32. Wakefield L, Kim SJ, Glick A, Winokur T, Coletta A; Sporn MB. Regulation of transforming growth factor-B subtypes by members of the steroid hormone superfamily. J Cell Sci 1990; 13(suppl):139–148.
33. Jakolew SB, Cubert J, Danielpour D, Sporn MB, Roberts AB. Differential regulation of the expression of transforming growth factor-β mRNAs by growth factors and retinoic acid in chicken embryo chondrocytes, myocytes and fibroblasts. J Cell Physiol 1992; 150:377-385.
34. Fujii D, Brissenden JE, Derynck R, Francke U. Transforming growth factor-β gene maps to human chromosome 19 long arm and to mouse chromosome 7. Somatic Cell Mol Genet 1986; 12:281–288.
35. Barton DE, Foellmer Be, Du J, Tamm J, Derynck R, Francke U. Chromosomal locations of TGFβs 2 and 3 in man and mouse: dispersion of the TGF-β family. Oncogene Res 1988; 3:323-331.
36. ten Dijke P, Guerts van Kessel AHM, Foulkes JG, LeBeau MM. Transforming growth factor-beta 3 maps to human chromosome 14, region q23-q24. Oncogene 1988; 3:721–724.

37. Kim SJ, Glick A, Sporn MB, Robert AB. Characterization of the promoter region of the human transforming growth factor-β1 gene. J Biol Chem 1989; 264:402–408.
38. Kim SJ, Jeang KT, Glick A, Sporn MB, Roberts AB. Promoter sequences of the human TFGβ gene responsive to TGF-β1 autoinduction. J Biol Chem 1989; 264:7041–7045.
39. Kim SJ, Denhez F, Kim KY, Holt JT, Sporn MB, Roberts AB. Activation of the second promoter of the TGF-β1 gene by TGF-β1 and phorbol ester occurs through the same target sequences. J Biol Chem 1989; 264:19373–19378.
40. Kim SJ, Angel P, Lafyatis R, Hattori K, Kim KY, Sporn MB, Karin M, Roberts AB. Autoinduction of transforming growth factor-β1 is mediated by the AP-1 complex. Mol Cell Biol 1990; 10:1492–1497.
41. Romeo DS, Park K, Roberts AB, Sporn MB, Kim SJ. An element of the transforming growth factor-β1 5' untranslated region represses translation and specifically binds a cytosolic factor. Mol Endocrinol 1993; 7:759–766.
42. Noma T, Glick AB, Geiser AG, O'Reilly MA, Miller J, Roberts AB, Sporn MB. Molecular cloning and structure of the human transforming growth factor-beta 2 gene promoter. Growth Factors 1991; 4(4):247–255.
43. Kim SJ, Wagner S, Liu F, O'Reilly MA, Robbins PD, Green MR. Retinoblastoma gene product activates expression of the human TGF-beta 2 gene through transcription factor ATF-2. Nature 1992; 358 (6384):331–334.
44. Lafyatis R, Lechleider R, Kim SJ, Jakowlew S, Roberts AB, Sporn MB. Structural and functional characterization of the transforming growth factor-β3 promoter: a cAMP response element regulates basal and induced transcription. J Biol Chem 1990; 265:19128–19136.
45. Geiser AG, Busam KJ, Kim SJ, Lafyatis R, O'Reilly MA, Webbink R, Roberts Sporn MB. Regulation of the transforming growth factor-beta 1 and -beta 3 promoters by transcription factor spl. Gene 1993; 129(2) 223–228.
46. Lafyatis R, Denhez F, Williams T, Sporn MB, Roberts AB. Sequence specific protein binding to and activation of the TGF-beta 3 promoter through a repeated TCCC motifiy. Nucleic Acid Res 1991; 19(23):6419–6425.
47. Arrick BA, Lee AL, Grendell RL, Derynck R. Inhibition of translation of transforming growth factor-beta 3 mRNA by its 5'untranslated region. Mol Cell Biol 1991; 11(9):4306–4313.
48. Kim SJ, Park K, Koeller D, Kim KY, Wakefield LM, Sporn MB, Roberts AB. Post-transcriptional regulation of the human transforming growth factor-β1 gene. J Biol Chem 1992; 267:13702–13707.
49. Dubois CM, Laprise MH, Blanchette F, Gentry LE, Ledue R. Processing of transforming growth factor β1 precursor by human furin convertase. J Biol Chem 1995; 270:10618–10624.
50. Wakefield LM, Smith DM, Broz S, Jackson M, Levinson AD, Sporn MB. Recombinant TGFβ1 is synthesized as a two component latent complex that shares structural features with the native platelet latent TGFβ1 complex. Growth Factors 1989; 1:203–218.

51 Rifkin DB, Kojima S. Abe M. Harpel JG. TGFβ1: structure, function and formation. Thromb Haemostasis 1993; 70(1):177–179.
52. Lawrence DA, Pircher R, Jullien P. Conversion of a high molecular weight latent beta-TGF under acidic conditions. Biochem Biophys Res Commun 1985; 133:1026–1034.
53. Keski-Oja JR, Lyons M, Moses HL. Inactive secreted form(s) of transforming growth factor-beta: activation by proteolysis. J Cell Biochem 1987; 11A (suppl.):60.
54. Lyons RM, Keski-Oja JR, and Moses HL. Proteolytic activation of latent transforming growth factor-β from fibroblast-conditional medium. J Cell Biol 1988; 106:1659–1665.
55. Sato Y, Rifkin DB. Inhibition of endothelial cell movement by pericytes and smooth muscle cells: activiation of a latent transforming growth factor-β1-like molecule by plasmin during co-culture. J Cell Biol 1989; 109: 309–315.
56. Miyazono K, Heldon CH. Role for carbohydrate structure in TGF-B1 latency. Nature (Lond.) 1989; 338:158–160.
57. Flaumenhaft R, Abe M, Mignatti P, Rifkin DB. Basic fibroblast growth factor-induced activation of latent transforming growth factor beta in endothelial cells: regulation of plasminogen activator activity. J Cell Biol 1992; 118:901–909.
58. Kojima S, Nara K, Rifkin DB. Requirement for transglutaminase in the activation of latent transforming growth factor-β in bovine endothelial cells. J Cell Biol 1993; 119:439–448.
59. Silver IA, Murrills RJ, Etherington DJ. Microelectrode studies on the acid microenvironment beneath adherent macrophages and osteoclasts. Exp Cell Res 1988; 175:266–276.
60. Pilatte Y, Bignon J, Lambre CR. Lysosomal and cytosolic sialidases in rabbit alveolar macrophages: demonstration of increased lysosomal activity after in vivo activation with bacillus Calmette-Guerin. Biochem Biophys Acta 1987; 923:150–155.
61. Purchio AF, Cooper JA, Brunner AM, Lioubin MN, Gentry LE, Kovacina KS, Roth RA, Marquardt H. Identification of mannose-6-phosphate in two asparagine-linked sugar chains on recombinant transforming growth factor-β1 precursor. J Biol Chem 1988; 263:14211–14214.
62. Koracina KS, Steele-Perkins G, Purchio AF, Lioubin M, Miyazono K, Heldin CL, Roth RA. Interactions of recombinant platelet transforming growth factor-β1 precursor with the insulin-like growth factor/mannose 6-phosphate receptor. Biochem Biophys Res Commun 1989; 160:393–403.
63. Dennis PA and Rifkin DB. Cellular activation of latent transforming growth factor beta requires binding to the cation-independent mannose 6-phosphate/insulin-like growth factor type II receptor. Proc Natl Acad Sci USA 1991; 88:580–584.
64. LeMarre J, Wollenberg GK, Gonias SL, Hayes MA. Biology of disease. Cytokine binding and clearance properties of proteinase-activated α2-macroglobulins. Lab Invest 1991; 65:3–14.

65. Huang SS, O'Grady P, Huang JS. Human transforming growth factor β· α2-macroglobulin complex is a latent form of transforming growth factor β. J Biol Chem 1988; 263:1535–1541.
66. Massagué J, Kelly B. Internalization of transforming growth factor-β and its receptor in BALB/c 3T3 fibroblasts. J Cell Physiol 1986; 128:216–222.
67. Massagué J. The transforming growth factor-beta family. Annu Rev Cell Biol 1990; 6:597–641.
68. Massagué J. Receptors for the TGFβ family. Cell 1992; 69:1067–1070.
69. Franzen P, ten Dijke p, Ichijo H, Yamashita H, Schulz P, Heldin CH, Miyazono K. Cloning of a TGFβ type I receptor that forms a heteromeric complex with the TGFβ type II receptor. Cell 1993; 75:681–692.
70. He WW, Gustafson ML, Hirobe S, Donahoe PK. Developmental expression of four serine threonine kinase receptors homologous to the activin transforming growth factor-β type II receptor family. Dev Dyn 1993; 196:133–142.
71. Lin HY, Wang XF, Ng-Eaton E, Weinberg RA, Lodish HF. Expression cloning of the TGF-β Type II receptor, a functional transmembrane serine/threonine kinase. Cell 1992; 68:775–785.
72. Lopez-Casillas F, Cheifetz S, Doody J, Andres JL, Lane WS, Massagué J. Structure and expression of the membrane proteoglycan betaglycan, a component of the TGF-β receptor system. Cell 1991; 67:785-795.
73. Wang XF, Lin HY, NG-Eaton E, Downward J, Lodish HF, Weinberg RA. Expression cloning and characterization of the TGF-β type III receptor. Cell 1991; 67:797–805.
74. Morén A, Ichijo, Mijazono K. Molecular cloning and characterization of the human and procine transforming growth factor-β type III receptors. Biochem Biophys Res Comm 1992; 189:356–362.
75. Segarini PR, Seyedin SM. The high molecular weight receptor to transforming growth factor-β contains glycosaminoglycan chains. J Biol Chem 1988; 263:8366–8370.
76. ten Dijke P, Ichijo H, Franzen P, Schulz P, Saras J, Toyoshima H, Heldin CH, Miyazono K. Activin receptor-like kinases: a novel subclass of cell-surface receptors with predicted serine/threonine kinase activity. Oncogene 1993; 8:2879–2887.
77. Massagué J, Attisano L, Wrana JL. The TGFβ family and its composite receptors. Trends Cell Biol 1994; 4:172–178.
78. ten Dijke P, Franzen P, Yamashita H, Ichijo H, Heldin CH, Miyazono K. Serine/threonine kinase receptors. Prog Growth Factor Res 1994; 5(1):55–72.
79. Massagué J, Cheifetz FTB, Andres JL. TGFβ receptors and TGFβ binding proteoglycans: recent progress in identifying their functional properties. Ann NY Acad Sci 1990; 593:243–258.
80. Segarini PR, Rosen DM, Seyedin SM. Binding of TGF-β to cell surface proteins varies with cell type. Mol Endocrinol 1989; 3:261–272.
81. Wakefield LM, Smith DM, Masui T, Harris CC, Sporn MB. Distribution and modulation of the cellular receptor for transforming growth factor-beta. J Cell Biol 1987; 195:965–975.

82. Rizzino A. Appearance of high affinity receptors for type β transforming growth factor during differentiation of murine embryonal carcinoma cells. Cancer Res 1987, 1987; 47:4386–4390.
83. Cochet C, Feige JJ, Chambaz EM. Bovine adrenocortical cells exhibit high affinity transforming growth factor β receptors which are regulated by adrenocorticotropin. J Biol Chem 1988; 263:5707–5713.
84. Ewton DZ, Spizz G. Olson EN, Florini JR. Decrease in transforming growth factor-beta binding and action during differentiation in muscle cells. J Biol Chem 1988; 263:4029–4032.
85. Goodman LV, Majack RA. Vascular smooth muscle cells express distinct transforming growth factor-beta receptor phenotypes as a function of cell density in culture. J Biol Chem 1989; 264:5241–5244.
86. Rizzano A, Kazakoff P, Ruff E, Kuszynski C, Nebelskick J. Regulatory effects of cell density on the binding of transforming growth factor-β, epidermal growth factor, platelet-derived growth factor and fibroblast growth factor. Cancer Res 1988; 48:4266–4271.
87. Fafeur V, Terman BI, Blum J, Bohlen P. Basic FGF treatment of endothelial cells down-regulates the 85kDa TGFβ receptor subtype and decreases the growth inhibitory response to TGFβ1. Growth Factors 1990; 3:237–245.
88. Centrella M, McCarthy TL, Canalis E. Parathyroid hormone modulates transforming growth factor activity and binding in osteoblastic cells. Proc Natl Acad Sci USA 1988; 85:5889–5893.
89. Centrella M, McCarthy TL, Canalis E. Glucocorticoid regulation of transforming growth factor β1 activity and binding in osteoblast-enriched cultures from fetal rat bone. Mol Cell Biol 1991; 11:4490-4496.
90. Centrella M, Casinghino S, Kim J, Pham T, Rosen V, Wozney J, McCarthy TL. Independent changes in type I and type II receptors for transforming growth factor β induced by bond morphogenetic protein 2 parallel expression of the osteoblast phonotype. Mol Cell Biol 1995; 3273–3281.
91. Frolick CA, Wakefield LM, Smith DM, Sporn MB. Characterization of a membrane receptor for transforming growth factor-β in normal rat kidney fibroblasts. J Biol Chem 1984; 259:10995–11000.
92. Kyprianou N, Isaacs JT. Identification of a cellular receptor for transforming growth factor-β in rat ventral prostate and its negative regulation by androgens. Endocrinology 1988; 123:2124–2131.
93. Barnett JV, Moustakas A, Lin W, Wang XF, Lin JY, Galper JB, Maas RL. Cloning and developmental expression of the chick type II and type III TGFβ receptors. Dev Dyn 1994; 199:12–27.
94. Roelen BAJ, Lin HY, Knezevic V, Freund E, Mummery CL. Expression of TGF-βs and their receptors during implantation and organogenesis of the mouse embryo. Dev Biol 1994; 166:716–728.
95. Cheifetz S, Bellon T, Cales C, Vera S, Bernabeu C, Massaqué J, Letarte M. Endoglin is a component of the transforming growth factor-β receptor system in human endothelial cells. J Biol Chem 1992; 267:19027–19030.
96. Sankar S, Mahooti-Brooks N, Centrella M, McCarthy TL, Madri JA. Expres-

sion of transforming growth factor type III receptor in vascular endothelial cells increases their responsiveness to transforming growth factor β2. J Biol Chem 1995; 270(22):13567–13572.
97. Wrana JL, Attisano L, Wieser R, Ventura F, Massaqué J. Mechanism of activation of the TGFβ receptor. Nature 1994; 370:341–347.
98. Chen F, Weinberg RA. Biochemical evidence for the autophosporylation and transphosphorylation of transforming growth factor β receptor kinases. Proc Natl Acad Sci 1995; 92:1565–1569.
99. Chen RH, Moses HL, Maruoka EM, Derynck R, Kawabata M. Phosphorylation-dependent interaction of the cytoplasmic domains of the type I and type II transforming growth factor-β receptors. J Biol Chem 1995; 270(20):12235–12241.
100. Chen RH, Ebner R, Derynck R. Inactivation of the type II receptor reveals two receptor pathways for the diverse TGFβ activities. Science 1993; 260:1335–1338.
101. Franzen P, Ichijo H, Miyazono K. Different signals mediate transforming growth factor-β1-induced growth inhibition and extracellular matrix production in prostatic carcinoma cells. Exp Cell Res 1993; 207:1–7.
102. Centrella M, Casinghino S, Kim J, Pham T, Rosen V, Wozney J, McCarthy TL. Bond morphogenetic protein (BMP-2) alters and defines the function of transforming growth factor-β (TGFβ) receptors on osteoblasts. J Bone Min Res 1994; 9 (suppl I):69A.
103. Graycar JL, Miller Da, Arrizk BA, Lyons RM, Moses HL, Derynck R. Human transforming growth factor-β3: recombinant expression, purification and biological activities in comparison with transforming growth factors-β1 and β2. Mol Endocrinol 1989; 3:1977–1986.
104. Merwin JR, Newman W, Beall D, Tucker A, Madri JA. Vascular cells respond differently to transforming growth factors beta 1 and beta 2. Am J Pathol 1991; 138:37–51.
105. Roberts AB, Kondaiah P, Rosa F, Watanabe S, Good P, Danielpour D, Roche NS, Rebbert ML, David IB, Sporn MB. Mesoderm induction in *Xenopus laevis* distinguishes has between the various TGF-β isoforms. Growth Factors 1990; 3:277–286.
106. Jennings JC, Mohan S, Lonkhart TA, Widstrom R, Baylink DJ. Comparison of the biological activity of TGF-beta 1 and TGF-beta 2: differential activity in endothelial cells. J Cell Physiol 1988; 137:167–172.
107. Jacobson SEW, Ruscetti FW, Roberts AB, Keller JR. TGF-β is a bidirectional modulator of cytokine receptor expression on murine bone marrow cells. J Immunology 1993; 151(9):4534–4544.
108. Madri JA, Bell L, Merwin JR. Modulation of vascular cell behavior by transforming growth factors β. Mol Reprod Dev 1992; 32:121–126.
109. Bell L, Romanic AM, Luthringer DJ, Tucker AM, Madri JA. Differential regulation of PAI-1 uPA and fibronectin expression by TGFβ1 and TGFβ2 in bovine aortic endothelial cells. J Biol Chem. Submitted.
110. Madri JA, Kocher O, Merwin JR, Bell L, Tucker A, Basson C. Interactions

of vascular cells with transforming growth factors-β. Ann NY Acad Sci 1990; 593:243–258.

111. Shah M, Foreman DM, Ferguson MWJ. Neutralisation of TGF-β1 and TGF-β2 or exogenous addition of TGF-β3 to cutaneous rat wounds reduces scarring. J Cell Sci 1995; 108:985–1002.
112. Assoian RK, Sporn MB. Type β transforming growth factor in human platelets: release during platelet degranulation and action on vascular smooth muscle cells. J Cell Biol 1986; 102:1217–1223.
113. Majack RA. Beta-type transforming growth factor specifies organizational behavior in vascular smooth muscle cell cultures. J Cell Biol 1987; 105:465–471.
114. Majack RA, Majesky MW, Goodman LV. Role of PDGF-A expression in the control of vascular smooth muscle cell growth by transforming growth factor-beta. J Cell Biol 1990; 111:239–247.
115. Battegay EJ, Raines EW, Siefert RA, Bowen-Pope DF, Ross R. TGF-β induces bimodal proliferation of connective tissue cells via complex control of an autocrine PDGF loop. Cell 1990; 63:515–524.
116. Stouffer GA, Owens GK. Angiotensin II induced mitogenesis of SHR derived cultured smooth muscle cells is dependent on transforming growth factor-β. Circ Res 1992; 70:820–828.
117. Stouffer GA, Owens GK. TGF-β promotes proliferation of cultured SMC via both PDGF-AA-dependent and PDGF-AA-independent mechanisms. J Clin Invest 1994; 93:2048–2055.
118. Ouchi Y, Hirosumi J, Watanabe M, Hattori A, Nakamura T, Orimo H. Inhibitory effect of transforming growth factor-β on epidermal growth factor-induced proliferation of cultured rat aortic smooth muscle cells. Biochem Biophys Res Commun 1988; 157:301–307.
119. Owens GK, Geisterfer AA, Yang YW, Komoriya A. Transforming growth factor-beta-induced growth inhibition and cellular hypertrophy in cultured vascular smooth muscle cells. J Cell Biol 1988; 107:771–780.
120. Nikol S, Bauriedel G, Pickering G, Heidemann P, Weir L, Höfling B. Role of transforming growth factor-β in human vascular smooth muscle cells in vitro. Abstracts of the American Heart Association Scientific Conference on the Molecular Cellular Biology of the Vascular Wall, 1993, p. 76.
121. Janat MF, Liau G. Transforming growth factor β1 is a powerful modulator of platelet-derived growth factor action in vascular smooth muscle cells. J Cell Physiol 1992; 150:232–242.
122. Saltis J, Agrotis A, Bobik A. TGF-β1 potentiates growth factor-stimulated proliferation of vascular smooth muscle cells in genetic hypertension. Am J Physiol 1992; 263(Cell Physiol 32):C420-C428.
123. Chen JK, Hoshi H, McKeehan WL. Transforming growth factor type β specifically stimulates synthesis of proteoglycan in human adult arterial smooth muscle cells. Proc Natl Acad Sci USA 1987; 84:5287–5291.
124. Merwin JR, Anderson JM, Kocher O, Itallie CM, Madri JA. Transforming growth factor beta 1 modulates extracaellular matrix organization and cell-

cell junctional complex formation during in vitro angiogenesis. J Cell Physiol 1990; 142:117 128.
125. Madri JA, Williams SK. Capillary endothelial cell cultures. Phenotypic modulation by matrix components J Cell Biol 1983; 97:152–165.
126. Merwin JR, Tucker A, Roberts A, Kondaiah P, Madri JA. Vascular cell responses to transforming growth factor beta 3 mimic those of transforming growth factor beta 1. In Vitro Growth Factors 1991; 5:149–158.
127. Madri JA, Pratt BM, Yannariello-Brown J. Matrix-driven cell size change modulates aortic endothelial cell proliferation and sheet migration. Am J Pathol 1988; 132:18–27.
128. Madri JA, Reidy MA, Kocher O, Bell L. Endothelial cell behavior after denudation injury is modulated by transforming growth factor-β1 and fibronectin. Lab Invest 1989; 60(6):755–765.
129. Heimark RL, Twardzik DR, Schwartz SM. Inhibition of endothelial regeneration by type-beta transforming growth factor from platelets. Science 1986; 233:1078–1080.
130. Frater-Schroder M, Muller G, Birchmeier W, Bohlen P. Transforming growth factor-beta inhibits endothelial cell proliferation. Biochem Biophys Res Commun 1986; 137:295–302.
131. Baird A, Durken T. Inhibition of endothelial cell proliferation by type-beta transforming growth factor: interactions with acidic and basic fibroblast growth factors. Biochem Biophys Res Comm 1986; 138:476–482.
132. Madri JA, Pratt BM, Tucker A. Phenotypic modulation of endothelial cells by transforming growth factor-β depends upon the composition and organization of the extracelllar matrix. J Cell Biol 1988; 106:1375–1384.
133. Basson CT, Kocher O, Basson MD, Asis A, Madri JA. Modulation of vascular cell integrin expression in vitro by TGF-β1 and PDGF. J Cell Physiol 1992; 153(1):118–128.
134. Kocher O, Kennedy S, Madri JA. Alternative splicing of fibronectin mRNA in the IIICS region in endothelial cells: functional significance Am J Pathol 1990; 137:1509–1524.
135. Schönherr E, Järveläinen HT, Sandell LJ, Wight TN, Effects of platelet-derived growth factor and transforming growth factor-β1 on the synthesis of a large versican-like chondroitan sulfate proteoglycan by arterial smooth muscle cells. J Biol Chem 1991; 266:17640–17647.
136. Schönherr E, Järveläinen HT, Kinsella MG, Sandell LJ, Wight TN. Platelet-derived growth factor and transforming growth factor-β1 differentially affect the synthesis of biglycan and decorin by monkey arterial smooth muscle cells. Arteroscler Thromb 1993; 13:1026–1036.
137. Cizmeci-Smith G, Asundi V, Stahl RC, Teichman LJ, Chernousov M, Cowan K, Carey DJ. Regulated expression of syndecan in vascular smooth muscle cells and cloning of rat syndecan core protein cDNA. J Biol Chem 1992; 267:15729-15736.
138. Lin J, Davidson JM. The elastogenic effect of recombinant transforming

growth factor-beta on porcine aortic smooth muscle cells. Biochem Biophys Res Comm 1988; 154(3):895–901.

139. Schlumberger W, Thie M, Rauterberg J, Robenek H. Collagen synthesis in cultured aortic smooth muscle cells. Modulation by collagen lattice culture, transforming growth factor-β1, and epidermal growth factor. Arterioscler Thromb 1991; 11:1660–1666.

140. Merrilees MJ, Scott L. Endothelial cell stimulation of smooth muscle glycosaminoglycan synthesis can be accounted for by transforming growth factor beta activity. Atherosclerosis 1990; 81:255–265.

141. Ignotz RA, Massagué J. Transforming growth factor-beta stimulates the expression of fibronectin and collagen and their incorporation into the extracellular matrix. J Biol Chem 1986; 4337–4345.

142. Saksela O, Moscatelli D, Rifkin DB. The opposing effects of basic fibroblast growth factor and transforming growth factor-beta on the regulation of plasminogen activator activity in capillary endothelial cells. J Cell Biol 1987; 105:957–963.

143. Reilly CF, McFall RC. Platelet-derived growth factor and transforming growth factors regulate plasminogen activator inhibitor-1 synthesis in vascular smooth muscle cells. J Biol Chem 1991; 266(15):9419–9427.

144. Basson CT, Knowles WJ, Abelda S, Bell L, Castronovo V, Liotta LA, Madri JA. Spatiotemporal segregation of endothelial cell integrin and non-integrin extracellular matrix binding proteins during adhesion events. J Cell Biol 1990; 110:789–802.

145. Majesky MN, Lindner V, Twardzik DR, Schwartz SM, Reidy MA. Production of transforming growth factor β1 during repair of arterial injury. J Clin Invest 1991; 88:904–910.

146. Nabel EG, Shum L, Pompili VJ, Yang Z, San H, Shu HB, Liptay S, Gold L, Gordon D, Derynck R. Direct transfer of the transforming growth factor β1 gene into arteries stimulates fibrocellular hyperplasia. Proc Natl Acad Sci USA 1993; 90:10759–10763.

147. Wolf YG, Rasmussen LM, Ruoslahti E. Antibodies against transforming growth factor-β1 suppress intimal hyperplasia in a rat model. J Clin Invest 1994; 93:1172–1178.

148. Yan EY, Moses HL. Transforming growth factor β1-induced changes in cell migration, proliferation, and angiogenesis in the chicken chorioallantoic membrane. J Cell Biol 1990; 111:731–741

149. Roberts AB, Sporn MB, Assoian RK, Smith DM, Roche NS, Wakefield LM, Heine UI, Liotta LA, Falanga V, Kehrl JH and Fauci AS. Transforming growth factor type β:Rapid induction of fibrosis and angiogenesis in vivo and stimulation of collagen formation in vitro. Proc Natl Acad Sci USA 1986; 83:4167–4171.

150. Phillips GD, Whitehead RA, Stone AM, Ruebel MW, Goodkin ML, Knighton DR. Transforming growth factor beta (TGF-β) stimulation of angiogenesis: an electron microscopic study. J Submicrosc Cytol Pathol 1993; 25(2):149–155

151. Raghow R. Role of transforming growth factor-β in repair and fibrosis. Chest 1991; 99(3):61S-65S.
152. Border WA, Ruoslahti E. Transforming growth factor-β in disease: the dark side of tissue repair. J Clin Invest 1992; 90:1–7.
153. Border WA, Noble NA. Transforming growth factorβ in tissue fibrosis. N Engl J Med 1994; 331(19):1286–1292.
154. Kane CJM, Hebda PA, Mansbridge JN, Hanawalt PC. Direct evidence for spatial and temporal regulation of transforming growth factor β1 during cutaneous wound healing. J Cell Physiol 1991; 148:157–173.
155. Van den Eijnden-van Raaij AJM, Koornneef I, van Zoelen EJJ. A new method for high yield purification of type beta transforming growth factor from human platelets. Biochem Biophys Res Commun 1988; 157:16–23
156. Chiefetz S, Weatherbee JA, Tsang MLS, Anderson JK, Mole JE, Lucas R, Massagué J. The transforming growth-factor beta system, a complex pattern of cross-reactive ligands and receptors. Cell 1987; 48:409–415.
157. Wahl SM, Hunt DA, Wakefield LM, McCartney-Francis N, Wahl LM, Roberts AB, Sporn MB. Transforming growth factor type β induces monocyte chemotaxis and growth factor products. Proc Natl Acad Sci USA 1987; 84:5788–5792.
158. Postlehwaite AE, Keski-Oja J, Moses H, Kang A. Stimulation of the chemotactic migration of human fibroblasts by transforming growth factor-β. J Exp Med 1987; 165:251–256.
159. Gold LI, Lee TC, Reibman J, Cronstien R, Weissmann G. TGF-β selectively induces neutrophil chemotaxis. J Cell Biochem 1990; (suppl)14C:294.
160. Ignotz RA, Massagué J. Cell adhesion protein receptors as targets for transforming growth factor-β action. Cell 1987; 51:189
161. Roberts CJ, Birkenmeier TM, McQuillan JJ, Akiyama SK, Yamada SS, Chen WT, Yamada KM, McDonald JA. Transforming growth factor-β stimulates the expression of fibronectin and both subunits of the human fibronectin receptor by cultured human lung fibroblasts. J Biol Chem 1988; 263:4586–4592.
162. Starksen NF, Harsh GR, Gibbs VC, Williams LT. Regulated expression of the platelet-derived growth factor A chain gene in microvascular endothelial cells. J Biol Chem 1987; 262:14381–14384.
163. Brogi E, Ferrera N, Isner JM. Transforming growth factor-beta1 increases the expression of vascular endothelial growth factor in human arterial smooth muscle cells. Circulation 1993; 88 (4, part 2):1736A.
164. Bell MR, Gersh BJ. Restenosis: a clinician's perspective. In: Schwartz RS, ed. Coronary Restenosis. Oxford: Blackwell Scientific Publications, 1993:15.54.
165. Hermans WRM, Rensing BJ, Strauss BH, Serruys PW. Prevention of restenosis after percutaneous transluminal coronary angioplasty: the search for a "magic bullet." Am Heart J 1991; (1,Pt 1):171–187.
166. Riessen R, Isner JM, Blessing E, Loushin C, Nikol S, Wight TN. Regional differences in the distribution of the proteoglycans biglycan and decorin in

the extracellular matrix of atherosclerotic and restenotic human coronary arteries. Am J Pathol 1994; 144(5):962–974.
167. Nikkari ST, Järveläinen HT, Wight TN, Ferguson M, Clowes AW. Smooth muscle cell expression of extracellular matrix genes after arterial injury. Am J Pathol 1994; 144(6):1348–1356.
168. Clowes AW, Reidy MA, Clowes MM. Mechanisms of stenosis after arterial injury. Lab Invest 1983; 49:208–215.
169. Miano JM, Vlasic N. Tota RR, Stemerman MB. Smooth muscle cell immediate-early gene and growth factor activation follows vascular injury: a putative in vivo mechanism for autocrine growth. Arteriosclerosis Thromb 1993; 13:211–219.
170. Wysocki SJ, Lamawansa MD, Zheng MH, Fan Yang, House AK, Norman PE. Transforming growth factor-β1 and type II receptor gene expression during arterial repair. Abstracts of the American Heart Association Scientific Conference on the Molecular Cellular Biology of the Vascular Wall, 1993, p. 27.
171. Nikol S, Weir L, Sullivan A, Sharaf B, White CJ, Zemel G, Hartzler G, Stack R, Leclerc G, Isner JM. Persistently increased expression of the transforming growth factor-β1 gene in human vascular restenosis: analysis of 62 patients with one or more episodes of restenosis. Cardiovasc Pathol 1994; 3(1):57–64.
172. Nikol S, Isner JM, Pickering JG, Kearney M, Leclerc G, Weir L. Expression of transforing growth factor-B1 is increased in human vascular restenosis lesions. J Clin Invest 1992; 90:1582–1592.
173. Shi Y, Pieniek M, Fard A, O'Brien, Zalewski. Myofibroblasts and adventitiail remodeling after coronary artery injury. Restenosis Summit VII 1995; 29 (Abstr.).
174. Koide M, Kawahara Y, Tsuda T, Nakayama I, Yokoyama M. Expression of nitric oxide synthase by cytokines in vascular smooth muscle cells. Hypertension 1194; 23(suppl 1):145–148.
175. Rakugi H, Gibbons G, Wang D, Billingham M, Vershave K, Ferguson J, Angellini P, Hogan P, Mussumy A, Buja LM, Clubb F, McAllister H, Willerson J, Dzau V. Expression of transforming growth factor beta 1 in human atherectomy specimens from primary and restenotic coronary artery lesions. J Am Coll Cardiol 1992; 19(3):329A.
176. Gruentzig A. Transluminal dilatation of coronary artery stenosis (letter). Lancet 1978; 1:263.
177. Muller DWM, Topol EJ. Trial design in restenosis: problems and solutions. In: Schwartz RS, ed. Coronary Restenosis. Boston: Blackwell Scientific Publications 1993:138–168.
178. Roberts AB, Heine UI, Flanders KC, Sporn MB. Transforming growth factor-β: major role in regulation of extracellular matrix. Ann NY Acad Sci 1990; 580:225–232.
179. Border WA, Noble NA, Yamamoto T, Harper JR, Yamaguchi Y, Pierschbacher MD, Ruoslahti E. Natural inhibitor of transforming growth factor-β

proteacts against scarring in experimental kidney disease. Nature 1992; 360:361–364.
180. Border WA, Noble NA, Yamamoto T, Harper JR, Yamaquchi Y, Pierschbacher MD, Ruoslahti E. Natural inhibitor of transforming growth factor-β protects against scarring in experimental glomerulonephritis by antiserum against transforming growth factor-β1. Nature 1990; 346:371–374.
181. Wahl SM, Allen JB, Costa GL, Wong HL, Dasch JR. Reversal of acute and chronic synovial inflammation by anti-transforming growth factor β. J Exp Med 1993; 177:225–230.
182. Givi SN, Hyde DM, Hollinger MA. Effect of antibody to transforming growth factor β on bleomycin induced accumulation of lung collagen in mice. Thorax 1993; 48:959–966
183. Logan A, Berry M, Gonzalez AM, Frautschy SA, Sporn MB, Baird A. Effects of transforming growth factor on scar production in the injured central nervous system of the rat. Eur J Neurosci 1994; 6:355–363.
184. Shah M, Foreman DM, Ferguson MWJ. Neutralising antibody to TGF-β1,2 reduces cutaneous scarring in adult rodents. J Cell Sci 1994; 107:1137–1157.

7

Endothelin and the Pathogenesis of Restenosis

Eliot H. Ohlstein and Stephen A. Douglas
SmithKline Beecham Pharmaceuticals, King of Prussia, Pennsylvania

I. INTRODUCTION

In 1988 Yanagisawa and colleagues demonstrated that supernatant from cultured porcine aortic endothelial cells produced endothelium-independent contraction of isolated porcine coronary arteries (1). An endothelial cell–derived peptide was purified and the amino acid sequence was determined. This peptide, now referred to as endothelin-1 (ET-1), is the most potent mammalian vasoconstrictor known to date, having potency an order of magnitude greater than that of either angiotensin II, vasopressin, or norepinephrine.

Since its initial isolation, ET-1 has been shown to be encoded in the genome of several mammalian species, including humans (1,2). The human genome also contains coding regions for two other endothelin isopeptides with a high degree of primary amino acid sequence identity, namely, endothelin-2 (ET-2) and endothelin-3 (ET-3).

The endothelins elicit their effects through activation of specific receptors of the G-protein coupled, seven transmembrane superfamily. Two human ET receptor subtypes, ET_A and ET_B, have been cloned, sequenced, and expressed (3,4). The ET_A receptor is characterized by high affinity and selectivity for ET-1 and ET-2 over ET-3, whereas the ET_B receptor has equivalent high affinity for all three peptides. The primary effects mediated by the ET_A receptor include vasoconstriction and vascular smooth muscle proliferation. In contrast, the ET_B receptor mediates vasodilation via the release of nitric oxide and mediates bronchoconstriction and vasoconstriction in certain vascular beds.

II. ENDOTHELIN AND THE MODULATION OF CARDIOVASCULAR STRUCTURE

Although the precise pathological mechanisms underlying experimental and clinical restenosis may differ substantially, it is widely accepted that several key processes are, to a greater or lesser extent, common to both, for example, thrombogenesis, cellular proliferation/migration, and matrix deposition. Consequently, there are several processes potentially subject to modulation by ET-1. The aim of this chapter is to discuss the ability of ET-1 to modulate these processes, and, as such, they will be discussed with reference to data obtained both in vitro and in vivo.

A. Endothelin-Induced Mitogenesis

The majority of studies concerning a putative role for ET-1 in the control of cardiovascular structure has centered around its ability to induce smooth muscle cell proliferation. ET-1 is a potent mitogen in several cultured cell lines of cardiovascular origin (5). In accordance with this observation, ET-1 also regulates the expression of several target genes involved in long-term cellular signalling through alternative transduction mechanisms, such as phosphorylation of cytosolic and membrane-bound proteins that are part of the signal-transduction pathway involved in mitogenesis, including mitogen-activated protein kinase ($p42^{MAPK}$), S6 kinase, and protein tyrosine kinase $pp60^{c\text{-}src}$ (6–8). ET-1 induces the expression of several proto-oncogenes (c-*fos*, c-*jun*, c-*myc*, VL-30, protooncogene/activator protein I complex, AP-1) and growth factors (PDGF, EGF, TGF-β, bFGF, insulin, insulin-like growth factor-I, vasopressin, and bombesin) (5).

In addition to stimulating vascular smooth muscle cell hypertrophy and protein synthesis (9,10), ET-1 directly stimulates an increase in both [^{3}H]thymidine incorporation and cell number in cultured vascular smooth muscle cells (11,12). This effect was originally reported to be the result of ET_A receptor activation since it was sensitive to the ET_A-selective antagonist BQ-123. However, several investigators failed to observe endothelin-induced mitogenesis in their own particular cell culture assays. While these findings may appear to be contradictory, it is important to consider the in vitro conditions under which such observations are performed. Early passaged rat aortic smooth muscle cells (contractile phenotype) express a single population of ET_A receptors. However, by repeatedly passaging cells (synthetic phenotype), ET_B receptor expression is increased, and ET-1–induced mitogenesis becomes refractory to BQ-123 (13,14).

Interestingly, when cultured rat aortic smooth muscle cells are transfected with an endothelin-1 expression plasmid, the cells (a) overexpress ET-1 mRNA, (b) secrete fivefold more mature, biologically active ET-1 into the culture supernatant, and (c) grow at a rate that is sixfold faster than wild-type cells (the latter response being sensitive to inhibition by BQ-123) (15). In addition to any direct mitogenic actions, ET-1 may also function as a co-mitogen (10,16,17). Indeed, a synergistic action exists between ET-1 and a wide variety of growth factors, including insulin, EGF, TGF-β, PDGF, bFGF, bombesin, and angiotensin II, in cells of both noncardiovascular (Swiss 3T3 fibroblasts) (18,19) and cardiovascular (rat aortic smooth muscle cells) origin (20).

B. Endothelin-Induced Matrix Synthesis

While it has been reported that ET-1 does not appear to promote extracellular matrix production in cultured smooth muscle cells (21), it is interesting to note that ET_A and ET_B receptor activation leads to type I and III collagen synthesis in cultured cardiac fibroblasts, and that ET_A receptor activation reduces collagenase activity in this cell line (22). In view of the sensitivity of cell culture assays to rapid phenotype changes, this is an area that warrants further examination (particularly considering the findings described below, where expression of endothelin-like immunoreactivity and related mRNA expression in the rat carotid artery model appear to be optimum at a time when matrix elaboration is peaking).

C. Endothelin-Induced Migration

It has been reported that ET-1 does not stimulate cultured smooth muscle or endothelial cell migration directly (23,24); however, Morbidelle et al. (25) have reported a promigratory role for the ET_B receptor in cultured endothelial cells. Endothelin is known to increase the release of numerous chemotactic factors, including TNF-α, MCP-1, and interleukins-1β, -6, and -8, from human monocytes and, therefore, may indirectly promote cellular migration (26,27). ET-1 influences cellular adhesion, inducing ICAM-1, VCAM-1, and E-selectin expression in human brain microvascular endothelial cell cultures (28,29). In addition, ET-1 may facilitate the infiltration of inflammatory cells into the vessel wall from the vessel lumen at sites adjacent to injury by modulating vascular permeability and fluid extravasation both directly, through dilation and constriction of resistance vessels, and indirectly, through mechanisms

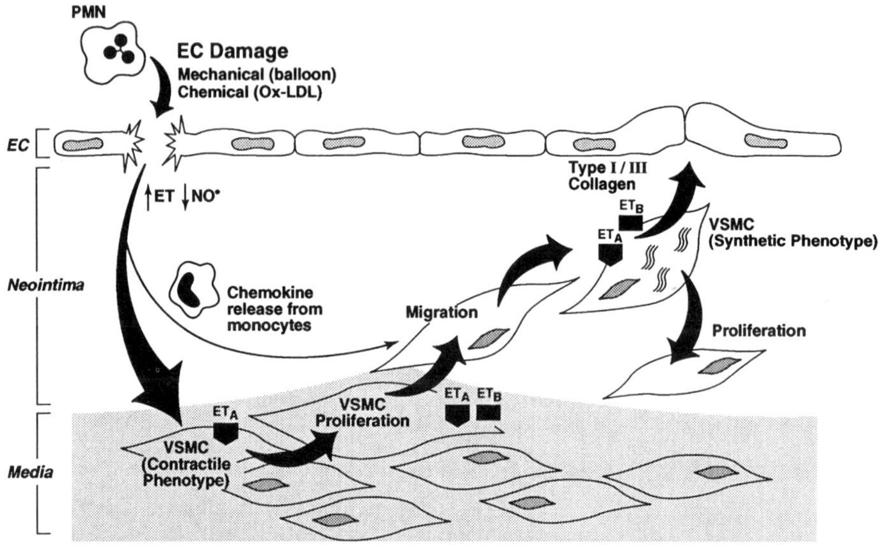

Figure 1 Potential sites of action for endothelin in neointima formation.

related to the peptides ability to stimulate the release of numerous vasoactive factors (30–33).

The putative role and potential sites of action for endothelin in neointima formation are summarized in Figure 1. Following endothelial wall injury, endothelin may promote cellular infiltration (PMN, monocytes, etc.), vascular smooth muscle proliferation, as well as matrix production. In addition, ET-1 mRNA is markedly upregulated in mononuclear cells in the atherosclerotic neointima following cardiac allograft transplantation (34). These effects, in combination with the its potent vasoconstrictor activity, may promote the vascular remodeling process.

III. THE ROLE OF ENDOTHELIN IN THE PATHOGENESIS OF VASCULAR RESTENOSIS

Indirect evidence obtained in both experimental animals and humans (changes in endothelin receptor kinetics and vascular reactivity to ET-1 and alterations in plasma/tissue levels of ET-1 immunoreactivity) has led to the proposition that ET-1 is involved in the etiology of numerous cardiovascular disorders characterized by abnormal vascular smooth muscle tone and growth. Not surprisingly, since ET-1 has been shown to promote cellular proliferation/migration and matrix synthesis in vitro, several research groups have begun to investigate whether such actions could translate into putative molecular mechanisms of pathological consequence in restenosis. The following section will describe recent studies performed to address this role for endothelin in an in vivo setting.

A. Effect of Exogenous Administration of Endothelin on Neointima Formation

Systemic administration of exogenous [^{125}I]endothelin-1 accumulates within the atherosclerotic plaques of hypercholesterolemic rabbits (35), and enhanced [^{125}I]endothelin-1 binding has been detected in hyperplastic lesions induced in pig femoral arteries and in atheromatous regions of human saphenous veins and coronary arteries (36,37). Based on the sensitivity of responses to ET-1 in atherosclerotic human coronary artery specimens to inhibition by FR 139317, it has been concluded that this tissue expresses both ET_A receptors and possible non-ET_A receptors (37). Moreover, both acute (38) and chronic (39) administration of exogenous ET-1 to rats augments, in a dose-dependent manner, the degree of neointima formation associated with carotid artery balloon angioplasty. Although a continuous systemic infusion of ET-1 was shown to augment neointima formation, the study was unable to discern between the mitogenic and pressor actions of this peptide since at the doses used the peptide was hypertensive (39). In contrast, however, an acute i.a. infusion of 500 pmol/kg ET-1 over a 30-min period immediately following balloon angioplasty produced a 73% increase in neointima cross-sectional area in the rat carotid artery model when assessed 1 week later, an effect obtained without any change in the morphometry of the contralateral carotid arteries (38). Subsequently, this phenomenon was shown to be dose dependent in vessels isolated from animals undergoing experimentation 14 days earlier. Indeed, a significant effect was observed with a dose as low as 50 pmol/kg, a dose that did not cause a significant hemodynamic response or an increase in systemic plasma levels of ET-1. The highest does of ET-1 studied (500 pmol/kg) increased the cross-sectional area of the neointima by 151%.

B. Evidence for Enhanced Levels of mRNA Species Encoding Endothelin-Related Proteins Following Angioplasty

Using quantitative reverse transcription and polymerase chain reaction (RT/PCR), Wang et al. (40) examined the temporal expression of mRNAs encoding endothelin-converting enzyme-1 (ECE-1), preproendothelin-1, and $ET_{A/B}$ receptors in the rat carotid artery balloon angioplasty model. A significant increase in ECE-1 and preproendothelin-1 mRNA is not observed until 6–24 h and 3–7 days, respectively, when levels are doubled. In contrast, both ET_A and ET_B receptor mRNAs are elevated approximately 20-fold, 3–7 and 1–3 days after angioplasty, respectively.

C. Evidence for Enhanced Endothelin Production in Atherosclerosis and Restenosis

Vasospasm and abnormal vascular smooth muscle proliferation are important complications of atherosclerosis and the vascular wall trauma seen following percutaneous transluminal coronary angioplasty (PTCA). Interestingly, oxidized LDL, a well-established atherogenic risk factor, stimulates ET-1 synthesis in human and porcine macrophage and endothelial cell cultures (5,41,42). Because atherosclerosis and PTCA are associated with reduced endothelial-nitric oxide release and enhanced ET-1 immunoreactivity (43–46), it has been proposed that this peptide may be involved in the etiology of these disorders since both basal and peptide-induced nitric oxide release will in turn attenuate endothelin-induced vasoconstriction and mitogenesis directly (through physiological antagonism) and indirectly (by promoting the dissociation of the ET-1 peptide-receptor complex or by attenuating ET-1 synthesis) (5,47). Indeed, both atherosclerosis and balloon angioplasty augment the contractile actions of ET-1 in blood vessels isolated from primates, rabbits, and rats (48–50).

Immunohistochemical studies clearly demonstrate a time-dependent increase in endothelin immunoreactivity as a consequence of balloon angioplasty in the rat (40). Enhanced expression of endothelin immunoreactivity is biphasic. Initially there is enhanced expression of endothelin immunoreactivity within the media of the vessel, a transient effect which peaks 3–7 days following injury and then rapidly declines as a neointima begins to form. This is followed by a more profound expression of endothelin immunoreactivity in the developing neointima, which is optimum 7–14 days following surgery, the neointimal smooth muscle cells representing the most likely cellular source of peptide synthesis within the lesion (34,40). Interestingly, immunoreactive expression of this mitogenic protein closely mimics that of PCNA, a marker of cellular proliferation. Furthermore, the temporal expression of endothelin immunoreactivity is in accord with the time-dependent, elevated levels of both ECE and ET-1 mRNA (see above). These data suggest that balloon catheter–induced vascular trauma results in the de novo synthesis of endothelin.

Initial clinical studies reported that PTCA induced a transient elevation of plasma endothelin immunoreactivity levels within the coronary sinus. This increase, however, likely resulted from endothelial cell destruction or transient ischemia, since a similar increase in endothelin levels within the systemic arterial circulation were not observed (46). However, a recent study has described a secondary, delayed increase in plasma endothelin levels within the coronary circulation several hours after balloon dilatation suggestive of local de novo production of this peptide in response to mechanical trauma to the vessel wall (51).

Thus, both experimental and clinical data indicate that balloon angioplasty results in the activation of the endothelin system at the site of vessel injury. The question remains, however, as to whether or not such an increase is of any pathological significance. This question has led to investigators examining the effects of endothelin receptor antagonist administration in laboratory animal models of restenosis.

D. Effect of Endothelin Receptor Antagonist Administration on Experimental Neointima Formation

The first report of an endothelin receptor antagonist exhibiting vasculoprotective efficacy in an animal model of restenosis came when Douglas et al. (38) described the effects of chronic administration of the nonpeptide $ET_{A/B}$ receptor antagonist SB 209670 in the rat carotid artery angioplasty model. SB 209670 (2.5 mg/kg, i.p., b.i.d—a regimen not associated with any pronounced hemodynamic effects in normotensive rat) attenuated neointima formation by approximately 53%. Subsequent studies by Tsujino et al. (52) and Wessale et al. (53) also reported a protective effect of both peptidic and nonpeptidic $ET_{A/B}$ antagonists: Ro 46–2005 (daily administration of 1.6 mg/kg, continuous i.v. infusion) and TAK-044 (daily administration of 5 mg/kg, u.i.d., s.c.) reduced lesion size by 38 and 79% in the rabbit iliac and rat carotid artery models, respectively.

Recently, Douglas et al. (54) have reported that administration of a dosage regimen of the ET_A-selective peptidic antagonist BQ-123 identical to that used in the SB 209670 study was devoid of any protective effect (38). Since this dosage regimen of BQ-123 was associated with a pronounced pharmacodymanic effect (assessed as a 90% inhibition of the pressor response to exogenous ET-1 administration), the authors postulated that inhibition of the ET_A receptor alone was insufficient to produce significant vasculoprotection. This hypothesis was forwarded in light of the in vitro observations described above where both ET_A and ET_B receptor subtypes had been associated with the ability of endothelin to promote cellular mitogenesis, migration, and matrix production. For example, it was known that the receptor subtype associated with mediating the mitogenic actions of ET-1 in vascular smooth muscle cells was extremely sensitive to phenotypic changes. Since, following rat aortic catheter-induced endothelium denudation, the vascular smooth muscle cells that migrate from the tunica media to form the neointima undergo an acute, yet profound, phenotype change (55), it was unclear whether such cells express either the ET_A and/or the ET_B receptors in vivo and hence could represent a plausible (if unsubstantiated, since an ET_B selective has not yet been examined in any model of restenosis) explanation for the reported failure of BQ-123 to attenuate neointima formation in the rat.

Support for this hypothesis came from the work of Azuma et al. (56), who reported that continuous i.v. administration of BQ-123 (5.3 mg/day, a dose shown to produce steady-state plasma levels one to two orders of magnitude greater than the K_d of this peptide for the ET_A receptor) failed to exhibit any vasculoprotective efficacy in the rabbit carotid artery model when assessed 4 weeks after injury. In addition, using autoradiography, these workers also demonstrated that the predominant receptor expressed in the neointima was the ET_B receptor subtype. In addition, this group has reported the presence of an atypical non-ET_A/ET_B receptors in the neointima (57).

However, more recent data indicate that the contribution made by the ET_A receptor to endothelin-induced neointima formation may show regional and/or species differences. Using a rat thoracic aorta model, Hele et al. (58) reported that oral administration of the $ET_{A/B}$ receptor antagonist bosentan and, more interestingly, the ET_A selective antagonist BMS 182874 (both 30 mg/kg, u.i.d.) reduced the degree of [^{3}H]thymidine incorporation at the site of injury (but not in other rapidly proliferating tissues such as testes) 2 days after injury by 36 and 55%, respectively. Although this study did not examine lesion formation per se (since the degree of [^{3}H]thymidine incorporation can be affected by numerous factors ranging from cellular uptake inhibitors to compounds that alter regional hemodynamics), the results were, nonetheless, interesting, suggesting that the ET_A receptor may play a significant role in lesion formation. This finding was supported by two subsequent studies, which showed that daily oral administration of BMS 182874 (100 mg/kg, p.o.) and FR 139317 (continuous i.v. infusion of 6 mg/kg/day) reduced lesion size in the rat carotid and rabbit iliac artery models, but only by 34 and 28%, respectively (59).

Thus, evidence clearly exists to support a pathogenic role for endothelin in the phenomenon of restenosis, at least in experimental animal models, although the precise significance of either receptor subtype requires further investigation. Furthermore, additional studies are required of alternate laboratory angioplasty models.

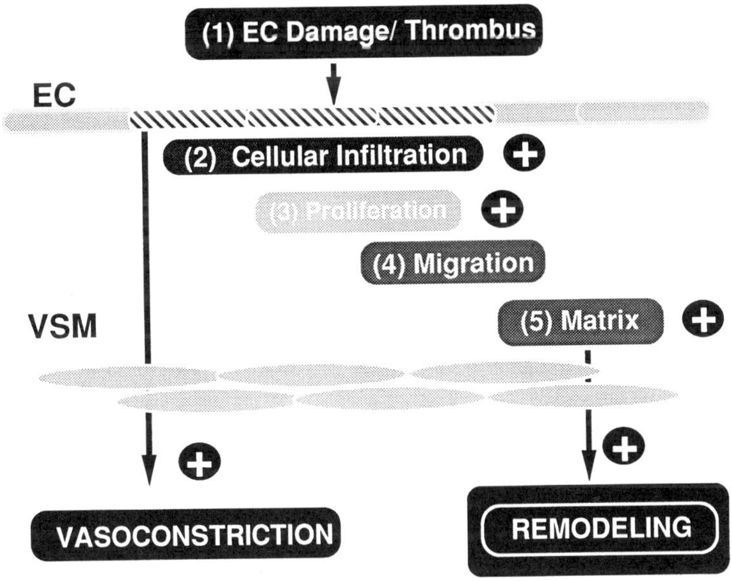

Figure 2 Potential involvement of endothelin receptors in response to vascular injury and neointima formation.

IV. SUMMARY

The role of endothelin and endothelin receptors in neointima formation may be summarized as shown in Figure 2. Following endothelial injury, ET-1 has the potential to interact with several key processes believed to be involved with the evolution of the neointimal lesion. ET-1 modulates vascular smooth muscle tone by exerting potent vasoconstrictor actions through the ET_A receptor subtype located on membrane of medial smooth muscle cells. This receptor subtype also mediates the growth-promoting actions of ET-1 in smooth muscle cells. The ET_A receptor is distinct from the ET_B receptor located on the endothelium, as the latter can mediate the release of the potent vasodilator endothelium-derived nitric oxide. Furthermore, endothelium-derived nitric oxide also promotes antimitogenic activity. Thus, under normal conditions a counterregulatory relationship exists between these endothelium-derived vasoactive agents ability to modulate the growth and tone characteristics of the vascular smooth muscle. As the vascular smooth muscle cells proliferate and migrate, phenotypic changes may occur and ET_B receptors appear that may be involved with matrix production as well as vascular smooth muscle proliferation. The consequences of these changes in endothelin receptor expression and function may contribute to the evolution of the neoinitmal lesion.

REFERENCES

1. Yanagisawa M, Kurihara H, Kimura S, Tomobe Y, Kobayashi M, Mitsui Y, Yazaki Y, Goto K, Masaki T. A novel potent vasoconstrictor peptide produced by vascular endothelial cells. Nature 1988; 332:411.
2. Kimura C, Itoh Y, Ohklubo S, Ogi K, Fujino M. Cloning and sequencing of a canine gene segment encoding mature endothelin. Nucleic Acids Res 1990; 17:3290.
3. Arai H, Hori S, Aramori I, Ohkubo H, Nakanishi S. Cloning and expression of a cDNA encoding an endothelin receptor. Nature (London) 1990; 348:730.
4. Sakurai T, Yanagisawa M, Takuwa Y, Miyazaki H, Kimura S, Goto K, Masaki T. Cloning of a cDNA encoding a non-isopeptide selective subtype of the endothelin receptor. Nature 1990; 348:732.
5. Ohlstein EH, Douglas SA. Endothelin-1 modulates vascular smooth muscle structure and vasomotion: implications in cardiovascular pathology. Drug Dev Res 1993; 29:108.
6. Wang Y, Simonson MS, Pouysségur J, Dunn MJ. Endothelin rapidly stimulates mitogen-activated protein kinase in rat mesangial cells. Biochem J 1992; 287:589.
7. Wang Y, Pousségur J, Dunn MJ. Endothelin stimulates mitogen-activated protein kinase p42 activity through the phosphorylation of the kinase in rat mesangial cells. J Cardiovasc Pharmacol 1993; 22 (suppl. 8):S164.
8. Simonson MS, Jones JM, Dunn MJ. Cytosolic and nuclear signaling by endothelin peptides: mesangial response to glomerular injury. Kidney Int 1992; 41:542.
9. Ito H, Hirata Y, Hiroe M, Tsujino J, Adachi S, Takamoto T, Nitta M, Taniguchi K, Marumo F. Endothelin-1 induces hypertrophy with enhanced expression of muscle specific genes in cultured neonatal rat cardiomyocytes. Circ Res 1991; 69:209.
10. Chua BHL, Krebs CJ, Chua CC, Diglio CA. Endothelin stimulates protein synthesis in smooth muscle cells. Am J Physiol 1992; 262:E412.
11. Ohlstein EH, Arleth A, Bryan H, Elliott JD, Sung C-P. The selective endothelin ET_A receptor antagonist BQ-123 antagonizes endothelin-1-mediated mitogenesis. Eur J Pharmacol 1992; 225:347.
12. Zamora MA, Dempsey EC, Walchak SJ, Stelzner TJ. BQ-123, an ET_A receptor antagonist, inhibits endothelin-1-mediated proliferation of human pulmonary artery smooth muscle cells. Am J Respir Cell Mol 1993; 9:429.
13. Eguchi S, Hirata Y, Imai T, Kanno K, Marumo F. Phenotypic change of endothelin receptor subtype in cultured rat vascular smooth muscle cells. Endocrinology 1994; 134:222.
14. Serradeil-Le Gal C, Herbert JM, Garcia C, Boutin M, Maffrand JP. Importance of the phenotypic state of vascular smooth muscle cells on the

binding and the mitogenic activity of endothelium. Peptides 1991; 12(3): 575–579.

15. Alberts GF, Peifley KA, Johns A, Kleha JF, Winkles JA. Constitutive endothelin-1 overexpression promotes smooth muscle proliferation via an external autocrine loop. J Biol Chem 1994; 269:10112.
16. Resink TJ, Scott-Burden T, Bühler FR. Activation of multiple signal transduction pathways by endothelin in cultured human vascular smooth muscle cells. Eur J Biochem 1990; 189:415.
17. Weissberg PL, Witchell C, Davenport AP, Hesketh TR, Metcalfe JC. The endothelin peptides ET-1, ET-2, ET-3 and sarafotoxin S6b are co-mitogenic with platelet-derived growth factor for vascular smooth muscle cells. Atherosclerosis 1990; 85:257.
18. Brown KD, Littlewood CJ. Endothelin stimulates DNA synthesis in Swiss 3T3 cells. Synergy with polypeptide growth factors. Biochem J 1989; 263:977.
19. Kusuhara M, Yamaguchi K, Ohnishi A, Abe K, Kimura S, Oono H, Hori S, Nakamura Y. Endothelin potentiates growth factor-stimulated DNA synthesis in Swiss 3T3 cells. Jpn J Cancer Res 1989; 80:302.
20. Weber H, Webb ML, Serafino R, Taylor DS, Moreland S, Norman J, Molloy CJ. Endothelin-1 and angiotensin-II stimulate delayed mitogenesis in cultured rat aortic smooth muscle cells: evidence for common signalling mechanisms. Mol Endocrinol 1994; 8:148.
21. Scott-Burden T, Resink TJ, Hahn AWA, Vanhoutte PM. Induction of endothelin secretion by angiotensin II: effects on growth and synthetic activity of vascular smooth muscle cells. J Cardiovasc Pharmacol 1991; 17 (suppl. 7):S96.
22. Guarda E, Katwa LC, Myers PR, Tyagi SC, Weber KT. Effects of endothelins on collagen turnover in cardiac fibroblasts, Cardiovasc Res 1993; 27:2130.
23. Wren A, Hiley CR, Fan T-P. Endothelin-3 mediated proliferation in wounded human umbilical vein endothelial cells. Biochem Biophys Res Commun 1993; 196:369.
24. Yue T-L, Wang X, Sung C-P, Olson B, McKenna PJ, Gu J-L, Feuerstein GZ. Interleukin-8: a mitogen and chemoattractant for vascular smooth muscle cells. Circ Res 1994; 75:1–7.
25. Morbidelli L, Orlando C, Maggi CA, Ledda F, Ziche M. Proliferation and migration of endothelial cells is promoted by endothelins via activatin of ET_B receptors. Am J Physiol 1995; 269:H686-H695.
26. Helset E, Sildnes T, Seljelid R, Konoski ZS. Endothelin-1 stimulates human monocytes in vitro to release TNF-α, IL-1β and IL-6. Mediat Inflamm 1993; 2:417.
27. Helset E, Sildnes T, Konopski ZS. Endothelin-1 stimulates monocytes in vitro to release chemotactic activity identified as interleukin-8 and monocyte chemotactic protein-1. Mediat Inflamm 1994; 3:155.
28. López-Farré A, Riesco A, Espinosa G, Digiuni E, Cernadas MR, Alvarez V, Montón M, Rivas F, Gallego MJ, Egido J, Casado S, Caramelo C. Effect of endothelin on neutrophil adhesion to endothelial cells and perfused heart. Circulation 1993; 88:1166.

29. McCarron RM, Wang L, Stanimirovic DB, Spatz M. Endothelin induction of adhesion molecule expression on human brain microvascular endothelial cells. Neurosci Lett 1993; 156:31.
30. McMurdo L, Lidbury PS, Corder R, Thiemermann C, Vane JR. Heterogeneous receptors mediate endothelin-1-induced changes in blood pressure, hematocrit, and platelet aggregation. J Cardiovasc Pharmacol 1993; 22(suppl. 8):S185.
31. Filep JG, Foldes-Filep E, Rousseau A, Fournier A, Sirois P, Yano M. Endothelin-1 enhances vascular permeability in the rat heart through the ET_A receptor. Eur J Pharmacol 1992; 219:343.
32. Kurose I, Miura S, Suematsu M, Fukumura D, Nagata H, Sekizuka E, Tsuchiya M. Involvement of platelet-activating factor in endothelin-induced vascular smooth muscle cell contraction. J Cardiovasc Pharmacol 1991; 17(suppl. 7):S279.
33. Zimmerman RS, Martinez AJ, Maymind M, Barbee RW. Effect of endothelin on plasma volume and albumin escape. Circ Res 1992; 70:1027.
34. Watschinger B, Sayegh MH, Hancock WW, Russell ME. Upregulation of endothelin-1 mRNA and peptide expression in rat cardiac allografts with rejection and arteriosclerosis. Am J Pathol 1995; 146(5):1065.
35. Prat L, Carrió I, Roca M, Riambau V, Berné L, Estorch M, Ferrer I, Garcia C. Polyclonal ^{111}In-IgG, ^{125}I-LDL and ^{125}I-endothelin-1 accumulation in experimental arterial wall injury. Eur J Nucl Med 1993; 20:1141.
36. Dashwood M, Barker SGE, Muddle JR, Yacoub MH, Martin JF. [^{125}I]-Endothelin-1 binding to vasa vasorum and regions of neovascularization in human and porcine blood vessels: a possible role for endothelin in intimal hyperplasia and atherosclerosis. J Cardiovasc Pharmacol 1993; 22(suppl. 8):S343.
37. Dashwood MR, Allen SP, Luu TN, Muddle JR. The effect of the ET_A receptor antagonist, FR 139317, on [^{125}I]-ET-1 binding to the atherosclerotic human coronary artery. Br J Pharmacol 1994; 112:386.
38. Douglas SA, Vickery-Clark LM, Storer BL, Hart T, Louden C, Elliott JD, Ohlstein, EH. A role for endogenous endothelin-1 in neointima formation following rat carotid artery balloon angioplasty: antiproliferative effects of the non-peptide endothelin receptor antagonist SB 209670. Circ Res 1994; 75:190.
39. Trachtenberg JD, Sun S, Choi ET, Callow AD, Ryan US. Effect of endothelin-1 infusion on the development of intimal hyperplasia after balloon catheter injury. J Cardiovasc Pharmacol 1993; 22(suppl. 8):S355.
40. Wang X, Douglas SA, Louden C, Vickery-Clark LM, Feuerstein GZ, Ohlstein EH. Expression of endothelin-1, endothelin-3, endothelin-converting enzyme-1, endothelin-A and endothelin-B receptor mRNA following angioplasty-induced neointima formation in the rat. Circ Res 1996; 78:322–328.
41. Martin-Nizard F, Houssaini HS, Lestavel-Delattre S, Duriez P, Fruchart J-C. Modified low density lipoproteins activate human macrophages to secrete immunoreactive endothelin. FEBS Lett 1991; 293:127.
42. Boulanger CM, Tanner FC, Beau M-L, Han AWA, Werner A, Lüscher TF.

Oxidized low density lipoproteins induce mRNA expression and release of endothelin from human and porcine endothelium. Circ Res 1992; 70:1191.
43. Lerman A, Edwards BS, Hallett JW, Heublein DM, Sandberg SM, Burnett JC, Jr. Circulating and tissue endothelin immunoreactivity in advanced atherosclerosis. N Engl J Med 1991; 325:997.
44. Bath PMW, Martin JF. Serum platelet-derived growth factor and endothelin concentrations in human hypercholesterolaemia. J Intern Med 1991; 230:313.
45. Ino T, Ohkubo M, Shimazaki S, Akimoto K, Nishimoto K, Iwahara M, Yabuta K, Hosoda Y. Plasma endothelin concentration: relation with vascular resistance and comparison before and after balloon dilatation procedures. Eur J Pediatr 1992; 151:416.
46. Tahara A, Kohno M, Yanagi S, Itagane H, Toda I, Akioka K, Teragaki M, Yasuda M, Takeuchi K, Takeda T. Circulating immunoreactive endothelin in patients undergoing percutaneous transluminal coronary angioplasty. Metabolism 1992; 40:1235.
47. Ohlstein EH, Douglas SA, Brooks DP, Hay DWP, Feuerstein GZ, Ruffolo RR, Jr. Functions mediated by peripheral endothelin receptors. In: Ruffolo RR, Jr., ed. Endothelin Receptors: From the Gene to the Human. Boca Rotan, FL: CRC Press, 1995:
48. Lopez JAG, Armstrong ML, Piegors DJ, Heistad DD. Vascular responses to endothelin-1 in atherosclerotic primates. Arteriosclerosis 1990; 10:1113.
49. Davies MG, Klyachkin ML, Kim JH, Hagen P-O. Endothelin and vein bypass grafts in experimental atherosclerosis. J Cardiovasc Pharmacol 1993; 22 (suppl. 8):S348.
50. Douglas SA, Vickery-Clark LM, Ohlstein EH. Functional evidence that angioplasty results in transient nitric oxide synthase induction. Eur J Pharmacol 1994; 255:81.
51. Malatino LS, Grassi R, Santicelli B. Release of immunoreactive endothelin from the heart during percutaneous transluminal coronary angioplasty. Am Heart J 1993; 126:700.
52. Tsujino M, Hirata Y, Eguchi S, Watanabe T, Chatani F, Marumoi F. Nonselective ETA/ETB receptor antagonits blockes proliferation of rat vasclar smooth muscle cells after balloon angioplasty. Life Sci 1995; 56:PL449.
53. Wessale J, Adler A, Novosad E, Burke S, Dayton B, Opgenorth T. Endothelin antagonism reduces neointima formed following balloon injury in rabbit. Fourth International Conference on Endothelin, London, U.K., 1995, p. 153.
54. Douglas SA, Vickery-Clark LM, Louden C, Ohlstein EH. Selective ET_A receptor antagonism with BQ-123 is insufficient to inhibit angioplasty induced neointima formation in the rat. Cardiovasc Res 1995; 29:641.
55. Orlandi A, Ehrlich HP, Ropraz P, Spagnoli LG, Gabbiani G. Rat aortic smooth muscle cells isolated from different layers at different times after endothelial denudation shows distinct biological features in vitro. Arterioscler Thromb 1994; 14:982.
56. Azuma H, Hamasaki H, Niimi Y, Terada T, Matsubara O. Rate of endothelin-1

in neointima formation after endothelial removal in rabbit cartoid arteries. Am J Physiol 1994; 267:H;2259.

57. Azuma H, Hamasaki H, Sato J, Isotani E, Obayashi S, Matsubara O. Different localization of ET_A and ET_B receptors in the hyperplastic vascular way. J Cardiovasc Pharmacol 1995; 25:802.
58. Hele DJ, Birrell M, Bush RC, Flynn DA, Brown TJ, Roach DJ. Selective ETA and mixed ETA/ETB receptor antagonist inhibit balloon catheter-induced smooth muscle cell proliferation in the rat thoracic aorta. Br J Pharmacol 1995; 114:
59. Jenkins-West T, Valentine M, Moreland S, Ferrer P. Intimal lesion development in balloon injured rat carotid arteries is suppressed by the endothelin receptor antagonists BMS-182874. FASEB J 1995; 9:A343.

8

Extracellular Matrix and Vascular Remodeling in Restenosis

Karen M. Anderson and Andrew J. Nichols
SmithKline Beecham Pharmaceuticals, King of Prussia, Pennsylvania

I. INTRODUCTION

Since its introduction in 1977 (1), percutaneous transluminal coronary angioplasty (PTCA) has been universally accepted as the interventional revascularization procedure of choice to relieve symptoms associated with atherosclerotic vascular disease. It is estimated that in 1995 approximately 500,000 PTCAs will be done in the United States alone (2). Ninety-five percent of patients can expect immediately successful revascularization (2,3). However, 30–50% of patients will experience significant restenosis within 6 months with at least 20% requiring subsequent intervention, including bypass surgery (3). Nearly two decades of intensive basic and clinical research have been devoted to identifying pharmaceuticals or new technologies to manage or prevent restenosis. Despite more than 50 clinical trials, no agent has been identified that is clearly effective in limiting restenosis in humans (3,4). The rates of restenosis following exciser laser angioplasty, directional coronary atherectomy, and rotational atherectomy are similar to those experienced with PTCA (2). Several (5–9), but not all (10), studies suggest that stents may produce less restenosis, but convincing data that clearly demonstrate long-term benefits of stenting are presently not available. Thus, restenosis remains the major limitation to interventional revascularization procedures.

Experimental animal models developed to examine the processes involved in restenosis have relied primarily on vascular responses to injury by balloon catheters. Based on numerous studies in these models, intimal vascular smooth muscle proliferation was considered the primary cause of restenosis. Accordingly, the majority of clinical trials were targeted at preventing or limiting vascular smooth muscle proliferation. It has been suggested that failure to identify an effective pharmacological agent in the clinic was due to poor experimental design (11). Alternatively, the assumption that restenosis results principally from intimal hyperplasia may be incorrect (12). Indeed, the role of intimal hyperplasia as the primary determinant of human restenosis has been challenged (13–16). Thus, an additional plausible explanation for failure in the clinic is that the trials have been aimed at the wrong target.

Recent provocative data suggest that restenosis may involve three major components: the lesion itself, the vascular wall (media), and the adventitia. Volumetrically, the greatest portion of a restenotic lesion consists of extracellular matrix (17–19). Increased attention has been paid recently to characterization of the processes involved in extracellular matrix deposition in developing lesions and their contribution to restenosis. Intriguing new data indicate that following vascular injury, medial enlargement occurs in response to both the initial injury and the developing lesion, and that restenosis may result from an inability of certain vessels to correctly undergo this form of vascular remodeling (20,21). Alternatively, reduction in vascular size or chronic constriction may underlie restenosis (22–32). Additional recent data indicate that myofibroblasts within the adventitia proliferate and synthesize extracellular matrix in response to vascular injury (33–36). Accumulation of sufficient adventitial extracellular matrix may result in scarlike contraction of the adventitia and compression of the underlying vascular wall. This compression itself could reduce chronic luminal diameter and/or impede the ability of an artery to enlarge normally, thereby contributing to restenosis. Clearly, remodeling in each of the three vascular components can affect vessel diameter or lumen area to influence development of restenosis. Extracellular matrix metabolism in each of these components is critically involved in the remodeling process. The purpose of this chapter is to review the data that implicate extracellular matrix metabolism and vascular remodeling (enlargement or constriction) as key processes involved in restenosis. We begin with a general description of the spectrum of vascular remodeling. This will be followed by brief synopses of the present literature concerning extracellular matrix composition of restenotic lesions, compensatory enlargement in atherosclerosis and restenosis, geometric remodeling or chronic constriction in restenosis, and the adventitial component of restenosis.

II. THE SPECTRUM OF VASCULAR REMODELING

Classically, vascular remodeling has been defined as either an adaptive thickening that occurs in hypertensive arteries in an effort to maintain constant wall tension despite elevated transmural pressure (37,38) or an adaptive compensatory enlargement of vessel diameter to preserve normal luminal diameter in the wake of developing atherosclerosis (39). Currently, vascular remodeling more broadly encompasses changes in the number, size, or orientation of vascular smooth muscle cells; altered quantity, composition, or orientation of extracellular matrix molecules; reduction in vessel mass or number (regression, rarefaction); and growth of vessels (angiogenesis) (40). Remodeling is an active process that involves changes in cell growth, cell death, cell migration, and extracellular matrix metabolism (41). Consistent with the classical definitions, remodeling is still considered an adaptive process, which occurs primarily in response to long-term changes in hemodynamics. But vascular remodeling is now recognized to be dependent on a dynamic interaction between hemodynamic stimuli and locally produced growth factors and vasoactive substances (41), and functional changes that are sustained for a number of days to weeks, rather than months to years, are considered long-term stimuli sufficient to initiate vascular structural changes (42). As summarized in Table 1, the various structural changes encompassed by this broader definition of vascular remodeling can be placed into five categories (40,41,43). The changes described in categories I–III are represented schematically in Figure 1.

III. THE COMPOSITION OF RESTENOTIC LESIONS

Kinetic analysis of the response of the rat carotid artery to balloon injury clearly determined that vascular smooth muscle proliferation constitutes an important component of "restenosis" in this animal model (17,18,44). Recently, however, controversy has arisen regarding the contribution of intimal hyperplasia to development of restenosis in humans. Both significant (45) and little-to-no (13–16) vascular smooth muscle proliferation has been documented in human restenotic atherectomy samples. Little smooth muscle proliferation was evident in a double-injury, non–cholesterol-fed rabbit iliac artery (46) or in normocholesterolemic balloon-injured porcine coronary artery (47), thus providing animal data in support of the concept that smooth muscle proliferation may be overestimated as the predominant mechanism in restenosis.

Regardless of the degree of smooth muscle proliferation that may occur following interventional procedures, there is a paradox between prolifera-

Table 1 The Spectrum of Vascular Remodeling

I. *Increased wall-to-lumen ratio with encroachment on lumen*
   A. *Increased wall thickness*
      Increased wall mass due to increased cell number or size
      May involve both medial and intimal layers
      May include medial to intimal migration of VSMCs
      Increased wall thickness and reduction in lumen contributes to increased wall-to-lumen ratio
      Myointimal hyperplasia (large- and medium-sized arteries, veins)
      Hypertensive vascular hypertrophy (small arteries, arterioles)
   B. *Decreased lumen diameter*
      Rearrangement of cellular and noncellular components of vascular wall resulting in primary reduction in luminal diameter
      No increase in smooth muscle mass
      Increased wall-to-lumen ratio solely due to decreased lumen diameter
      Occurs primarily in hypertensive resistance vessels

II. *Decreased wall-to-lumen ratio: enlargement or dilation of the blood vessel*
   Both inner and outer diameters increase significantly
   Active restructuring of both cellular and noncellular components of vessel wall
   Not necessarily accompanied by increase in cell mass
   Decreased wall-to-lumen ratio due to decreased wall thickness and increased lumen diameter
   Primarily in large vessels
   Vascular compensatory enlargement associated with high blood flow states, developing atherosclerotic/restenotic lesions
   Aneurysms

III. *No change in wall-to-lumen ratio: regression or atrophy*
   Both outer and inner diameters are reduced with no change in wall-to-lumen ratio
   Substantial reduction in both vascular mass and caliber
   Response to chronic reduction in blood flow
   Occurs in large and medium sized arteries

IV. *Rarefaction*
   Loss of capillary surface area
   Microcirculation of hypertensive vascular beds

V. *Angiogenesis*

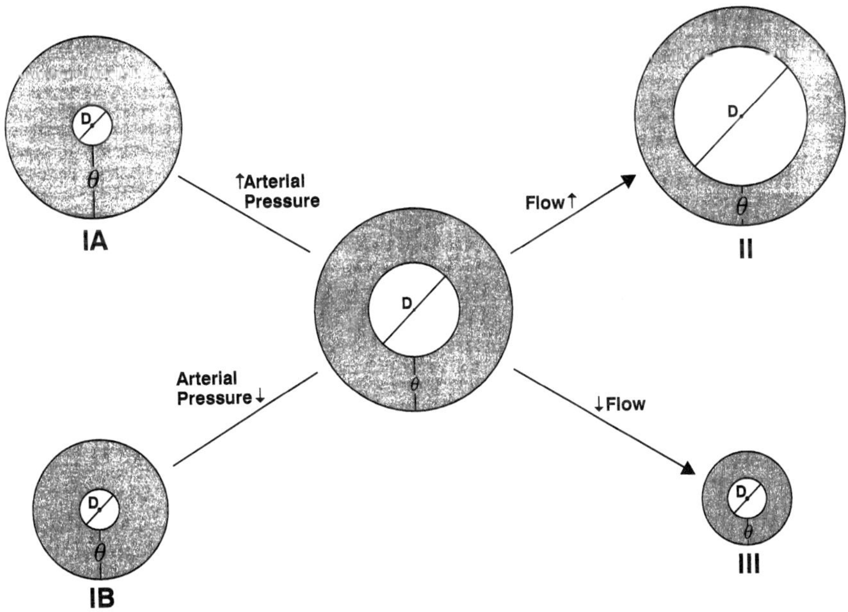

Figure 1 Schematic representation of vascular remodeling, which occurs following changes in arterial pressure or blood flow. (IA) Increased wall-to-lumen ratio as a result of both medial hypertrophy and reduced lumen diameter; (IB) increased wall-to-lumen ratio without medial hypertrophy, but reduced luminal diameter subsequent to rearrangement of cellular and noncellular vascular wall components; (II) compensatory enlargement—reduced wall-to-lumen ratio resulting from both decreased medial thickness and increased luminal diameter; (III) regression—reduction in vascular mass and caliber without a change in wall-to-lumen ratio; (D) lumen diameter; θ: medial wall thickness; roman numerals refer to classifications detailed in Table 1 and text.

tion occurring early (1–2 weeks) and late (3–12 months) clinical restenosis. In both rat (17,18) and human (19) restenotic samples, it has been determined that by 3 months after intervention, more than 80% of the restenotic lesion volume consists of extracellular matrix. This recognition that extracellular matrix constitutes the vast majority of the volume of a space-occupying lesion which may impinge on the arterial lumen indicated the potential relevance of extracellular matrix accumulation to restenosis.

The extracellular matrix molecules that comprise the major structural components of the vascular wall include collagen types I, III, IV, and V, elastin, proteoglycans, and glycoproteins. Numerous studies in experimental animal models provided evidence of increased extracellular matrix proteins including collagen types I and II (46,48–53), elastin (46,51,54,55), proteoglycans (50–52,54,56–60), and fibronectin (46,48,49,56) in restenotic lesions. Generally, the data indicated that induction of elevated extracellular matrix expression began approximately 1 week following vascular injury, that it peaked at 2–4 weeks, and that it remained elevated for months. Thus, the induction of matrix deposition was a relatively late event in the response to vascular injury. Importantly, the significant and persistent increase in extracellular matrix accumulation corresponded to that time at which vascular smooth muscle proliferation had ceased and correlated temporally to the period over which restenotic lesions gained much of their mass (51,52,54). Strauss et al. (51) demonstrated in a double-injury, non–cholesterol-fed rabbit iliac artery model of restenosis that there was a lag between early increased collagen and elastin synthesis and delayed increased collagen and elastin content. Thus, variable rates of matrix degradation during growth of the lesion may be an important mechanism in the regulation of extracellular matrix protein content (51). Other reports (61,62) support this concept.

To date, a limited number of studies have been done to characterize the extracellular matrix constituents within developing human restenotic lesions. Immunohistochemical examination of atherectomy samples of restenotic coronary artery lesions confirmed substantial accumulation of proteoglycans following PTCA (54,63). Specifically, biglycan expression increased substantially, whereas there was no evidence for decorin expression (54,63); versican expression exceeded that of biglycan (64). Preliminary studies suggest that tranilast, a compound that reportedly reduces collagen deposition, significantly attenuated restenosis 3 months after PTCA or directional coronary atherectomy (65,66). Thus, the importance of extracellular matrix accumulation in human restenosis is just emerging.

Together with the data from experimental models, the human studies indicate that the expression of extracellular matrix protein genes and the accumulation of extracellular matrix have an important role in the pathogenesis of intimal lesions. The potential importance of extracellular matrix molecules is heightened by the recognition that, in addition to occupying space, extracellular matrix molecules may also modify other biological functions in the artery wall, including lipid retention, smooth muscle cell migration and proliferation, and release of growth factors (54,67). Matrix accumulation itself occurs in response to growth factors. As reviewed in Chapter 6, transforming growth factor-beta (TGF-β) is the most potent stimulus for extracellular matrix accumulation identified to date, and TGF-β_1 expression correlates with increased matrix deposition in both animal models of restenosis and human atherectomy samples of restenotic lesions.

IV. ACTIVE REMODELING OF THE VASCULAR WALL FOLLOWING REVASCULARIZATION

A. Compensatory Enlargement

Glagov and colleagues (39,68) first described compensatory vessel enlargement, a process by which human arteries enlarge as atherosclerotic plaques develop and progress. By histological examination of sections of coronary arteries from hearts obtained at autopsy, they demonstrated that human coronary arteries enlarge in relation to plaque area and that functionally important lesion stenosis can be delayed until the lesion occupies 40% of the potential lumen area (Fig. 2A). Arterial enlargement thus preserves near-normal lumen cross-sectional area despite the presence of rather large plaques. Compensatory enlargement of coronary arteries has also been documented by epicardial echocardiography (69). Most recently, intravascular ultrasound has confirmed that this active remodeling process occurs in both coronary (70,71) and peripheral (72) atherosclerotic arteries.

Two recent studies in the hypercholesterolemic rabbit (20,21) suggested that compensatory enlargement may be an important determinant of chronic lumen area following angioplasty (Fig. 2B). Kakuta et al. (20) demonstrated that in the iliac artery, the area defined by the internal elastic lamina was increased 20% 4 weeks after angioplasty, and that this enlargement of the vessel accommodated nearly 60% of the neointimal formation to effectively limit lumen narrowing despite lesion progression. Interestingly, both restenotic and nonrestenotic vessels had equivalent lesion areas; the difference in lumen area between the two groups could be accounted for completely by significantly greater internal elastic lamina and external elastic lamina areas in the nonrestenotic group. Guzman et al. (21) determined in their rabbit femoral artery model that the external elastic lamina area was the most important and reliable predictor of lumen area. These studies indicated that vessels can remodel (enlarge) in response to neointimal lesion formation (Fig. 2B) and suggested that vessels that do not, or cannot, enlarge adequately to preserve lumen diameter in the face of increasing lesion size will likely show evidence of restenosis after angioplasty or other interventions (Fig. 2C).

B. Chronic Constriction

In contrast to vascular enlargement following angioplasty, several groups (22–32) reported evidence of chronic vascular constriction (referred to as "geometric remodeling" by some investigators) following revascularization. Such constriction has been documented by both angiography (22,23) and intravascular ultrasound (30) following balloon angioplasty of normal rabbit iliac artery (23,30), atherosclerotic rabbit femoral artery (22), and

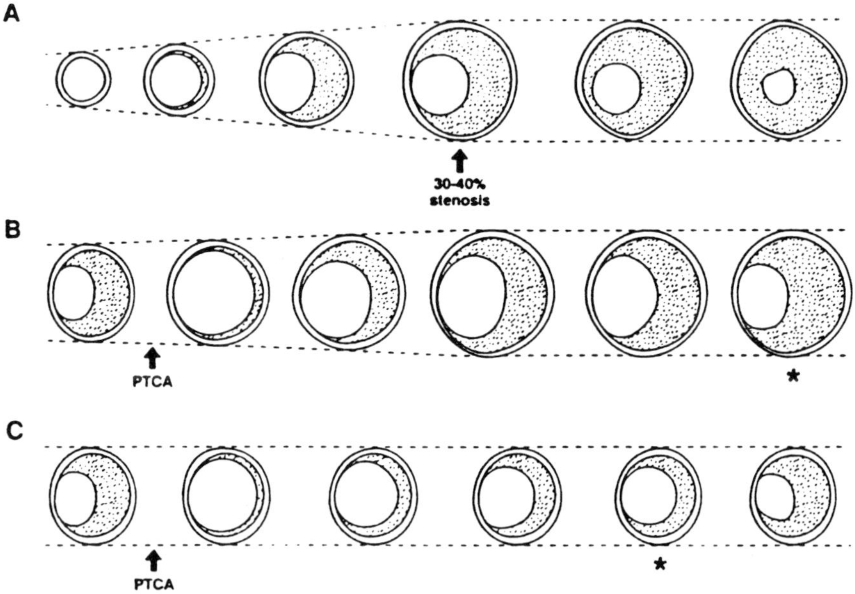

Figure 2 Schematic representation of compensatory enlargement during development and progression of atherosclerotic and restenotic lesions. (A) In atherosclerotic arteries, both inner and outer arterial diameters increase significantly in relation to plaque area to preserve normal or adequate lumen. Enlargement is limited—once the atherosclerotic plaque comprises 30–40% of the potential lumen area, enlargement cannot adequately compensate and lumen area begins to decrease. (B) Compensatory enlargement also may be an important determinant of chronic lumen area following angioplasty. Enlargement of the vessel accommodates post-PTCA neointimal formation to effectively limit lumen narrowing despite lesion progression. (C) Vessels that do not enlarge adequately to preserve lumen diameter in the face of increasing lesion size show evidence of restenosis after angioplasty or other interventions. (*) Lumen area is equivalent to lumen area before PTCA was performed.

both normal and atherosclerotic Yucatan micropig iliac arteries (23). Estimates of the contribution of geometric remodeling to restenosis in these animal models ranged from 11 to 67%. The reduction in arterial size was noted to progress over the course of weeks (23) and to represent an important correlate of restenosis 3–4 weeks after balloon dilation (22). Importantly, a recent series of preliminary studies using both quantitative coronary angiography and intravascular ultrasound suggested that this form of vascular remodeling contributed significantly (60–84%) to late lumen loss following PTCA or directional coronary atherectomy in humans (24–27,29,33). Intravascular ultrasound studies suggested that human femoral arteries also experienced chronic reductions in circumference following angioplasty (28).

C. Mechanisms Responsible for Remodeling of the Vascular Wall

The mechanisms of arterial remodeling after interventional revascularization are not currently understood. The basis for compensatory enlargement is likely analogous to mechanisms operating to produce enlargement during progression of atherosclerosis. Two general mechanisms have been proposed (39,42,43,73): (a) formation of an eccentric plaque leading to increased flow velocity subjecting the noninvolved vascular segment to high shear stress, a known stimulus for remodeling, and (b) atrophy or rearrangement of vascular tissue underlying the lesion due possibly to compression, necrosis, or release of degradative substances by the plaque itself. Geometic remodeling or chronic constriction may be analogous to the reduction in mass and caliber seen in some nonhypertrophied hypertensive vessels as a result to rearrangement of the cellular and noncellular components (74). Alternatively, constriction may result from the physical pressure imparted by scar contraction of an enveloping fibrotic adventitia as described below.

Interesting new data suggest that the mechanisms that produce restenosis may depend on the intervention used. Although not completely consistent with all the data presented above, DiMario et al. (75) recently provided data obtained by intracoronary ultrasound that indicated that restenosis after PTCA resulted from constriction, whereas restenosis following directional coronary atherectomy was predominantly due to proliferation. In a comparison of stented versus nonstented lesions, Leon and Mintz (76) demonstrated that stented lesions were associated with excessive tissue growth and proliferation, whereas restenosis in nonstented vessels was due to chronic constriction. Thus, the task of identifying mechanisms for vascular remodeling in restenosis is further complicated by the plethora of stenting devices and procedures now being used clinically.

V. ADVENTITIAL RESPONSE FOLLOWING VASCULAR INJURY: POTENTIAL ROLE FOR SCAR CONTRACTION AS MEDIATOR OF RESTENOSIS

To date, little attention has been placed on examination of adventitial responses to vascular injury. Several preliminary studies suggested that balloon angioplasty or stent:artery size ratios that exceed 1.3:1.0 produced stretch injury of the adventitia, and that deep medial injury potentially exposed portions of the adventitia to circulating elements or factors released by injured medial cells. These stimuli elicited an adventitial inflammatory and reparative response characterized by myofibroblast differentiation and proliferation, leukocyte infiltration, and increased extracellular matrix deposition (22,33–36,74,77,78). In the cholesterol-fed atherosclerotic rabbit femoral artery model of restenosis, the ratio of adventitial area to the combined intima-media area correlated positively with chronic constriction, which in turn correlated with late stenosis (22). In porcine coronary arteries, the adventitial response to vascular injury included myofibroblast proliferation (PCNA, bromodeoxyurindine), fibronectin and collagen accumulation, and elevated TGF-β_1 expression (33–36). It was proposed that adventitial fibrosis may result in scarlike contraction of the adventitia and circumferential compression of the underlying vascular wall. This compression could prevent arterial compensatory enlargement (Fig. 3A). Alternatively—or additionally—it may cause chronic constriction to effectively reduce chronic luminal diameter (Fig. 3B). Schwartz (33) reported that heat injury to the porcine coronary artery rapidly produced a dense fibrous rim in the adventitia, whereas placement of a copper stent into the artery produced an inflammatory response without adventitial fibrosis. Despite producing a lesion six times greater in volume than that produced by heating, stent placement resulted in comparable degrees of stenosis. Reportedly, adventitial fibrosis prevented arterial enlargement in response to intimal hyperplasia. In contrast, the inflammatory nature of the adventitial response to the stent did not lead to inhibition of compensatory enlargement; the stent itself also likely physically opposed vessel constriction. Thus, the adventitial response to injury appears to be dependent on the interventional procedure used, and the adventitial contribution to restenosis appears related to the degree to which a fibrotic would healing response is elicited. Overall, these data suggest a potentially crucial role of the adventitia in mechanisms of restenosis in certain circumstances and indicate that additional examination of adventitial reactivity is warranted.

VI. SUMMARY

The purpose of this chapter was to review the present understanding of vascular remodeling in general and to summarize the role of remodeling in restenosis. As it applies to restenosis, remodeling includes changes in plaque area, changes in total vessel area, or changes in the area circumscribed by the internal elastic lumina. Increasing evidence suggests that vascular remodel-

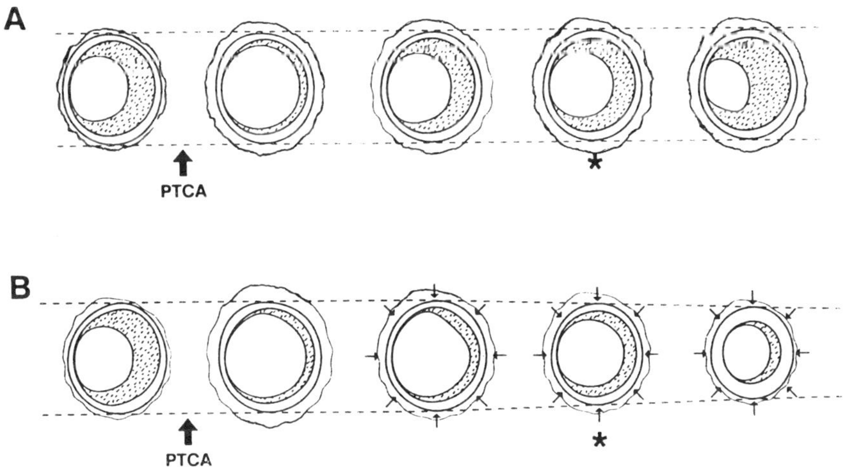

Figure 3 Adventitial response to vascular injury. Accumulation of sufficient adventitial extracellular matrix may result in scarlike contraction of the adventitia and compression of the underlying vascular wall. This compression could impede the ability of an artery to enlarge normally (A), or the compression itself could actively reduce chronic luminal diameter (B), thereby contributing to restenosis.

ing occurs after angioplasty and other interventional revascularization procedures. Restenosis may occur because of substantial encroachment of the space-occupying lesion on the lumen, chronic constriction, or failure of the vessel to undergo compensatory enlargement in response to developing lesions. It is now clear that consideration of mechanisms for restenosis must include examination of active-reactive changes within multiple vascular components: the lesion, the vascular wall, and the adventitia The mechanisms responsible for vascular remodeling are not understood. However, it is now clear that alterations in extracellular matrix turnover or arrangement of extracellular matrix proteins within the vessel are involved in the response of all three vascular components to various interventions. Thus, extracellular matrix metabolism is a major factor in vascular remodeling and may impart subsequent development of restenotic lesions, chronic constriction, or comparatory enlargement. Numerous previous clinical trials targeted to prevent vascular smooth muscle proliferation have failed to prevent restenosis, and recently the prevalence of proliferation in human restenotic lesions has been questioned. Thus, it is critical that future research into effective restenotic therapies move beyond inhibition of vascular smooth muscle proliferation as a site target. With the increased recognition of the role of extracellular matrix metabolism in vascular remodeling, inhibition of mechanisms controlling extracellular matrix production and/or stimulation of mechanisms responsible for extracellular matrix degradation may prove useful methods for the prevention of restenosis.

REFERENCES

1. Greuntzig A. Transluminal dilatation of coronary artery stenosis (letter). Lancet 1978; 1:263.
2. Bell MR, Gersh BJ. Restenosis: a clinician's perspective. In: Schwartz RS, ed. Coronary Restenosis. Boston: Blackwell Scientific Publications, 1993:15–54.
3. Hermans WRM, Rensing BJ, Strauss BH, Serruys PW. Prevention of restenosis after percutaneous transluminal coronary angioplasty: The search for a "magic bullet." Am Heart J 1991; 122(1, Pt1):171–187.
4. Franklin SM, Faxon DP. Pharmacologic prevention of restenosis after coronary angioplasty: review of the randomized clinical trials. Coronary Art Dis 1993; 4:232–242.
5. Laham RJ, Carrozza JP, Berger CJ, Cohen DJ, Baim DS. Long-term (4–6 year) outcome of Palmaz-Schatz coronary stenting. Circulation 1995; 92(8): I-281.
6. Wong SC, Zidar JP, Chuang YC, Schatz RA, Goldberg S, Baim DS, Leon MB. Stents improve late clinical outcomes: results from the combined (I+II) REStenosis study. Circulation 1995; 92(8):I-281.
7. Debbas N, Sigwart U, Eeckhout E, Stauffer JC, Vogt P, Goy JJ. Late clinical follow-up 9 years after intra-coronary stenting with the Wallstent. Circulation 1995; 92(8):I-280.
8. Hermiller JB, Fry ET, Berkompas DC, Saltiel FS, Peters TF, Ness BK, Orr CM, Van Tassel J, Pinkerton A. Five-year clinical follow-up of the Gianturco-Roubin stent: no late stent restenosis. Circulation 1995; 92(8):I-280.
9. Penn IM, Ricci DR, Almond DG, Lazzam C, Marquis JF, Webb JG, Roy L, Barbeau G, O'Neill BJ, Rake R, Wong C, Foley JB, Brown RIG, Sridhar K, Fischman DL. Coronary artery stenting reduces restenosis: Final results from the trial of angioplasty and stents in Canada (TASC)I. Circulation 1995; 92(8):I-279.
10. Sturm M, Jost S, Nolte CWT, Hausleiter J, Amende I, Lichtlen PR. Development of restenosis beyond 6 months after Palmaz-Schatz stent implantation. Circulation 1995; 92(8):I-281.
11. Muller DWM, Topol EJ. Trial design in restenosis: problems and solutions. In: Schwartz RS, ed. Coronary Restenosis. Boston: Blackwell Scientific Publications, 1993:138–168.
12. Currier JW, Faxon DP. Restenosis after percutaneous transluminal coronary angioplasty: Have we been aiming at the wrong target? J Am Coll Cardiol 1995; 25:516–520.
13. Strauss BH, van Suylen RJ, Umans VA, deFeyter PJ, Marco J, Robertson GC, Wijns W, Heyndrickx GR, Vuzevski VD, Bosman FT, Serruys PW. Direc-

tional atherectomy for treatment of restenosis within coronary stents: clinical angiographic and histologic results. J Am Coll Cardiol 1992; 20:1465–1473.
14. O'Brien E, Alpers C, Stewart D, Ferguson M, Tran N, Gordon D, Benditt EP, Hinohara T, Simpson J, Schwartz S. Proliferation in primary and restenotic coronary atherectomy tissue: implications for antiproliferative therapy. Circ Res 1993; 73:223–231.
15. Leclerc G, Kearney M, Schneider D, Rosenfield K, Losordo DW, Isner JM. Assessment of cell kinetics in human restenotic lesions by in vitro bromodeoxyuridine labeling of excised atherectomy specimens. Clin Res 1993; 41:343A.
16. Waller BF, Pinkerton CA, Orr CM, Slack JD, Van Tassel JW, Peters T. Morphological observations late (>30 days) after clinically successful coronary balloon angioplasty. Circulation 1991; 83:I-28.
17. Clowes AW, Reidy MA, Clowes MM. Kinetics of cellular proliferation after arterial injury: smooth muscle growth in the absence of endothelium. Lab Invest 1983; 49:327–333.
18. Clowes AW, Reidy MA, Clowes MM. Mechanisms of stenosis after arterial injury. Lab Invest 1983; 49:208–215.
19. Schwartz RS, Holmes DR, Topol EJ. The restenosis paradigm revisited: an alternative proposal for cellular mechanisms. J Am Coll Cardiol 1992; 20:1284-1293.
20. Kakuta T, Currier JW, Haudenschild CC, Ryan TJ, Faxon DP. Differences in compensatory vessel enlargement, not intimal formation, account for restenosis after angioplasty in the hypercholesterolemic rabbit model. Circulation 1994; 89:2809–2815.
21. Guzman LA, Mick MJ, Arnold AM, Forudi F, Whitlow PL. Role of intimal hyperplasia and arterial remodeling after balloon angioplasty: an experimental study in the rabbit atherosclerotic model. Restenosis Summit VII 1995; 28.
22. Lafont A, Guzman LA, Whitlow PL, Goormastic M, Cornhill JF, Chisolm GM. Restenosis after experimental angioplasty: intimal, medial and adventitial changes associated with constrictive remodeling. Circ Res 1995; 76:996–1002.
23. Post MJ, Bvorst C, Kuntz RE. The relative importance of arterial remodeling compared with intimal hyperplasia in lumen renarrowing after balloon angioplasty. Circulation 1994; 89:2816–2821.
24. Kovach JA, Mintz GS, Kent KM, Pichard AD, Satler LF, Popma JJ, Leon MB. Serial intravascular ultrasound studies indicate that chronic recoil is an important mechanism of restenosis following transcatheter therapy. J Am Coll Cardiol 1993; 21:484A.
25. Mintz GS, Kovach JA, Javier SP, Ditrano CJ, Leon MB. Geometric remodeling is the predominant mechanism of late lumen loss after coronary angioplasty. Circulation 1993; 88:I-654.
26. Mintz GS, Kovach JA, Pichard AD, Kent KM, Satler LF, Popma JJ, Painter JA, Morgan K, Leon MB. Geometric remodeling is the predominant mechanism of clinical restenosis after coronary angioplasty. J Am Coll Cardiol 1994; 23:138A.

27. Bier JD, Kakuta T, Currier JW, Mukjurjee S, Levine GN, Chodes AP, Ryan TJ, Faxon DP. Arterial remodeling: importance in primary versus restenotic lesions. J Am Coll Cardiol 1994; 23:139A.
28. Pasterkamp G, Wensing PJW, Post MJ, Hillen B, Mali WPTM, Borst C. Paradoxical vessel wall shrinkage as an important mechanism of femoral artery stenosis: an intravascular ultrasound study. J Am Coll Cardiol 1994; 23:242A.
29. Luo H, Nishioka T, Forrester J, Kim CJ. Comparison of de novo and restenosis coronary artery lesions: an intravascular ultrasound study. Circulation 1995; 92(8):I-17.
30. Makkar RR, Sheth S, Yhip P, Luo H, Fishbein MC, Dev V, Eigler NL, Litvach FI. Geometric remodeling predominantly accounts for luminal loss in rabbit iliac artery injury model: a serial intravascular ultrasound study. Circulation 1995; 92(8):I-93.
31. Mintz GS, Fitgerald PJ, Kuntz RE, Simonton CA, Bersin RM, Yock PG, Baim DM, Leon MB. Lesion site and reference segment remodeling after directional coronary atherectomy: an analysis from the optimal atherectomy restenosis study. Circulation 1995; 92(8):I-93.
32. Kimura T, Kaburagi S, Tashima Y, Nobuyoshi M, Mintz GS, Popma JJ. Geometric remodeling and intimal regrowth as mechanisms of restenosis: observations from serial ultrasound analysis of restenosis (SURE) trial. Circulation 1995; 92(8):I-76.
33. Schwartz RS. Restenosis: attention to adventitial injury. Restenosis Summit VII 1995; 120–123.
34. Shi Y, Pieniek M, Fard A, O'Brien J, Zalewski A. Myofibroblasts and remodeling after coronary artery injury. Restenosis Summit VII 1995; 29.
35. Shi Y, Pieniek M, Fard A, O'Brien J, Zalewski A. Phenotypic modulation of adventitial myofibroblasts following vascular injury. Circulation 1995; 92(8): I-34.
36. Shi Y, O'Brien J. Fard A, Zalewski A. Adventitial myofibroblasts contribute to neointimal formation following coronary arterial injury. Circulation 1995; 92(8):I-34.
37. Mulvany MJ. The structure of the resistance vasculature in essential hypertension. J Hypertension 1987; 5:129–136.
38. Baumbach GL, Heistad DD. Remodeling of cerebral arterioles in chronic hypertension. Hypertension. 1989; 13:968–972.
39. Glagov S, Weisenberg E, Zarins CK, Stankunavicius R, Kolettis GJ. Compensatory enlargement of human atherosclerotic coronary arteries. NEJM 1987; 316(22):1371–1375.
40. Struijker-Boudier HA, Smits JFM and DeMey JGR. Pharmacology of cardiac and vascular remodeling. Annu Rev Pharmcol Toxicol 1995; 35:509–539.
41. Gibbons GH, Dzau VJ. The emerging concept of vascular remodeling. NEJM 1994; 330(20):1431–1437.
42. Langille BL. Remodeling of developing and mature arteries: Endothelium, smooth muscle, and matrix. J Cardiovasc Pharmacol 1993; 21(suppl. 1):S11-S17.

43. Dzau VJ, Gibbons GH. Vascular remodeling: mechanisms and implications. J Cardiovasc Pharmacol 1993; 21(suppl. 1):S1-S5.
44. Clowes Aw, Clowes MM. Kinetics of cellular proliferation after arterial injury, IV: heparin inhibits rat smooth muscle mitogenesis and migration. Circ Res 1986; 58:839–845.
45. Pickering JG, Weir L, Jekanowski J, Kearney MA, Isner JM. Proliferation activity in peripheral and coronary atherosclerotic plaque among patients undergoing percutaneous revascularization. J Clin Invest 1993; 91:1469–1480.
46. Strauss BH, Chisholm RJ, Keeley FW, Gotlieb AI, Logan RA, Armstrong PW. Extracellular matrix remodeling after balloon angioplasty injury in a rabbit model of restenosis. Circ Res 1994; 75:650–658.
47. Schwartz RS, Edwards WD, Huber KC, Antoniades LC, Bailey KR, Camrud AR, Jorgenson MA, Holmes DR. Coronary Restenosis: prospects for solution and new perspectives from a porcine model. Mayo Clin Proc 1993; 68:54–62
48. Madri JA, Reidy MA, Kocher O, Bell L. Endothelial cell behavior after denndation injury in modulated by transforming growth factor-β1 and fibronectin. Lab Invest 1989; 60(6):755–765
49. Majesky MN, Lindner V, Twardzik DR, Schwartz SM, Reidy MA. Production of transforming growth factor β1 during repair of arterial injury. J Clin Invest 1991; 88:904–910.
50. Nabel EG, Shum L, Pompili VJ, Yang Z, San H, Shu HB, Liptay S, Gold L, Gordon D, Derynck R. Direct transfer of the transforming growth factor $\varepsilon\beta$1 gene into arteries stimulates fibrocellular hyperplasia. Proc Natl Acad Sci USA 1993; 90:10759–10763.
51. Wysocki SJ, Lamawansa MD, Zheng MH, Fan Yang, House AK, Norman PE. Transforming growth factor-β1 and type II receptor gene expression during arterial repair. Abstracts of the American Heart Association Scientific Conference on the Molecular and Cellular Biology of the Vascular Wall, 1993, p. 27.
52. Helin P, Lorenzen I, Garbarsch C, Matthiessen ME. Repair in arterial tissues: morphological and biochemical changes in rabbit aorta after a single dilatation injury. Circ Res 1991; 29:542–554.
53. Snow A, Bolender R, Wight TN, Clowes A. Heparin modulates the composition of the extracellular matrix domain surrounding arterial smooth muscle cells. Am J Pathol 1990; 137:313–330.
54. Nikkari ST, Jarvelainen HT, Wight TN, Ferguson M, Clowes AW. Smooth muscle cell expression of extracellular matrix genes after arterial injury. Am J Pathol 1994; 144(6):1348–1356.
55. Boyd CD, Kniep AC, Pierce RA, Deak SB, Karboski C, Miller DC, Parker MI, Mackenzie JW, Rosenbloom J, Scott GE. Increased elastin mRNA levels associated with surgically induced intimal injury. Connect Tiss Res 1988; 18:65-78.
56. Wolf YG, Rasmussen LM, Ruoslahti E. Antibodies against transforming growth factor-β1 suppress initmal hyperplasia in a rat model. J Clin Invest 1994; 93:1172–1178.

57. Richardson M, Ihnatowytez I, Moore S. Glycosaminoglycan distribution in rabbit aortic wall following balloon catheter deendothelialization. An ultrastructural study. Lab Invest 1980; 43:509–516.
58. Wight TN, Curwen KD, Litrenta MM, Alonso DR, Minick CR. Effect of endothelium on glycosaminoglycan accumulation in injured rabbit aorta. Am J Pathol 1983; 113:156–164.
59. Salisbury BGJ, Hajjar DP, Minick CR. Atlered glycosaminoglycan metabolism in injured arterial wall. Exp Mol Pathol 1985; 42:306–319.
60. Merrilees MJ, Scott LJ. Effects of endothelial removal and regeneration on smooth muscle glycosaminoglycan synthesis and growth in rat carotid artery in organ culture. Lab Invest 1985; 52:409–419.
61. Laurent GJ. Dynamic state of collagen: pathways of collagen degradation in vivo and their possible role in regulation of collagen mass. Am J Physiol 1987; 252(Cell Physiol 21):C1-C9.
62. Dollery CM, McEwan JR, Henney AM. Matrix metalloproteinases and cardiovascular disease. Circ Res 1995; 77:863–868.
63. Riessen R, Isner JM, Blessing E, Loushin C, Nikol S, Wight TN. Regional differences in the distribution of the proteoglycans biglycan and decorin in the extracellular matrix of atherosclerotic and restenotic human coronary arteries. Am J Pathol 1994; 144(5):962–974.
64. Lin H, McManus BM, Kanda T. Prominence of versican in the early neointimal response to injury by balloon dilation of coronary arteries: analysis of primary and restenotic lesions obtained by directional atherectomy. Circulation 1995; 92(8):I-424.
65. Kosuga K, Tamai H, Ueda K, Hsu Y-S, Ono S, Tanaka S, Doi T, Wang M, Motohara S, Uehata H. Efficacy of tranilast on restenosis after directional coronary atherectomy (DCA). Circulation 1995; 92(8):I-346.
66. Ueda K, Tamai H, Hsu Y-S. Efficacy of tranilast on restenosis after percutaneous transluminal coronary angioplasty in small sized coronary arteries. Circulation 1995; 92(8):I-347.
67. Wight TN. Cell biology of arterial proteoglycans. Arteriosclerosis 1989; 9:1–20.
68. Zarins CK, Weisenberg E, Kolettis G, Stankunavicius R, Glagov S. Differential enlargement of artery segments in response to enlarging atherosclerotic plaques. J Vasc Surg 1988; 7:386–394.
69. McPherson DD, Sirna SJ, Hiratzkja LF. Coronary arterial remodeling studied by high-frequency epicardial echocardiography: an early compensatory mechanism in patients with obstructive coronary atherosclerosis. J Am Coll Cardiol 1991; 17:79–86.
70. Hermiller JB, Tenaglia AN, Kisslo KB, Phillips HR, Bashore TM, Stack RS, Davidson CJ. In vivo validation of compensatory enlargement of atherosclerotic coronary arteries. Am J Cardiol 1993; 71:665–668.
71. Di Mario C, Ruygrok PN, Serruys PW. Vascular remodeling in coronary artery disease. J Cardiovasc Pharmacol 1994; 24(suppl. 3):S5-S15.
72. Losordo DW, Rosenfiled K, Kaufman J, Pieczek A, Isner JM. Focal compen-

satory enlargement of human arteries in response to progressive atherosclerosis: in vivo documentation using intravascular ultrasound. Circulation 1994; 89:2570–2577.
73. Glagov S. Intimal hyperplasia, vascular modeling, and the restenosis problem. Circulation 1994; 89:2888–2891.
74. Dzau VJ, Milner P, Gibbons GH. Vascular remodeling in human coronary restenosis. Restenosis Summit VII 1995; 84–85.
75. DiMario C, Gil R, Camenzind E, Ozaki Y, von Birgden C, Umans V, de Jaegere P, de Feyter PJ, Roelandt JRTC, Serruys PW. Quantitative assessment with intracoronary ultrasound of the mechanisms of restenosis after percutaneous transluminal coronary angioplasty and directional coronary atherectomy. Am J Cardiol 1995; 75:772–777.
76. Leon MB, Mintz GS. Patterns of arterial responses after transcatheter therapies. Restenosis Summit VII 1995; 158–159.
77. Anderson HR, Maeng M, Thorwest M, Falk E. Constrictive vascular remodeling rather than neointima formation explains luminal narrowing after deep vessel wall injury. Insights from a new porcine coronary (re)stenosis model. Circulation 1995; 92(8)I-346.
78. Brott BC, Labinaz M, Culp SC, Fortin DF, Virmani R, Phillips HR, Stack RS. Vessel remodeling after angioplasty: comparative anatomic studies. Circulation 1994; 23:138A.

9

Thrombin: A Versatile Protease in Restenosis

Jeffrey M. Stadel
SmithKline Beecham Pharmaceuticals, King of Prussia, Pennsylvania

I. INTRODUCTION

The leading cause of morbidity and mortality in industrialized societies is vascular disease. The underlying pathology in the vast majority of patients with vascular disease is atherosclerosis. Atherosclerosis is a long-term progressive disease that results in the build-up of plaque in the lumen of blood vessels restricting blood flow. This plaque consists of lipids and cells, such as macrophages, lymphocytes, and smooth muscle cells, which are encompassed by extracellular matrix. The major pathological event that gives rise to symptoms of vascular disease is occlusion of a major artery by a thrombus or an embolism formed on the surface of a plaque resulting in ischemic compromise of tissues supplied by the vessel. Thrombosis is the pathological extension of the normal homeostasis process required to prevent blood loss following damage to the vessel wall. Thrombi are often associated with endothelial injury in regions of high shear stress, such as the surface of a disrupted atherosclerotic plaque in coronary arteries.

A widespread clinical approach to atherosclerosis is percutaneous transluminal coronary angioplasty (PTCA). Current estimates indicate that nearly half a million procedures are performed annually in the United States alone. Despite a high initial success rate (~ 95%) in restoring blood flow in stenosed blood vessels, PTCA is plagued by long-term (3–6 months) restenosis in more than one-third of the patients treated (1). The problem of restenosis has triggered research by both clinicians and basic scientists to alleviate this enigma. However, over the course of the past 10 years no successful therapy has emerged, and the basic mechanisms underlying restenosis remain controversial (2–4). Currently there is a need for new paradigms or identification of additional therapeutic targets to promote progress in this arena. The subject of this chapter is a possible role for the multifunctional serine protease, thrombin, in the progression of vascular disease and restenosis. Thrombin is an attractive therapeutic target, and identification of specific inhibitors is currently under very active investigation.

II. CURRENT CONCEPTS OF RESTENOSIS

For the past 20 years a theory proposed by Ross and colleagues (5–7) to explain the initiation and progression of atherosclerosis has dominated our concepts and experiments toward alleviating cardiovascular disease. This hypothesis, termed "response to injury," has evolved over a 20-year period as new data have come to light. The basic tenents of the hypothesis hold that the initiation of atherosclerosis results from an insult/injury to the vascular endothelium resulting in increased vascular permeability and trafficking of leukocytes. This initial inflammatory event triggers a fibroproliferative repair process that may become excessive if the initial source of injury is not curtailed. The initial inflammatory event promotes the permeability of lipids, particularly in the form of low-density lipoprotein (LDL), into the subendothelial intima and the margination of monocytes and T lymphocytes into the intima as well. Differentiated macrophages accumulate cholesterol from ingested LDL, becoming foam cells that constitute the first observable lesion of atherosclerosis, the fatty streak. Cytokines and growth factors from activated cells promote the migration and proliferation of smooth muscle cells in the intima, and these smooth muscle cells elaborate an extracellular matrix that leads to the formation of the fibrous atherosclerotic plaque with a necrotic lipid core. As this plaque continues to grow, the blood flow through the artery decreases. Unstable plaques can rupture in the face of stress exerted by this turbulent blood flow providing a surface for occlusive thrombus formation.

The basic postulates of the response-to-injury hypothesis have strongly influenced the concepts underlying restenosis following PTCA. It is clear that the inflation of a balloon in a stenotic artery injures the vessel wall beyond denuding the vessel of endothelial cells. Both atherosclerosis and restenosis share the fibroproliferative formation of a neointima that impinges on arterial blood flow. Therefore, many of the cell types and apparent pathological processes associated with atherosclerosis appear also to be players in restenosis following PTCA. However, there are clear differences between the two pathologies: for example, there is no apparent role for lipids in restenosis, and restenosis occurs over a period of months compared to the decades of progressive atherosclerosis.

The initial research into restenosis concentrated on the mechanism of neointima formation with the intent to identify molecular targets for therapeutic intervention. Investigators have focused their attention on growth factors and inflammatory cytokines as well as their receptors as therapeutic targets to inhibit smooth muscle proliferation and thus control neointima formation. Although we have learned much about the temporal process and putative mediators of neointimal formation (1, 8), no agents derived from these studies have translated to clinical therapies. Some have argued that the problem lies in the use of animal models that may not accurately reflect disease processes in humans. Much of the research has utilized balloon angioplasty of a normal carotid artery in a rat model that is readily accessible, but does not include a stenotic atherosclerotic lesion prior to angioplasty. Others have suggested that neointimal formation may not be the major pathology, but that elastic recoil of the dilated artery and/or remodeling of vessel wall mass are major contributors to restenosis (3, 4).

Thrombin has recently received attention because its multifunctional nature impinges on a number of the processes outlined above. As described in detail below, thrombin plays a critical role in thrombus formation, and the recently described cellular effects of thrombin have thrust it to the forefront as a therapeutic target. Clinical trials with thrombin inhibitors are ongoing and will be discussed later.

III. THROMBIN: AN ENZYMATIC CHAMELEON

Thrombin was first identified as the final enzyme produced by the coagulation cascade. The conversion of catalytically inert prothrombin to catalytically competent thrombin leads to cleavage of peptides from the serum protein fibrinogen, which allows the monomers to polymerize to form fibrin, the meshwork of a blood clot. Thrombin also activates, by proteolysis, factor XIII, which possesses transglutaminase activity and thus cross-links fibrin, stabilizing the clot. Thrombin also promotes its own formation by activating cofactors in blood: factor V and factor VIII. The procoagulant activity of thrombin is modulated in two ways. Antithrombin III and heparin cofactor II selectively bind and inhibit thrombin, and the activity of these serpins is enhanced by the presence of heparin. Thus, heparin has become a standard anticoagulant therapy, but it is limited by the fact that serpins cannot inhibit thrombin when it is associated with the fibrin matrix, a point we will return to later.

The second way in which the prothrombotic activity of thrombin is curbed involves a fascinating twist in the enzymatic activity of thrombin itself. Once activated, thrombin can bind to a protein, thrombomodulin, that is expressed on the surface of vascular endothelial cells (10). When associated with thrombomodulin, thrombin no longer recognizes fibrinogen or factors V, VIII, and XIII in the clotting cascade. Thrombin now efficiently activates protein C. Protein C in turn promotes the degradation of the activated forms of factors V and VIII and thereby inhibits coagulation. Thus thrombin plays an essential role in initiating clot formation, but at the same time this multifunctional protease displays an altered substrate specificity when complexed with thrombomodulin on the surface of endothelial cells leading to the shut down of the coagulation cascade. Recent mutational analysis of thrombin indicates that it is possible to engineer thrombin to display selectivity for protein C over fibrinogen and thus act as an anticoagulant (11).

Although thrombin shares structural homology to other serine proteases, including trypsin, its substrate specificity is relatively restricted. The reason for the substrate selectivity of thrombin compared to trypsin is the structure of its active site and the use of exosites or additional binding domains on the protease to enhance affinity and properly align substrates for cleavage. Crystal structures of thrombin in combination with inhibitors have helped define the selective action of thrombin (12–14). The major exosite regulating binding specificity is a surface groove whose composition is relatively enriched in basic amino acids. This site has been termed the anion exosite or the fibrinogen exosite. This site has been implicated in the binding recognition of fibrinogen, the serpins, thrombomodulin, and the specific thrombin inhibitor hirudin. Hirudin is a protein isolated from the medicinal leech that inhibits blood coagulation by specifically binding to and inhibiting thrombin, allowing the leech to ingest its blood meal. Crystal structures of the thrombin-hirudin complex (13) reveal that the inhibitor protein binds to both the active site and the anion exosite of thrombin explaining both its specificity and high affinity. The interaction of the C-terminus of hirudin with the exosite involves both electrostatic as well as hydrophobic interactions, which then aligns the N-terminus to engage the active site of thrombin. These x-ray structures of thrombin have aided in the design of selective novel inhibitors of the protease.

IV. CHARACTERIZATION OF THROMBIN RECEPTORS ON VASCULAR CELLS

Over the past 20 years there has been a growing literature describing the effects of thrombin on various cell types (for reviews, see Refs. 15, 16). Thrombin has been reported to have multiple effects on vascular cells, both those in the circulation and those making up the vessel architecture. First and foremost, thrombin is the most potent activator of platelets leading to aggregation and thrombus formation (17). Several studies show that thrombin plays a critical role in arterial thrombosis in animal models (18–20). Depending on the degree of stenosis, platelet aggregation can lead to a mural thrombus or an occlusive thrombus, which results in catastrophic ischemia for the organs supplied by the affected blood vessels. A mural thrombus may also feed the progression of neointimal formation. Activated platelets release a variety of cytokines, such as PDGF, TGF-β, and IGF-1, which can promote smooth muscle cell migration and proliferation, as well as matrix deposition. Moreover, thrombin itself becomes trapped in the fibrin clot and is slowly released over time by fibrinolysis. As described below, thrombin can have direct effects on the cells making up the vascular wall.

Thrombin is also reported to be chemotactic for leukocytes (21), such as monocytes, and to be mitogenic for lymphocytes (22). Thrombin can also promote leukocyte trafficking at sites of injury by promoting upregulation of adhesion molecules, e.g., P-selectin, on the surface of endothelial cells (23). These adhesion molecules arrest circulating leukocytes and allow them to migrate toward sites of injury or infection in the subendothelial space where they initiate an inflammatory response necessary for repair. The significance of thrombin's proinflammatory action in vivo remains to be defined.

Thrombin has both direct and indirect effects on cells that make up the vascular wall that could be related to the process of restenosis. In addition to the modulation of adhesion receptors on endothelial cells, thrombin causes these cells to change shape leading to increased vascular permeability. Thrombin also contributes to a proinflammatory state by promoting secretion of lipid-derived mediators such as platelet activating factor and leukotrienes from endothelial cells (24). Thrombin also modulates vascular tone by stimulating the production of prostacyclin and nitric oxide from endothelial cells, which promotes vascular smooth muscle relaxation (25). The proinflammatory environment promoted by thrombin is a prerequisite for wound repair but also likely contributes to the pathology of restenosis.

Thrombin itself has been reported to be a mitogen for mesenchymal cells. These proliferative effects of the protease have been most extensively characterized in fibroblasts (26, 27) and vascular smooth muscle cells (28). Proliferation of both of these cell types is thought to be key to neointima formation and for vascular remodeling. The stimulation of smooth muscle cell mitosis appears to be both direct (28) and indirect, as antibodies to bFGF attenuate the mitogenic effect of thrombin on these cells isolated in vitro (29). In addition, thrombin also stimulates endothelial cells to secrete

PDGF, which is a potent smooth muscle cell mitogen and chemotactic agent (30). One further activity of thrombin on smooth muscle cells is to cause contraction, which could play a role in blood vessel recoil subsequent to PTCA. Thrombin-mediated contraction may become important in restenosis when the vessel wall is denuded of endothelium following balloon angioplasty and the smooth muscle cells become directly exposed to blood components.

When one takes into account the varied activities of thrombin on vascular cells, thrombin appears to be a vital coordinator of the response to vascular injury, promoting both the inflammatory and proliferative responses necessary for wound repair. Thrombin has direct and indirect effects on nearly all of the cell types implicated in the response-to-injury hypothesis associated with atherosclerosis and restenosis. As stated above, if the injury is severe and/or if the initiating insult is continuous, the wound repair processes may become excessive and lead to pathologies. Thrombin could also be involved in the newly emerging concepts in restenosis of elastic recoil and vascular wall remodeling by affecting vascular tone, its proliferative effects on vascular cells, and its potential effects on remodeling of the extracellular matrix providing a new "context" for cell responsiveness (31, 32).

How does thrombin promote such diverse activities in varied cell types? It was not always clear if the effects of a protease like thrombin on cellular functions were direct or indirect. This raised the question: Is the proteolytic activity of thrombin necessary or is another domain of the enzyme recognized by a cell surface receptor? A major leap forward in our understanding of how thrombin affects cells occurred with the simultaneous cloning of a thrombin receptor in two laboratories (33, 34). Examination of the translated amino acid sequence revealed some shared as well as unique characteristics. First of all, the hydrophilic sequences of the receptor were interspersed between seven hydrophobic stretches that likely represent transmembrane helixes. This seven-transmembrane motif is the signature of the G protein–coupled receptor superfamily (35). This is consistent with the observation that the signaling events associated with cellular activation by thrombin can often be inhibited by pretreating cells with pertussis toxin. This toxin covalently modifies a subset of G proteins preventing association with their agonist-occupied receptor and thus interrupts signal transduction. Additional inspection of the thrombin receptor primary sequence led to a proposed novel mechanism for receptor activation. Coughlin and colleagues (33, 36) identified in the extracellular N-terminal domain of the receptor a potential thrombin cleavage site and a downstream amino acid sequence that showed remarkable homology to the hirudin C-terminal domain involved in binding to the thrombin anion exosite. This group of investigators proposed that thrombin could bind with high affinity through these two sites and that thrombin could activate the receptor by proteolytic cleavage. Experimental evidence in support of this model relies on three observations. First, amino acid substitution at the proposed thrombin cleavage site to prevent proteolysis also prevented receptor activation (33). Second, substitution at the thrombin cleavage site with an amino acid sequence specific for a different protease altered the specificity for receptor activation to the second protease, while thrombin was now inactive toward the mutant receptor (36). Third, peptides were synthesized based on the predicted sequence of the neo-N-terminus following thrombin cleavage of the receptor (33, 36). These peptides proved to be full agonists for the thrombin effects on varied cell types, although they were several orders of magnitude less potent than thrombin itself. These peptides are now universally accepted as surrogate agonists for thrombin. The model generated from these experiments is termed the "tethered ligand model," in which the agonist is covalently attached to the receptor, but is only available following appropriate proteolytic cleavage. Apparently the neo-N-terminus folds back, intramolecularly, on the receptor to activate it. Although data surface from time to time that can be interpreted as evidence for an additional and distinct thrombin receptor, only the original cloned receptor has been found to be associated with thrombin's effects on varied cell types, and no genetic data support a second thrombin receptor subtype at this time.

The tethered ligand model is novel and intriguing, but it also raises a number of mechanistic questions. Thrombin's effects on target cells are concentration dependent, similar to that observed for classical soluble agonists acting at their receptors. How does an enzyme behave this way, and since the activated receptor also contains the agonist on a covalent leash, how does the receptor turn off? Results from a study by Ishii et al. (37) showed that the rate of cell surface receptor cleavage by thrombin is proportional to the accumulation of the intracelluar second messenger phosphoinositol. These authors propose that activated thrombin receptors promote release of a quantum of second messengers and that the receptor is then rapidly turned off or desensitized. Thrombin concentration determines the rate of receptor activation and therefore the release of second messengers. This proposal differs from classical receptor theory since there is no apparent equilibrium binding or graded receptor occupancy.

For other G protein–coupled receptors, desensitization has been closely correlated with phosphorylation of the receptor on intracellular hydrophilic domains. Phosphorylation of the thrombin receptor subsequent to activation has also been observed (38). These results provide a possible mechanism for rapid receptor shut-down. Following receptor activation by either thrombin or peptide mimetics of the neo-N-terminus, thrombin receptors are also rapidly internalized from the cell surface. Internalized receptors are either recycled to the plasma membrane or targeted to lysozomes for degradation (for review, see Ref. 39). Interestingly, the extent of thrombin receptor internalization as well as the mechanisms of recyling and degradation appear to be distinct in different cell types. The requirement for distinct mechanisms for handling thrombin receptor intracellular processing may relate to the diverse functional responses generated by thrombin challenge in varied cell types.

To date, few tools exist, such as neutralizing antibodies against the thrombin receptor or potent receptor antagonists, to probe the role of thrombin receptors in inflammatory or wound repair processes. However, using antibodies that recognize the receptor and probes generated from the cloned receptor cDNA for in situ hybridization, it has been possible to show that thrombin receptor expression is relatively low in normal blood vessels but is rapidly and strongly upregulated in both the media and neointimal layers following PTCA (40). The enhanced receptor expression was associated with both smooth muscle cells and endothelial cells. Thrombin receptors are also strongly expressed in atherosclerotic plaques compared to adjacent normal artery sections (41). These results strongly indicate a role for thrombin and its receptor in vascular pathology.

V. THROMBIN INHIBITORS MOVE INTO THE CLINIC

In the clinic today there are currently two classes of antithrombotic drugs: coumarins and heparins. Coumarins act by inhibiting the vitamin K–dependent formation of γ-carboxylglutamic acid on a variety of proteins in the cogulation cascade. These include factors VII, IX, and X as well as prothrombin and protein C. The posttranslational modification of these factors and proteins is necessary for their activity. The major limitations on coumarins as anticoagulants are the slow onset of the therapeutic effect (several days) and the variability of patient response, requiring chronic monitoring to determine that the level of anticogulation is appropriate without the liability of excessive bleeding.

Heparin is the most widely used anticoagulant, but it too suffers from several drawbacks. As seen with the coumarins, the response to heparin is also variable and requires surveillance to maintain the appropriate balance between anticoagulation and untoward bleeding. Heparin binds to circulating antithrombin III and promotes a 1000-fold acceleration of the binding to thrombin, thus inhibiting its activity. The complex of heparin with serpin also inhibits other serine proteases in the coagulation cascade. The availability of heparin in the circulation is modulated by its binding to serum proteins, such as vitronectin and fibronectin, and its inactivation by heparinase and platelet factor 4, which are secreted from activated platelets. A major liability for heparin is its failure to promote inhibition of thrombin when the protease is bound to the fibrin clot (42). Thrombin becomes tightly associated with the matrix of the clot and maintains catalytic activity and thus its procoagulant activities toward fibrinogen and platelets. Recently, more defined low molecular weight heparins are under investigation, but there appears to be no improvement in activity toward clot-bound thrombin by the low molecular weight heparins. Thrombin is also slowly released from the clot during thrombolysis, and therefore its activities toward cells of the vasculature can be sustained over time at the site of injury, which may impact on the process of restenosis.

Initial attempts to discover thrombin inhibitors as therapeutics focused on mechanism-based active site inhibitors. The archetype compound identified by this approach is PPACK (D-phenylanyl-L-prolyl-L-arginyl-chloromethyl ketone). PPACK covalently binds to the active site of thrombin to inhibit catalytic activity. Although infusion of PPACK has been shown to inhibit thrombosis and platelet deposition following angioplasty (43), this agent is not a viable clinical candidate because of its irreversible binding and the potential of nonspecific modification of cysteines on other proteins. However, the co-crystal structure of PPACK with thrombin has been instructive in the design of the next generation of thrombin active site inhibitors. Boronic acid derivatives of the basic D-Phe-Pro-Arg backbone represent potent, selective, and reversible inhibitors of thrombin. Probably the best studied example of this class of inhibitors is DUP714 (44), which has been shown to be an effective antithrombotic agent in animal models of arterial and venous thrombosis. However, DUP714 does possess significant inhibitory activity toward plasmin. Modification of the peptide backbone is currently being explored to enhance the specificity of this class of inhibitor toward thrombin.

Another variation on the theme of active site–directed thrombin inhibitors is the discovery of argatroban ([2R,4R]-4-methyl-1-[N^2-[(3-methyl-1,2,3,4-tetrahydro-8-quinolonyl) sulphonyl]-L-arginyl]-2-piperidinecarboxylic acid) (45). This arylsulfonylarginine amide was discovered by screening a series of related compounds. Argatroban binds tightly and competitively at the active site of thrombin, but does not engage the catalytic residues at the site. Argatroban takes advantage of the additional amino acid residues defining substrate specificity adjacent to the active site to achieve a K_i in the nanomolar range. In vivo, argatroban has been shown to be more effective than heparin in preventing coronary thrombosis in animal models of coronary thrombolysis and vessel wall injury (46).

Argatroban has been infused in patients with angina and following PTCA (47). The infusion resulted in a dose-dependent increase in prothrombin time and was effective against recurring ischemic events. Argatroban has recently been approved in Japan for use in various thrombotic indications.

The major disadvantage of active site inhibitors of thrombin is the potential to interact with other serine proteases and therefore compromising selectivity. An alternative approach to achieving thrombin specificity is to take advantage of the exosites on thrombin. Hirudin, as described above, is a naturally occurring 65-amino-acid leech protein that binds to the active site of thrombin and shows high potency and specificity by engaging the anion exosite. Hirudin can now be produced recombinantly in large quantities for clinical investigation. The recombinant protein differs only in that it lacks the posttranslational modification of sulfation of Tyr-63 and is thus often referred to desulfato hirudin. The protein appears to have very low antigenicity and is small enough to inhibit thrombin when the protease is bound up in the fibrin matrix of the clot. Seizing on the advantage of duel site inhibitors of thrombin, a 20-amino-acid synthetic peptide was produced connecting the structural features of the N-terminus of hirudin that binds to the active site of thrombin to the salient amino acids in the C-terminus of hirudin that bind to the anion exosite by a polyglycine spacer. This potent and selective thrombin inhibitor is termed hirulog (48).

Both hirudin and hirulog have been shown to be effective antithrombotic agents in animal models of arterial and venous thrombosis. Hirudin has also been shown to be effective in significantly limiting restenosis in a rabbit model that included development of an atherosclerotic lesion prior to the angiography (49). The animals given hirudin showed significantly less restenosis 28 days following angioplasty as assessed by angiography. Hirudin was also found to significantly inhibit platelet and fibrin deposition after angioplasty (50) or stent implantation (51) in pig models.

The promising effects of direct thrombin inhibitors in animal models of thrombosis and restenosis have cleared the way for these agents to be tested in humans. To date the most widely studied thrombin inhibitors are hirudin and hirulog, although many of the trials have been relatively small, precluding the possibility of definitive conclusions on safety and efficacy. The effect of recombinant hirudin in patients with angina pectoris who were treated with angioplasty has recently been reported (52). A patient population of 113 was randomized, 2:1, receiving either hirudin or heparin as an initial bolus followed by infusion over 24 h. At the end of the infusions angiography was performed and showed complete perfusion in all patients from the hirudin-treated group, compared to 92% in the heparin-treated group. This evaluation of the short-term effects of hirudin indicated that the safety and tolerance of the thrombin inhibitor were similar to heparin. A subsequent clinical study using 163 patients showed hirudin to be better than heparin in reducing the size of coronary thrombi and to decrease myocardial infarction in patients with unstable angina treated with PTCA (53). Similarly, small trials with hirulog showed it to be superior to heparin in treating patients with unstable angina (54).

Antithrombotics are often administered as adjunctive agents with thrombolytic enzymes to increase the rate of vessel reperfusion and to inhibit spontaneous reocclusion. In preliminary trials, both hirudin and hirulog showed a significant increase in the rate of coronary patency compared to heparin. These data encouraged the use of hirudin in larger ongoing clinical trials to obtain definitive evaluation of safety and efficacy. These trials cover a variety of acute and chronic coronary syndromes as endpoints. In addition, a prospective randomized multicenter trial comparing heparin and recombinant hirudin in over 1100 patients with unstable angina and subsequently undergoing angioplasty is currently underway. In this trial, termed HELVETICA (hirudin in a European restenosis prevention trial versus heparin treatment in PTCA patients), the definition of angioplasty is extended to include atherectomy and laser therapy to extend the blood vessel lumen (55). All of these procedures suffer from significant restenosis. Several of these studies, however, have been interrupted because of increased rates of hemorrage, and the dose of hirudin has been scaled back allowing the trials to continue (56–58). We now await the final results to see if there is sufficient therapeutic index for hirudin's beneficial antithrombotic effects compared to its promotion of unwanted bleeding complications.

VI. CONCLUSIONS

The conceptual framework underpinning the experimental approaches to restenosis continues to evolve, driven in large part by the need for effective therapeutic agents. The response-to-injury hypothesis focused early attention on the growth of the neointima. The improved resolution of existing technologies and the emergence of novel techniques have expanded our horizons beyond neointimal formation to include elastic recoil and sustained remodeling of the vessel wall following injury. Clearly restenosis is a complex pathology and new approaches must be entertained to encompass these new concepts.

The recent availability of highly selective and potent inhibitors of thrombin have allowed the investigation of the potential role of this multifunctional serine protease in vascular pathologies, such as restenosis. Through its critical position in the coagulation cascade and through its direct and indirect effects on vascular cells, thrombin is an important orchestrator of wound repair following injury. The early success of thrombin inhibitors in animal models of arterial and venous thrombosis raised expectations that antithrombins could become clinically relevant therapeutic agents. This enthusiasm was heightened by small clinical trials that demonstrated a clear benefit over heparin. However, in large clinical trials to address definitively the safety and efficacy of thrombin inhibitors, hemorrhage has emerged as a potential limitation on these agents. We will have to await publication of the results of these long-term trials to determine if therapeutic benefit will be clearly differentiated from unwanted bleeding complications. A future approach that also holds promise is to target the newly identified thrombin receptor. Thrombin receptor antagonists would presumably spare thrombin's role in the coagulation cascade while blocking the versatile effects of thrombin on the cell types that appear to contribute directly to the processes of restenosis.

REFERENCES

1. O'Brien ER, Schwartz SM. Update on the biology and clinical study of restenosis. Trends Cardiovasc Med 1994; 4:169–178.
2. Schwartz SM, deBlois D, O'Brien ERM. The intima: soil for atherosclerosis and restenosis. Circ Res 1995; 77:445–465.
3. Currier JW, Faxon DP. Restenosis after percutaneous transluminal coronary angioplasty: Have we been aiming at the wrong target? J Am Coll Cardiol 1995; 25:516–520.
4. Mattsson E, Clowes A. Current concepts in restenosis following balloon angioplasty. Trends Cardiovasc Res 1995; 5:200–204.
5. Ross R, Glomset JA. The pathogenesis of atherosclerosis. N Engl J Med 1976; 295:420–425.
6. Ross R. The pathogenesis of atherosclerosis—an update. N Engl J Med 1986; 314:488–300.
7. Ross R. The pathogenesis of atherosclerosis: a perspective for the 1990s. Nature 1993; 362:801–809.
8. Schwartz SM, Liaw L. Growth control and morphogenesis in the development and pathology of arteries. J Cardiovasc Pharmacol 1993; 21:S31–S49.
9. Davies EW, Fujikawa K, Kisiel W. The coagulation cascade: interaction, maintenance and regulation. Biochemistry 1991; 30:10,363–10,370.
10. Esmon CT. Cell mediated events that control blood coagulation and vascular injury. Annu Rev Cell Biol 1993; 9:1–26.
11. Gibbs CS, Coutre SE, Tsiang M, Li W-X, Jain AK, Dunn KE, Law VS, Mao CT, Matsumura SY, Mejza SJ, Paborsky LR, Leung LLK, Conversion of thrombin to an anticoagulant by protein engineering. Nature 1995; 378:413–415.
12. Bode W, Turk D, Karshikov A. The refined 1.9 Å x-ray crystal structure of D-PheProArg chloromethyl ketone inhibited human α-thrombin: structure analysis, overall structure, electrostatic properties, detailed active site geometry, structure-function relationships. Protein Sci 1992; 1:426–471.

13. Rydel TJ, Tulinsky A, Bode W, Huber R. Refined structure of the hirudin-thrombin complex. J Mol Biol 1991; 221:583–601.
14. Qiu X, Padmanabhan KP, Carperos VE, Tulinsky A, Kline T, Maraganore JM, Fenton JW. Structure of the hirulog 3-thrombin complex and nature of the S' subsites of substrates and inhibitors. Biochemistry 1992; 31:11,689–11,697.
15. Coughlin SR, Vu T-K, Hung DT, Wheaton VI. Characterization of a functional thrombin receptor: issues and opportunities. J Clin Invest 1992; 89:351–305.
16. Coughlin SR. Thrombin receptor function and cardiovascular disease. Trends Cardiovasc Med 1994; 4:77–83.
17. Davey M, Luscher E. Action of thrombin and other coagulant and proteolytic enzymes on blood platelets. Nature 1967; 216:857–858.
18. Eidt J, Allison P, Nobel S, Ashton J, Golino P, McNatt J, Buja LM, Willerson JT. Thrombin is an important mediator of platelet aggregation in stenosed canine coronary arteries with endothelial injury. J Clin Invest 1989; 84:18–27.
19. Fitzgerald D, Fitzgerald G. Role of thrombin and thromboxane A_2 in reocclusion following coronary thrombolysis. Proc Natl Acad Sci USA 1989; 86:7585–7589.
20. Hansen S, Harker L. Interruption of acute platelet-dependent thrombosis by the synthetic antithrombin PPACK. Proc Natl Acad Sci USA 1988; 85:3184–3188.
21. Bar-Shavit R, Kahn A, Wilner GD, Fenton JW. Monocyte chemotaxis: stimulation by specific exosite region in thrombin. Science 1983; 220:728–731.
22. Chen LB, Buchanan JM. Mitogenic activity of blood components: thrombin and prothrombin. Proc Natl Acad Sci USA 1975; 72:131–135.
23. Zimmerman GA, McIntyre TM, Prescott SM. Thrombin stimulates neutrophil adherence by an endothelial cell-dependent mechanism. Ann NY Acad Sci 1986; 485:349–368.
24. Prescott SM, Zimmerman GA, McIntyre TM. Human endothelial cells in culture produce platelet-activating factor when stimulated by thrombin. Proc Natl Acad Sci USA 1984; 81:3534–3538.
25. Weksler BB, Ley CW, Jaffe EA. Stimulation of endothelial cell prostacyclin by thrombin, typsin, and ionophore A23187. J Clin Invest 1982; 62: 923–930.
26. Chen LB, Teng NNH, Buchanan JM. Mitogenicity of thrombin and surface alterations on mouse splenocytes. Exp Cell Res 1976; 101:41–46.
27. Pouyssegur J, Seuwen K. Transmembrane receptors and intracellular pathways that control cell proliferation. Annu Rev Physiol 1992; 54:195–210.
28. McNamara CA, Sarembok IJ, Gimple LW, Fenton JW, Coughlin SR, Owen GK. Thrombin stimulation of smooth muscle cell proliferation is mediated by a proteolytic, receptor-mediated mechanism. J Clin Invest 1992; 91:94–98.
29. Weiss RH, Maduri M. The mitogenic effect of thrombin in vascular smooth muscle cells is largely due to the basic fibroblastic growth factor. J Biol Chem 1993; 268:5724–5727.

30. Daniel TO, Gibbs VC, Milfay DF, Garavoy M, Williams LT. Thrombin stimulates c-sis gene expression in microvascular endothelial cells. J Biol Chem 1986; 261:9579–9582.
31. Senger DR, Perruzzi CA, Papadopoulos-Sergiou A, Van De Walter L. Adhesive properties of osteopontin: regulation by a naturally occurring thrombin-cleavage site in close proximity to the GRGD cell-binding domain. Mol Biol Cell 1994; 5:565–574.
32. Nathan C, Sporn M. Cytokines in context. J Cell Biol 1991; 113:981–986.
33. Vu -TK, Hung DT, Wheaton VI, Coughlin SR. Molecular cloning of a functional thrombin receptor reveals a novel proteolytic mechanism of receptor activation. Cell 1991a; 64:1057–1068.
34. Rasmussen UB, Vouret-Craviari V, Jallet S, Schlesinger Y, Pages G, Pavirini A, Lecocq J-P, Pouyssegur J, Van Obberghen-Schilling E. cDNA cloning and expression of a hamster α-thrombin receptor coupled to Ca^{2+} mobilization. FEBS Lett 1991; 288:123–128.
35. Dohlman HG, Thorner J, Caron MG, Lefkowitz RJ. Model systems for the study of seven-transmembrane segment receptors. Annu Rev Biochem 1991; 60:653–688.
36. Vu T-KH, Wheaton VI, Hung DT, Coughlin SR. Domains specifying thrombin-receptor interaction. Nature 1991b; 353:674–677.
37. Ishii K, Hein L, Kobilka BK, Coughlin SR. Kinetics of thrombin receptor cleavage on intact cells: relation to signalling. J Biol Chem 1993; 268: 9780–9786.
38. Ishii K, Chen J, Ishii M. Inhibition of thrombin receptor signalling by a G-protein coupled receptor kinase: functional specificity among G-protein coupled receptor kinases. J Biol Chem 1994; 269:1125–1130.
39. Brass LF, Wookalis MJ, Hoxie JA. Trafficking thrombin receptors: biodiversity on the receptor superhighway. Trends Cardiovasc Med 1995; 5:123–128.
40. Wilcox JN, Rodriguez J. Subramanian R, et al. Characterization of thrombin receptor expression during vascular lesion formation. Circ Res 1994; 75: 1029–1038.
41. Nelken NA, Soifer SJ, O'Keefe J, Vu TK, Charo IF, Coughlin SR. Thrombin receptor expression in normal and atherosclerotic human arteries. J Clin Invest 1992; 90:1614–1621.
42. Weitz JI, Hudoba M, Massel D, Maraganore J, Hirsch J. Clot-bound thrombin is protected from inhibition by heparin-antithrombin III but is susceptible to inactivation by antithrombin III-independent inhibitors. J Clin Invest 1990; 86:385–391.
43. Kaplan AV, Leung LL, Leung WH, Grant GW, McDougall IR, Fischell TA. Roles of thrombin and platelet membrane glycoprotein IIb/IIIa in platelet subendothelial deposition after angioplasty in an ex-vivo whole artery model. Circulation 1991; 84:1279–1288.
44. Kettner C, Mersinger L, Knabb R. The selective inhibition of thrombin by peptides of boroarginine. J Biol Chem 1990; 265:18,289–18,297.
45. Kikumoto R, Tomao Y, Tezuka T Selective inhibition of thrombin by (2R,4R)-

4-methyl-1-{N2-[(3-methyl-1,2,3,4-tetrahydro-8-quinolinyl)-sulfonyl]-L-arginyl]-2-piperidinecarboxylic acid. Biochemistry 1984; 23:85–90.
46. Jang IK, Gold HK, Leinbach RC. Persistent inhibition of arterial thrombosis by a 1-hour intravenous infusion of Argatroban, a selective thrombin inhibitor. Coronary Artery Dis 1992; 3:407–414.
47. Gold HK, Torres FW, Garabedian HD, Werner W, Jang I-K, Kahn A, Hagstrom JN, Yasuda T, Leinbach RC, Newell JB, Bovill EG, Stump DC, Collen D. Evidence for a rebound coagulation phenomenon after cessation of a 4-hour infusion of a specific thrombin inhibitor in patients with unstable angina pectoris. J Am Coll Cardiol 1993; 21:1039–1047.
48. Maraganore JM, Bourdon P, Jablonski J, Ramachandran KI, Fenton JW. Design and characterization of hirulogs: a novel class of bivalent peptide inhibitors of thrombin. Biochemistry 1990; 29:7095–7101.
49. Saremblock IJ, Gertz SD, Gimple LW, Owen RM, Powers ER, Roberts WC. Effectiveness of recombinant desulphatohirudin in reducing restenosis after balloon angioplasty of atherosclerotic femoral arteries in rabbits. Circulation 1991; 84:232–243.
50. Heras M, Chesebro JH, Webster MWI, Hirudin, heparin, and placebo during deep arterial injury in the pig. The in vivo role of thrombin in platelet mediated thrombosis. Circulation 1990; 82:1476–1484.
51. Buchwald AB, Sandrock D, Unterberg C, Ebbecke M, Nebendahl K, Luders S, Munz DL, Wiengand V. Platelet and fibrin deposition on coronary artery stents in minipigs: effect of hirudin versus heparin. J Am Coll Cardiol 1993; 21:249–254.
52. van den Bos AA, Deckers JW, Heyndrickx GR, Laarman G-J, Suryapranata H, Zijlstra F, Close P, Rijnierse JJMM, Buller HR, Serruys PW. Safety and efficacy of recombinant hirudin (CGP 39 393) versus heparin in patients with stable angina undergoing coronary angioplasty. Circulation 1993; 88:2058–2066.
53. Topol EJ, Fuster V, Harrington RA, Califf RM, Kleiman DJ, Cohen M, Chpekis A, Gold HK, Tennanbaum MA, Rao AK, Debouer D, Schwartz D, Henis M, Chesebro J. Recombinant hirudin for unstable angina pectoris: a multicenter, randomized angiographic trial. Circulation 1994; 89:1557–1567.
54. Topol EJ, Bonan R, Jewitt D, Sigwart U, Kakkar VV, Rothman M, de Bono D, Ferguson J, Willerson JT, Strony J, Ganz P, Cohen MD, Raymond R, Fox I, Maraganore J, Adelman B. Use of a direct antithrombin, hirulog, in place of heparin during coronary angioplasty. Circulation 1993; 87:1622–1629.
55. Serruys PW, Fox KAA, Herrman J-PR, Bach D, Close, P, Decker JW, HELVETICA Investigators. Recombinant hirudin (CGP 39 393) reduces the incidence of major adverse cardiac events, reported within the first 96 hours post-angioplasty in unstable patients (Braunwald classification) pretreated by heparin. Restenosis Summit 1995; VII:256.
56. Antman EM. Hirudin in acute myocardial infarction: safety report from the Thrombolysis and Thrombin Inhibition in Myocardial Infraction (TIMI) 9A trial. Circulation 1994; 90:1624–1630.

57. Neuhaus K-L, v Essen R, Tebbe U, Jessel A, Heindrick H, Maurer W, Doring W, Harmjanz D, Kotter V, Kalhammer E, Simon H, Horacek T. Safety observations from the pilot phase of the randomized r-hirudin for improvement of thrombolysis (HIT-III) study. Circulation 1994; 90:1638–1642.
58. GUSTO IIa Investigators. Randomized trial of intravenous heparin versus recombinant hirudin for acute coronary syndromes. Circulation 1994;90:1631–1637.

10

The Role of Herpesviruses in Atherosclerosis and Thrombosis

Andrew C. Nicholson, Robert J. Kaner, and David P. Hajjar
Cornell University Medical College, New York, New York

I. INTRODUCTION

The etiological role of viruses in the pathogenesis of atherosclerosis remains unclear, however, circumstantial evidence continues to accumulate suggesting a role for herpesvirus infections in the initiation and/or progression of this disease. Atherosclerosis is a multifactorial process that involves a complex interplay of genetic and environmental factors. The premise of the "response-to-injury" hypothesis formulated by Drs. Russell Ross and John Glomset of the University of Washington in 1973 is that atherosclerosis is initiated by injury to the endothelium. Since the proposal of this theory, there has been a vast amount of research in the field of experimental atherosclerosis in an attempt to define the biochemical and molecular mechanisms responsible for this initial injury and the subsequent progression of the disease process. Hypercholesterolemia, cigarette smoking, hypertension, and diabetes are clear risk factors for the development of the disease but do not account for all cases of atherosclerosis. Infectious agents and viruses in particular have been proposed as potential initiators of the atherosclerotic process since the late 1970s, when it was shown that an avian virus could cause atherosclerosis in chickens, which had many morphological and biochemical features of the human disease (1–4). Coupled with the epidemiological association between viral infection and accelerated atherosclerosis in heart transplant patients (5,6), the observation of viral nucleic acids in the atherosclerotic vessel wall and the association of cytomegalovirus with restenosis following coronary angioplasty led to a resurgence in interest in a possible link between viruses and either the etiology or the pathogenesis of atherosclerosis (7–10). This chapter will review the evidence supporting the hypothesis that herpesviruses may be involved as initiating or secondary factors in the pathogenesis of atherosclerosis and thrombosis.

II. EPIDEMIOLOGICAL EVIDENCE LINKING HERPESVIRUSES AND ATHEROSCLEROSIS

Seven members of the herpesvirus family are now known to infect humans (11). Of these, herpes simplex virus type 1 (HSV-1), herpes simplex virus type 2 (HSV-2), and human cytomegalovirus (CMV) have been the primary candidate viruses whose potential relationship to atherosclerosis has been studied. Herpes simplex viral infections are widespread in the general population (12). More than half of children demonstrate antibodies to HSV-1 by 10 years of age (13). The frequency of HSV-2 infection is less certain, but various studies cite a prevalence of 0.3–22% (14). In the 35- to 44-year age group, well over 10% of the general population demonstrates antibodies to HSV-2 (13). A more recent study concluded the incidence to be 16.4% in the population of those aged 15–74 (15). Antibodies to CMV are even more widespread in the population, indicating previous infection in greater than 50% of adults (16).

A seroepidemiological association between CMV infection and atherosclerosis was originally suggested by Adam et al. (17). This was based on a case-control study of cardiovascular surgery patients, who were compared with a control group of subjects not undergoing surgery but matched for similar cholesterol levels and other atherosclerosis risk factors. In the 157 pairs evaluated, the incidence of positive CMV antibodies was higher in the surgical group than in the control group (90 and 74%, respectively; $p < 0.001$). A greater percentage of surgical cases than controls had high titers of CMV antibodies (57 and 26%, respectively). There was no correlation between antibody titers and serum cholesterol or triglycerides.

A study in a subgroup of the Framingham patients failed to find an overall association between a history of fever blisters or cold sores with the prevalence or 6-year incidence of coronary heart disease (angina pectoris, coronary insufficiency, or myocardial infarction) in the Framingham Heart Study in patients 58–89 years old (18). Previous work in this group of patients had shown a strong correlation of the self-reported history with serological evidence of previous HSV-1 infection. This study does not completely rule out the possibility of such a relationship, particularly since a subgroup of women with recurrent cold sores had a 1.5-fold relative risk (95% confidence interval 1.0–2.1) of developing coronary heart disease (18).

A recent seroepidemiological study compared HSV-1, HSV-2, and CMV antibody status to the results of B-mode ultrasonography of the carotid arteries, used as a marker of asymptomatic carotid artery thickening, a manifestation of early atherosclerosis (19). Three hundred and forty matched case-control pairs from the Atherosclerosis Risk in Communities (ARIC) Study were evaluated. This study found a modest (odds ratio = 1.55), though significant ($p = 0.03$), positive association between CMV antibodies and asymptomatic carotid artery thickening.

The strongest epidemiological link between infection with herpesviruses and atherosclerosis in humans is in the heart transplant population. Several studies have demonstrated a strong correlation between CMV infection and accelerated atherosclerosis in this population. At Stanford University, 300 cardiac transplant patients were treated with immunosuppression and followed prospectively for the occurrence of CMV infection and the development of atherosclerosis. Of those tested, 91 patients developed CMV infections based on (a) positive cultures for CMV, (b) demonstration of characteristic CMV inclusion bodies in tissue samples, and/or (c) a fourfold rise in IgG cytomegalovirus antibodies. After 5 years of follow-up, the rate of graft loss due to accelerated atherosclerosis (with an endpoint of death or retransplantation) was 69% in CMV-infected patients but only 37% in the non–CMV-infected group (5). Furthermore, there was a 10-fold greater incidence of patients who died with greater than 50% luminal obstruction in their coronary arteries in the CMV-positive as compared with the non–CMV-infected patients (5). Interestingly, similar results were reported from a somewhat smaller study at the University of Minnesota (6), which compared rates of CMV infection and atherosclerosis in 102 immunosuppressed patients who had received a cardiac transplant and survived for at least one year. At 2 years posttransplant, 32% of the CMV-positive patients had coronary artery disease as opposed to 10% of the CMV-negative patients.

These results have been reproduced by investigators from other transplant centers with carefully documented coronary angiography and endomyocardial biopsies (20). Moreover, pathological studies have demonstrated an endothelialitis associated with the accelerated atherosclerosis (21), which correlated with quantitation of the virus in endomyocardial biopsies (22). There are also in vitro data suggesting that CMV infection of endothelial cells upregulates MHC class II expression, which may enhance T-cell–mediated inflammatory processes in the vessel wall (23).

III. PATHOBIOLOGICAL EVIDENCE LINKING HERPESVIRUSES AND ATHEROSCLEROSIS

In 1984, Gyorkey et al. (24) reported the detection of virions of the herpesvirus family in electron microscopic sections from the aortas of 10 of 60 patients with atherosclerosis undergoing cardiovascular surgery. These viral particles were in various stages of viral replication and included empty nucleocapsids and virions with dense cores. They were present in rare smooth muscle and endothelial cells. Of the 1360 grids examined, only 35 showed evidence of virus. Benditt et al. (25) showed evidence of HSV nucleic acids in the ascending aorta in tissue removed during coronary bypass surgery by in situ hybridization. Eleven of 160 tissue samples were positive. In most cases, the tissue was histologically normal. In a second series of experiments examining tissues that contained abnormally thickened intima, two of four reacted positively with an HSV-2 probe. The positive staining occurred in cells located in discrete foci of increased cellularity within or adjacent to the intima. Melnick et al. (26) reported the detection of CMV antigen in cells cultured from arterial tissue surgically removed from patients with severe arterial disease. Petrie et al. (27) showed that in situ hybridization techniques would increase the frequency of detection of CMV in cultured smooth muscle cells from arterial plaques relative to immunohistochemical staining. More recently, Hendrix et al. (28) showed that the detection of CMV nucleic acids by polymerase chain reaction (PCR) was possible in 90% of samples obtained from patients with severe atherosclerosis as compared to only 53% in patients with minimal or no atherosclerosis. The presence of the complete viral genome was demonstrated in these samples by both dot blot DNA hybridization and PCR using probes and primers derived from the immediate early and late genomic regions. Messenger RNA from the immediate early but not the late genomic regions could be demonstrated by in situ DNA hybridization. This suggested to the authors that CMV exists in the vessel wall primarily in a latent state where expression of immediate early messenger RNA transcripts may occur (29) without expression of messenger RNA coding for structural capsid proteins. Indeed, CMV DNA is widely distributed throughout the arterial tree (30), lending credence to the possibility that the vascular system may be the site of latency for this virus. We speculate that this may lead to an alteration in the factors that control growth in the vessel wall predisposing to intimal thickening.

To look for evidence of viral antigens or nucleic acids in the vessel wall at an earlier stage in the formation of the atherosclerotic lesion, Yamashiroya et al. (31) performed immunohistochemical and DNA hybridization studies on the coronary arteries and aortas of young trauma victims using fresh autopsy material. Evidence for HSV or CMV was detected in 8 of 20 specimens of coronary arteries. Viral DNA or antigens were found in cells both in the intact luminal surface and in focal clusters of spindle-shaped or foam cells in the intimal layer. This study adds circumstantial evidence to support the hypothesis that viruses might be involved in the early events in atherogenesis.

The pathogenesis of inflammatory abdominal aortic aneurysms in humans (32) has been linked to CMV (33). In this study PCR was used to detect CMV DNA in 41 aortic lesions excised at surgery and 16 aortic tissues obtained at autopsy. CMV DNA was detected in 88% (7/8) of inflammatory aortic lesions with periaortic fibrosis, including 5/6 aortic aneurysms, 61% (20/33) of atherosclerotic aneurysms, but only 31% (5/16) of autopsy samples without inflammation or atherosclerosis. This subendothelial inflammation associated with CMV infection can also be seen in human hearts during atherosclerosis of coronary allografts (34). Of considerable mechanistic interest in this regard is a report of T-lymphocyte activation by CMV-infected allogeneic cultured human endothelial cells (35). Peripheral blood mononuclear cells exhibit enhanced lysis of CMV- or HSV-infected vascular smooth muscle cells, perhaps contributing to cell turnover in an active vascular lesion (36).

IV. ANIMAL MODELS OF HERPESVIRUS-INDUCED ATHEROSCLEROSIS

The development of an animal model for atherosclerosis induced by a herpesvirus infection by Fabricant et al. (1–3) has provided considerable experimental evidence to support the hypothesis that herpesviruses are involved in the pathogenesis of atherosclerosis. Pathogen-free normocholesterolemic chickens were infected with 100 PFU of Marek's disease virus (MDV), a herpesvirus that causes malignant lymphomas of T-cell origin in chickens (37). Uninfected pathogen-free chickens served as a control. At 30 weeks, the virally infected chickens demonstrated grossly visible atherosclerotic lesions in the large coronary arteries, the aorta, and the major aortic branches (1). Detailed histological examination of these atherosclerotic lesions showed a fibroproliferative lesion similar to the proliferative lesions of human atherosclerosis (2). Of interest, the atherosclerotic lesions could be prevented by preimmunizing the animals with a related herpesvirus of turkeys (4). Feeding the chickens a high-cholesterol diet produced a synergistic effect by increasing cholesterol accumulation (3). Biochemical analysis of the samples of aortic tissue from the normocholesterolemic, MDV-infected group by Hajjar et al. (3) revealed a significantly higher content of choles-

gene. HSV-1 also increases CE synthesis and HMG-CoA reductase activity but concomitantly reduces CE hydrolysis and cholesterol efflux. Viral infection was associated with a time-dependent decrease in protein kinase A activity and an increase in viral-induced protein kinase (VPK) activity commensurate with the accumulation of esterified cholesterol. The relationship between increased VPK activity and alterations in CE accumulation in virally infected cells was explored using an HSV-1 VPK^- mutant in which the portion of the HSV-1 genome encoding VPK had been deleted. CE accumulation was significantly increased (>50-fold) in HSV-1–infected cells compared to uninfected cells. However, the HSV-1 VPK^- mutant had no significant effect on CE accumulation, implying that viral kinase activity is necessary in order for HSV-1 to induce CE accumulation in vascular smooth muscle (58).

The mechanism by which VPK alters cellular host cholesterol trafficking is unknown. Although VPK possesses similarities to eukaryotic protein kinases A and C, the cellular substrates for VPK are unknown. It has been shown that VPK can phosphorylate viral substrates, but it has also been speculated that VPK may phosphorylate some host proteins (59). This is the first demonstration that increased VPK activity is associated with altered activities of kinase-dependent proteins involved in cholesterol trafficking. We have not conclusively demonstrated that VPK specifically phosphorylated serine/threonine residues on those proteins involved in cholesterol metabolism. However, since CE accumulation following HSV-1 infection in vascular smooth muscle cells was abrogated in cells infected with an HSV-1 VPK^- mutant, this kinase is clearly implicated in altered lipid metabolism following herpesvirus infection (58).

VI. VIRAL INDUCTION OF CYTOKINES AND GROWTH FACTORS: ROLE IN CHOLESTEROL TRAFFICKING

Recent studies have suggested that the immune system may be important in atherosclerotic lesion development since T lymphocytes accumulate within the atherosclerotic lesion (60–62). Viral infection could induce the production and/or release of mediators (cytokines or growth factors) by vascular or immune cells, which might modulate cholesterol metabolism in vascular smooth cells or macrophages. In addition, cytokines could induce the expression of adhesion molecules by the endothelium and affect the ability of the endothelium to bind monocytes or inflammatory cells as discussed below. CMV infection in vitro induces macrophages to increase the expression of RNA for interleukin-1β (IL-1β), tumor necrosis factor-α (TNF-α), and colony-stimulating factor-1 (CSF-1) (63). In a mouse model of herpetic keratitis there is increased expression of IL-1β and interleukin-6 (IL-6) (64). HSV-1 infection of monocytes strongly upregulates TNF-α release (65). CMV infection of monocytes induces release of TNF-α in vitro and in vivo (66). The role of TNF as an antiviral cytokine is unclear. TNF-α appears to play a role in host defense against CMV in vivo (67). While TNF-α is an inducer of interferon messenger RNA transcripts, a well-documented cytokine that has antiherpesviral activity, others have shown that TNF's antiviral activity is not abolished in the presence of antiserum to interferon (68). Wong and Goeddel (69) have postulated that the antiviral activity of TNF is attributable to lysis of virally infected cells rather than induction of interferon. However, TNF has also been shown to promote replication and pathogenicity of rat cytomegalovirus (70). The immediate-early genes of human CMV are capable of specifically activating transcription of the monocyte macrophage IL-1β gene as detected in a CAT assay system (71). This is of interest in light of the increased expression IL-1β in atherosclerotic lesions as compared to normal vessel wall (72–74). Alternatively, CMV may upregulate cytokine mRNA expression via activation of specific transcription factors such as NF-kB, AP-1, and CRE/B (75). Pseudorabies virus, another herpes family virus, induces the expression of IL-6 mRNA in infected human fibroblasts (76). CMV upregulates IL-6 mRNA expression and protein release from human endothelial cells (77). Other members of the herpesvirus family, such as Epstein-Barr virus, contain genes that appear to have important regulatory effects on host cell cytokine synthesis (78). CMV infection also enhances mRNA expression of platelet-derived growth factor-BB and TGF-β_1 in rat aortic allografts (39).

Production of cytokines within the atherosclerotic lesion could affect lipid uptake and metabolism by vascular smooth muscle cells or macrophages. We have shown that TNF and IL-1 can modulate LDL receptor–mediated cholesterol metabolism by increasing LDL receptor gene transcription (79). TNF can also inhibit macrophage expression of the scavenger receptor (80). In addition, both TGF-β (81) and PDGF (82,83) can upregulate LDL receptor expression in vascular smooth muscle cells.

VII. PROTHROMBOTIC EFFECTS OF VIRAL INFECTION OF THE VASCULAR ENDOTHELIUM

When the vascular endothelium is injured or activated, it undergoes a phenotypic modulation resulting in the loss of anticoagulant properties and the acquisition of procoagulant properties. Endothelial cell injury is a common feature of viral infection and can alter hemostasis in two ways: directly, by altering endothelial cell function, and indirectly, via activation of immune and inflammatory pathways (84). Herpesvirus infection of the endothelium can shift endothelial cell properties from an antithrombotic to a prothrombotic state. Data from our laboratory and others demonstrate that herpesvirus infection of endothelial cells in vitro can inhibit anticoagulant functions and induce a procoagulant phenotype.

Viral infection can alter hemostatic balance resulting in either hemorrhage or coagulation. Thrombocytopenia is an occasional symptom of common viral infections and is most likely immune mediated (85). Severe hemorrhage is a hallmark of the hemorrhagic fever viruses. These viruses cause hemorrhage by multiple mechanisms, including thrombocytopenia, platelet dysfunction, hepatic insult and reduction in the levels of coagulation factors, and direct and indirect endothelial cell damage (84). Endothelial cell infection may represent a common pathway by which viruses alter hemostasis. Many human viruses have been shown to infect human endothelial cells in vitro. These include HSV-1, adenovirus type 7, measles virus, parainfluenza type 3, mumps virus, poliovirus type 1, echovirus type 9, CMV, coxsackievirus B3, and dengue and Junin viruses (43,86,87). However, the in vivo consequences of endothelial cell infection by most of these viruses is undetermined.

Herpesviral infection alters the normal thromboresistant surface formed by intact vascular endothelium by three mechanisms: (a) inhibition of anticoagulant/antithrombotic properties, (b) induction of procoagulant/prothrombotic properties, and (c) indirectly, by secreting prothrombotic cytokines, which increase binding sites for inflammatory cells. Although most experimental evidence demonstrating these effects is derived from in vitro studies using endothelial cells in monolayer culture, there is histological evidence supportive of these phenomena in vivo. For example, HSV-1 can induce mucosal lesions, which are often accompanied by a local vasculitis with fibrin deposition (88). Disseminated intravascular coagulation (DIC) is seen in fatal systemic neonatal HSV infections (89). DIC is thought to result, in part, from direct damage to the vessel wall and exposure of subendothelial collagen (89).

One mechanism by which herpesvirus induces a prothrombotic endothelium is by inhibiting normal anticoagulant and antithrombotic properties. Endothelial cells normally synthesize and express heparan sulfate proteoglycan (HSPG) on their surface. HSPG is a critical element for recruiting and binding antithrombin III, which is responsible for the inactivation of several coagulation proteases (thrombin and activated factors IX, X, XI, and XII). HSV infection of the endothelium markedly reduces HSPG synthesis and surface expression by endothelial cells (90). The expression of thrombomodulin on the endothelial surface is also reduced as a result of HSV-1 and HSV-2 infection (91). Loss of thrombomodulin is concomitant with a reduction in thrombin-dependent protein C activation. Inhibition of the protein C/protein S/thrombomodulin pathway is, therefore, another mechanism that could lead to thrombin generation by reducing the ability of protein C to inactivate factors Va and XIIIa.

In addition to inhibiting anticoagulant mechanisms, herpesviruses can induce procoagulant/prothrombotic properties of the endothelium. Visser and colleagues have demonstrated altered membrane topography on HSV-infected endothelial cells, i.e., they have shown that the outer leaflet membrane conformation may be abnormal in HSV-infected endothelium (92). They hypothesized that viral-induced changes in endothelial cell phospholipid may alter the efficiency of assembly of the prothrombinase complex. To test this hypothesis, they assessed the ability of HSV-infected endothelium to support prothrombinase complex assembly using purified prothrombin and factors Va and Xa and demonstrated enhanced (two to threefold) thrombin generation. They further demonstrated enhanced thrombin-induced platelet accumulation on HSV-infected endothelium. Thrombin-induced PGI_2 production by the infected endothelium was reduced by a factor of 20 (92). Since thrombin-induced PGI_2 synthesis and release is thought to be a mechanism by which the endothelial cell may diminish thrombin-induced platelet adherence and aggregation, this may further compound platelet adhesion to the HSV-infected endothelium. HSV can also induce the transient expression of tissue factor on the endothelial cell surface. Tissue factor is not normally expressed by endothelial cells but can be induced by endotoxin or cytokines (93,94). Tissue factor expression in response to HSV was dependent on the magnitude of infection and increased linearly with increasing multiplicity of infection (MOI). Maximal expression (three- to fourfold greater than mock-infected cells) was seen at 4 h, but expression returned to baseline by 20 h (91). Tissue factor mRNA was also transiently induced (95). Tissue factor expression did not require viral replication since replication defective virus could also produce tissue factor procoagulant activity (95). In addition, CMV also has the capacity to induce procoagulant activity on human endothelial cells as measured by a reduction in clotting time (96), suggesting a facilitated formation of the prothrombinase complex.

Our laboratory has extended these findings, showing that HSV infection of endothelial cells induces von Willebrand factor (vWF) secretion and that vWF mediates platelet adhesion to virally infected endothelial cells (97). Other types of endothelial cell injury—rickettsial infection (98) and endotoxin (99)—also cause vWF release. We hypothesize that thrombin is generated following assembly of the prothrombinase complex on the virally infected endothelium and subsequently mobilizes vWF from the Weibel-Palade body to the endothelial cell surface, where it acts as a platelet receptor. In contrast, CMV infection causes the disappearance of vWF from endothelial cells (100). We have shown that specific virally encoded glycoproteins expressed on the surface of HSV-infected endothelium bind and promote activation of factor X, thereby contributing to thrombin generation (101). We found that HSV infection of endothelial cells promoted enhanced monocyte adhesion (101) and that this enhanced adhesion was dependent on EC surface expression of HSV glycoprotein C (gC). Adhesion was blocked by monoclonal antibodies to gC but not by antibodies to glycoprotein D (gD) or glycoprotein E (gE) (101). Adhesion was dependent on local generation of thrombin and was blocked by treating endothelial cells with specific thrombin inhibitors or by growing cells in prothrombin-depleted serum. To support the hypothesis that gC was indeed involved in monocyte adhesion and could potentially be involved in thrombin activation, we used murine L cells, which were stably transfected with the gene for herpesvirus gC (101). We found that factor X bound to the transfected L cells but not to the nontransfected cells (101). Furthermore, cross-linking and immunoprecipitation studies demonstrated that factor X and gC formed a complex on the cell surface. In order to identify a site in factor X which bound to gC, we utilized a group of partially overlapping peptides representative of different regions of the factor X molecule (102). Three synthetic factor X peptides (provided by Drs. Dario Altieri and Thomas Edgington of the Scripps Research Institute) blocked factor X mediated procoagulant activity and suppressed monocyte adhesion to HSV-infected endothelium. The three blocking peptides are in the catalytic domain of factor X (102). In summary, our data suggest that interaction of factor X with gC on the surface of HSV-infected cells leads to formation of factor Xa, activation of thrombin, and enhanced binding of monocytes.

The third mechanism by which herpesvirus infection could contribute to a prothrombotic endothelium involves an increase in the number of binding sites for inflammatory cells. Adhesion of inflammatory cells (neutrophils and monocyte/macrophages) and the release of inflammatory cytokines could shift the endothelial surface balance further from thromboresistance to a more prothrombotic state. HSV infection of the endothelium induces the expression of two important neoantigens on the endothelial surface: HSV gE and HSV gC. These virally encoded glycoproteins function as Fc and complement (C3b) receptors, respectively (103). The presence of these receptors suggested that the HSV-infected endothelium could bind Fc and C3b-bearing granulocytes. In fact, granulocyte adherence was increased by about twofold to HSV-infected endothelial cells (42,104) This increased adherence did not require antibody or complement, as increased adherence could be demonstrated when the granulocytes were suspended in serum-free media (42). However, addition of IgG containing anti-HSV antibody further increased granulocyte adherence (105). These data suggest that Fc or C3b receptors may act as granulocyte receptors on the HSV-infected endothelium but also that receptors other than Fc or C3b (i.e., adhesion molecules) are acting as granulocyte receptors (105).

Enhanced attachment of granulocytes to the virally infected endothelium was associated with increased granulocyte-mediated lysis of HSV-infected endothelial cells (105). CMV infection of endothelial cells also increases the adherence of granulocytes (106). In fact, adherence was greater to the CMV-infected endothelium (500% of control adherence) than had been reported for HSV infection (200% of control adherence). Tunicamycin, an agent that prevents glycosylation, abolished the effect of CMV infection on the increase of PMN adherence, suggesting that glycoproteins play a role in adhesion of granulocytes to the CMV-infected endothelium (106). The increased binding of granulocytes could not be induced by supernatants from the CMV-infected cells, suggesting that adherence is a cell-bound phenomenon not induced by an adherence-stimulation factor (106). This is in contrast to the increased binding of monocytes to the HSV-1–infected endothelium, which can be stimulated by a factor secreted into the medium (107).

Endothelial cells express several leukocyte receptors on their surface, including E-selectin (ELAM-1), ICAM-1, VCAM-1, and P-selectin (GMP140, PADGEM, CD62), in response to cytokines, phorbol esters, or exposure to other agonists (108). E-selectin, ICAM-1, and VCAM-1 expression is induced in response to cytokines (TNF and IL-1) in a process requiring protein synthesis. P-selectin is a cytoplasmic protein found on the membrane of Weibel-Palade bodies of resting endothelial cells (109). After stimulation by thrombin, histamine, or complement proteins, the Weibel-Palade body is rapidly translocated, and its membrane becomes incorporated into the plasma membrane of the cell, resulting in surface expression (109). This translocation from a preformed intracellular membrane compartment to the cell surface does not require de novo protein synthesis (109). Our recent data support the model that herpes infection induces endothelial cell surface expression of P-selectin and increased monocyte adhesion (101) (Fig. 1). We propose the following mechanism. HSV gC acts as a binding site for factor X. Concomitant generation of tissue factor converts bound factor X to factor Xa in an active prothrombinase complex, leading to generation of thrombin. Thrombin then can act in an autocrine manner to induce expression of a leukocyte receptor, P-selectin (110). This concept is supported by data demonstrating that increased binding of monocytes to the HSV-1–infected endothelium can be stimulated by a factor secreted into the medium (107). Our data indicate that monocyte

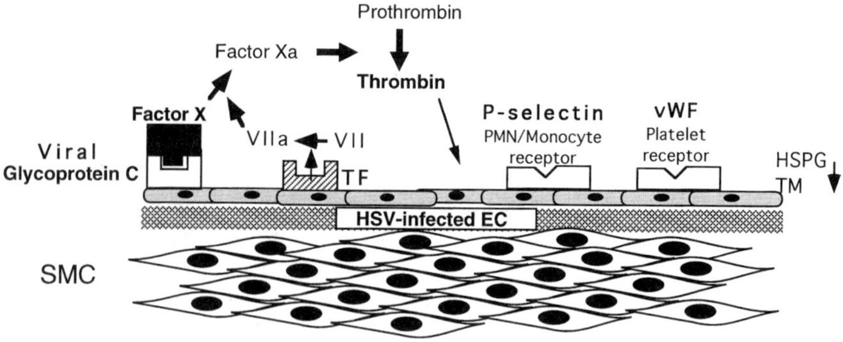

Figure 1 HSV induction of endothelial procoagulant activity. This model illustrates mechanisms by which herpes simplex virus (HSV) infection of the vascular endothelium can shift the hemostatic balance from an antithrombotic to a prothrombotic state. HSV infection induces the synthesis and expression of viral glycoprotein (C). This glycoprotein can serve as an Fc and C3b receptor and, in addition, a binding site for factor X. Increased binding of factor X and its subsequent conversion to the active form, factor Xa, can lead to the conversion of prothrombin to thrombin. HSV can also increase surface expression of tissue factor and facilitate activation of the extrinsic pathway of the coagulation cascade. Thrombin can induce surface expression of P-selectin, a monocyte and neutrophil (PMN) receptor, and von Willebrand factor (vWF), which acts as a platelet receptor. The binding of inflammatory cells and platelets and the release of cytokines and inflammatory mediators can further amplify this cascade. HSV can also reduce surface expression of heparan sulfate proteoglycan (HSPG) and thrombomodulin (TM), which, in turn, can lead to reduced antithrombin III (ATIII) binding and thrombin-dependent protein C activation and inhibit normal anticoagulant surface properties.

adhesion induced by herpes infection is blocked by anti-P selectin but not by anti-ELAM or antibodies to other adhesive leukocyte integrins (LFA-1, MAC-1, and P150,95) (110). This suggests that P-selectin is a major receptor for monocytes on the herpes-infected endothelium (110). The adhesion of inflammatory cells to the HSV-infected endothelium can further amplify the prothrombotic phenotype of the endothelium. Release of cytokines such as IL-1 and TNF from adherent and activated inflammatory cells can induce tissue factor expression by endothelial cells (93,111).

VIII. MOLECULAR GENETICS OF ATHEROSCLEROSIS

The monoclonal hypothesis of Benditt and Benditt (112) is based on the observation that 75% of atherosclerotic plaques from human tissues removed at surgery or at autopsy demonstrated a monoclonal phenotype of the glucose-6-phosphate dehydrogenase enzyme (G-6-PD), based on electrophoretic mobility. This technique takes advantage of the fact that the polymorphic forms of this enzyme are expressed in an X-linked fashion. Medial cells from regions adjacent to atherosclerotic plaques and from nonplaque areas display equal amounts of each polymorphic form of the enzyme as would be expected in an X-linked gene, since one of the two X chromosomes is inactivated early in embryonic development. Similar results were obtained by other laboratories (114,115). Nevertheless, the interpretation of these experiments in supporting the monoclonal hypothesis has been challenged (116), the principal argument being that the G-6-PD marker may be linked to some other gene that gives these cells a selective growth advantage, i.e., a "phenotype-selective advantage hypothesis," without the proliferative lesion being truly monoclonal in origin.

The monoclonal hypothesis suggests that the smooth muscle cell proliferation seen in the atherosclerotic lesion is similar to a benign tumor as, for example, in uterine leiomyomas (117). A logical extension of this hypothesis is to infer that alterations in the smooth muscle cell genome by chemical mutagens or viruses might be involved in the smooth muscle cell proliferation characteristic of human atherosclerosis. Supporting such an idea is the experimental observation of focal smooth cell proliferation induced in the aortic intima of chickens treated with a chemical mutagen initiation-promotion sequence (118). This may be a reasonable explanation linking cigarette smoking with the development of atherosclerosis (119–121), since the urine of smokers is known to contain excessive amounts of mutagenic or premutagenic substances (122).

Penn et al. (123) reported the presence of transforming DNA in samples derived from human coronary artery atherosclerotic plaques. Plaque-derived DNA had the capacity to transform NIH 3T3 cells in vitro. The transformed cell lines were capable of forming tumors in nude mice. These observations regarding the presence of a transforming gene element have been extended into an animal model of early arterial plaques induced by administration of the carcinogen 7,12,dimethylbenz(a)anthracene (DMBA) to cockerels (124). Further studies on vascular smooth muscle derived from human plaques show enhanced expression of the proto-oncogene *myc* (125), although this could be a marker of enhanced cellular replication without true transformation. Whether the presence of a transforming gene is a generalized phenomenon in atherosclerotic lesions has been challenged by Yew et al., who were unable to detect transforming activity in DNA isolated from atherosclerotic plaques of human carotid arteries (126). Nevertheless, other laboratories have detected evidence of a similar transforming gene in atherosclerotic plaques (127). This study reported the correlation of transformation with the absence of a 140 kDa protein normally secreted by these cells. Interestingly, other studies have identified a 140 kDa antitumorigenic glycoprotein that acts as an antiangiogenesis factor (128,129). The loss of this protein correlates with a transformed phenotype. This study (127) raises the possibility that the transforming gene activity may represent the loss of a normal antioncogene or gene controlling cellular proliferation. The identity of the transforming gene(s) remains elusive.

Although no transforming gene of viral origin has been identified as causing human atherosclerosis, the results of recent studies demonstrate that vascular cells, like other cells, have the potential to be transformed by viral genes. Nachtigal and colleagues have shown vascular smooth muscle cells were transformed following transfection with a plasmid containing the SV40 early region (130). They also showed that rabbit arterial smooth muscle cells were immortalized following transfection with a plasmid containing the BglII N fragment (MTRII) of HSV-2 (131). Immortalization is probably the most important attribute of transformation, since these cells normally have a finite life span in vitro (131). The transformed cells did not retain the viral DNA sequences, consistent with the findings noted above in HSV-induced transformation. Transformation of rat embryo cells by SV40 can result in marked accumulation of cholesteryl esters apparently due to an alteration in the regulation of LDL receptors (132). These studies provide circumstantial evidence that virally induced transformation can predispose to some of the characteristic features of atherogenesis.

The transforming potential of herpesviruses (133–135) is well established in a large number of studies. These studies do not demonstrate a single viral oncogene, a virus-coded transforming protein, or any genomic DNA sequences that directly transform cells by a "single-hit" kinetic model (135), but they do suggest that the mechanism of transformation is complex. The fact that genomic viral sequences are not retained in the transformed cells makes the elucidation of the transformation mechanism more problematic (136,137). Despite this, the genetic elements involved in transformation have been mapped to specific subsegments of the viral genome (138,139). This was done by cleaving the viral genomic DNA into small fragments, isolating the fragments, and testing which ones retained the capacity to transform target cells into which they were transfected. These experiments led to the designation of specific regions of the viral genome as responsible for this transforming property. There is a single morphological transformation region of HSV-1 (MTRI) (139). Two morphological transforming regions are found in HSV-2: MTRII (127) and MTRIII (140,141). A specific fragment of the HSV-1 genome mediates the degradation of host mRNA responsible in part for the suppression of host protein synthesis noted above (142). Of interest, this fragment overlaps the MTRII of HSV-2 and is within an open reading frame encoding a 1.9 kb RNA leading to synthesis of a 58 kDa protein (143). The authors proposed two possible interpretations for the co-mapping of the transforming and host shut-off functions: (a) the two functions could involve different gene products, e.g., if the mechanism of transformation involved a gene insertion into a promoter, or (b) transformation could be an indirect consequence of the inhibition of host protein synthesis (142). This inhibition might lead to transient stress alterations, causing rearrangements of genes regulating the cell cycle (142). They also suggested that the more efficient shut-off by HSV-2 (139,144) might explain why this region appears to be transforming only in HSV-2, but not in the homologous region of HSV-1 (139). Since shut-off of host cell protein synthesis is incompatible with long-term survival, the authors also point out (142) that this may explain why viral DNA is not retained in the transformed cells and is lost in daughter generations (136,137). Very small DNA fragments of a size unable to code for a transforming protein are also capable of inducing morphological transformation (145). As noted above, the DNA used to induce the morphological transformation is not retained within the transformed cell, and there is no evidence for an HSV-coded transforming protein (137).

The mechanism of transformation by these herpesvirus DNA fragments has not been elucidated. Proposals have been made to implicate DNA stem loop structures, ribonucleotide reductase activity, mutagenesis, gene amplification, increased or altered expression of cellular genes, activation of endogenous viruses, protein kinase activity, and the possible interaction between latency of the virus and transformation (133). However, no conclusive proof exists for any of these mechanisms (133). Recently, shuttle vectors have been employed to study sequence analysis of the mutations induced in cellular DNA by HSV-1 (146). Of interest, the maximal increase in mutation frequency was noted at 4 h after HSV-1 infection, implicating an immediate-early or early viral protein. Sequence analysis of the chromosomal fragments may lead to information about putative cellular targets for the virally induced mutagenesis. Mutagenesis (146) could be a possible explanation for a "hit-and-run" mechanism (138) of virally induced transformation. Since vascular smooth muscle cells can be transformed by HSV-2 (132), we speculate that herpesvirus-induced transformation may be a contributory mechanism to loss of growth control in the atherosclerotic vessel wall. The fact that specific regions of viral DNA can be isolated that are consistently capable of transforming target cells opens the speculative possibility that viruses may transform cells in vivo without viral replication.

Herpesviral genes have been linked to the development of atherosclerosis in an animal model. Japanese quail genetically susceptible to atherosclerosis were found to have specific DNA segments of Marek's disease herpesvirus incorporated into their genome (147). Two lines of Japanese quail, one highly susceptible and the other resistant to atherosclerosis, were developed through genetic selection (148). The susceptible quail developed severe aortic lesions, which resembled human atherosclerosis (149), within 9 weeks when fed a high-cholesterol diet. When the genomic DNA from these susceptible animals was hybridized with DNA probes prepared by restriction endonuclease digestion of MDV DNA representing about 30% of the total MDV genome, a strong signal was detected in all genetically susceptible animals. In addition, the amount of DNA detected appeared to be proportional to the degree of atherosclerosis in the aortas. Of interest, the restriction patterns developed from endonuclease digestion of the cellular DNA showed that only a limited number of specific endonuclease restriction fragments hybridized to the MDV total probe. These results suggested that a specific part of the MDV genome, but not the total genome, was detectable in atherosclerotic tissue. Functional MDV was not detected by virus isolation, serology, or exposure of other chicks to susceptible quail. Examination of embryos from these different strains suggested that the viral genes were passed through the germline. The authors concluded that this indicated that either the viral gene or one very closely linked to it was responsible for the susceptibility to atherosclerosis. These conclusions regarding retention of viral DNA in the germline are quite different from the results observed with HSV-1 transformation in vitro. In addition, vertical transmission of viral DNA in vivo has not been observed previously. It remains to be determined if the MDV probes can cross-hybridize with a normal cellular gene, and if the signals detected may be due to cross-hybridization with a quail gene that exhibits pleomorphism in the DNA of the two strains of quail. If this were the case, the conclusions of the study would have to be altered.

Human CMV also has two morphological transforming regions (150, 151). Viral DNA is not retained in cells transformed by the human CMV strain AD-169; however, there is one report of viral DNA being retained in cells transformed by human CMV strain Towne (152). A potential link between CMV and p53 inactivation in coronary restenosis was recently proposed by Steven Epstein and colleagues at the National Institutes of Health (113). They demonstrated that IE84, a CMV protein, binds to and inhibits p53 function. Mutations in p53 that lead to loss of function are often accompanied by enhanced stability, which allows the protein to be detectable by immunostaining. It was demonstrated that there was a significant concordance between p53 immunoreactivity in human restenotic lesions and the presence of CMV DNA; viral DNA was detected in 11 of 13 (85%) of the p53 immunopositive lesions but only 3 of 11 (27%) of the p53 immunonegative lesions. Conversely, almost 80% of the CMV-positive lesions (11 of 14) were p53-immunopositive. It was speculated that latent CMV could be reactivated following a procedure such as balloon angioplasty, IE84 could inhibit the function of p53, and the inhibition of p53 could contribute to the smooth muscle cell proliferation seen in some postangioplasty patients (113). Another potential mechanism by which CMV infection of vascular smooth muscle cells could increase smooth muscle cell mass within an atherosclerotic or restenotic lesion would not be by increasing smooth muscle cell proliferation, but by inhibiting apoptosis (programmed cell death) (153). Human CMV-infected fibroblasts have been shown to be resistant to the induction of apoptosis (154). Two CMV gene products that block apoptosis were identified:IE1 and IE2. Whether these two gene products can inhibit vascular SMC proliferation in vivo or in vitro has yet to be tested.

IX. SUMMARY

A possible role for herpesviruses in the etiology and/or pathogenesis of atherosclerosis has been based upon:

1. Evidence of widespread and often systemic infection with these viruses in the general population
2. The presence of antigens and nucleic acid sequences of herpesviruses in atherosclerotic lesions
3. The association between CMV infection and accelerated atherosclerosis and in cardiac allograft recipients
4. The observation of herpesvirus-induced atherosclerosis occurring in animal models of the disease
5. Profound effects upon cholesteryl metabolism in vascular smooth muscle cells infected with herpesviruses in vitro leading to cholesteryl ester accumulation
6. Loss of anticoagulant properties by vascular endothelial cells and the acquisition of procoagulant properties when infected by herpesviruses in vitro
7. Increased binding of inflammatory cells to herpesvirus-infected endothelial cells
8. The ability of herpesviruses to induce expression of cytokines by vascular and inflammatory cells
9. The transforming potential of herpesviruses, the ability of vascular smooth muscle cells to be transformed by viruses, and the recognition of transforming gene elements in atherosclerotic lesions

However, despite all of this circumstantial evidence, a cause-and-effect relationship between viruses and human atherosclerosis has not been definitively established. Further research is necessary to solidify or refute the hypothesis that viruses cause or contribute to the development of atherosclerosis.

REFERENCES

1. Fabricant CG, Fabricant J, Litrenta M, Minick C. Virus induced atherosclerosis. J Exp Med 1978; 148:335–340.
2. Minick CR, Fabricant CG, Fabricant J, Litrenta MM. Atheroarteriosclerosis induced by infection by herpesvirus. Am J Pathol 1978; 96:673–706.
3. Hajjar D, Fabricant C, Minick C, Fabricant J. Virus-induced atherosclerosis. Herpesvirus infection alters arterial cholesterol metabolism and accumulation. Am J Pathol 1986; 122:62–70.
4. Fabricant C, Fabricant J, Minick CR, Litrenta M. Herpes virus induced atherosclerosis in chickens. Fed Proc 1983; 42:2476–2479.
5. Grattan M, Moreno-Cabral C, Starnes V, Oyer P, Stinson E, Shumway N. Cytomegalovirus infection is associated with cardiac allograft rejection and atherosclerosis. JAMA 1989; 261:3561–3566.
6. MacDonald K, Rector T, Braunlan E, Coubo S, Olivari M. Association of coronary artery disease in cardiac transplant recipients with cytomegalovirus infection. Am J Pathol 1989; 64:359–362.
7. Cunningham M, Pasternak R. The potential role of viruses in the pathogenesis of atherosclerosis. Circulation 1988; 77:964–966.
8. Melnick J, Adam E, DeBakey M. Cytomegalovirus and atherosclerosis. BioEssays 1995; 17:899–903.
9. Hajjar D. Viral pathogenesis of atherosclerosis: impact of molecular mimicry and viral genes. Am J Pathol 1991; 139:1195–1211.
10. Visser M, Vercellotti G. Herpes simplex virus and atherosclerosis. Eur Heart J 1993; 14(suppl K):39–42.
11. Frenkel N, Schirmer E, Wyatt L, Katsofanas G, Roffman E, Danovich R, June C. Isolation of a new herpesvirus from human $CD4^+$ T cells. Proc Natl Acad Sci USA 1990; 87:748–752.
12. Corey L, Spear P. Infections with herpes simplex viruses. N Engl J Med 1986; 314:686–691.
13. Nahmias A, Josey K. Epidemiology of herpes simplex 1 and 2. In: Viral Infection of Humans—Epidemiology and Control. New York: Plenum, 1978: 253–271.
14. Rooney JF. Epidemiology of herpes simplex. Ann Intern Med 1985; 103: 404–419.
15. Johnson R, Nahmias A, Magder L, Lee F, Brooks C, Snowden M. A seroepidemiologic survey of the prevalence of herpes simplex virus type 2 in the United States. N Engl J Med 1986; 321:7–12.
16. Marshall G, Rabalais G, Stewart J, Dobbins J. Cytomegalovirus seroprevalence in women bearing children in Jefferson County, Kentucky. Am J Med Sci 1993; 305:292–296.

17. Adam E, Melnick J, Probesfield J, Petrie B, Burek J, Bailey K, McCollum C, DeBakey M. High levels of cytomegalovirus antibody in patients requiring vascular surgery for atherosclerosis. Lancet 1987; 2:291.
18. Havlik R, Blackwelder W, Kaslow R, Castelli W. Unlikely association between clinically apparent herpesvirus infection and coronary incidence at older ages: the Framingham Heart Study. Arteriosclerosis 1989; 9:877–880.
19. Sorlie PD, Adam E, Melnick SL, Folsom A, Skelton T, Chambless LE, Barnes R, Melnick JL. Cytomegalovirus herpesvirus and carotid atherosclerosis—the ARIC study. J Med Virol 1994; 42:33–37.
20. Koskinen P, Nieminen M, Krogerus L, Lemstrom K, Mattila S, Hayry P. Cytomegalovirus infection and accelerated cardiac allograft vasculopathy in human cardiac allografts. J Heart Lung Transplant 1993; 12:724–729.
21. Paavonen T, Mennander A, Lautenschlager I, Mattila S, Hayry P. Endothelialitis and accelerated atherosclerosis in human heart transplant coronaries. J Heart Lung Transplant 1993; 12:117–122.
22. Koskinen P, Krogerus L, Nieminen M, Mattila S, Hayry P, Lautenschlager I. Quantitation of cytomegalovirus infection-associated histologic findings in endomyocardial biopsies of heart allografts. J Heart Lung Transplant 1993; 12:343–354.
23. Ustinov J, Loginov R, Bruggeman C, van der Meide P, Hayry P, Lautenschlager I. Cytomegalovirus induces class II expression in rat heart endothelial cells. J Heart Lung Transplant 1993; 12:644–651.
24. Gyorkey F, Melnick J, Guinn G, Gyorkey P, DeBakey M. Herpes viridae in endothelial cells of the proximal aorta of atherosclerotic patients. Expt Mol Pathol 1984; 40:328–339.
25. Benditt E, Barrett T, McDougall J. Viruses in the etiology of atherosclerosis. Proc Natl Acad Sci USA 1983; 80:6386–6389.
26. Melnick J, Dreesman G, McCollum C, Petrie B, Burek J, DeBakey M. Cytomegalovirus antigen within human arterial smooth muscle cells. Lancet 1983; 2:644–646.
27. Petrie B, Melnick J, Adam E, Burek J, McCollum C, DeBakey M. Nucleic acid sequence of cytomegalovirus in cells cultured from human arterial tissue. J Infect Dis 1987; 155:158–159.
28. Hendrix M, Salimans M, van Boven C, Bruggeman C. High prevalence of latently present cytomegalovirus in artery walls of patients suffering grade III atherosclerosis. Am J Pathol 1990; 136:23–28.
29. Stinski M, Thomsen D, Stenberg R, Goldstein L. Organization and expression of immediate early genes of the human cytomegalovirus. J Virol 1983; 46:1–14.
30. Hendrix M, Daemen M, Bruggeman C. Cytomegalovirus nucleic acid distribution within the human vascular tree. Am J Pathol 1991; 138:563–567.
31. Yamashiroya H, Ghosh L, Yang R, Robertson A. Herpesviridae in the coronary arteries and aorta of young trauma victims. Am J Pathol 1988; 130:71–79.
32. Walker DI, Bloor K, Williams G, Gillie I. Inflammatory aneurisms of the abdominal aorta. Br J Surg 1972; 59:609–614.

33. Tanaka S, Toh Y, Mori R, Komori K, Okadome K, Sugimachi K. Possible role of cytomegalovirus in the pathogenesis of inflammatory aortic diseases: a preliminary report. J Vasc Surg 1992; 16:274–279.
34. Koskinen P, Lemstrom K, Bruggeman C, Lautenschlager I, Hayry P. Acute cytomegalovirus infection induces a subendothelial inflammation (endothelialitis) in the allograft vascular wall—a possible linkage with enhanced allograft arteriosclerosis. Am J Pathol 1994; 144:41–50.
35. Waldman WJ, Adams PW, Orosz CG, Sedmak D. T lymphocyte activation by cytomegalovirus-infected allogeneic cultured human cells. Transplant 1992; 54:887–896.
36. Datta SK, Tumilowicz JJ, Trentin JJ. Lysis of human arterial cells infected with herpesviridae by peripheral blood mononuclear cells: implications for atherosclerosis. Viral Immunol 1993; 6:153–160.
37. Paterson JC, Cottral GE. Experimental coronary sclerosis III. Lymphomatosis as a cause of coronary sclerosis in chickens. Arch Pathol 1950; 49:669–707.
38. Lemstrom K, Bruning J, Bruggeman C, Lautenschlager I, Hayry P. Cytomegalovirus infection enhances smooth muscle cell proliferation and intimal thickening of rat aortic allografts. J Clin Invest 1993; 92:549–558.
39. Lemstrom K, Aho P, Bruggeman C, Hayry P. Cytomegalovirus infection enhances mRNA expression of platelet derived growth factor-BB and transforming growth factor-beta 1 in rat aortic allografts. Arterioscler Thromb 1994; 14:2043–2052.
40. Persoons M, Daemen M, Bruning J, Bruggeman C. Active cytomegalovirus infection of arterial smooth muscle cells in immunocompromised rats. A clue to herpes virus associated atherosclerosis. Circ Res 1994; 75:214–220.
41. Kaner RJ, Medina J, Nicholson AC, Ursea R, Schwartz SM, Hajjar DP. Developmentally regulated herpesvirus plaque formation in arterial smooth muscle cells. Circ Res 1993; 73:10–14.
42. Macgregor RR, Friedman HM, Macarak EJ, Kefalides NA. Virus infection of endothelial cells increases granulocyte adherence. J Clin Invest 1980; 65:1469–1477.
43. Friedman H, Macarak E, MacGregor R, Wolfe J, Kefalides N. Virus infection of endothelial cells. J Infect Dis 1981; 143:266–273.
44. Lashgari M, Friedman H, Kefalides N. Suppression of matrix protein synthesis by herpes simplex virus in bovine smooth muscle cells. Biochem Biophys Res Commun 1987; 143:145–151.
45. Ho DD, Rota TR, Andrews CA, Hirsch MS. Replication of cytomegalovirus in endothelial cells. J Infect Dis 1984; 150:956–957.
46. Tumilowicz JJ, Gawlik ME, Powell B, Trenton J. Replication of cytomegalovirus in human arterial smooth muscle cells. J Virol 1985; 56:839–845.
47. Sydiskis RJ, Roizman B. Polysomes and protein synthesis in cells infected with a DNA virus. Science 1966; 153:76–78.
48. Fenwick ML, Clark J. Early shut off of host protein synthesis in cells infected with herpes simplex virus. J Gen Virol 1982; 61:121–125.
49. Kefalides NA, Ziaie Z. Herpes simplex virus suppression of human endo-

thelial matrix protein synthesis is independent of viral protein synthesis. Lab Invest 1986; 55:328–336.
50. London FS, Brinker J, Ziaie Z, Kefalides NA. Suppression of host mRNA in human smooth muscle cells by a virion competent factor in herpes simplex virus type 1. Lab Invest 1990; 62:189–195.
51. Nishiola Y, Silverstein S. Degradation of cellular mRNA during infection by herpes simplex virus. Proc Natl Acad Sci USA 1977; 74:2370–2374.
52. Fabricant CG, Krook L, Gillespie J. Virus-induced cholesterol crystals. Science 1973; 181:566–557.
53. Hajjar D, Falcone D, Fabricant C, Fabricant J. Altered cholesteryl ester cycle is associated with lipid accumulation in herpesvirus-infected arterial smooth muscle cells. J Biol Chem 1985; 260:6124–6128.
54. Hajjar D. Herpesvirus infection prevents activation of cytoplasmic cholesteryl esterase in arterial smooth muscle cells. J Biol Chem 1986; 261:7611–7614.
55. Hajjar D, Pomerantz K, Falcone D, Weksler B, Grant A. Herpes simplex virus infection in human arterial cells: implications in arteriosclerosis. J Clin Invest 1987; 80:1317–1321.
56. Hajjar D, Pomerantz K, Snow J. Analysis of the physical state of cholesteryl esters in arterial smooth muscle—derived foam cells by differential scanning calorimetry. Biochem J 1990; 268:693–697.
57. Hajjar D, Nicholson A, Hajjar K, Sando G, Summers B. Decreased messenger RNA translation in herpesvirus-infected arterial cells: effects on cholesteryl ester hydrolase. Proc Natl Acad Sci USA 1989; 86:3366–3370.
58. Hsu H-Y, Nicholson AC, Pomerantz K, Kaner RJ, Hajjar DP. Altered cholesterol trafficking in herpesvirus-infected arterial cells. Evidence for viral protein kinase-mediated cholesterol accumulation. J Biol Chem 1995; 270:19630–19637.
59. Purves FC, Longnecker R, Leader D, Roizman B. Herpes simplex virus 1 protein kinase is encoded by open reading frame US3 which is not essential for virus growth in cell culture. J Virol 1987; 61:2896–2901.
60. Munro J, Cotran R. Biology of Disease: The pathogenesis of atherosclerosis: atherogenesis and inflammation. Lab Invest 1988; 58:249–261.
61. Hansson G, Jonasson, L, Seifert P, Stemme S. Immune mechanisms in atherosclerosis. Arteriosclerosis 1989; 9:567–578.
62. Hansson G, Holm J, Jonasson L. Detection of activated T lymphocytes in the human atherosclerotic plaque. Am J Pathol 1989; 135:169–175.
63. Dudding L, Haskel S, Clark BD, Auron PE, Sporn S, Huang ES. Cytomegalovirus infection stimulates expression of monocyte associated mediator genes. J Immunol 1989; 143:3343–3352.
64. Staats HF, Lausch RN. Cytokine expression in vivo during murine herpetic keratitis. J Immunol 1993; 151:277–283.
65. Gosselin J, Flamand L, D'Addario M, Hiscott J, Menezes J. Infection of peripheral blood mononuclear cells by herpes simplex and Epstein-Barr viruses. Differential induction of interleukin 6 and tumor necrosis factor-alpha. J Clin Invest 1992; 89:1849–1856.

66. Smith PD, Saini SS, Raffeld M, Manischewitz JF, Wahl SM. Cytomegalovirus induction of tumor necrosis factor-alpha by human monocytes and mucosal macrophages. J Clin Invest 1992; 90:1642–1648.
67. Pavic I, Polic B, Crnkovic I, Lucin P, Jonjic S, Koszinowski UH. Participation of endogenous tumor necrosis factor in host resistance to cytomegalovirus infection. J Gen Virol 1993; 74:2215–2223.
68. Kohase M, Henriksen-DeStefano D, May T, Vilcek J, Sehgal P. Induction of β_2-interferon by tumor necrosis factor; a homeostatic mechanism in the control of cell proliferation. Cell 1986; 45:659–666.
69. Wong GHW, Goeddel DV. Tumor necrosis factors α and β inhibit virus replication and synergize with interferons. Nature 1986; 323:819–822.
70. Haagmans B, Stals F, van der Meide P, Bruggeman C, Horzinek M, Schijns V. Tumor necrosis factor alpha promotes replication and pathogenicity of rat cytomegalovirus. J Virol 1994; 68:2297–2304.
71. Iwamoto GK, Monick MM, Clark BD, Auron PE, Stinsky MF, Hunninghake GW. Modulation of interleukin 1 beta gene expression by the immediate early genes of human cytomegalovirus. J Clin Invest 1990; 85:1853–1857.
72. Wang A, Doyle M, Mark D. Quantitation of mRNA by the polymerase chain reaction. Proc Natl Acad Sci USA 1989;86:9717–9721.
73. Clinton S, Fleet J, Loppnow H, Salomon R, Clark B, Cannon J, Shaw A, Dinarello C, Libby P. Interleukin-1 gene expression in rabbit vascular tissue in vivo. Am J Pathol 1991; 138:1005–1014.
74. Moyer C, Sajuthi D, Tulli H, Williams J. Synthesis of IL-1 alpha and IL-1 beta by arterial cells in atherosclerosis. Am J Pathol 1991; 138:951–960.
75. Boldogh I, Fons MP, Albrecht T. Increased levels of sequence specific DNA-binding proteins in human cytomegalovirus-infected cells. Biochem Biophys Res Commun 1993; 197:1505–1510.
76. Sehgal P, Helfgott DC, Santhinam U, Tatter S, Clerick R, Ghrayeb J, May LT. Regulation of the acute phase and immune responses in viral disease enhance expression of the beta 2 interferon hepatocyte stimulating factor interleukin 6 gene in virus infected human fibroblasts. J Exp Med 1988; 167:1951–1956.
77. Almeida GD, Porada CD, St Jeor S, Ascensao J. Human cytomegalovirus alters interleukin-6 production by endothelial cells. Blood 1994; 83:370–376.
78. Moore KW, Vieira P, Fiorentino DF, Trounstein ML, Khan TA, Mosmann TR. Homology of cytokine synthesis inhibitory factor (IL-10) to the Epstein-Barr virus gene BCRFI. Science 1990; 248:1230–1234.
79. Stopeck A, Nicholson A, Mancini F, Hajjar D. Cytokine regulation of LDL receptor gene transcription in HEP G2 cells. J Biol Chem 1993; 268:17489–17494.
80. Van Lenten B, Fogelman A. Lipopolysacchride-induced inhibition of scavenger receptor expression in human monocyte-macrophages is mediated through tumor necrosis factor-alpha. J Immunol 1992; 148:112–116.
81. Nicholson A, Hajjar D. Transforming growth factor-beta up-regulates low density lipoprotein receptor-mediated cholesterol metabolism in vascular smooth muscle cells. J Biol Chem 1992;267:25982–25987.

82. Chait A, Ross R, Albers J, Bierman E. Platelet-derived growth factor stimulates activity of low density lipoprotein receptors. Proc Natl Acad Sci USA 1980; 77:4084–4088.
83. Roth M, Emmons L, Perruchoud A, Block L. Expressions of the low density lipoprotein receptor and 3-hydroxy-3-methylglutaryl coenzyme A reductase genes are stimulated by recombinant platelet-derived growth factor enzymes. Proc Natl Acad Sci USA 1991; 88:1888–1892.
84. Cosgriff T. Viruses and hemostasis. Rev Infect Dis 1989; 11:5672–5688.
85. Kelton J, Neame P. Hemorrhagic complications of infection. In: Homeostasis and Thrombosis. Philadelphia: J.B. Lippincott, 1987:965–974.
86. Friedman H, Wolfe J, Kefalides N, Macarak E. Susceptibility of endothelial cells derived from different blood vessels to common viruses. In Vitro Cell Dev Biol 1986; 22:397–401.
87. Friedman H. Infection of endothelial cells by common human viruses. Rev Infect Dis 1989; 11:S700–S704.
88. McSorley J, Shapiro L, Brownstein M, Hsu K. Herpes simplex virus and varicella-zoster: comparative histology of 77 cases. Int J Dermatol 1974; 13:69–75.
89. Phinney P, Fligiel S, Bryson Y, Porter D. Necrotizing vasculitis in a case of disseminated neonatal herpes simplex infection. Arch Path Lab Med 1982; 106:64–67.
90. Kaner R, Iozzo R, Ziaie Z, Kefalides N. Inhibition of proteoglycan synthesis in human endothelial cells after infection with herpes virus type 1 in vitro. Am J Respir Cell Mol Biol 1990; 2:423–431.
91. Key N, Vercellotti G, Winkelmann J, Moldow C, Goodman J, Esmon N, Esmon C, Jacob H. Infection of vascular endothelial cells with herpes simplex virus enhances tissue factor activity and reduces thrombomodulin expression. Proc Natl Acad Sci USA 1990; 87:7095–7097.
92. Visser M, Tracy P, Vercellotti G, Goodman J, White J, Jacob H. Enhanced thrombin generation and platelet binding on herpes simplex virus-infected endothelium. Proc Natl Acad Sci USA 1988; 85:8227–8230.
93. Bevilacqua M, Pober J, Wheeler M, Cotran R, Gimbrone M. Interleukin-1 activation of vascular endothelium. Effects on procoagulant activity and leukocyte adhesion. Amer J Pathol 1985; 121:393–403.
94. Adams DH, Wyner LR, Karnovsky MJ. Experimental graft arteriosclerosis. 2. immunocytochemical analysis of lesion development. Transplant 1993; 56:794–799.
95. Key N, Bach R, Vercellotti G, Moldow C. Herpes simplex virus type 1 does not require productive infection to induce tissue factor in human umbilical vein endothelial cells. Lab Invest 1993; 68:645–651.
96. van Dam-Mieras M, Muller A, van Hinsbergh V, Mullers W, Bomans P, Bruggeman C. The procoagulant response of cytomegalovirus infected endothelial cells. Thromb Haemost 1992; 68:364–370.
97. Etingin O, Silverstein R, Hajjar D. von Willeband factor mediates platelet adhesion to virally infected endothelial cells. Proc Natl Acad Sci USA 1993; 90:5153–5156.

98. Sporn L, Shi R, Silverman D, Marder V. Rickettsia rickettsia infection of cultured endothelial cells induces release of large von Willebrand factor multimers from Weibel-Palade bodies. Blood 1991; 78:2595–2602.
99. Schorer A, Moldow C, Rick M. Interleukin 1 or endotoxin increases the release of von Willebrand factor from human endothelial cells. Br J Hematol 1987; 67:193–197.
100. Bruggeman C, Debie W, Muller A, Schutte B, van Dam-Mieras M. Cytomegalovirus alters the von Willebrand factor content in human endothelial cells. Thromb Haemost 1988; 59:264–268.
101. Etingin O, Silverstein R, Friedman H, Hajjar D. Viral activation of the coagulation cascade: molecular interactions at the surface of the infected endothelial cell. Cell 1990; 61:657–662.
102. Altieri D, Etingin O, Fair D, Brunck T, Geltosky J, Hajjar D, Edgington T. Structural homogolous ligand binding of integrin mac-1 and viral glycoprotein C receptors. Science 1991; 254:1200–1203.
103. Cines DB, Lyss AP, Bina M, Corkey R, Kefalides NA. Fc and C3 receptors induced by Herpes simplex virus infection in cultured endothelial cells. J Clin Invest 1982; 69:123.
104. Zajac B, O'Neill K, Friedman H, MacGregor R. Increased adherence of human granulocytes to herpes simplex type 1 infected endothelial cells. In Vitro Cell Dev Biol 1988; 24:321–325.
105. Visser M, Jacob H, Goodman J, McCarthy J, Furcht L, Vercellotti G. Granulocyte-mediated injury to herpes simplex virus-infected human endothelium. Lab Invest 1989; 60:296–304.
106. Span A, van Boven C, Bruggeman C. The effect of cytomegalovirus infection on the adherence of polymorphonuclear leukocytes to endothelial cells. Eur J Clin Invest 1989; 19:542–548.
107. Span A, Endert J, van Boven C, Bruggeman C. Virus induced adherence of monocytes to endothelial cells. FEMS Microbiol Immunol 1989; 47:237–244.
108. McEver R. GMP-140: A receptor for neutrophils and monocytes on activated platelets and endothelium. J Cell Biochem 1991; 45:156–161.
109. Hattori R, Hamilton K, Fugate R, McEver R, Sims P. Stimulated secretion of endothelial cell von Willebrand factor is accompanied by rapid distribution of the intracellular granule membrane protein, GMP-140. J Cell Biochem 1989; 264:7768–7771.
110. Etingin O, Silverstein R, Hajjar D. Identification of a monocyte receptor on herpesvirus-infected endothelial cells. Proc Natl Acad Sci USA 1991; 88: 7200–7203.
111. Schorer A, Kaplan M, Rao G, Moldow C. Interleukin 1 stimulates endothelial cell tissue factor production and expression by a prostaglandin-independent mechanism. Thromb Haemo 1986; 56:256–259.
112. Benditt EP, Benditt JM. Evidence for a monoclonal origin of human atherosclerotic plaque. Proc Natl Acad Sci USA 1973; 70:1753–1756.
113. Speir E, Modali R, Huang E, Leon M, Shawl F, Finkel T, Epstein S. Potential role of human cytomegalovirus and p53 interaction in coronary atherosclerosis. Science 1994; 265:391–394.

114. Pearson TA, Wang A, Solez K, Heptinstall RH: Clonal characteristics of fibrous plaques and fatty streaks from human aortas. Am J Pathol 1975; 81:379–385.
115. Thomas WA, Reiner JM, Janakidevi K, Lee KT. Population dynamics of arterial cells during atherogenesis: X. Study of monotrypism in atherosclerotic lesions of black women heterozygous for glucose-6-phosphate dehydrogenase (G6PD). Exp Mol Pathol 1979; 31:367–386.
116. Thomas WA, Kim DN. Biology of disease: atherosclerosis as a hyperplastic and/or neoplastic process. Lab Invest 1983; 48:245–255.
117. Linder D, Gartler SM. Glucose-6-phosphate dehydrogenase mosaicism: utilization as a cell marker in the study of leiomyomas. Science 1965; 150:67–68.
118. Majesky MW, Reidy MA, Benditt EP, Juchau MR. Focal smooth muscle proliferation in the aortic intima produced by an initiation promotion sequence. Proc Natl Acad Sci USA 1985; 82:3450–3454.
119. Strong JP, Richards ML, McGill HC Jr., et al. The association of cigarette smoking with coronary and aortic atherosclerosis. Atherosclerosis 1969; 10:303–317.
120. Albert RE, Vanderlaan M, Burns F, Nishezume M. Effect of carcinogens on chicken atherosclerosis. Cancer Res 1977; 37:2232–2235.
121. Penn A, Batestini G, Solomon J, Burns F, Albert RE. Dose-dependent size increase of aortic lesions following chronic exposure to 7,12-Dimethylbenz(*a*)anthracene. Cancer Res 1981;41:588–592.
122. Yamasaki E, Aimes BN. Concentration of mutagens from urine by absorption with a nonpolar resin XID2: Cigarette smokers have mutagenic urine. Proc Natl Acad Sci USA 1977; 74:3555–3559.
123. Penn A, Garte SJ, Warren L, Nesta D, Mindich B. Transforming gene in human atherosclerotic plaque DNA. Proc Natl Acad Sci USA 1986; 83:7951–7955.
124. Penn A, Snyder C. Arteriosclerotic plaque development is promoted by polynuclear aromatic hydrocarbons. Carcinogenesis 1988; 9:2185–2189.
125. Parkes JL, Cardell RR, Hubbard FC, Hubbard D, Meltzer A, Penn A. Cultured human atherosclerotic plaque smooth muscle cells retain transforming potential and display enhanced expression of the *myc* protooncogene. Am J Pathol 1991; 138:765–775.
126. Yew PR, Rajavashisth TB, Forrester J, Barath P, Lusis AJ. NIH 3T3 transforming gene not a general feature of atherosclerotic plaque DNA. Biochem Biophys Res Comm 1989; 165:1067–1071.
127. Ahmed AJ, O'Malley BW, Yatsu FM. Presence of a putative transforming gene in human atherosclerotic plaques. Circulation 1990;III-35 (Abstr.)
128. Rastinejad F, Polverini PJ, Bouck NP. Regulation of the activity of a new inhibitor of angiogenesis by a cancer suppressor gene. Cell 1990; 56:345–355.
129. Good DJ, Polverini PJ, Rastinejad F, Le-Beau MM, Lemons RS, Frazier WA, Bouck NP. A tumor suppressor-dependent inhibitor of angiogenesis is immunologically and functionally indistinguishable from a fragment of thrombospondin. Proc Natl Acad Sci USA 1990; 87:6624–6628.
130. Nachtigal M, Legrand A, Nagpal ML, Nachtigal SA, Greenspan P. Transfor-

mation of rabbit vascular smooth muscle cells by transfection with the early region of SV40 DNA. Am J Pathol 1990; 136:297–306.
131. Nachtigal M, Legrand A, Greenspan P, Nachtigal SA, Nagpal ML. Immortalization of rabbit vascular smooth muscle cells after transfection with a fragment of the BglII N region of herpes simplex virus type 2 DNA. Intervirology 1990; 31:166–174.
132. Chen JK, Lee L, McClure DB. Altered low density lipoprotein receptor regulation is associated with cholesteryl ester accumulation in simian virus 40 transformed rodent fibroblast cell lines. In Vitro Cell Dev Biol 1988; 24:353–358.
133. Macnab JCM. Herpes simplex virus and human cytomegalovirus, their roles and morphological transformation in genital cancer. J Gen Virol 1987; 68:2525–2550.
134. Duff R, Rapp F. Oncogenic transformation of hamster embryo cells after exposure to herpes simplex virus type 2. Nature 1971; 233:48–50.
135. Duff R, Rapp F. Oncogenic transformation of hamster embryo cells after exposure to inactivated herpes simplex virus type 1. J Virol 1973; 12:209–217.
136. Galloway DA, McDougall JK. The oncogenic potential of herpes simplex viruses: evidence for a "hit and run" mechanism. Nature (London) 1983; 302:21–24.
137. Cameron IR, Park M, Dutia BM, Ore A, Macnab JCM. Herpes simplex virus sequences involved in the initiation of oncogenic morphological transformation of rat cells are not required for maintenance of the transformed state. J Gen Virol 1985;66:517–527.
138. Camacho A, Spear PG. Transformation of hamster embryo fibroblasts by a specific fragment of the herpes simplex virus genome. Cell 1978; 15:993–1002.
139. Reyes GR, Lafemina R, Hayward SD, Hayward GS. Morphological transformation by DNA fragments of human herpes viruses: Evidence for two distinct transforming regions in herpes simplex virus types 1 and 2, and lack of correlation with biochemical transfer of the thymidine kinase gene. Cold Spring Harbor Symp Quant Biol 1980; 44:629–641.
140. Peden K, Mounts P, Hayward GS. Homology between mammalian cell DNA sequences and human herpesvirus genomes detected by a hybridisation procedure with high complexity probe. Cell 1982; 31:71–80.
141. Jariwalla RJ, Aurelian L, Ts'o POP. Immortalization and neoplastic transformation of normal diploid cells by defined cloned DNA fragments of herpes simplex virus type 2. Proc Natl Acad Sci USA 1980; 80:5902–5906.
142. Kwong AD, Kruper JA. Frenkel N. Herpes simples virus virion host shutoff function. J Virol 1988; 62:912–921.
143. Frink RJ, Anderson KP, Wagner MJ. Herpes simplex virus type 1 HindIII fragment L encodes spliced and complementary mRNA species. J Virol 1981; 39:559–572.
144. Powell KL, Courtney RJ. Polypeptides synthesized in herpes simplex virus type 2-infected HEp-2 cells. Virology 1975; 66:217–228.

145. Galloway DA, Nelson JA, McDougal JK. Small fragments of herpes virus DNA with transforming activity contained insertion sequence like structures. Proc Natl Acad Sci USA 1984; 81:4736–4740.
146. Hwang CBC, Shillitoe EJ. DNA sequence of mutations induced in cells by herpes simplex virus type-1. Virology 1990; 178:180–188.
147. Pyrzak R, Shih JCH. Detection of specific DNA segments of Marek's disease herpesvirus in Japanese quails susceptible to atherosclerosis. Atherosclerosis 1987; 68:77–85.
148. Shih JCH, Pomen EP, Kao KJ. Genetic selection, general characterization and histology of atherosclerosis-susceptible and resistant Japanese quail. Atherosclerosis 1983; 49:41.
149. Shih JCH, Pyrzak R, Guy JS. Discovery of noninfectious viral genes complementary to Marek's disease herpes virus in quail susceptible to cholesterol-induced atherosclerosis. J Nutr 1989; 119:294–298.
150. Oram JD, Downing RG, Akrigg A, Dollery AA, Duggleby CJ, Wilkenson GWG, Greenaway P. Use of recombinant plasmids to investigate the structure of the human cytomegalovirus genome. J Gen Virol 1982; 59:111–129.
151. Clanton C, Jariwalla RJ, Krejas C, Rosenthal LJ. Neoplastic transformation by cloned human cytomegalovirus DNA fragment uniquely homologies to one of the transforming regions of herpes simplex virus type 2. Proc Natl Acad Sci USA 1983; 80:3826–3830.
152. El-Beik T, Razzaque A, Jariwalla RJ, Cihlar RL, Rosenthal LJ. Multiple transforming regions of human cytomegalovirus DNA. J Virol 1986; 60:645–652.
153. Schwartz S, Bennett M. Death by any other name. Am J Pathol 1995; 147:229–234.
154. Zhu H, Shen Y, Shenk T. Human cytomegalovirus IE1 and IE2 proteins block apoptosis. J Virol 1995; 69:7960–7970.

11

Anticoagulants and Antithrombotics in the Prevention of Vascular Restenosis

Robert G. Johnson, Jr., and William R. Huckle
Merck Research Laboratories, West Point, Pennsylvania

Robert S. Schwartz
Mayo Clinic and Mayo Foundation, Rochester, Minnesota

I. INTRODUCTION

Arterial injury results in the ongoing formation of mural thrombus rich in fibrin and platelets. One type of arterial injury is that observed after percutaneous transluminal coronary angioplasty (PTCA), now widely accepted as a therapy for coronary artery disease. During the procedure, not only is the vessel wall injured, presenting a potent stimulus for activation of the coagulation cascade and platelet activation, but also exposure of the atheromatous core of the plaque is in itself a highly thrombogenic stimulus. The acceptance and use of intravascular stent placement during angioplasty probably provides an even greater contribution to thrombus formation. The major iatrogenic complication of angioplasty with or without stent placement is the net development of restenosis produced by the contributions of elastic recoil, remodeling, and neointimal hyperplasia (1–3). While stent implantation has limited the contribution of elastic recoil, no pharmacological agent or mechanical intervention has reliably limited the hyperplastic response (4,5).

At issue from the perspective of pathogenesis (and therefore with implications for therapeutic and pharmacological targets) is the relationship between the early thrombotic events and the thickness of the eventual neointima. Working from first principles, it is a realistic hypothesis that the formation of a fibrin- and platelet-rich thrombus results in the release of growth factors and cytokines from platelets and that the clot recruits lymphocytes and macrophages and provides the framework for smooth muscle cell migration and proliferation. Moreover, it cannot be ruled out that the thrombus may contribute to additional plaque growth by acting as a scaffold for incorporation of new material into the plaque. While a definitive cause-and-effect relationship between thrombus and neointimal formation has not been clearly established, mural thrombus has been detected in the coronary arteries of humans after PTCA (6). An increased restenosis risk is observed in ischemic syndromes known to be associated with mural thrombus (7).

As thrombus is the earliest event in the response to angioplasty, inhibition of thrombus formation has been a goal of clinical and preclinical studies, not only for prevention of acute occlusion but also for the potential inhibition of restenosis. The approach has focused on both potent anticoagulants and antiplatelet drugs. Several comprehensive reviews in this area have been published (8–10).

II. REVIEW OF THE COAGULATION CASCADE AND THE ROLE OF PLATELETS

Thrombosis is a complex, multifactorial process dependent upon a variety of bloodborne and tissue elements (for reviews, see Refs. 11–13). It is explosive due to the rapid turnover of sequential enzymatic steps and is dependent upon platelets.

Deep arterial injury results in a series of events that activate the intrinsic and extrinsic coagulation pathways (Fig. 1). In the extrinsic pathway, tissue exudate [mainly tissue factor (thromboplastin)] activates the coagulation pathway through its binding to factor VII/VIIa. Tissue factor is particularly abundant in the atherosclerotic vessel wall. The intrinsic pathway is initiated by contact of the blood with a negatively charged surface (e.g., collagen, foreign bodies, fissure in an atherosclerotic plaque). It is called the intrinsic pathway since all of the factors are present in the blood.

Thromboplastin released from the damaged cells is a lipoprotein that, when released into the blood, fixes factor X through gamma-carboxyglutamic acid to a phospholipid moiety in the presence of calcium. Factor VII slowly activates factor X to factor Xa, a reaction that accelerates when factor Xa converts factor VII to VIIa. In the intrinsic pathway, prekallikrein and factor Xa converts factor VII to VIIa. In the intrinsic pathway, prekallikrein and factor XI are bound to negatively charged surfaces via a high molecular weight kininogen. The complex is activated by factor XIIa, which in turn activates factor XI to factor XIa. Factor IX in the presence of a

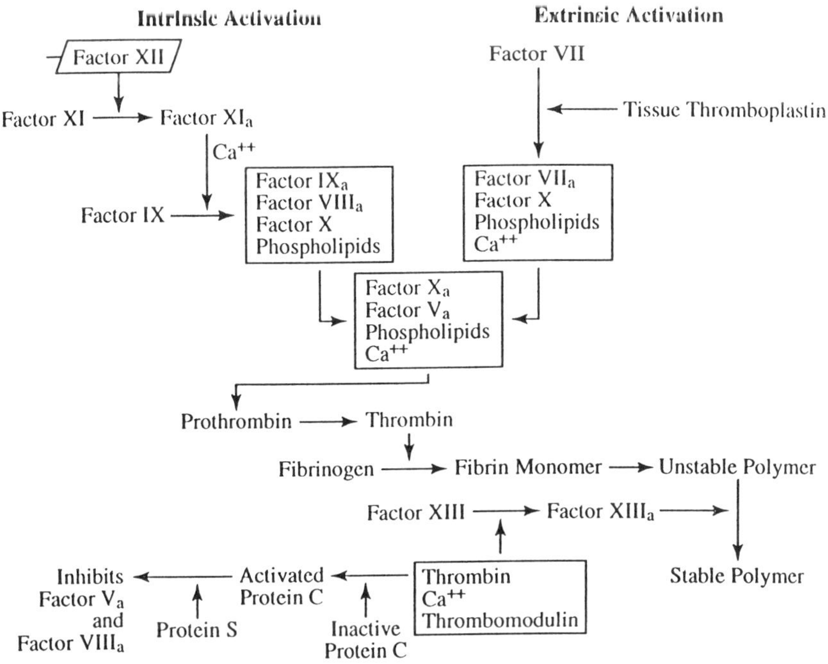

Figure 1 Schematic of the intrinsic and extrinsic pathways in the coagulation cascade. The intrinsic pathway relies only upon factors within the blood, the cascade is initiated by interaction with a negatively charged surface (e.g., collagen, foreign body, fissure in an atheroma), and the phospholipid is furnished by platelets. In the extrinsic pathway, the cascade is initiated by the release of tissue factor (thromboplastin) from the damaged cells. The pathways converge at the level of factor X activation to factor Xa. This a simplified schematic of a complicated pathway presented as a framework for the discussion of pharmacological therapy. For a more complete review of the coagulation pathways, see Refs. 11–13.

negative surface and the other factors noted, particularly factor VIII, activates factor X to factor Xa, presumably on the platelet surface.

The pathways converge at factor Xa, which converts prothrombin to thrombin. The reaction is greatly enhanced by factor Va, which is bound to the phospholipid of platelets and tissue factor. Thus, factors Xa and Va, phospholipid, and calcium form the "prothrombinase complex," which activates prothrombin to thrombin. Free thrombin acts upon fibrinogen by cleaving the arginine-glycine bond in the Aα and Bβ chains, allowing binding of the fibrin monomers end to end and side to side. Precipitation of the

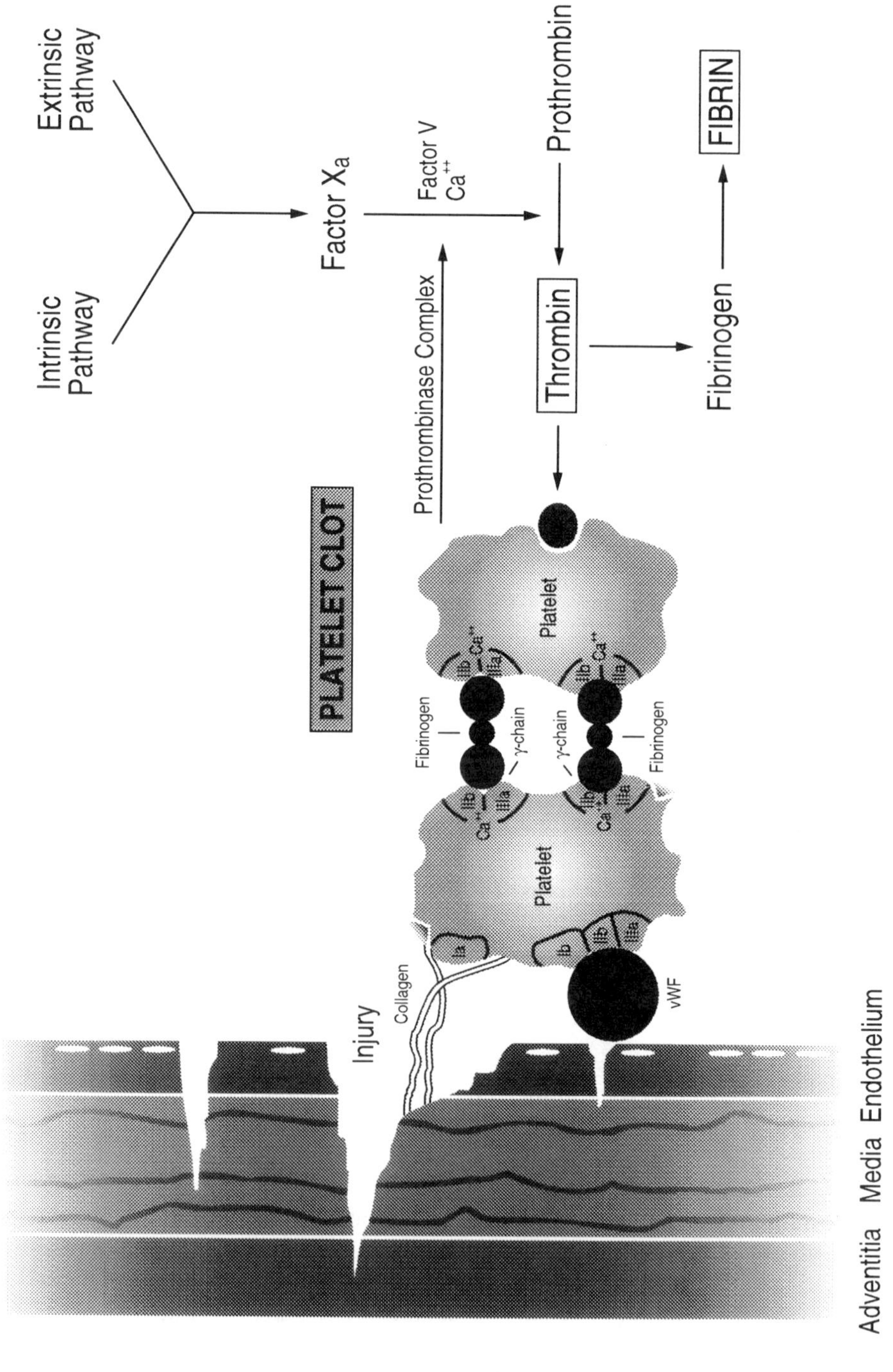
Intrinsic Pathway
Extrinsic Pathway
Factor Xa
Factor V
Ca++
Prothrombin
Prothrombinase Complex
Thrombin
Fibrinogen
FIBRIN
PLATELET CLOT
Platelet
Platelet
Fibrinogen
γ-chain
γ-chain
Fibrinogen
IIb
IIIa
Ca++
Ia
Ib
vWF
Collagen
Injury
Adventitia
Media
Endothelium

coupled monomers forms a gel, which becomes the skeleton of the thrombus. The fibrin gel is stabilized by factor XIII, which cross-links lysine residues.

Activation of factor Xa generates thrombin in large quantities at the site of the injury. Thrombin plays a central role in the thrombotic event through a variety of actions (14). First, it enzymatically drives the reaction that converts fibrinogen to fibrin. Second, thrombin is the most potent stimulator of platelet activation and aggregation. Third, it may induce vasoconstriction through the local release of endothelin and other vasoactive substances. Fourth, thrombin is a putative mitogen for vascular smooth muscle cells. Thrombin's actions may be additionally magnified by the loss of endothelium in the injured area, which normally contributes an anticoagulant effect. The lack of endothelium and presence of deep medial injury also result in the exposure of blood to collagen and other mediators, such as ADP, serotonin, epinephrine, and thromboxane A_2, which are stimulators of platelet adhesion and aggregation. Release of thromboplastin from the atheroma also ultimately contributes to thrombin generation. Significant thrombin generation in human coronary arteries after PTCA has been measured (15) (Fig. 2). As can be appreciated, the orderly and controlled nature of this cascade may be perturbed upon abrupt injury to an atherosclerotic vessel.

Figure 2 Schematic of the interrelationships between thrombosis and vascular injury after percutaneous transluminal coronary angioplasty (PTCA). Inflation of the PTCA balloon ± stent results in denudation of the endothelium and fissuring into the medial wall of the coronary artery. Removal of the endothelium results in loss of inhibitory factors of the coagulation cascade and exposure of the negative surfaces. Injury of the media releases tissue factor and exposes collagen. As evidenced in this diagram, there is a close interplay between platelets and the coagulation cascade, particularly the contributions to the prothrombinase complex and the large number of mediators released by platelets (ADP, serotonin, thromboxane, etc.). Thrombin occupies a central role in the explosive cascade. It enzymatically cleaves fibrinogen to form fibrin and is also a very potent stimulator of platelet aggregation and secretion. Therefore, agents that either decrease its activity (thrombin inhibitors) or decrease its production (factor Xa inhibitor or higher in the cascade) have been popular drug targets.

Table 1 Potential Anticoagulant and Antithrombotic Targets for Prevention of Restenosis

Coagulative	Platelet activation
Tissue factor	GPIIb/IIIa receptor[a]
Factor VII_a	Thrombin receptor
Factor X_a[a]	GPIb receptor
Thrombin[a]	Von Willebrand factor
Protein C	

[a]Major efforts in these areas.

III. STRATEGY FOR PHARMACOLOGICAL THERAPY OF RESTENOSIS BY INHIBITION OF ANTICOAGULANT AND ANTITHROMBOTIC PATHWAYS

The history of strategies for limiting restenosis with anticoagulant or antithrombotic agents has been determined largely by two factors: the availability of existing (and clinically utilized) antithrombotics and anticoagulants (e.g., heparin and aspirin) and the development of newer agents that specifically inhibit the critical proteins within the coagulation cascade and on the surface of platelets. These include inhibition of thrombin generation (by factor Xa inhibitors) (16), thrombin action (by direct thrombin inhibitors) (17), or platelet aggregation (GP IIb/IIIa receptor antagonists) (18) (Table 1). Since acute occlusion remains a serious complication of angioplasty, many early clinical studies were focused on inhibiting catastrophic thrombosis with a secondary interest in restenosis.

IV. CLINICAL STUDIES OF RESTENOSIS USING ANTITHROMBOTICS AND ANTICOAGULANTS

To date, no clinical intervention using antithrombotics or anticoagulant therapy has resulted in a decrease in the clinical angiographic restenosis rate (Table 2). However, several factors confound the interpretation of these studies. In some cases the index compound either is not sufficiently potent to predict inhibition of the appropriate events, an inappropriate dose was administered, or its target is not a significant factor in the pathogenesis of restenosis. For example, the clinical restenosis data on aspirin is quite clear-cut, suggesting that aspirin alone is not sufficient to significantly

Table 2 Clinical Restenosis Angiographic Trials Using Anticoagulants/Antithrombotics

Agent	Study	Result	Ref.
Anticoagulants			
Coumadin	Multiple	No effect	*Circ.* 69:721 (1984) *Br.H.J.* 60:485 (1988)
Heparin	Multiple	No effect	*Am.H.J.* 117:777 (1989)
Hirudin	HELVETICA	No effect	*NEJM.* 333:757 (1995)
Hirulog		No effect	*Circ.* 92:I-608 (1995)
LMW heparin			
Enoxaparin	ERA	No effect	*Circ.* 90:908 (1994)
Enoxaparin	EMPAR	No effect	*Circ.* 90:2651 (1994)
Antiplatelet agents			
Aspirin	Multiple	No effect	*JACC.* 17:2B (1991)
GR32191B	CARPORT	No effect	*Circ.* 84:1568 (1991)
Ketanserin		No effect	*Circ.* 88:1588 (1993)
Sulotroban	M-HEART II	No effect	*JACC.* 19:209A (1992)
Dipyridamole		No effect	*NEJM.* 318:1714 (1988)
Ticlopidine	Multiple	No effect	*Circ.* 75:IV-400 (1987)
Omega -3 fatty acids	EMPAR	No effect	*Circ.* 90:I-651 (1994)
7E3 [ReoPro]	EPILOG	Pending	
Integrelin	IMPACT-II	No effect	*Circ.* 92:I-606 (1995)
MK-383	RESTORE	Pending	

inhibit thrombus formation or restenosis (19). Conversely, even very effective inhibitors of platelet aggregation may not be sufficient to block the cascade of events leading to intimal hyperplasia. An example is the potent antagonist of the platelet GPIIb/IIIa receptors, Integrelin. The first angiographic study of Integrelin (IMPACT II) indicated no effect upon lumen diameter at 6-month follow-up (20). Since this agent affects only platelet aggregation and not adhesion or release, its mechanism of action may not be sufficient to block the events leading to the cascade. [Another clinical trial, EPILOG, has been initiated to study the effects of the monoclonal anti-GPIIb/IIIa antibody c7E3 [ReoPro] on angiographic restenosis (21).] Moreover, while the magnitude of injury and therefore thrombus formation in animal models appears to correlate with the degree of neointimal formation, the relationship between thrombus mass and degree of restenosis is by no means established. For example, in arterial stenosis associated with heart transplant, the insult that initiates the pathophysiological process leading to intimal hyperplasia is primarily immunological, with minimal contribution of thrombus. Nevertheless, transplant restenosis is one of the most severe forms of neointimal hyperplasia observed in humans. Despite these caveats, there is sufficient rationale for continuing to evaluate anticoagulants and antithrombotics in restenosis.

Another difficulty with the clinical trials has been the protocol design. For example, the potent thrombin inhibitor hirudin failed to reduce the occurrence of restenosis (HELVETICA study) (22). However, its route of administration and dosage may not have permitted sufficient inhibition of thrombin to achieve the desired result.

As small, highly potent low molecular weight compounds with oral bioavailability become available that affect factor Xa, thrombin, and GP IIb/IIIa pathways (16–18,23,24) more definitive clinical protocols can be designed. The underlying concern is that antithrombotic or antirestenotic efficacy and bleeding complications may go hand in hand. However, the availability of local delivery devices may allow adequate local concentrations of inhibitor to be achieved and systemic toxicity to be circumvented.

V. THE EFFECT OF ANTICOAGULANTS AND ANTITHROMBOTICS IN PRECLINICAL RESTENOSIS MODELS

A. Animal Models

Unfortunately, there is no universally accepted animal model of restenosis. Popular models include the rat carotid artery balloon injury model (25,26), the rabbit femoral or iliac artery balloon injury model (with or without cholesterol feeding) (27), and porcine coronary artery models (28).

The rat model has proved to be very permissive in terms of demonstrating efficacy of pharmacological interventions. A number of compounds that have failed to show an effect upon angiographically measured luminal diameters in large clinical trials have demonstrated a significant effect in the rat. The rat model is based on an extremely elastic noncoronary artery with an injury that produces only a small amount of thrombus. This model is no longer used by these authors. Criticisms of the cholesterol-fed rabbit model include the large macrophage component, the presence of fatty streaks rather than complex atheromatous lesions, and the potential augmentation of the extrinsic coagulation pathway mediators.

We have chosen the porcine coronary balloon angioplasty model for our research (29). It has been chosen because (a) the pig has a coronary artery size and distribution similar to humans, (b) clinical catheters and stents may be used, (c) the morphology of the porcine neointima is similar to that in humans, and (d) quantification of injury and neointimal response is readily performed. The severity of vessel injury and neointimal responses are measured by histomorphometry of elastin-van Gieson–stained sections. An ordinal vessel injury score is obtained and neointimal thickness measured at each wire site. Mean injury scores and intimal thicknesses then are calculated for each injured vessel. A wide range of compounds has been tested in this model, with each study confirming the high correlation between the degree of injury and the magnitude of neointimal thickness. Many of the agents tested in the pig coronary model demonstrated efficacy in the rat model but showed no effect in the pig or in clinical studies (for review, see Ref. 29).

B. Data in the Rabbit Atherosclerotic Model

There is a great deal of activity and enthusiasm for testing anticoagulants and antithrombotics in preclinical animal models (Table 3). (Experiments using the rat model will not be included here.) In the rabbit atherosclerotic model several important studies have been performed. In the first (27), two factor Xa inhibitors, recombinant antistasin (r-ATS) or tick anticoagulant peptide (r-TAP), were tested in the atherosclerosis-forming rabbit. Antistasin is a 119-amino-acid polypeptide originally isolated from the leech. Tick anticoagulant peptide is a 60-amino-acid polypeptide purified initially from the soft tick *Ornithodoros moubata* (Fig. 3). Both proteins are highly selective, competitive, reversible inhibitors of factor Xa with subnanomolar dissociation constants (30–34). r-ATS has a plasma half-life of many hours, while TAP's half-life is short (<60 min). Neither inhibitor has direct effects on platelets or other proteins in the coagulation pathway. Factor Xa is the serine protease that catalyzes the conversion of prothrombin to thrombin in the prothrombinase complex. The overall complex stimulates the reaction rate more than 280,000-fold. Since thrombin itself is the catalyst for fibrin production, inhibition of factor Xa and therefore thrombin generation may be a more effective mechanism than inhibiting thrombin activity once it is formed. Despite a mere 2-h i.v. infusion of either r-ATS or TAP around the time of angioplasty, treatment resulted in a larger luminal diameter measured by quantitative angiography at day 28 after the procedure (1.0 ± 0.3 mm for control vs 1.2 ± 0.3 for r-ATS, and 1.2 ± 0.3 for r-TAP, $p = 0.09$). In addition, there was decreased percentage cross-sectional narrowing by plaque measured by histomorphometric analysis in both the r-ATS– and r-TAP–treated arteries compared with the control (42 ± 21%, 47 ± 18%, and 63 ± 14%, respectively). The presence (or absence) of mural thrombus and the effect of these inhibitors at early times postangioplasty were not investigated in this study.

Table 3 Preclinical Restenosis Studies Using Anticoagulants/Antithrombotics

Animal	Agent	Mechanism	Result	Ref.
Anticoagulants				
Pig	Heparin	Antithrombin III Factor X_a inhibitor Antiproliferative	No effect	*Circ.* 92:I-785 (1995)
Pig	Tick anticoagulant peptide	Factor X_a inhibitor	40% ↓ in NIT	*Circ.* 93:1542 (1996)
Pig	Hirudin	Thrombin inhibitor	20% ↓ in NIT	*JACC.* 25:302A (1995)
Rabbit, atherosclerotic	Heparin	As above	No effect	*Circ.* 86:1536 (1992) *Circ.* 92:I-847 (1995)
Rabbit, atherosclerotic	Antistasin	Factor X_a inhibitor	50% ↓ in lumen diam.	*Circ.* 89:1262 (1994)
Rabbit, atherosclerotic	Tick anticoagulant peptide	Factor X_a inhibitor	20% ↓ NIT	*Circ.* 89:1262 (1994)
Rabbit, atherosclerotic	DEGR-VII_a	Factor VII_a inhibitor	↑ MLD (0.50 mm)	*Circ.* 92:3041 (1995)
Rabbit, atherosclerotic	TFPI[a]	Factor VII_a inhibitor Factor X_a inhibitor	↑ MLD (0.44 mm)	*Circ.* 92:3041 (1995)
Rabbit, atherosclerotic	Tick anticoagulant peptide	Factor X_a inhibitor	No effect	*Circ.* 92:3041 (1995)
Rabbit, atherosclerotic	Hirudin	Thrombin inhibitor	No effect	*Circ.* 92:3041 (1995)
Baboon	Heparin	As above	No effect	*Circ.* 91:2972 (1995)
Antithrombotics				
Rabbit, atherosclerotic	AZ-1	GPIIb/IIIa antagonist	↑ MLD (0.40 mm)	*Circ. Res.* 75:268 (1994)
Syrian hamster	G4120	GPIIb/IIIa antagonist $\alpha_v\beta_3$ antagonist	20% ↓ in NIT	*Circ.* 90:2203 (1994)

[a]Tissue factor pathway inhibitor.

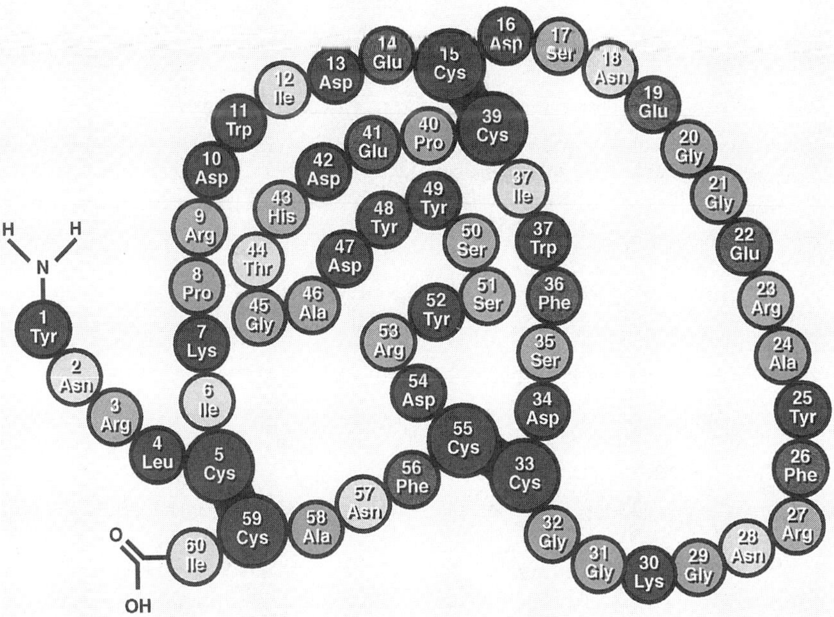

Figure 3 Sequence of tick anticoagulant peptide (TAP). TAP used in the described studies was made by recombinant techniques in yeast and has been shown to be identical to the native peptide (30,31). It is a 60-amino-acid single-chain polypeptide including six cysteine residues.

In an excellent recent study (35), four inhibitors that block specific factors within the coagulation cascade were tested: (a) DEGR-VIIa, an active site–inactivated form of factor VIIa that blocks the binding of factor VIIa to tissue factor; (b) TFPI, recombinat tissue factor pathway inhibitor, which binds factor Xa and inhibits the tissue factor-VIIa complex; (c) TAP; and (d) hirudin, a potent and specific thrombin inhibitor. These inhibitors were compared with the control (saline infusion) by continuous infusion for 3 days. Two endpoints were measured. The mean minimal luminal diameter measured 21 days after angioplasty was found to be significantly different between control and the DEGR-VIIa–treated groups (0.74 mm ± 0.25 vs. 1.24 ± 0.27 mm; $p = 0.0001$) and between controls and TFPI group (0.88 mm ± 0.21 vs. 1.32 mm ± 0.21; $p = 0.001$). The ratio of neointimal cross-sectional area compared with the area of internal elastic lamina in the DEGR-VIIa–tested group was less than for the control (0.48 ± 0.12 vs 0.67 ± 0.12; $p = 0.001$) and the ratio for the TFPI group was also less than for the control (0.46 ± 0.20 vs. 0.64 ± 0.13; $p = 0.003$).

Interestingly, while the factor Xa inhibitor was given for a longer period of time in this study than in the former study, the dose was less than half and no effect on restenosis was observed in the latter study. The results indicate that early blockade of the extrinsic coagulant pathway is important for inhibition of the response to arterial injury in this animal model. Whether the extrinsic coagulation pathway contributes a greater role to mural thrombus in this particular model compared to humans remains to be established.

C. Data from the Porcine Coronary Artery Model

TAP, hirudin, and heparin have been tested in the porcine coronary artery model. On the day of the procedure, the study animals were given either r-TAP (6.5 mg) or heparin (10,000 U) and then underwent oversized metallic coil injury using the standard method the right, circumflex, and/or left anterior descending coronary arteries (36). Thereafter, continuous infusion of r-TAP (average dose 194 μg/kg/min) or heparin was given to the study pigs for 60 h, with a goal of maintaining the activated clotting time (ACT) at 200 s (36). The average ACT in the study animals was 189 $\pm$ 26 s (vs. a control of 109 $\pm$ 27 s) and the aPTT values were 20 $\pm$ 8 s in the r-TAP group and 20 $\pm$ 3.9 s in the control group. The average r-TAP concentration in serum was 274 $\pm$ 59 μM.

Neointimal thicknesses and injury scores were measured in these studies as described in Section V.A. The mean neointimal thickness in the r-TAP group was 0.30 $\pm$ 0.08 vs. 0.48 $\pm$ 0.12 mm in the control group, while the mean injury scores for the two groups were not different (1.98 $\pm$ 0.31 and 1.98 $\pm$ 0.19, respectively). When the treatments were compared using the difference between the intercepts of regression lines for plots of neointimal thickness vs. injury score (Fig. 4), the estimated mean difference between r-TAP and control groups was -36.2% ($p < 0.001$). The average distal luminal diameter did not differ between the control and treatment groups. Since the cumulative percentage of injury scores was similar, the neointimal thickness could be represented as a function of the cumulative percent (Fig. 5). As indicated, over the entire range, neointimal thickness was inhibited in the group receiving r-TAP. Differences in neointimal areas calculated by planarimetry were also highly significant.

Similar studies have been reported in abstract form using a constant infusion of heparin (35.8 $\pm$ 9.9 U/kg/h) for 60 h (37) or PEG-hirudin (38) (0.1 mg/kg/h i.v. after a 1 mg/kg i.v. bolus) for 72 h. In the heparin study, there was no beneficial effect on neointimal thickness. The hirudin study showed a 38% decrease in neointimal thickness.

Cumulatively, these data in the porcine model suggest that early intervention with potent anticoagulants primarily affecting thrombus produc-

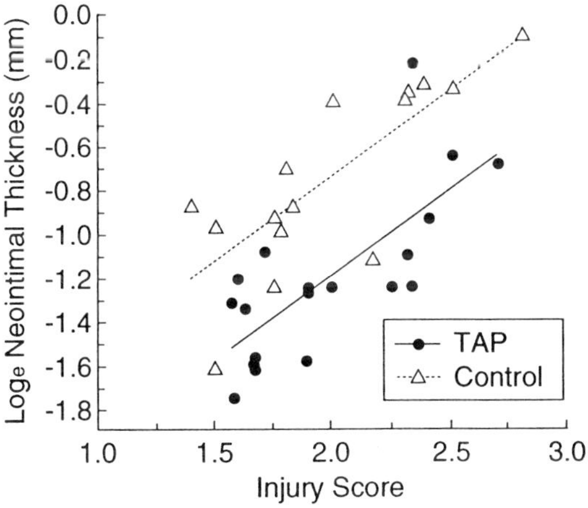

Figure 4 Graph of the relationship between neointimal thickness and injury score. The neointimal thickness is shown to be proportional to the depth of the injury (measured as the ordinal injury score; see text) for both the porcine arterial segments in the r-TAP (open circles) and control (closed triangles) animals. However, the degree of neointimal thickness is less in the r-TAP group for the same magnitude of arterial injury. The results of the regression analyses are listed in the text. Each plotted point represents one lesion. (From Ref. 36.)

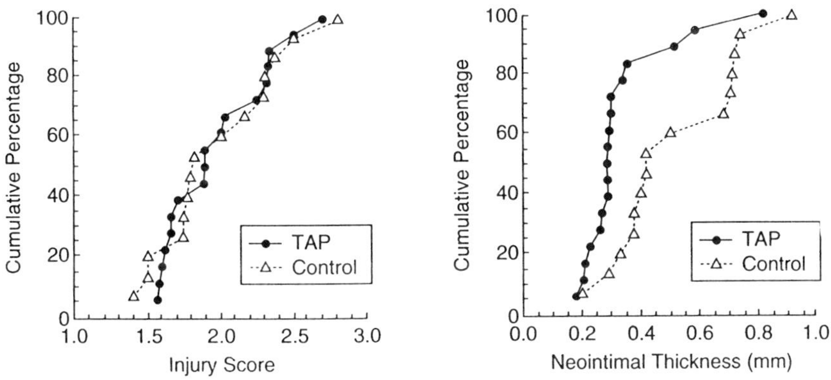

Figure 5 Graph of the cumulative percentage for the injury scores and neointimal thicknesses for r-TAP (open circles) and control (closed circles). No significant differences between the injury scores in the two groups were observed; however, a 36% decrease in the neointimal thickness was observed in the r-TAP group. (From Ref. 36.)

tion and to a lesser extent thrombin generation influences late-outcome, vascular stenosis. The findings are consistent with the observation that fibrin deposition is an early event in neointimal formation. That heparin administration has not influenced neointimal formation in this model or a primate model (39) suggests that anticoagulants more effective than heparin may be required. A variety of factors may be responsible for the observed heparin resistance, including insensitivity of clot-bound factor Xa and thrombin to inhibition by antithrombin III–dependent inhibitors (40), presence of heparin-neutralizing proteins (e.g., platelet factor 4 or thrombospondin), heparin-induced platelet activation, and fibrin II monomer–mediated heparin neutralization.

Since thrombin is an important stimulator of platelet aggregation and secretion, r-TAP and PEG-hirudin may significantly decrease platelet recruitment. Data reported in abstract form on ^{111}indium-labeled platelet deposition after balloon angioplasty and stent placement in the porcine coronary artery indicate that r-TAP is very effective in reducing platelet deposition at the site of the injury compared to heparin (41). Hirudin effects on platelet deposition following angioplasty have also been reported (42).

There have been no reported studies on the effect of GPIIb/IIIa antagonists performed in the pig coronary restenosis model. However, recent studies of intimal hyperplasia after balloon/stent injury in pigs deficient in von Willebrand factor, in which significantly less neointimal thickening occurred in the von Willebrand pigs compared to normal animals despite similar degrees of arterial injury, suggest a platelet contribution to the process (43). Studies using a monoclonal antibody against GPIIb/IIIa (AZ-1) showed no effect on neointimal formation after angioplasty in cholesterol-fed rabbit femoral arteries (44). Nevertheless, inhibition of platelet adhesion, aggregation, and/or secretion remains a rational approach for inhibition of intimal hyperplasia in animal studies, especially in view of the ongoing clinical trials of GPIIb/IIIa inhibitors.

VI. FUTURE DIRECTIONS

As already noted, the utility of potent antithrombotics and anticoagulants may be limited by bleeding complications associated with their systemic administration. An exciting area of current investigation involves the development of delivery devices, including modified stents and infusion catheters, which may allow controlled, local administration of these agents. For example, the anti-GP IIb/IIIa antibody AZ-1 has been adsorbed onto stents coated with a cellulose polymer for evaluation of antiplatelet efficacy in rabbit iliac arteries (45). Effects of coating stents with heparin have been studied in rat arteriovenous shunts (46), as well as rabbit iliac (47), pig coronary (48), and baboon carotid arteries (49). In pilot clinical studies, local infusion of heparin immediately after angioplasty is being evaluated as a preventive measure for restenosis (50). Results using these emerging delivery technologies likely will reveal the full potential of antithrombotics and anticoagulants in the prevention of restenosis after angioplasty.

REFERENCES

1. Anderson H. Restenosis after coronary angioplasty. Disease-a-Month 1993; 39:613–670.
2. Holmes DR Jr., Schwartz RS. Restenosis: the clinical problem. Coronary Artery Dis 1993; 4(3):229–231.
3. Lee PC, Gibbons GH, Dzau VJ. Cellular and molecular mechanisms of coronary artery restenosis. Coronary Artery Dis 1993; 4:254–259.
4. Herrman JPR, Hermans WRM, Vos J, Serruys PW. Pharmacological approaches to the prevention of restenosis following angioplasty. The search for the Holy Grail? (Part I). Drugs 1993; 46:18–52.
5. Herrman JP, Hermans WR, Vos J, Surruys PW. Pharmacological approaches to the prevention of restenosis following angioplasty. The search for the Holy Grail? (Part II). Drugs 1993, 46(2):249–262.
6. den Heijer P, van Dijk RB, Hillege HL, Pentinga ML, Serruys PW, Lie KI. Serial Angioscopic and angiographic observations during the first hour after successful coronary angioplasty: a preamble to a multicenter trial addressing angioscopic markers for restenosis. Am Heart J 1994; 128:656–663.
7. Rupprecht HJ, Brenneke R, Bernhard G, Erbel R, PopT, Meyer J. Analysis of risk factors for restenosis after PTCA. Cathet Cardiovasc Diagn 1990; 19:151–159.
8. Herrman J-PR, Serruys PW. Thrombin and antithrombotic therapy in interventional cardiology. Texas Heart Inst J 1994; 21:138–147.
9. Schwartz L, Seidelin PH. Antithrombotic and thrombolytic therapy in patients undergoing coronary artery interventions: A review. Prog Cardiovasc Dis 1995; XXXVIII(1):67–86.
10. Barry WL, Sarembock IJ. Antiplatelet and anticoagulant therapy in patients undergoing percutaneous transluminal coronary angioplasty. Cardiol Clin 1994; 12:517–535.
11. Verstraete M. Biology and chemistry of thrombosis. In: Haber E, Braunwald E, eds. Thrombolysis. Basic contributions and Clinical Progress, St. Louis: Mosby Year Book, 1991:
12. Colman RW et al., eds. Hemostasis and Thrombosis: Basic Principles and Clinical Practice, 3rd ed. Philadelphia, Lippincott, 1993.
13. Handin RI et al., eds. Blood: Principles and Practice of Hematology and Hematologic Oncology, 4th ed. Philadelphia, Lippincott 1993.
14. Harker LA, Hanson SR, Runge MS. Thrombin hypothesis of thrombus generation and vascular lesion formation. Am J Cardiol 1995; 75:12B-17B.
15. Marmur JD, Merlini PA, Sharma SK, Khaghan N, Torre SR, Israel DH,

Ardissino D, Ambrose JA. Thrombin generation in human coronary arteries after percutaneous transluminal balloon angioplasty. J Am Coll Cardiol 1994; 24(6):1484–1491.
16. Yamazaki M. Factor Xa inhibitors. Drugs of the Future 1995; 20(9):911–918.
17. Deutsch E, Rao AK, Colman RW. Selective thrombin inhibitors: The next generation of anticoagulants. JACC 1993; 22:1089–1092.
18. Fitzgerald GA, Meagher EA. Antiplatelet drugs. Eur J Clin Invest 1994; 24:46–49.
19. Schwartz RS, Murphy JG, Edwards WD, Camrud AR, Garratt KN, Vlietstra RE, Holmes DR. Coronary artery restenosis and the "virginal membrane": smooth muscle cell proliferation and the intact internal elastic lamina. J Invasive Cardiol 1991; 3(1):3–9.
20. Lincoff AM, Tcheng JE, Ellis SG, Moliterno DJ, Kitt MM, Debowey D, Topol EJ. Randomized trial of platelet glycoprotein IIb/IIIa inhibition with Integrelin for preventin of restenosis following coronary intervention: the IMPACT II angiographic substudy. Circulation 1995; 92(suppl.):I-607.
21. Topol EJ, Califf RM, Weisman HF et al. Randomised trial of coronary intervention with antibody against platelet IIb/IIIa integrin for reduction of clinical restenosis: results at six months. Lancet 1994; 343:881–6.
22. Serruys, PW, Herrman JP, Simon R, Rutsch W, Bode C, Laarman GJ, van Dijk R, van den Bos AA, Umans VA, Fox KA, et al. A comparison of hirudin with heparin in the prevention of restenosis after coronary angioplasty. N Engl J Med 1995; 333:757–763.
23. Becker RC. Thrombin antagonists and antiplatelet agents. Am J Cardiol 1992; 69:39A–51A.
24. Harker LA. Strategies for inhibiting the effects of thrombin. Blood Coag Fibrinol 1994; 5(1):S47–S58.
25. Prescott MF, Webb RL, Reidy MA. Angiotensin-converting enzyme inhibitor versus angiotensin II, AT1 receptor antagonist. Effects on smooth muscle cell migration and proliferation after balloon catheter injury. Am J Pathol 1991; 139:1291–1296.
26. Olson LV, Clowes AW, Reidy MA. Inhibition of smooth muscle cell proliferation in injured rat arteries. J Clin Invest 1992; 90:2044–2049.
27. Ragosta M, Gimple LW, Gertz SD, Dunwiddie CT, Vlasuk GP, Haber HL, Powers ER, Roberts WC, Sarembock IJ. Specific factor Xa inhibition reduces restenosis after balloon angioplasty of atherosclerotic femoral arteries in rabbits. Circulation 1994; 89:1262–1271.
28. Schwartz RS, Murphy JG, Edwards WD, Camrud AR, Vlietstra RE, Holmes DR Jr. Restenosis after balloon angioplasty: A practical proliferative model in porcine coronary arteries. Circulation 1990; 82:2190–2200.
29. Schwartz RS, Edward WD, Huber KC, et al. Coronary restenosis: prospects for solution and new perspectives from a porcine model. Mayo Clin Proc 1993; 68(1):54–62.
30. Neeper MP, Waxman L. Smith De, et al. Characterization of recombinant tick anticoagulant peptide: A highly selective inhibitor of blood coagulation factor Xa. J Biol Chem 1990; 265:17746–17752.

31. Lehman ED, Shaefer TF, Przysiecki CT et al. Large-scale purification and characterization of recombinant tick anticoagulant peptide. Chromatographia 1992; 574:225-35.
32. Dunwiddie C, Thornberry NA, Bull HG, et al. Antistasin, a leech-derived inhibitor of factor Xa. Kinetic analysis of enzyme inhibition and identification of the reactive site. J Biol Chem 1989; 264(28):16694–16699.
33. Jordan SP, Waxman L, Smith DE, Vlasuk GP. Tick anticoagulant peptide: kinetic analysis of the recombinant inhibitor with blood coagulation factor Xa. Biochemistry 1990; 29(50):11095–11100.
34. Jordan SP, Mao SS, Lewis SD, Shafer JA. Reaction pathway for inhibition of blood coagulation factor Xa by tick anticoagulant peptide. Biochemistry 1992; 31(23):5374–5380.
35. Jang Y, Guzman LA, Lincoff M, Gottsauner-Wolf M, Forudi F, Hart CE, Courtman DW, Ezban M, Ellis SG, Topol EJ. Influence of blockade at specific levels of the coagulant cascae on restenosis in a rabbit atherosclerotic femoral artery injury model. Circulation 1995; 92:3041–3049.
36. Schwartz RS, Holder DJ, Holmes DR Jr, Veinot JP, Camrud AR, Jorgeson MA, Johnson RG JR. Neointimal thickening after severe coronary artery injury is limited by short-term administration of a factor Xa inhibitor results in a porcine model. Circulation 1996; 93:1542–1548.
37. Johnson RG, Huckle WR, McFall RC, Fujita T, Holder DJ, Powers M, Acker WR, Schwartz RS, Drag MD. Aggressive heparin administration and neointimal formation in a porcine coronary artery model of restenosis. Circulation 1995; 92(8):I-785.
38. Srivatsa SS, Edwards WD, Simari RD, Holmes DR, Schwartz RS. Chronic hirudin infusion reduces neointimal thickening after injury in a porcine coronary model. J Am Coll Cardiol 1995(Feb.):302A (abst).
39. Geary RL, Koyama N, Wang TW, Vergel S, Clowes AW. Failure of heparin to inhibit intimal hyperplasia in injured baboon arteries. The role of heparin-sensitive and -insensitive pathways in the stimulation of smooth muscle cell migration and proliferation. Circulation 1995; 91:2972–2981.
40. Eisenberg PR, Siegel JE, Abendschein DR, Miletich JP. Importance of factor Xa in determining the procoagulant activity of whole-blood clots. J Clin Invest 1993; 91:1877–1883.
41. Huckle WR, Rogers IT, Acker WR, Lodge KE, Holder DJ, Johnson RG Jr. Inhibition of acute platelet deposition in porcine coronary arteries after percutaneous transluminal coronary angioplasty (PTCA) by a factor Xa inhibitor. Circulation 1995; 92(8):I-684.
42. Heras M, Chesebro JH, Penny WJ, Bailey KB, Badimon L, Fuster V. Effects of thrombin inhibition on the development of acute platelet-thrombus deposition during angioplasty in pigs. Circulation 1989; 79:657–665.
43. Schwartz RS, Bowie EJW, Nichols WL, Edwards WD, Camrud AR, Jorgenson MA, Holmes DR. The effect of homozygous von Willebrand disease on neointimal formation following coronary artery injury: a quantitative study in pigs. Atherosclerosis (submitted).
44. Azrin MA, Ling FS, Chen QS, Pawashe A, Migliaccio F, Homer R, Todd M,

Ezekowitz MD. Preparation, characterization and evaluation of a monoclonal antibody against the rabbit platelet glycoprotein IIb/IIIa in an experimental angioplasty model. Circ Res 1994; 75:268–277.
45. Aggarwal RK, Ireland DFC, Azrin MA, Ezekowitz MD, deBono DP, Gershlick AH. Antithrombotic properties of stents eluting platelet glycoprotein IIb/IIIa antibody. Circulation 1995; 92(suppl 1):I-488.
46. DeScheerder IK, Wang K, Wilczec KL, Meuleman D, Piessens JH. Heparin coating of metallic stents decrease their thrombogenicity but does not decrease neointimal hyperplasia. Circulation 1995; 92(suppl. 1):I-537.
47. Stratienko AA, Zhu D, Lambert CR, Palmaz J, Schatz RA, Santamore WP. Improved thromboresistance of heparin-coated Palmaz-Schatz stents in an animal model. Circulation 1993; 88(suppl 1):I-596.
48. van der Giessen WJ, Hardhammar PA, van Beusekom HMM, Emanuelsson HU, Tang ZH, Verdouw PD, Serruys PW. Prevention of (sub)acute thrombosis using heparin-coated stents. Circulation 1994; 90(suppl 1):I-650.
49. Chronos NAF, Robinson KA, Kelly AB, Yoklavich M, Rowland SM, Narayan PN, Harker LA, Hanson SR. Thrombogenicity of tantalum stents is decreased by surface heparin bonding: scintigraphy of 111-In-platelet deposition in baboon carotid arteries. Circulation 1995; 92(suppl 1):I-490.
50. Camenzind E, Kint PP, Dimario C, Ligthart J, van der Giessen W, Boersma E, Serruys PW. Intracoronary heparin delivery in humans, acute feasibility and long-term results. Circulation 1995;92:2463–2472.

12

Insights into Vascular Biology via Targeted Gene Inactivation and Adenovirus-Mediated Gene Transfer of the Plasminogen System

Peter Carmeliet and Désiré Collen
Flanders Interuniversity Institute for Biotechnology, Leuven, Belgium

I. THE PLASMINOGEN SYSTEM

The plasminogen system is composed of the inactive proenzyme plasminogen (Plg), which can be converted to plasmin by either of two plasminogen activators: tissue-type plasminogen activator (t-PA) and urokinase-type plasminogen activator (u-PA) (1). This system is controlled at the level of plasminogen activators by plasminogen activator inhibitors (PAIs), of which PAI-1 is believed to be physiologically the most important (2), and at the level of plasmin by α_2-antiplasmin (1,2). Other inhibitors include PAI-2, proteinase nexin-1, and α_2-macroglobulin (1). Due to its fibrin specificity, t-PA is primarily involved in clot dissolution, although it has also been involved in ovulation, bone remodeling, and brain function (3). u-PA, on the other hand, binds a cellular receptor, the urokinase receptor (u-PAR), and has been implicated in pericellular proteolysis during cell migration and tissue remodeling in a variety of normal and pathological processes, including ovulation, trophoblast invasion, angiogenesis, keratinocyte migration, inflammation, and cancer (4,5). Binding of u-PA to u-PAR, which has been identified on many diverse cell types, including monocytes, endothelial, and smooth muscle cells (4–6), can localize u-PA on the cell surface, thereby accelerating the conversion of plasminogen to plasmin and possibly reducing its susceptibility to inhibition by PAIs (7).

Despite circumstantial evidence, it is as yet unclear whether or in what conditions binding of u-PA to its receptor is (absolutely) required for plasminogen activation and cellular migration in vivo. Plasmin is a broad substrate-specific proteinase that is able to degrade fibrin and a variety of extracellular matrix proteins either directly or indirectly via activation of other matrix-degrading enzymes such as the metalloproteinases (8). Cell-specific clearance of plasminogen activators by LDL receptor-related protein (LRP) or gp330 may modulate pericellular plasmin proteolysis (9).

II. TARGETED INACTIVATION AND ADENOVIRUS-MEDIATED TRANSFER OF GENES IN MICE

Two gene technologies developed over the last decade have made possible the manipulation of the genetic balance of candidate molecules in a controllable manner such that novel insights into their in vivo role can be obtained. Targeted inactivation of genes via homologous recombination in embryonic stem cells allows us to study the consequences of single or combined deficiencies of gene products in transgenic "knock-out" mice (10), whereas adenovirus-mediated gene transfer makes it possible to obtain transient but significant overexpression of target genes (11). In mice, systemic administration of recombinant adenoviruses can induce the expression of target genes to plasma levels of >10 μg/ml. By combining these technologies, e.g., adenovirus-mediated gene transfer in knock-out mice, expression of the inactivated target gene can be restored. Such studies do not only allow us to generate disease models, but in addition offer the possibility of rescuing a pathological phenotype and evaluating gene therapeutic strategies. Homologous recombination was used to generate transgenic mice with single or combined deficiencies of t-PA (12), u-PA (12), PAI-1 (13,14), u-PAR (15–17), and Plg (18,19), whereas recombinant adenoviruses expressing t-PA (20) or PAI-1 (Carmeliet, Gerard, and Collen, unpublished observations) were constructed to induce overexpression of these genes.

III. HEALTH AND SURVIVAL

No effects on health and survival were observed in t-PA–, u-PAR–, or PAI-1–deficient mice (12,13,15). A small percentage of u-PA–deficient mice developed chronic (nonhealing) ulcerations and rectal prolapse but without effect on survival (12). Plg-deficient (18,19) and combined t-PA:u-PA–deficient (12) but not combined t-PA:u-PAR–deficient mice (17) developed chronic ulcerations and rectal prolapse, but, in addition, these mice suffered significant growth retardation, developed a wasting syndrome with anemia, dyspnea, lethargia, and cachexia, and had a significantly shorter life span. Generalized thrombosis in the gastrointestinal tract, in the lungs, and in other organs (including gonads, liver, and kidney) might, at least in part, explain their increased morbidity and mortality. The difference in phenotypes between combined t-PA:u-PAR–deficient and t-PA:u-PA–deficient mice indicates that sufficient pericellular plasmin proteolysis can occur, even in the absence of u-PAR, and suggests, therefore, that binding of u-PA is not required for these processes. That the phenotype of the Plg-deficient and combined t-PA:u-PA–deficient mice is very familiar suggests that t-PA and u-PA are the only important physiological plasminogen activators in vivo.

IV. NEOINTIMA FORMATION

Cardiovascular ischemia due to atherothrombosis is a leading cause of morbidity and mortality. Widely used therapeutic interventions such as bypass surgery, percutaneous transluminal balloon angioplasty, atherectomy, or the in situ application of vascular stents restore blood flow and improve tissue oxygenation, but "restenosis" of the vessel occurs in 30–50% of treated patients within 3–6 months. This may result from remodeling of the vessel wall (21) and/or accumulation of cells and extracellular matrix in the intimal or adventitial layer. Several mechanisms are believed to participate in the intimal thickening as part of a hyperactive wound-healing response, including intraluminal thrombosis, proliferation, apoptosis, or migration of smooth muscle cells (22–25). Experimental animal studies have documented the role of various growth factors and cytokines in the proliferation or migration of smooth muscle cells (26,27). In addition, proteinases might be involved in the degradation of the extracellular basement membrane surrounding the smooth muscle cells, allowing them to migrate to distant sites. Two proteinase systems have been implicated, the plasminogen (or fibrinolytic) system (28–32) and the metalloproteinase system (33–37), which in concert can degrade most extracellular matrix proteins.

The constitutive expression of t-PA by endothelial cells and of PAI-1 by medial vascular smooth muscle cells suggests a role of the plasminogen system in maintaining vascular patency and hemostasis (38,39). Following transient reduction of t-PA as a result of endothelial cell damage (28), u-PA and t-PA activity in the vessel wall are significantly increased, coincident with the time of smooth muscle cell proliferation and migration (28–31). This increase in plasmin proteolysis is counterbalanced by increased expression of PAI-1 in injured smooth muscle and endothelial cells and by its release from accumulating platelets (40). Expression of components of the fibrinolytic system is also induced in cultured endothelial cells, smooth muscle cells, or macrophages as a result of wounding or treatment with growth factors and cytokines that are released after injury (4,41). t-PA has also been proposed to act as an autocrine mitogen after injury (42). Thus, although these observations suggest a role of the plasminogen system in matrix remodeling, such as occurs during plaque ulceration and the formation of aneurysms (43,44), in thrombosis (39,45,46), passivation of the injured luminal vessel surface, and migration or proliferation of vascular cells, its precise and causative role in these in vivo processes remain to be determined.

A. Models to Study Vascular Wound Healing and Neointima Formation in Mice

Several models of arterial injury have been used to induce arterial neointima formation in different species. Extensively investigated models involve the use of a balloon catheter or stents to overextend and/or denude the vessel (47,48). They have gained much attention not only for their reproducibility and feasibility but also because such injury resembles the injury inflicted in patients undergoing balloon angioplasty or stenting. Balloon catheters or stents of the appropriate size are, however, not available for use in mice. Although intraluminal application of a curved flexible wire was used in one study to induce neointima formation in carotid arteries of mice (49), the small dimensions of the arteries render such manipulations a technical challenge.

We have compared two different techniques to induce neointima formation in the mouse: a clinically relevant model based on the use of a guidewire to overextend and abrade the vessel, which resembles the mechanical injury that occurs after balloon angioplasty in patients and in existing animal models, and an experimental model based on the use of an electric current, which allowed us to examine the molecular mechanisms of neointima formation in a technically less challenging way (P. Carmeliet et al., unpublished). The electric current induces a more severe injury across the vessel wall than the balloon catheter– or the filament loop–induced injury ("gentle injury") in the rat carotid artery (22,27,50), resulting in necrosis of all viable medial cells. This has implications for the understanding of vascular wound healing following electric injury. In the mechanically injured arteries, residual viable smooth muscle cells over the entire injury start to proliferate and migrate across the elastic membrane and, consequently, form a uniform neointima over the entire injured length (22,28). In the electrically injured arteries, the death of all viable medial cells makes it necessary for wound healing to start from the adjacent uninjured segments. Presumably, smooth muscle cells in these adjacent regions proliferate and migrate, resulting in the progression of a neointima from the uninjured borders into the central necrotic region. Although the electric current model does not have a direct clinical correlate, similar genotype-specific differences in neointima formation between the electric and mechanical model were observed, indicating that the observations are not model-dependent (51).

B. u-PA–Induced Plasmin Proteolysis Mediates Smooth Muscle Cell Migration

Microscopic and morphometric analysis, both in the mechanical as well as in the electric injury model, revealed that the rate and degree of neointima formation (determined by the percent luminal stenosis or the cross-sectional neointimal area) and the amount of accumulated neointimal cells were similar after injury in wild-type, t-PA–, and u-PAR–deficient arteries (51). However, neointima formation in PAI-1–deficient arteries occurred sooner postinjury and was characterized by a greater smooth muscle cell accumulation, which more frequently occluded the lumen (51). In contrast, both the degree and the rate of arterial neointima formation in u-PA–, Plg-, and combined t-PA:u-PA–deficient arteries was significantly reduced up to 6 weeks postinjury (51). In the electrically injured arteries, a small neointima developed only at the borders of the injury with residual necrosis in the center, suggesting that smooth muscle cells did not migrate into the necrotic center. Evaluation of the possible mechanisms responsible for these genotype-specific differences in neointima formation revealed that remodeling of the vessel wall (defined as a change in the size of the cross-sectional area within the external elastic laminae) was not different for the genotypes, nor was the degree of cellular proliferation in the media and neointima (51). Rather, impaired migration of smooth muscle cells appeared to cause reduced neointima formation in mice lacking u-PA–mediated plasmin proteolysis, since the progression of the neointima from the borders of the injured segment toward the necrotic center (quantified by determining the percentage of sections throughout the injured region revealing a neointima) occurred at a rate that was similar in wild-type, t-PA–, and u-PAR–deficient mice, enhanced in PAI-1–deficient mice but reduced in u-PA–, Plg-, and combined t-PA:u-PA–deficient mice (51). Table 1 summarizes the observations of vascular wound healing in the different knock-out mice.

These studies demonstrate that plasmin proteolysis promotes vascular wound healing and neointima formation, whereas inhibition of plasminogen activation by PAI-1 significantly impairs and delays this process.

Table 1 Effects of Targeted Gene Inactivation and Adenovirus-Mediated Gene Transfer of the Plasminogen System on Vascular Wound Healing and Fibrin Surveillance

Mice	Neointima formation	Fibrin deposition		Fibrin degradation	
		Spontaneous	Induced	Plasma clot lysis	Matrix breakdown
Wild type	++	−	++	+++	++++
t-PA$^{-/-}$	++	−	++++	+	++++
Ad.t-PA in t-PA$^{-/-}$	N.D	N.D.	N.D.	++++	N.D.
u-PA$^{-/-}$	−[a]	+	++++	+++	−
TU$^{-/-}$	−[a]	++++	++++	−[b]	−
u-PAR$^{-/-}$	++	−	++	+++	+++[c]
TR$^{-/-}$	N.D.	+	N.D.	N.D.	N.D.
PAI-1$^{-/-}$	++++	−	−	++++	++++
Ad.PAI-1 in PAI$^{-/-}$	−[a]	N.D.	N.D.	−	N.D.
Plg$^{-/-}$	−[a]	++++	++++	−[b]	−

Overview of the consequences of targeted gene inactivation or rescue by adenovirus-mediated gene transfer on neointima formation, fibrin deposition (thrombosis), and fibrin degradation (thrombolysis) semi-quantitatively expressed on a scale from "−" (very little to absent response) to "++++" (maximal response).

[a]Neointima formation in these mice is reduced but not absent (51). Intra- and extravascular fibrin deposition was examined in knock-out mice without (spontaneous) or with (induced) endotoxin challenge, locally injected in the footpad as described in Refs. 12 and 14. Fibrin degradation was evaluated by monitoring lysis of a ^{125}I-labeled fibrin pulmonary plasma clot or degradation of a ^{125}I-labeled fibrin matrix, as described in Refs. 12 and 14.

[b]Spontaneous lysis in these knock-out mice occurs at a very slow rate and only becomes significant after 72 h (12,18).

[c]Degradation by u-PAR$^{-/-}$ macrophages occurred at a somewhat slower initial rate, but was similar after 8 h (15,51).

t-PA-/-: t-PA deficient; u-PA deficient: u-PAR-/-: u-PAR deficient; PAI-1/-/-: PAI-1 deficient; TU-/-: combined t-PA and u-PA deficient; TR-/-: combined t-PA and u-PAR deficient; Plg-/-: plasminogen deficient; Ad.t-PA in t-PA-/-: intravenous injection of recombinant adenovirus expressing human t-PA in t-PA–deficient mice; Ad.PAI-1 in PAI-1-/-: intravenous injection of recombinant adenovirus expressing human PAI-1 in PAI-1–deficient mice; N.D.: not done.

They are consistent with other observations that the plasmin inhibitor tranexamic acid inhibits migration of smooth muscle cells across the internal elastic lamina in the rat carotid balloon injury model (29) and with initial results that transgenic mice overexpressing human PAI-1 show reduced neointima formation following cold-induced vascular injury (Di Scullio et al., personal communication). Immunoneutralization of u-PA has been shown to reduce migration of cultured smooth muscle cells and endothelial cells in rat (4,52). Unpublished studies further demonstrate that migration of cultured u-PA–deficient smooth muscle cells (Herbert et al., personal communication) and of u-PA–deficient endothelial cells (van Hinsbergh et al., personal communication) is reduced. A role for u PA in cellular migration has also been documented for a variety of other cell types, including tumor cells, keratinocytes, corneal epithelial cells, and monocytes/macrophages (4,53,54).

A surprising observation was that deficiency of u-PA, but not of u-PAR, reduced neointima formation in vivo. Since u-PAR is expressed by smooth muscle cells and endothelial cells (5,6,51), binding of u-PA to its cellular receptor is not required for migration of these cells. Such a conclusion is supported by previous observations that an increase in soluble (not membrane-bound) human u-PA in murine tumor cells enhances their invasiveness (55) and that scavenging of soluble u-PA by a truncated (non–membrane-anchored) u-PAR impairs cellular invasion (56). Furthermore, a membrane-anchored form of u-PA catalyzes plasminogen activation on the cell surface with characteristics, comparable to those of u-PAR–bound u-PA (57), suggesting that cell surface localization rather than binding to u-PAR is important. The kinetic advantage resulting from u-PAR–accelerated plasminogen activation may be irrelevant for certain u-PA–dependent phenomena that develop over long time periods, or u-PA may be localized to the cell surface via binding to other molecules, such as fibrin, plasminogen, extracellular matrix, or cell-adhesion molecules (58–60). Whatever the mechanism, pericellular proteolysis can still occur in the absence of u-PAR. This is also evidenced by our observations that degradation of ^{125}I-labeled fibrin over 8 h is only transiently affected by u-PAR deficiency (15,51) and that thrombosis, sterility, and organ dysfunction in combined t-PA:u-PAR–deficient mice is significantly less severe than in combined t-PA:u-PA–deficient mice (12,17). It should be noticed, however, that the lack of an appreciable effect on neointima formation in u-PAR knock-out mice does not exclude a role for this receptor in other biological processes (e.g., cancer), since the relevance of u-PAR may depend on the amount and the cell-specific, temporal, and spatial expression of u-PAR. Whether, to what extent, and under which conditions u-PAR may contribute to its importance in other u-PA–dependent phenomena such as cancer (61,62) or antiogenesis (Rosenberg et al., personal communication) remains to be determined.

C. Inhibition of Neointima Formation by Adenovirus-Mediated PAI-1 Gene Transfer

The involvement of plasmin proteolysis in neointima formation was supported by intravenous injection in PAI-1–deficient mice of a replication-defective adenovirus that expresses human PAI-1, which resulted in more than 1000-fold increased plasma PAI-1 levels and in a similar degree of inhibition of neointima formation as observed in u-PA–deficient mice (51). Proteinase-inhibitors have been suggested as anti-restenosis drugs and recently, the short-term benefit of a metalloproteinase inhibitor in reducing neointima formation in balloon-injured rat carotid arteries was demonstrated (34). Induction of PAI-1 has also been reported to reduce neointima formation in cold-injured arteries (Di Scullio et al., personal communication). Our studies suggest that strategies aimed at reducing u-PA–mediated plasmin proteolysis may be beneficial for reduction or prevention of restenosis. However, antifibrinolytic strategies should be targeted at inhibiting plasmin proteolysis and not at preventing the interaction of u-PA with its receptor.

V. THROMBOSIS AND THROMBOLYSIS

t-PA is believed to be primarily responsible for removal of fibrin from the vascular tree, as mediated by specific affinity for fibrin, resulting in clot-restricted plasminogen activation (1). The role of u-PA in thrombolysis is less well defined. It lacks affinity for fibrin and requires conversion from a single-chain precursor to a catalytically active two-chain derivative (1). Whether, to what extent, and under which conditions u-PA might participate in fibrin clot dissolution in vivo remain to be identified. Other plasminogen activation pathways, such as the "intrinsic" pathway (involving blood coagulation factor XII, high molecular weight kininogen, prekallikrein, and possibly u-PA) (63) as well as plasminogen-independent mechanisms (64) have been proposed to contribute to clot lysis, but their role in vivo remained to be defined.

Deficient fibrinolytic activity, e.g., resulting from increased plasma PAI-1 levels or reduced plasma t-PA or plasminogen levels, might contribute to the development of thrombotic events (65–68). Elevated plasma PAI-1 levels have indeed been correlated with a higher risk of deep venous thrombosis and of thrombosis during hemolytic uremic syndrome, disseminated intravascular coagulation, sepsis, surgery, and trauma (67–70). PAI-1 plasma levels have also been elevated in patients with ischemic heart disease, angina pectoris, and recurrent myocardial infarction (71,72). However, the acute phase reactant behavior of PAI-1 (73) does not make it possible to deduce whether increased PAI-1 levels are a cause or consequence of thrombosis. To date, abnormal fibrin clot surveillance resulting from genetic deficiencies of t-PA or u-PA has not been reported in humans, but quantitative and qualitative deficiencies of plasminogen have been associated with increased thrombotic tendency (65,66).

A. Fibrin Deposits and Pulmonary Plasma Clot Lysis in Transgenic Mice

Microscopic analysis of tissues from u-PA–deficient mice revealed occasional minor fibrin deposits in liver and intestines and excessive fibrin deposition in chronic nonhealing skin ulcerations (12), whereas in t-PA–, u-PAR–, or PAI-1–deficient mice, no spontaneous fibrin deposits were observed (12–16). Mice with a single deficiency of Plg or a combined deficiency of t-PA and u-PA, however, revealed extensive fibrin deposits in several organs associated with ischemic necrosis, possibly resulting from thrombotic occlusions (12,18,19). Interestingly, mice with a combined deficiency of t-PA and u-PAR did not display such excessive fibrin deposits (17), indicating that u-PA–mediated plasmin proteolysis can still occur in the absence of u-PAR, and that binding of u-PA to u-PAR is not required for pericellular proteolysis in these processes. Mice with a single deficiency of t-PA or u-PA were significantly more susceptible to development of venous thrombosis following local injection of proinflammatory endotoxin in the footpad (12). Hypoxia has also been demonstrated to induce ^{125}I-fibrin–labeled deposition in the lung arteries of t-PA– or u-PA–deficient mice, but not in wild-type or PAI-1–deficient mice (Stern et al., personal communication). The increased susceptibility of t-PA–deficient mice to endotoxin and the severe spontaneous thrombotic phenotype of Plg-deficient and combined t-PA:u-PA–deficient mice could be explained by their significantly reduced rate of spontaneous lysis of ^{125}I-fibrin–labeled plasma clots, injected via the jugular vein and embolized into the pulmonary arteries (12,18). Notably, spontaneous lysis of pulmonary plasma clots was most reduced in Plg-deficient or combined t-PA:u-PA–deficient mice, suggesting cooperation between both activators. On the contrary, PAI-1–deficient mice were virtually protected against development of venous thrombosis following injection of endotoxin, consistent with their ability to lyse ^{125}I-fibrin–labeled plasma clots at a significantly higher rate than wild-type mice (14). This difference in clot lysis became even more significant after pretreatment of the mice with endotoxin (14) or by incorporating increasing amounts of platelets in the pulmonary plasma clots (Carmeliet et al., unpublished observations). Recent data demonstrate that the resistance of platelet-enriched plasma clots to spontaneous lysis in wild-type mice is reduced in PAI-1–deficient mice (Carmeliet et al., unpublished data). The increased susceptibility of u-PA–deficient mice to thrombosis associated with inflammation or injury, might be due to their impaired macrophage function. Indeed, thioglycolate-stimulated macrophages (known to express cell-associated u-PA) isolated from u-PA–deficient mice, lacked plasminogen-dependent breakdown of ^{125}I-labeled fibrin (fibrinolysis) or of ^{3}H-labeled subendothelial matrix (mostly collagenolysis), whereas macrophages from t-PA−, u-PAR−, or PAI-1–deficient mice did not (12,15). An overview of the thrombosis/thrombolysis phenotypes in the different knock out mice is displayed in Table 1.

B. Adenovirus-Mediated Transfer of t-PA or PAI-1

More recently, we have used adenovirus-mediated transfer of fibrinolytic system components in knock-out mice in an attempt to revert their phenotypes. Intravenous injection of adenoviruses, expressing a recombinant PAI-1–resistant human t-PA (rt-PA) gene in t-PA–deficient mice increased plasma rt-PA levels 100-to 1000-fold above normal and restored their impaired thrombolytic potential in a dose-related way (20). Conversely, adenoviral-mediated transfer of recombinant human PAI-1 in PAI-1–deficient mice reduced the increased thrombolytic potential of PAI-1–deficient mice (P. Carmeliet et al., unpublished). The model of adenovirus-mediated t-PA transfer is currently being used as a reporter bioassay system to evaluate the immunological aspects of adenovirus-mediated gene transfer or the regulation of gene expression by tissue-specific or inducible promoters.

Collectively, these gene targeting and gene transfer studies confirm the importance of the plasminogen system in maintaining vascular patency and indicate that both plasminogen activators significantly cooperate in this process. Interestingly, u-PA appears to play a more significant role than previously anticipated in the prevention of fibrin deposition during conditions of inflammation or injury. A surprising finding, however, is that u-PA can still exert significant pericellular proteolysis in the absence of u-PAR, suggesting that binding of u-PA to u-PAR is not required. Furthermore, t-PA and u-PA appear to be the only significant physiological plasminogen activators.

VI. HEMOSTASIS

Hemostasis involves platelet deposition and coagulation to stabilize hemostatic plug. Failure to stabilize the clot, e.g., as a result of hyperfibrinolytic activity, might result in delayed rebleeding. A hemorrhagic tendency has indeed been observed in patients with increased plasma t-PA or reduced plasma a_2-antiplasmin or PAI-1 activity levels (2,74,75). Delayed rebleeding might explain the hemorrhagic tendency in transgenic mice, expressing high levels of plasma u-PA (76), and in transgenic mice, overexpressing GM-CSF, with increased production of u-PA by peritoneal macrophages (77). In contrast to patients with low or absent plasma PAI-1 levels, PAI-1–deficient mice did not reveal spontaneous or delayed rebleeding, even after trauma

(14). Lower plasma PAI-1 levels and the occurrence of alternative PAIs in murine plasma (unpublished data) might explain the less pronounced hyperfibrinolytic phenotype and the species-specific difference in plasmin proteolysis control.

VII. CONCLUSIONS

Targeted gene inactivation and adenovirus-mediated gene transfer in mice are valuable tools to investigate the molecular mechanisms underlying neointima formation, thrombosis, and hemostasis. Such studies have provided novel insights in the role of the plasminogen system components in vascular biology and, as discussed elsewhere, in the role of the plasminogen and coagulation system in development, reproduction, glomerulonephritis, skin healing, lung inflammation, corneal ulceration, bone remodeling, cancer, blood vessel development, atherosclerosis, and brain function (78).

ACKNOWLEDGMENTS

The authors are grateful to the members of the Center for Transgene Technology and Gene Therapy and Drs. V. Ploplis, E. Plow, and R. C. Mulligan for their contribution to these studies.

REFERENCES

1. Collen D, Lijnen HR. Basic and clinical aspects of fibrinolysis and thrombolysis. Blood 1991; 78:3114–3124.
2. Schneiderman J, Loskutoff DJ. Plasminogen activator inhibitors. Trends Cardiovasc Med 1991; 1:99–102.
3. Vassalli JD, Sappino AP, Belin D. The plasminogen activator/plasmin system. J Clin Invest 1991; 88:1067–1072.
4. Blasi F, Conese M, Moller LB, Pedersen N, Cavallaro U, Cubellis MV, Fazioli F, Hernandez-Marrero L, Limongi P, Munoz-Canoves P, Resnati M, Rüttininen L, Sidenius N, Soravia E, Soria MR, Stoppelli MP, Talarico D, Teesalu T, Valcamonica S. The urokinase receptor: structure, regulation and inhibitor-mediated internalization. Fibrinolysis 1994; 1(suppl. 1):182–188.
5. Vassalli JD. The urokinase receptor. Fibrinolysis 1994; 8(suppl. 1):172–181.
6. Reuning U, Bang NU. Regulation of the urokinase-type plasminogen activator receptor on vascular smooth muscle cells is under the control of thrombin and other mitogens. Arteriosclerosis Thromb 1992; 12:1161–1170.
7. Behrendt N, Ronne E, Dano K. The structure and function of the urokinase receptor, a membrane protein governing plasminogen activation on the cell surface. Biol Chem Hoppe-Seyler 1995; 376:276–279.
8. Saksela O, Rifkin D. Rev. Cell. Biol. 1988; 4:93–126.

9. Andreasen PA, Sottrup-Jensen Li, et al. Receptor-mediated endocytosis of plasminogen activators and activator/inhibitor complexes. FEBS Lett 1994; 338:239–245.
10. Soriano P. Gene targeting in embryonic stem cells. Ann Rev Neurosci 1995; 18:1–18.
11. Schneider MD, Frech BA. The advent of adenovirus: gene therapy for cardiovascular disease. Circulation 1995; 88:1937–1942.
12. Carmeliet P, Schoonjans L, Kieckens L, Ream B, Degen J, Bronson R, De Vos R, van den Oord JJ, Collen D, Mulligan RCM. Physiological consequences of loss of plasminogen activator gene function in mice. Nature 1994; 368:419–424.
13. Carmeliet P, Kieckens L, Schoonjans L, Ream B, Van Nuffelen A, Prendergast G, Cole M, Bronson R, Collen D, Mulligan RCM. Plasminogen activator inhibitor-1 gene-deficient mice. I. Generation by homologous recombination and characterization. J Clin Invest 1993; 92:2746–2755.
14. Carmeliet P, Stassen JM, Schoonjans L, Ream B, van den Oord JJ, De Mol M, Mulligan RC, Collen D. Plasminogen activator inhibitor-1 gene-deficient mice. II. Effects on hemostasis, thrombosis and thrombolysis. J Clin Invest 1993; 92:2756–2760.
15. Dewerchin M, Van Nuffelen, Wallays G, Bouché A, Moons L, Carmeliet P, Mulligan RCM, Collen D. Generation and characterization of urokinase receptor-deficient mice. J Clin Invest. In press.
16. Bugge TH, Suh TT, Flick MJ, Daugherty CC, Romer J, Solberg H, Ellis V, Dano K, Degen JL. The receptor for urokinase-type plasminogen activator is not essential for mouse development or fertility. J Biol Chem 1995; 270:16886–16894.
17. Bugge TH, Flick MJ, Danton MJ, Daugherty CC, Dano K, Carmeliet P, Collen D, Degen JL. Urokinase-type plasminogen activator contributes to fibrin clearance by receptor-dependent and receptor-independent pathways. Submitted.
18. Ploplis V, Carmeliet P, Vazirzadeh S, Van Vlaenderen I, Moons L, Plow E, Collen D. Effects of disruption of the plasminogen gene on thrombosis, growth and health in mice. Circulation 1995; 92:2585–2593.
19. Bugge TH, Flick MJ, Daugherty CC, Degen JL. Plasminogen deficiency causes severe thrombosis but is compatible with development and reproduction. Genes Dev 1995; 9:794–807.
20. Carmeliet P, Stassen JM, Collen D, Meidell R, Gerard R. Adenovirus-mediated gene transfer of rt-PA restores thrombolysis in t-PA deficient mice. Submitted.
21. Kakuta T, Currier JW, Haudenschild CC, Ryan TJ, Faxon DP. Differences in compensatory vessel enlargement, not intimal formation, account for restenosis after angioplasty in the hypercholesterolemic rabbit model. Circulation 1994; 89:2809–2815.
22. Clowes AW, Reidy MA. Prevention of stenosis after vascular reconstruction: pharmacologic control of intimal hyperplasia—a review. J Vasc Surg 1991; 13:885–891.

23. Lee PC, Gibbons GH, Dzau VJ. Cellular and molecular mechanisms of coronary artery restenosis. Coronary Artery Dis 1993; 4:254–259.
24. Casscells W. Migration of smooth muscle and endothelial cells. Critical events in restenosis. Circulation 1992; 86:723–729.
25. Schwartz SM, Reidy MA, O'Brien ERM. Assessment of factors important in atherosclerotic occlusion and restenosis. Thromb Haemost 1995; 74:541–551.
26. Libby P, Schwartz D, Brogi E, Tanaka H, Clinton SK. A cascade model for restenosis. A special case of atherosclerotic progression. Circulation 1992; 86(suppl. III):47–52.
27. Reidy MA, Fingerle J, Lindner V. Factors controlling the development of arterial lesions after injury. Circulation 1992; 86(suppl. III):43–46.
28. Clowes AW, Clowes MM, Au YPT, Reidy MA, Belin D. Smooth muscle cells express urokinase during mitogenesis and tissue-type plasminogen activator during migration in injured rat carotid artery. Circ Res 1990; 67:61–67.
29. Jackson CL, Raines EW, Ross R, Reidy MA. Role of endogenous platelet-derived growth factor in arterial smooth muscle cell migration after balloon catheter injury. Arterioscler Thromb 1993; 13:1218–1226.
30. Jackson CL, Reidy MA. The role of plasminogen activation in smooth muscle cell migration after arterial injury. Ann NY Acad Sci 1992; 667:141–150.
31. Reidy MA, Jackson C, Lindner V. Neointimal proliferation: control of vascular smooth muscle cell growth. Vasc Med Rev 1992; 3:156–167.
32. Clowes AW, Clowes MM, Kirkman TR, Jackson CL, Au YP, Kenagy R. Heparin inhibits the expression of tissue-type plasminogen activator by smooth muscle cells in injured rat carotid artery. Circ Res 1992; 70:1128–1136.
33. Dollery CM, McEwan JR, Henney AM. Matrix metalloproteinases and cardiovascular disease. Circ Res 1995; 77:863–868.
34. Bendeck MP, Zempo N, Clowes AW, Galardy RE, Reidy MA. Smooth muscle cell migration and matrix metalloproteinase expression after arterial injury in the rat. Circ Res 1994; 75:539–545.
35. Galis ZS, Muszynski M, Sukhova GK, Simon-Morrissey E, Unemori EN, Lark MW, Amento E, Libby P. Cytokine-stimulated human vascular smooth muscle cells synthesize a complement of enzymes required for extracellular matrix digestion. Circ Res 1994; 95:181–189.
36. Libby P. Molecular bases of the acute coronary syndromes. Circulation 1995; 91:2844–2850.
37. Newby AC, Southgate KM, Davies M. Extracellular matrix degrading metalloproteinases in the pathogenesis of arteriosclerosis. Basic Res Cardiol 1994; 89:59–70.
38. Simpson AJ, Booth NA, Moore NR, Bennett B. Distribution of plasminogen activator inhibitor (PAI-1) in tissues. J Clin Pathol 1991; 44:139–143.
39. Chomiki N, Henry M, Alessi MC, Anfosso F, Juhan-Vague I. Plasminogen activator inhibitor-1 expression in human liver and healthy or atherosclerotic vessel walls. Thromb Haemost 1994; 72:44–53.
40. Sawa H, Fujii S, Sobel BE. Augmented arterial wall expression of type-1 plasminogen activator inhibitor induced by thrombosis. Arterioscler Thromb 1992; 12:1507–1515.

41. Carmeliet P, Collen D. Physiological consequences of over-or underexpression of fibrinolytic system components in transgenic mice. In: Vascular Control of Hemostasis; Advances of Vascular Biology (Vadas M, Harlan J, eds.). In press.
42. Herbert JM, Lamarche I, Prabonnaud V, Dol F, Gauthier T. Tissue-type plasminogen activator is a potent mitogen for human aortic smooth muscle cells. J Biol Chem 1994; 269:3076–3080.
43. Lupu F, Heim DA, Bachmann F, Hurni M, Kakkar VV, Kruithof EKO. Plasminogen activator expression in human atherosclerotic lesions. Arterioscler Thromb Vasc Biol 1995; 15:1444–1455.
44. Schneiderman J, Sawdey MS, Keeton MR, Bordin GM, Bernstein EF, Dilley RB, Loskutoff DJ. Increased type 1 plasminogen activator inhibitor gene expression in atherosclerotic human arteries. Proc Natl Acad Sci USA 1992; 89:6998–7002.
45. Schneiderman J, Bordin GM, Engelberg I, Adar R, Seiffert D, Thinnes T, Bernstein EF, Dilley RB, Loskutoff DJ. Expression of fibrinolytic genes in atherosclerotic abdominal aortic aneurysm wall. A possible mechanism for aneurysm expansion. J Clin Invest 1995; 96:639–645.
46. Lupu F, Bergonzelli GE, Heim DA, Cousin E, Genton CY, Bachmann F, Kruithof EKO. Localization and production of plasminogen activator inhibitor-1 in human healthy and atherosclerotic arteries. Arterioscler Thromb 1993; 13:1098–1100.
47. Muller DWM, Ellis SG, Topol AJ. Experimental models of coronary artery restenosis. J Am Coll Cardiol 1992; 19:418–432.
48. Jackson CL. Animal model of restenosis. Trends Cardiovasc Med 1994; 4:122–130.
49. Lindner V, Fingerle J, Reidy M. Mouse model of arterial injury. Circ Res 1993; 73:792–796.
50. Fingerle J, Au YPT, Clowes AW, Reidy MA. Intimal lesion formation in rat carotid arteries after endothelial denudation in absence of medial injury. Arteriosclerosis 1990; 10:1082–1087.
51. Carmeliet P, Moons L, Stassen JM, Declercq C, De Mol M, Dewerchin M, Ploplis V, van den Oord JJ, Mulligan RC, Plow E, Gerard R, Collen D. Receptor-independent plasminogen activation by urokinase-type plasminogen activator (u-PA) mediates arterial neointima formation. A gene targeting and gene therapy study in mice. Submitted.
52. Quax PHA, Khouw IMSL, Bakker TR, van Leeuwen RTJ, Verheijen JH. Urokinase-type plasminogen activator is involved in smooth muscle cell migration in wounded cultures. Fibrinolysis 1994; 8(suppl. 1):148.
53. Hearing VJ, Law LW, Corti A, Appella E, Blasi F. Modulation of metastatic potential by cell surface urokinase of murine melanoma cells. Cancer Res 1988; 48:1270–1278.
54. Ossowski L, Russo-Payne H, Wilson EL. Inhibition of urokinase-type plasminogen activator by antibodies: the effect on dissemination of a human tumor in the nude mouse. Cancer Res 1991; 51:274–281.

55. Yu HR, Schultz RM. Relationship between secreted urokinase plasminogen activator activity and metastatic potential in murine B16 cells transfected with human urokinase sense and antisense genes. Cancer Res 1990; 50:7623–7633.
56. Wilhelm O, Weidle U, Hohl S, Rettenberger P, Schmitt M, Graeff H. Recombinant soluble urokinase receptor as a scavenger for urokinase-type plasminogen activator. Inhibition of proliferation and invasion of human ovarian cancer cells. FEBS Lett 1994; 337:131–134.
57. Lee SW, Kahn ML, Dichek DA. Expression of an anchored urokinase in the apical endothelial cell membrane. J Biol Chem 1992; 267:13020–13029.
58. Plow EF, Herren T, Redlitz A, Miles LA, Hoover-Plow JL. The cell biology of the plasminogen system. FASEB J 1995; 9:939–945.
59. Wei Y, Waltz DA, Rao N, Drummond RJ, Rosenberg S, Chapman HA. Identification of the urokinase receptor as an adhesion receptor for vitronectin. J Biol Chem 1994; 269:32380–32388.
60. Stephens RW, Bokman AM, Myöhänen HT, Reisberg T, Tapiovaara H, Pedersen N, Grondahl-Hansen J, Llinas M, Vaheri A. Heparin binding to the urokinase kringle domain. Biochemistry 1992; 31:7572–7579.
61. Crowley CW, Cohen RL, Lucas BK, Liu G, Shuman MA, Levinson AD. Prevention of metastasis by inhibition of the urokinase receptor. Proc Natl Acad Sci USA 1993; 90:5021–5025.
62. Kook YH, Adamski J, Zelent A, Ossowski L. The effect of antisense inhibition of urokinase receptor in human squamous cell carcinoma on malignancy. EMBO J 1994; 13:3983–3991.
63. Kluft C, Dooijewaard G, Emeis JJ. (1987) Role of the contact system in fibrinolysis. Sem Thromb Hemost 13, 50–68.
64. Simon DI, Ezratty AM, Francis SA, Rehnke H, Loscalzo J. Fibrinogen is internalized and degraded by activated human monocytoid cells via Mac-1 (CD11b/CD18): a nonplasmin fibrinolytic pathway. Blood 1993; 82:2414–2422.
65. Aoki N, Moroi M, Sakata Y, Yoshida N, Matsuda M. Abnormal plasminogen—a hereditary molecular abnormality found in a patient with recurrent thrombosis. J Clin Invest 1978; 61:1186–1195.
66. Robbins KC. Dysplasminogenemias. Prog Cardiovasc Dis 1992; 34:295–308.
67. Nilsson IM, Ljungner H, Tengborn L. Two different mechanisms in patients with venous thrombosis and defective fibrinolysis: low concentration of plasminogen activator or increased concentration of plasminogen activator inhibitor. Br Med J 1985; 290:1453–1455.
68. Aillaud MF, Juhan-Vague I, Alessi MC, Maracal M, Vinson MF, Arnoud D, Vague PH, Collen D. Increased PA-inhibitor levels in the postoperative period. No cause-effect relation with increased cortisol. Thromb Haemost 1985; 54:466–468.
69. Colucci M, Paramo JA, Collen D. Generation in plasma of a fast-acting inhibitor of plasminogen activator in response to endotoxin stimulation. J Clin Invest 1985; 75:818–824.

70. Sprengers ED, Kluft C. Plasminogen activator inhibitors. Blood 1987; 69: 382–387.
71. Paramo J, Colucci AM, Collen D. Plasminogen activator inhibitor in the blood of patients with coronary artery disease. Br Med J 1985; 291:573–574.
72. Hamsten A, de Faire U, Walldius G, et al. Plasminogen activator inhibitor in plasma: risk factor for recurrent myocardial infarction. Lancet 1987; 2:3–9.
73. Juhan-Vague I, Aillaud MF, De Cock F, Philip-Joet C, Arnaud A, Serradimigni A, Collen D. The fast-acting inhibitor of tissue-type plasminogen activator is an acute phase reactant protein. Prog Fibrinol 1985; 7:146–149.
74. Fay WP, Shapiro AD, Shih JL, Schleef RR, Ginsburg D. Complete deficiency of plasminogen activator inhibitor type 1 due to frameshift mutation. N Engl J Med 1992; 327:1729–1733.
75. Schleef RR, Higgins DL, Pillemer E, Levitt LJ. Bleeding diathesis due to decreased functional activity of type 1 plasminogen activator inhibitor. J Clin Invest 1989; 83:1747–1752.
76. Heckel JL, Sandgren EP, Degen, JL, Palmiter RD, Brinster RI. Neonatal bleeding in transgenic mice expressing urokinase-type plasminogen activator. Cell 1990; 62:447–456.
77. Elliott MJ, Faulkner-Jones BE, Stanton H, Hamilton JA, Metcalf D. Plasminogen activator in granulocyte-macrophage-CSF transgenic mice. J Immunol 1992; 149:3678–3681.
78. Carmeliet P, Collen, D. Insights in the in vivo role of the coagulation and fibrinolytic system via gene targeting and gene transfer in transgenic mice. A comparison with genetic alterations in man. Submitted.

13

The Role of Thrombosis in Restenosis

Richard Gallo, Richard Hayes, Lina Badimon, James H. Chesebro, Valentin Fuster, and Juan J. Badimon
The Cardiovascular Institute, Mount Sinai Medical Center, New York, New York

Coronary angioplasty has gained wide acceptance as the procedure of choice in many patients with coronary artery disease since its introduction in 1977 by Gruntzig. Despite improvements in equipment and technique, acute reocclusion after successful angioplasty occurs in approximately 5% of patients, and late restenosis, the most important problem after coronary angioplasty, occurs in 30–35% of patients. In this chapter we summarize our current understanding of the process of postangioplasty restenosis, with special attention to the contributory role of platelets, thrombin, and thrombosis and subsequent intimal proliferation.

I. PATHOLOGY OF RESTENOSIS

Coronary angioscopy, tissue specimens from atherectomy, and postmortem examination have provided valuable information about the nature of the arterial injury and its morphological sequelae. Coronary angioscopy immediately after angioplasty has documented plaque fissures, tears, and cracks with mural thrombus in 70–80% of cases in spite of antithrombotic therapy (1).

Postmortem examination after balloon angioplasty documents incomplete dissolution of atherosclerotic plaques, tears, medial dissections into and around the plaque (accompanied by eccentric and serpigeonous residual

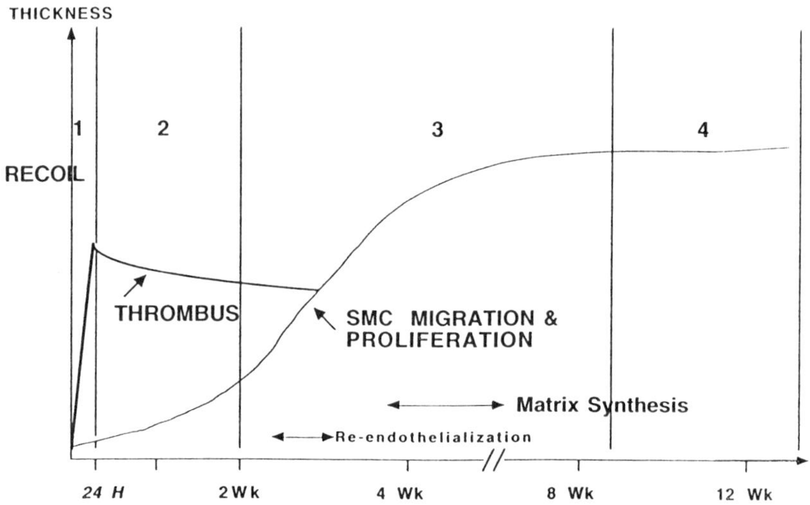

Figure 1 Natural history of balloon angioplasty in a porcine model of coronary angioplasty. The three sequential phases of vascular response are demonstrated.

lumens), and residual thrombus extruding from fissures in the vessel wall. Additionally extensive injury associated with thrombus is seen in areas of the vessel wall opposite and adjacent to an eccentric plaque. Turbulent flow and stasis of blood flow is inevitable within these arteries (2).

Arterial tissue from atherectomy confirms the presence of mural thrombus, intimal smooth muscle cells (SMC), and fibroblast proliferation within the first 15–30 days after the intervention in a high proportion of cases. Furthermore, atherectomy specimens from peripheral arteries of patients with restenosis show intimal hyperplasia in 75% of cases, large amounts of thrombus (>20% of specimen) in 25% of cases, and lesser amounts of thrombus in over 65% of cases (3).

II. PROCESSES LEADING TO RESTENOSIS

Restenosis is a reparative process that is activated in response to injury induced by angioplasty. This process can be temporally classified into three phases (Fig. 1):

Phase I—Recoil, which tends to occur within the first 24 h.
Phase II—Mural thrombus formation with subsequent organization by connective tissue, which occurs within the first 2–3 weeks.

Phase III—Smooth muscle cell activation, migration, proliferation along with increased synthesis of extracellular matrix, which occurs within the first 3 months.

The sequence of events resulting in restenosis are depicted in Figure 2 (4).

A. Phase I: Recoil

An immediate increase in the size of the vascular lumen is observed after percutaneous coronary interventions. The mechanism responsible for the

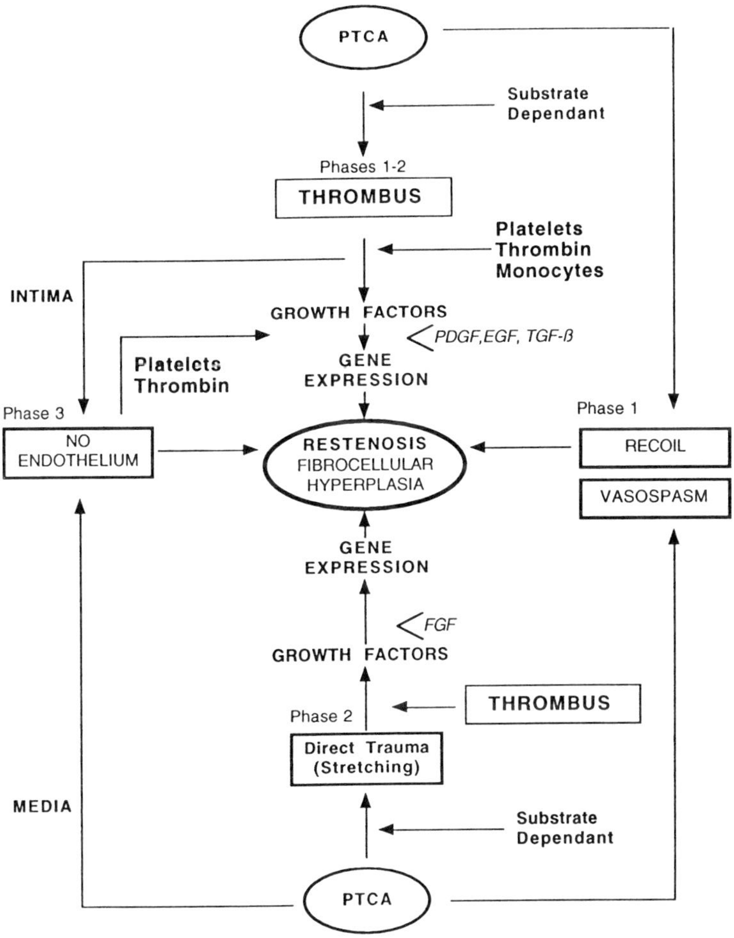

Figure 2 Sequence of events resulting in restenosis after PTCA.

acute luminal loss observed in some patients is termed "recoil." Recoil develops within minutes or hours of the intervention and is a consequence of the inherent elastic properties of vascular cells and extracellular matrix reacting to overstretching. It has been reported that the immediate elastic recoil that follows arterial stretching accounts for the acute decrease in lumen cross-sectional area just after balloon angioplasty (5). Recoil may be the predominant contributor to restenosis in vessels where the dilated plaque is composed mainly of fibrotic or sclerotic tissue. However, recoil may play a lesser role than thrombosis in restenosis of lipid rich plaques where high content of tissue factor and increased thrombogenicity make them more prone to develop luminal and intra-mural thrombi.

B. Phase II: Mural Thrombus Formation

Balloon angioplasty causes significant vascular injury, as evidenced by the significant fracture and compression seen in the atherosclerotic plaque. Similarly, there are areas of endothelial denudation, intimal disruption, medial disruption, and necrosis of smooth muscle cells. Exposure of subendothelial and medial constituents to flowing blood leads to activation of the hemostatic system resulting in platelet deposition and extensive fibrin deposition (6).

1. The Role of Platelets

Arterial thrombus formation is initiated mainly by platelet adhesion to disrupted atherosclerotic plaques or exposed subendothelium (severe injury) and, to lesser degree, to areas of mild injury. Platelet adhesion effectively coats the newly injured vessel wall with a platelet-rich thrombus. This process involves the interaction of adhesive membrane glycoproteins and numerous platelet receptors. The initial bond is usually between the platelet glycoprotein Ia/IIa complex and collagen. This bond is strengthened by the interaction with other glycoproteins, principally glycoprotein IIa/IIb and von Willebrand factor (vWF), and between fibronectin and Gp Ic/IIa. vWF binds to a second platelet receptor site on GpIIb/IIIa, facilitating the stabilization of platelet–vessel wall adhesion and platelet-platelet aggregation (Fig. 3). Exposed smooth muscle cells, vessel wall collagen, circulating α_2-agonists, tissue factor from both atherosclerotic plaque and vessel wall, along with newly generated thrombin are powerful platelet activators. Occupation of platelet receptors by these agonists ultimately results in discharge of numerous factors from alpha granules, such as ADP, serotonin, thromboxane A_2, as well as various growth factors further enhancing platelet activation and aggregation and local vasoconstriction (7).

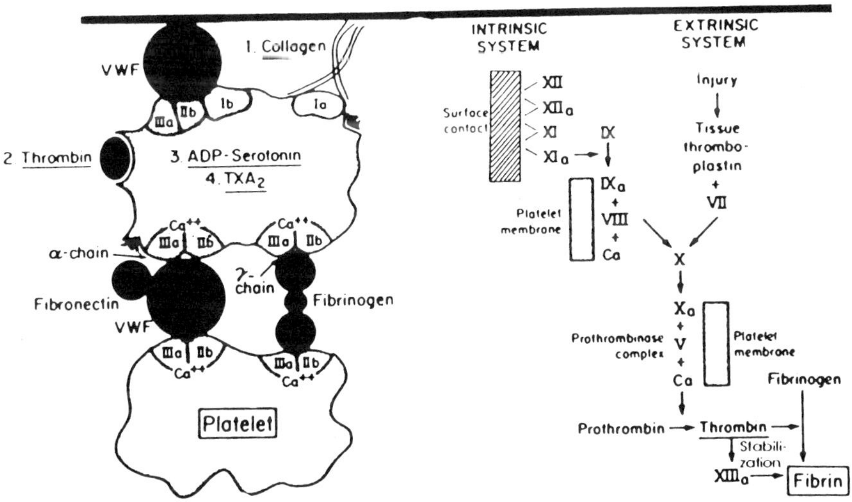

Figure 3 Diagram showing the biochemical interactions between platelet membrane receptors, vessel wall, and adhesive macromolecules during platelet adhesion and aggregation. Also depicted are the intrinsic and extrinsic pathways of coagulation with activator complexes, which amplify and accelerate thrombin generation and resultant thrombosis.

After activation, previously quiescent platelet receptors undergo measurable conformational changes. Activated platelets express new receptors (e.g., GpIIb/IIIa and p-selectins), permitting them to become competent receptors for numerous adhesive proteins. The simultaneous binding of fibrinogen molecules to clusters of adjacent platelets results in platelet aggregation and subsequent thrombus formation (Fig. 3) (7).

Experimental evidence supports the hypothesis that platelets are involved early in the cascade of cellular responses leading to restenosis. Platelet deposition occurs almost instantaneously after injury, peaks in 4–12 h, and is sustained for at least 24–48 h (8). Attenuation of platelet deposition has been shown to inhibit vascular lesion formation in animal models of von Willebrand's disease and antibody-mediated thrombocytopenia. As will be discussed later, platelets are a rich source of platelet-derived growth factor (PDGF), a powerful chemoattractant and mitogen for smooth muscle cells in vitro (9).

2. *The Role of Thrombin*

Thrombin expression is upregulated in smooth muscle cells after severe arterial injury. Thrombin has been shown to mediate many cellular activities involved in the restenosis process, including smooth muscle cell migration and proliferation (10).

Thrombin is generated via the intrinsic and extrinsic coagulation systems. After arterial injury, exposed tissue factor originating from the atherosclerotic plaque, media, or adventitia interacts with factor VII with subsequent activation of factor X resulting in the conversion of prothrombin to thrombin (Fig. 3).

Thrombin is the most potent activator of platelets; furthermore, it converts fibrinogen to fibrin, activates several coagulation factors, and stabilizes the thrombus by cross-linking fibrin. Active thrombin binds to the subendothelial extracellular matrix, where it is protected from inactivation by antithrombin III and heparin but not by direct thrombin inhibitors such as hirudin. Platelet and smooth muscle cell lipid membranes also provide binding sites for the prothrombinase complex, which is capable of enhancing thrombin generation 300,000 times. Thrombin may bind to the deeply injured vessel wall and markedly increase platelet deposition and thrombus formation at this level (11).

Thrombin has also been shown to stimulate growth factor release (including PDGF) and smooth muscle cell proliferation (10). Thrombin shares with other growth factors, especially PDGF, the ability to activate numerous transmembrane signaling pathways.

Other evidence for the role of thrombin in restenosis comes from experimental work in which the effects of direct thrombin inhibition have been studied. We have recently shown that hirudin infusion can reduce histological restenosis at 28 days after balloon angioplasty of porcine coronary arteries. Similar work by Sarembock and colleagues has also shown a reduction in histological and angiographic restenosis in a hypercholesterolemic rabbit model of restenosis (12).

Monocytes, macrophages, and other leukocytes are activated within hours of arterial injury. Numerous cytokines and chemotactic and mitogenic factors are released locally and contribute to smooth muscle cell activation, migration, and replication (6). By analyzing samples obtained at atherectomy, it has recently been reported that there is an increased macrophage content at sites of plaque disruption and thrombosis in patients with unstable angina or non–Q-wave myocardial infarctions (13).

3. *The Role of Vascular Injury and Substrate*

The principal determinants of the severity of the thrombogenic response include the degree of vascular injury, the surface area of exposure, the types of substrates in the underlying vessel wall (collagen, tissue factor, smooth muscle cells, atheromatous core), and rheological conditions such as shear stress and time of exposure.

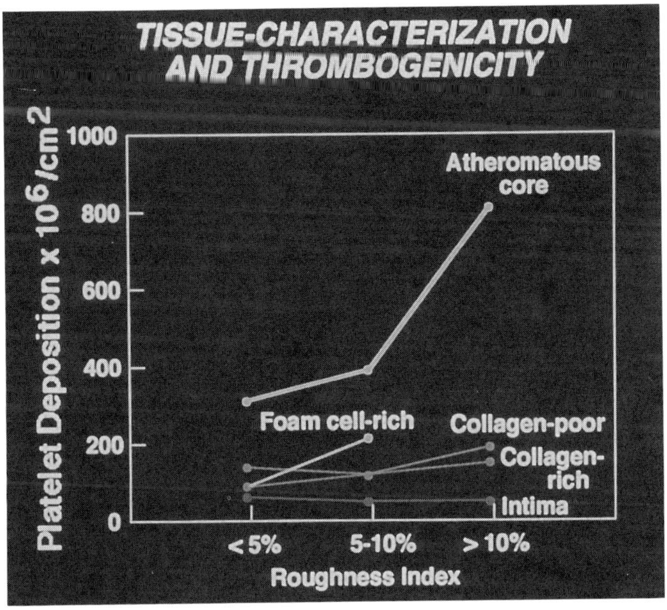

Figure 4 Graph of different levels of thrombogenicity of various atherosclerotic plaque components. (From Ref. 14.)

Coronary atherosclerotic lesions display diverse morphology and composition, varying from highly lipid-rich to fibrotic. We and others have recently compared the thrombogenicity of the different types of atherosclerotic plaques. Thrombus formation on fatty streaks, sclerotic plaques, lipid-rich atheroma and segments of normal intima derived from human aortas obtained at autopsy were studied. The atheromatous lipid-rich core is the most thrombogenic component of human atherosclerotic plaques. Therefore, percutaneous transluminal coronary angioplasty (PTCA) of plaques with a high content of lipid material will be associated with a significant higher acute thrombotic response as compared with the other plaque types (Fig. 4) (14). In a separate experiment we also demonstrated that the increased thrombogenicity of lipid-rich atheromatous plaques was due to the extremely high content of tissue factor (15). Additionally residual mural thrombus, because of its high content in fibrin-bound thrombin, is one of the most thrombogenic surfaces demonstrated. This is extremely important when balloon angioplasty is performed in patients with an acute coronary syndrome such as unstable angina or myocardial infarction. Rheological conditions induced by geometrical changes to the vessel wall after the invasive procedure will also modulate thrombus formation (16). Normal coronary arteries respond to increased shear stress by vasodilating. This compensatory endothelium-dependent vasodilation does not occur in atherosclerotic segments. With high shear force, red cells force platelets to the periphery and enhance their deposition.

Acute arterial injury is associated with acute vasoconstriction. Vasoconstriction is endothelium-dependent, platelet-dependent, and cholesterol-endothelin dependent. Experimental data suggest that platelets contribute to reduction of blood flow. Platelet-dependent vasoconstriction occurs in the absence of endothelium, suggesting a direct effect of platelet-secreted vasoconstrictors on the underlying muscle cells (17,18). Although inhibition of platelet deposition may reduce vasospasm, it does not totally prevent it, suggesting the presence of a secondary platelet-independent pathway. Angioplasty disrupts the antithrombotic properties of intact endothelium. Production of nitric oxide or endothelial-derived relaxation factor (EDRF), a potent antiplatelet and vasorelaxant, is affected. Other local antithrombotic and growth inhibitors, such as heparan sulfate, are no longer produced sufficiently to counter the effects of platelets, thrombin, and fibrin at the site of arterial injury (19).

C. Phase III: Smooth Muscle Cell Activation and Extracellular Matrix Synthesis

This phase can be further divided into three distinct phases. The first, characterized histopathologically by acute thrombosis followed by the activation and replication of medial smooth muscle cells, occurs during the first week following arterial injury. The second phase begins during the first week after injury and lasts approximately 14 days, being distinguished by the migration of medial smooth muscle cells into the neointima. The third and final phase is represented by a more chronic phase (weeks to months) of intimal proliferation and extracellular matrix deposition (4).

1. First Phase: Medial Smooth Muscle Cell Activation

Numerous vasoconstrictors (including thromboxane A_2, serotonin, and prostaglandins) and mitogenic factors are released by activated platelets. The most important growth factors released by platelets are PDGF, epidermal growth factor (EGF), and transforming growth factor-β (TGF-β) (9). Stretching of the arterial wall by itself induces smooth muscle cell activation and growth by stimulating the release of growth factors, specifically fibroblast growth factor (FGF) from endothelial and medial smooth muscle cells (Fig. 2). Additionally, the existence of an active thrombotic stimulus will increase the local concentration of growth factors such as thrombin and PDGF (6). As a consequence of all these potent growth factors, a high number of medial smooth muscle cells will become activated within the first 4 days after balloon injury. These cells undergo a transformation, resulting in increased protein synthesis and soon leading to a period of rapid replication (9,19).

2. *Second Phase: Medial Smooth Muscle Cell Migration*

The migration of smooth muscle cells across the internal elastic lamina to form the neointima represents the beginning of the second phase (4). Following angioplasty the smooth muscle cells observed in the neointima may originate from either plaque, remnant intima, media, or a combination of all three. In a porcine model of restenosis, smooth muscle cells are perceived in the neointima from 3 days to 1 week after injury. (8). The duration of migration is not known, nor is it known whether a phase of cellular replication is required before smooth muscle cells can begin migration. In vitro data suggest that PDGF is a potent smooth muscle cell mitogen more than a chemoattractant (20). PDGF is produced by a variety of cells in the vessel wall, including endothelium and medial smooth muscle cells (PDGF-AA) in addition to the platelet (PDGF-BB) (21). Other growth factors, including TGF-β, FGF, and angiotensin II, have also been implicated in smooth muscle cell migration after injury (22).

PDGF-BB also stimulates the release of plasmin from smooth muscle cells. Plasmin is an important protein involved in the digestion of extracellular matrix creating space for the migration of smooth muscle cells from the media to the intima. Increased plasmin activity has been detected in rat arteries following deep arterial injury, and the importance of plasmin in the restenotic process has been shown by the significant reduction of smooth muscle cell migration by transamic acid in rat carotids after angioplasty (23).

3. *Third Phase: Intimal Proliferation and Synthesis of Extracellular Matrix*

Approximately 50% of the smooth muscle cells arriving into the intima undergo replication for weeks to months following balloon angioplasty (19). In porcine coronary arteries we have found that peak neointimal thickness occurs by days 21–28 due primarily to fibromuscular hyperplasia (8). Cellular proliferation in the intima is identifiable in human histological sections as soon as 5 days after angioplasty and stabilizes by the third to fourth month after balloon angioplasty (24).

As smooth muscle cells lose their capacity to proliferate, they begin to deposit large quantities of extracellular matrix, including proteoglycans, collagen, and elastin. Heparan sulfate is the predominant proteoglycan deposited initially. The neointima of vessels undergoing balloon angioplasty lacks or is poor in heparan sulfate. Absence of normally functioning endothelium contributes to the decreased production of heparan sulfate. Additionally platelets, monocytes, and other leukocytes release proteolytic enzymes that cleave heparan sulfate, which has an inhibitory effect on smooth muscle cells (25). As the third wave progresses and proliferation winds down, there is gradual replacement of proteoglycans by collagen and elastin. The majority of reendothelialization occurs during the final phase, and the new endothelium begins to produce larger quantities of heparan sulfate and nitric oxide, both of which have inhibitory properties on smooth muscle cells (6). Deendothelialization following balloon angioplasty permits constant interaction of platelets and PDGF with the vessel wall. Furthermore, lack of a physiologically normal endothelium for an undetermined time after angioplasty leads to a decrease in local nitric oxide generation, resulting in increased platelet aggregability and decreased smooth muscle cell inhibition. Whether intimal smooth muscle cell proliferation and/or synthesis of extracellular matrix ceases after normal endothelium covers the injury site remains unknown at this time.

III. CLINICAL TRIALS OF ANTITHROMBOTICS TO PREVENT RESTENOSIS IN ANGIOPLASTY

A. Antiplatelet Agents

Aspirin is used in angioplasty both to prevent acute vessel closure and to prevent restenosis. The evidence is clear from three randomized controlled trials, a retrospective analysis, and a meta-analysis that 80 mg of aspirin produces a significant decrease in complication rates when given one day prior to angioplasty (26). However, the evidence that aspirin reduces restenosis is more conflicting. Many of the trials that tried to evaluate the efficacy of aspirin in preventing restenosis had very small sample sizes. The largest such trial, performed by Schwartz and colleagues (27), showed no statistically significant difference with aspirin at a dose of 990 mg/day when compared with placebo. A meta-analysis (28) that pooled results from 608 patients showed a trend toward reduced restenosis in patients treated with aspirin that was not statistically significant. Two other smaller studies report conflicting results, one showing a reduction in restenosis in patients taking 100 mg/day of aspirin (29), while a second showed no difference in restenosis in spite of a larger dose (30).

Despite its proven benefits in reducing acute complications, aspirin does not effectively inhibit platelet-vessel wall interactions after severe arterial injury. Monoclonal antibodies against GpIIb/IIIa have been shown to be more effective than aspirin in inhibiting arterial thrombosis in animal models of coronary angioplasty. The recent EPIC trial (31) evaluated 2099 patients who were to undergo angioplasty or atherectomy and were at high risk for ischemic complications (severe unstable angina, acute myocardial infarction (MI), or high-risk morphology). All patients received aspirin and non–weight-adjusted heparin. Patients were then randomized to receive the monoclonal antibody c7E3 (as a bolus alone or as a bolus plus 12-h infusion) or placebo. Patients randomized to bolus plus 12-h infusion showed a statistically significant 37% decrease in the primary 30-day endpoint of death, nonfatal MI, coronary artery bypass grafting, or repeat intervention. The trade-off was a 50% increase in major bleeding (14 vs. 7%) primarily at the puncture site or during coronary artery bypass grafting; however, there was no increase in intracerebral bleeding. Six-month follow-up of the EPIC study (32) revealed a similarly impressive 23% reduction in ischemic events (death, nonfatal MI, need for revascularization).

The IMPACT II study (33) evaluated integrelin, a cyclic peptide blocker of the GpIIb/IIIa receptor, in patients undergoing balloon angioplasty. All patients received aspirin 325 mg and weight-adjusted heparin. Patients were then randomized to placebo or to two different doses of integrelin. At 24 h there were significantly fewer events in both groups of patients randomized to receive the GpIIb/IIIa antagonist. At 30 days there was only a trend toward lower event rates in all patients randomized. It was concluded that there was no clear-cut dose effect with integrelin, no increased efficacy in the high-risk group versus the low-risk group, and a larger benefit at 24 h, which was reduced at 30 days. Therefore, it appears, at least on the basis of these two studies, that c7E3 is more effective than integrelin in preventing restenosis. It may be that the difference between these two agents is that c7E3, unlike integrelin, binds not only to the GpIIb/IIIa, but also to the vitronectin receptor ($\alpha_v \beta_3$), which is involved in platelet adhesion to the vessel wall (34).

B. Antithrombins

Few studies to date have looked at heparin versus placebo in the prevention of restenosis after balloon angioplasty. Ellis and colleagues (35) randomized 416 patients with an uncomplicated intervention to heparin for 18–24 h versus placebo and found no difference in restenosis at follow-up at a mean of 180 days later. Despite the effectiveness of low molecular weight heparin in inhibiting smooth muscle cell proliferation in vitro and in the reduction of restenosis in animal models, no benefit has been reported in humans (36). Two other large-scale trials with low molecular weight heparin are currently being performed (FACT and EMPAR).

Two randomized studies have evaluated coumadin postangioplasty. Thornton and colleagues (37) randomized 248 patients after successful angioplasty to either coumadin or aspirin started on the day of procedure. Follow-up angiography revealed no difference in restenosis. Urban et al. (38) also detected no difference in restenosis in patients treated with coumadin; however, there was a delay of several days in achieving a therapeutic INR at a time when platelet deposition has been shown to be most evident.

Two large-scale randomized trials have investigated direct thrombin inhibitors in the prevention of restenosis after angioplasty. In the HELVETICA trial (39), 1141 patients with unstable angina were randomized to either heparin as a bolus of 10,000 units followed by a weight-adjusted 24-h infusion or hirudin as a 40-mg bolus, followed by a 0.2 mg/kg infusion, and then either further subcutaneous hirudin or placebo for an additional 3 days. All patients received aspirin. The primary endpoint of event-free survival at 30 weeks was no different in any of the three groups (67.3, 63.5, and 68%, respectively). However, the secondary endpoint of cardiac event rate within 96 hours of intervention was significantly reduced in the patients receiving hirudin. Of note, levels of F1.2, a marker of thrombin generation, remained elevated immediately postangioplasty only in patients on hirudin and not those on heparin, suggesting that although hirudin blocked thrombin activity it was not effective in inhibiting the generation of thrombin. Bittl and colleagues (40) randomized 4098 patients with either unstable or postinfarction angina to heparin as a bolus followed by an infusion over 18–24 h versus Hirulog as a 1 mg/kg bolus followed by a 2.5 mg/kg infusion over 4 h and then a 0.2 mg/kg infusion over 14–20 h. Again, all patients received aspirin. Hirulog did not reduce the incidence of the in-hospital primary endpoint (death, MI, abrupt closure of the treated vessel, or rapid clinical deterioration requiring acute intervention) versus heparin (11.4 vs. 12.2%), although the bleeding risk was significantly reduced. In patients with postinfarct angina, although the primary endpoint was significantly reduced (9.1 vs. 14.2%), the 6-month follow-up showed no subsequent difference in the incidence of death, MI, or repeated revascularization.

Neither of these two trials of direct thrombin inhibitors showed a reduction in the incidence of restenosis at 6–7 months, although early event rates were significantly reduced. Hypotheses as to why no benefit was observed include that the administered dose was too low (animal studies utilized infusion rates many times higher) and that the treatment interval was too short—variables that could be adjusted in future trials. However, past studies have shown that higher doses of hirudin may increase bleeding complications; therefore, there may be a fine line between increased efficacy and increased risk of bleeding (41).

REFERENCES

1. Uchida Y, Hasegawa K, Kawamura K, Shibuya I. Angioscopic observation of the coronary luminal changes induced by percutaneous transluminal coronary angioplasty. Am Heart J 1989; 117:769–776.
2. Farb A, Virmani R, Atkinson JB, Kolodgie FD. Plaque morphology and pathologic changes in arteries from patients dying after coronary balloon angioplasty. J Am Coll Cardiol 1990; 16:1421–1429.
3. Johnson DE, Hinohara T, Selmon MR, Braden LJ, Simpson JB. Primary peripheral arterial stenosis and restenosis excised by transluminal atherectomy: a histopathologic study. J Am Coll Cardiol 1990; 15:419–425.
4. Fuster V, Falk E, Fallon JT, Badimon L, Chesebro JH, Badimon JJ. The three processes leading to post PTCA restenosis: dependence on the lesion substrate. Thromb Hemost 1995; 74:552–559.
5. Hanet C, Wijns W, Michel X, Schroeder E. Influence of balloon size and stenosis morphology on immediate and delayed elastic recoil after PTCA. JACC 1991; 18:506–511.
6. Ip J, Fuster V, Israel D, Badimon L, Badimon JJ, Stein B, Chesebro J. The role of platelets, thrombin and hyperplasia in restenosis after coronary angioplasty. J Am Coll Cardiol 1991; 17:77B-88.
7. Coleman RW, Cook JJ, Niewiarowski S. Mechanisms of platelet aggregation. In: Hemostasis and Thrombosis, Basic Principles and Clinical Practice. Coleman R, Hirsh J, Marder V, Salzman EW, eds. J.B. Lippincott, 1994:508–523.
8. Steele PM, Chesebro JH, Stanson AW, Holmes DR, Dewanjee MK, Badimon L, Fuster V. Balloon angioplasty: natural history of the pathological response to injury in a pig model. Circ Res 1985; 57:105–112.
9. Schwartz SM, Reidy MA, O'Brian ERM. Assessment of factors important in atherosclerotic occlusion and restenosis. Hemost Thromb 1995; 74:541–551.
10. Fagar G. Thrombin and proliferation and vascular smooth muscle cells. Circ Res 1995; 77:645–650.
11. Chesebro JH, Webster MWI, Zoldhelyi P, Roche PC, Badimon L, Badimon JJ. Antithrombotic therapy and progression of coronary artery disease: antiplatelets versus antithrombins. Circulation 1992; 86:III100–III111.
12. Sarembock I, Gertz SD, Gimple LW, Owen RM, Powers ER, Roberts WC. Effectiveness of recombinant desulphatohirudin in reducing restenosis after balloon angioplasty of atherosclerotic femoral arteries in rabbits. Circulation 1991; 84:232–243.
13. Moreno P, Falk E, Palacios I, Newell JB, Fuster V, Fallon JT. Macrophage infiltration in acute coronary syndromes. Implications for plaque rupture. Circulation 1994; 90:988–996.
14. Fernandez-Ortiz A, Badimon JJ, Falk E, Fuster V, Meyer B, Mailhac A, Weng D, Shah PK, Badimon L. Characterization of the relative throm-

bogenicity of atherosclerotic plaque components: Implications for consequences of plaque rupture. J Am Coll Cardiol 1994; 23:1562–1569.

15. Toschi V, Fallon JT, Gallo R, Lettino M, Fernandez Ortiz, A, Badimon, Chesebro JH, Nemerson, Fuster V, Badimon JJ. Tissue factor predicts the thrombogenicity of human atherosclerotic plaque components. Circulation 1995; 92:I-112(abs).
16. Badimon L, Badimon JJ. Mechanism of arterial thrombosis in non-parallel streamlines: platelet-thrombi grow on the apex of stenotic severely injured vessel wall. J Clin Invest 1989; 84:1134–1144.
17. Lam JYT, Chesebro JH, Steele PM, Badimon L, Fuster V: Is vasospasm related to platelet deposition? Relationship in a porcine preparation of arterial injury in vivo. Circulation 1987; 75:243–248.
18. Lam JYT, Chesebro JH, Badimon L, Fuster V. Serotonin and thromboxane A_2 receptor blockage decrease vasoconstriction but not platelet deposition after deep arterial injury. Circulation 1986; 74(suppl II):II-97.
19. Lee PC, Gibbons GH, Dzau VJ. Cellular and molecular mechanisms of coronary restenosis. Coronary Artery Dis 1993; 4:254–259.
20. Ross R. Platelet-derived growth factor. Lancet 1989; i:1179–1182.
21. Ross R, Raines EW, Bowen-Pope DF. The biology of PDGF. Cell 1986; 46:155–169.
22. Scott-Burden T, Vanhoutte PM. Regulation of smooth muscle cell growth by endothelium-derived growth factors. Tex Heart Inst J 1994; 21:91–97.
23. Austin D, Ratliff NB, Hollman J, Tabei S, Phillips DF. Intimal proliferation of smooth muscle cells as an explanation for recurrent coronary artery stenosis after percutaneous transluminal coronary angioplasty. J Am Coll Cardiol 1985; 6:369–375.
24. Gravans MB, Roubin GS. Histopathologic phenomena at the site of percutaneous transluminal coronary angioplasty. Hum Pathol 1989; 20:477–485.
25. Clowes AW, Karnovsky MJ. Suppression by heparin of smooth muscle cell proliferation in injured arteries. Nature 1977; 265:625–626.
26. Barry WL, Sarembock IJ. Antiplatelet and anticoagulant therapy in patients undergoing percutaneous transluminal coronary angioplasty. Cardiol Clin 1994; 12:517–535.
27. Schwartz L, Bourassa MG, Lesperance JL, et al. Aspirin and dipyridamole in the prevention of restenosis after percutaneous transluminal coronary angioplasty. N Engl J Med 1988; 318:1714–1719.
28. Ohman EM, Califf RM, Lee KL, et al. Restenosis after angioplasty: overview of clinical trials using aspirin and omega-3 fatty acids [abstact]. J Am Coll Cardiol 1988; 15:88A.
29. Taylor RR, Gibbons FA, Cope GD, et al. Effects of low dose aspirin on restenosis after coronary angioplasty. Am J Cardiol 1991; 68:874–878.
30. Pepine C, Macdonald R, Bass T, et al. Effect of selective and nonselective TxA_2 blockade on events after PTCA: M-Heart II [abstract]. J Am Coll Cardiol 1988; 11:238A.
31. EPIC investigators. Use of a monoclonal antibody directed against the plate-

let glycoprotein IIb/IIIa receptor in high-risk coronary angioplasty. N Engl J Med 1994; 330:956–961.
32. Topol EJ, Califf RM, Weisman HF, Ellis SG, et al. Randomised trial of coronary intervention with antibody against platelet IIb/IIIa integrin for reduction of clinical restenosis: results at six months. Lancet 1994; 343:881–886.
33. Tcheng J, Lincoff M. IMPACT II. Presented at the 17th Congress of the European Society of Cardiology, August 20–24, 1995, Amsterdam.
34. Jang Y, Lincoff AM, Flow E, Topol EJ. Cell adhesion molecules in coronary artery disease. J Am Coll Cardiol 1994; 24:1591–1501.
35. Ellis SG, Roubin JW, Willentz J, et al. Effect of 18–24 hour heparin administration for prevention of restenosis after uncomplicated coronary angioplasty. Am Heart J 1989; 117:777–782.
36. Faxon DP, Spiro TE, Minor S, Cote G et al. Low molecular weight heparin in prevention of restenosis after angioplasty: results of enoxaparin restenosis ERA trial. Circulation 1994; 90:908–914.
37. Karsch K. REDUCE. Presented at the 17th congress of the European Society of Cardiology, August 20–24, 1995, Amsterdam.
37. Thornton MA, Gruentzig AR, Hollman J, et al. Coumadin and aspirin in prevention of recurrence after transluminal coronary angioplasty: a randomized study. Circulation 1984; 69:721–727.
38. Urban P, Buller N, Fox K, et al. Lack of effect of warfarin on restenosis rate or on clinical outcome after balloon coronary angioplasty. Br Heart J 1988; 60:485.
39. Surruys PW, Herrman JP, Simon R, et al. A comparison of hirudin with heparin in the prevention of restenosis after coronary angioplasty. N Engl J Med 1995; 333:757–763.
40. Bittl JA, Strony J, Brinker JA, et al. Treatment with bivalirudin (hirulog) as compared with heparin during coronary angioplasty for unstable or post-infarction angina. N Engl J Med 1995; 333:764–769.
41. Sobel BE. Intracranial bleeding, fibrinolysis, and anticoagulation: causal connections and clinical implications. Circulation 1994; 90:2147–2152.

14

Porcine Models of Coronary Restenosis

Robert N. Willette, Calvert Louden, and Robert K. Jackson
SmithKline Beecham Pharmaceuticals, King of Prussia, Pennsylvania

I. INTRODUCTION

The use of swine to study the vascular response to intraluminal injury has gained wide acceptance over the past 10 years. Our group's approach to the porcine model has been focused on the evaluation of novel therapeutic approaches to the treatment of arterial restenosis. It is from this perspective that the following discussion was prepared. Thus, the purpose of this review is to present the rationale for the use of the pig, describe the general technique, compare and contrast some of the variations in the use of the model, and highlight significant similarities to the human problem of coronary restenosis.

II. RATIONALE AND PRACTICAL CONSIDERATIONS

Swine are the one readily available animal species whose cardiovascular anatomy and physiology resembles that of humans. There are many similarities between the species. In humans and pigs, size and distribution of arteries are similar (1), with blood flow through the right and left anterior descending coronary arteries supplying nearly 80% of the myocardium in swine (2).

Similarities in end-artery coronary anatomy also make the pig an excellent model for the study of regional myocardial ischemia (3). In the 25- to 30-kg pig, the heart-to-body size ratio is identical to that of humans (2). Blood pressure values (4), heart rate (4), and lipoprotein patterns (5) are also similar. Swine have a platelet-coagulation system that is more closely related to that of humans than most other mammalian species used in cardiovascular research (6,7). One notable exception is that a number of cyclic peptide and nonpeptide glycoprotein IIb/IIIa (fibrinogen receptor) antagonists are powerful inhibitors of platelet aggregation in the dog, nonhuman primate, and human, but not in pig (A. J. Nichols, personal communication).

Pigs are one of the few animals that develop atherosclerosis naturally and have a significant incidence of end-organ lesions (8). Like humans, the severity of atherosclerosis can be dramatically increased by feeding diets high in fat and cholesterol. Atherosclerotic plaques observed in domestic pigs (9) and miniature pigs (10) bear a strikingly close resemblance to the human condition. It has been reported that the combination of an atherogenic diet and arterial injury in the pig creates a lesion more typical of human atherosclerosis than diet alone (8,11).

There are also some very practical considerations that favor the use of pigs for restenosis studies. First, the size of the vasculature and heart of miniature swine and juvenile domestic breeds makes pigs ideal for developing and testing intravascular device prototypes similar in size and configuration to the model that may be used in humans. Second, standard interventional cardiac techniques can be applied in the pig using the same catheters and equipment used for human procedures.

Although the pig is not the most widely used model of restenosis, it has become the model of choice for studying the effects of vascular injury on the neointimal response in coronary arteries. The response to injury in elastic arteries, e.g., the carotid artery, can be effectively studied in rats, rabbits, and dogs, however, coronary artery size in pigs allows the response to be investigated in a muscular artery. It has also been reported that the local proliferative response elicited by interventional techniques, i.e., percutaneous transluminal coronary angioplasty (PTCA) and stenting, is identical in appearance in both pig and human coronary vessels (12). In particular, human and porcine proliferative coronary lesions have a similar matrix and cellular density. In the pig, neointimal thickness resulting from vascular injury is directly proportional to the depth of the arterial injury, similar to the relationship that is thought to exist in human coronary arteries (12,13). This proportionality can be useful when quantifying the efficacy of drug effect on the neointimal response to injury.

As has been established, pig anatomy and physiology make it an excellent animal model to study cardiovascular disease in humans; however, the size of swine and the cost of maintaining them in a laboratory setting can provide definite drawbacks. For example, domestic breeds have been bred for meat production, gaining up to 1 kg per day and reaching weights of over 500 kg. Animals of this size are difficult to handle and house in a standard biomedical research facility.

Fortunately, most cardiovascular research can be accomplished in pigs of a much smaller size. Young domestic pigs weighing between 23 and 55 kg and miniature and micro breeds are routinely used. Because of their size, the miniature (25–40 kg at 6 months of age) and micro (16–20 kg at 6 months of age) breeds are becoming a standard for atherosclerosis research and other longer term studies. For short-term studies, juvenile domestic pigs in the 25- to 30-kg range are used.

In our laboratories we have conducted a number of studies using specific pathogen-free (SPF) pigs, and although the purchase price is higher than conventionally raised farm pigs for research ($275 vs. $170) there are certain advantages. SPF swine were developed in the pork industry to produce a healthier animal that would achieve market weight faster than those in conventional production operations. The primary advantage to cardiovascular researchers is that the SPF pig is free of respiratory and pulmonary pathogens such as *Mycoplasma hyopneumoniae*, which could confound research results. To maintain registry as an SPF herd, periodic testing and necropsies are performed on the herd and the results recorded. If SPF pigs are used, it must be considered that they cannot be housed in the same area with conventionally raised swine. SPF pigs may be highly susceptible to organisms carried asymptomatically by the conventional farm animal.

III. PORCINE MODELS OF RESTENOSIS

A. Technique

The following is a discription of the technique employing the placement of oversized stents in normal pig coronary arteries. The procedure is essentially that described by Schwartz et al. (12,14) and Rodgers et al. (11), who have demonstrated the utility of the model for the study of restenotic events. Relevant modifications of the general technique will also be highlighted.

Juvenile domestic pigs (we use a Yorkshire cross-bred from a specific pathogen-free stock—Barton Farms, NJ) weighing 25–30 kg are sedated with ketamine (33 mg/kg, i.m.) and atropine sulfate (60 μg/kg, i.m.). The central ear vein is then cannulated for the induction of anesthesia with thiamylal sodium (8 mg/kg, i.v.). Each animal is intubated, placed in a dorsal recumbent position, and ventilated with isoflurane in oxygen sufficient to maintain surgical anesthesia. Coronary angiography is accomplished by first isolating the right common carotid artery and introducing an 8–9F hemostatic sheath. Under fluoroscopic guidance, common Judkin PTCA guides are reversed for engaging the LAD and the RCA, e.g., JR4 for the LAD and JL4 for the RCA. The guide catheter diameter is useful for estimating vessel diameter. Following identification by the injection of contrast media, a 0.014-in. guidewire is then passed into the target artery, and a deflated 3.0-mm PCTA balloon carrying a compressed tantalum or stainless steel stent is delivered to a predetermined coronary site based on size. The stent is deployed by a single 9–10 atm inflation (~30% > artery diameter), and the PTCA balloon is deflated and removed. Subsequent angiography is used to confirm successful stent deployment. The right common carotid artery is usually ligated, all other wounds are repaired, and the pig is prepared for recovery and observation. Various combinations of anticoagulant, antiplatelet, vasodilator, and antiarrhythmic agents are routinely used in this procedure (12,14,15). In our laboratory, one day prior to the stent/angioplasty procedure all animals received verapamil (60 mg) and aspirin (500 mg) orally and are fasted for 16–18 h. Fifteen minutes prior to coronary catheterization, heparin (200 IU/kg, i.v.), aspirin (5 mg/kg, i.v.), and bretylium (50 mg, i.v.) are administered. Nitroglycerine (100 μg) is administered into the coronary artery just prior to removing the guide catheter. Heparin is again administered (200 IU/kg, i.v.) at the end of the procedure and buprenorphine (0.1 mg/kg, i.m.) is administered as a postoperative analgesic to smooth recovery. Using this procedure >90% of the animals prepared may survive ≥30 days. Most mortalities occur within the postoperative period (<48 h).

Four weeks after stenting, the animals are sacrificed and the hearts are perfuse fixed with neutral buffered formalin at systemic pressures for 1 h. The hearts are immersed in fixative for 24 h. The stented coronary arteries are then carefully removed into 70% ethanol and prepared for histological sectioning and staining. If the vessels are to be prepared with the stents in situ, then special embedding, sectioning, and staining techniques are required. One method, based on that described by Karas et al. (15), is to harden the tissue by embedding in glycol methacrylate (GMA). The infiltration and polymerization procedure can take up to 4 days to attain the adequate hardness. The tissue is then cut into four equal pieces with a diamond wafering saw, reembedded, and cut at 5 μm with a tungsten carbide knife. Sections prepared this way are routinely stained with toluidine blue (Fig. 1C). Once histological sections are prepared for microscopic examination, standard digital image analysis techniques can be used to quantify the neointimal response (area or thickness), the lumen area, and the degree of stent injury based on strut position in the vessel wall (14).

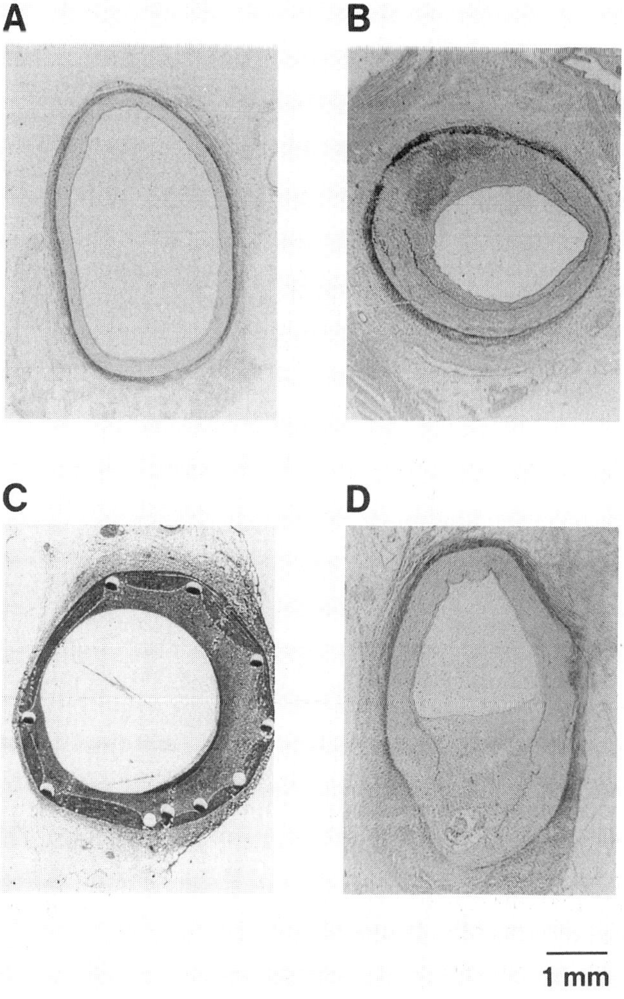

Figure 1 Histological sections obtained from representative coronary arteries in four separate studies were prepared 28 days after injury. The normal (sham; A), balloon overinflation (B) and the platinum single strut stent (D) were stained using the Verhoeff–Van Giesen technique. Histological sections from the traditional, multistrut stent design (platinum) were embedded in glycol methacrylate and stained with toluidine (C). This allowed for processing of the tissue with the stent embedded in the vessel wall.

To address issues of stent cost and availability, we have used the procedure described above to deliver multiple-strut and single-strut platinum stents (0.01 in.) to produce coronary injury (NuMed Inc., Hopkinton, NY). The lesions observed with these experimental platinum stents are qualitatively and quantitatively similar to those produced by tantalum and stainless steel stents (see Fig. 1C,D). In addition, the single-strut stent was easily removed from fixed vessels and therefore required no special histological preparation (Fig. 1D). Because no metal remains in the vessels following removal of the single strut, magnetic resonance imaging (MRI) microscopy can also be used for lesion analysis (Fig. 2).

Another variation in the technique has been the use of simple balloon overinflation as a method for producing coronary injury (12,16,17). Typically, the vessel is intentionally overinflated approximately 25–100% with a 3.5-mm PTCA balloon catheter for approximately 20 s at 10 atm and repeated two or three times. With this technique, neointimal formation occurs only when the internal elastic lamina is ruptured (Fig. 1B). Acute mortality increases when using a 4.0-mm PTCA balloon in 30-kg pigs (personal observation). In our laboratory, the overall incidence of neointimal formation following overinflation is 45% (n = 33) vs. 100% (n = 68) in stented coronary arteries.

Other variations in the model include coronary stenting following preinjury (endothelial abrasion) of the target coronary vessel and in the setting of prolonged hypercholesterolemia (11,18). However, in a much-needed study by the Baylor group (19), it was found that the degree and character of neointimal thickening observed 4 weeks after stenting in normolipemic swine is similar to that observed in swine on a high-cholesterol diet with and without prior endothelial abrasion. In all cases the neointima consisted primarily of smooth muscle cells and matrix (collagen). It was concluded that intracoronary stenting (not cholesterol levels or underlying vascular injury) is the major stimulus to induce neointimal thickening in porcine models of restenosis.

B. Lesion Characterization

In the porcine stent model of coronary restenosis, each stent strut represents a discrete site of vessel injury capable of initiating a neointimal response. This is illustrated by the uniform neointimal formation evoked by the introduction of a single stent strut (Fig. 2). It has been demonstrated that at 4 weeks following "stenting" the neointimal response (thickening) is related to the stent-induced injury of the vessel wall. Specifically, the deeper the stent strut is driven into the vessel wall, the greater is the neointimal response (14). A simplified injury scoring scheme (14) has al-

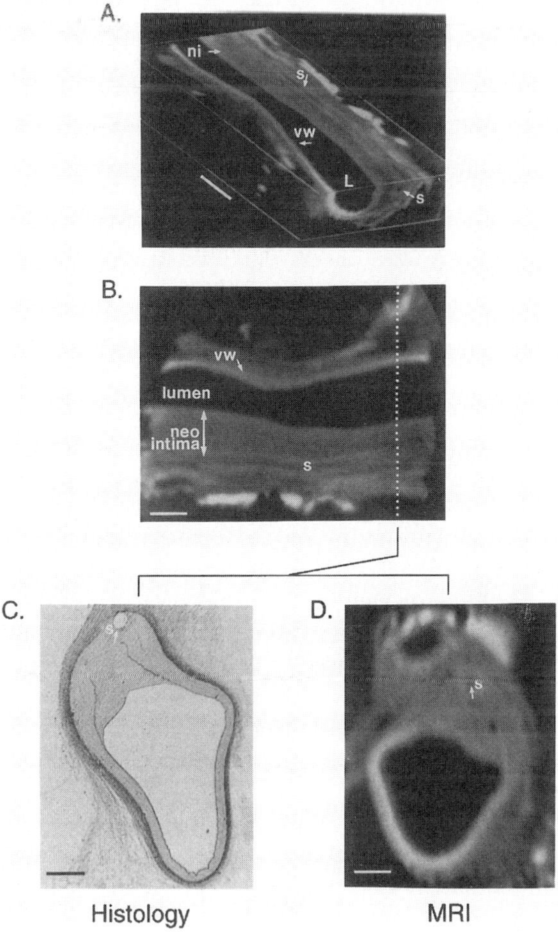

Figure 2 Ex vivo magnetic resonance image (MRI) obtained from a porcine left anterior descending coronary artery following removal of a platinum single strut research stent. Note longitudinal strut canal (S). Oblique (A) and longitudinal (B) renderings illustrate the uniform profile of the neointima (bar=1 mm) formed after 28 days. The relative neointimal thickness obtained from MRI (D) and histological (C) sections correlated well (bar=0.6 mm).

lowed the neointimal response to injury to be normalized, quantified, and compared for the evaluation of potential antirestenotic agents in this model. A significant injury-response relationship has been observed with tantalum, stainless steel, and platinum stents in the porcine stent model of coronary restenosis (personal observations). Consistent with these observations in the pig, histopathological evidence in humans suggests that the depth of angioplasty injury increases the likelihood of restenosis (13). It is interesting that the injury-response relationship does not exist in the canine stent model of coronary restenosis, where the neointimal response to stenting is minimal (20).

A significant injury-response relationship has also been described at 4 weeks in the porcine overinflation model of coronary restenosis (17). In this model, the distance between the ruptured ends of the internal elastic lamina is linearly related to the resultant neointimal area. These authors also found that there was essentially no difference in the injury-response relationship in Feeder pigs and Yucatan minipigs following balloon overinflation.

The neointima formed in the stent model of coronary restenosis is often referred to as a proliferative lesion. Various investigators have attempted to define the genesis of this lesion (12,15,16,21–23). Four overlapping stages of development are generally appreciated. The first stage has been referred to as *thrombotic*, in which platelets accumulate and mural thombi from within the first hour at injury sites (16,21). These mural thrombi containing platelets, fibrin, and erythrocytes become less prevalent after 24–48 h. An occlusive thrombus is rarely observed, most likely because of the effective antiplatelet and anticoagulant protocols used in this model. The second stage, *cellular recruitment*, commences 3–4 days after injury. At this time endothelial regrowth along the luminal borders is apparent and is complete by approximately day 7. Numerous monocytes and lymphocytes then attach to the endothelium and migrate deeply into the thrombus. Monocytes are thought to be responsible for the subsequent resorption of the thrombus. The third stage, *cellular proliferation*, overlaps cellular recruitment and is thought to be initiated by the release of cytokines and growth factors from activated monocytes. By day 7 approximately 28% of the cells accumulating within the lesion are PCNA (proliferating cell nuclear antigen)–positive smooth muscle cells (23). The number of PCNA-positive cells declines steadily over the next 4 weeks. Thus, the maximum proliferative phase precedes the maximum lesion size by 2–3 weeks. However, PCNA-positive smooth muscle cells with a distinct secretory phenotype are still present in the lesion at 4 weeks (Fig. 3). The precise origin of proliferating smooth muscle cells remains unclear; with possible sites including normal adjacent media, injured media, and adventitia. The final phase accounting for the production of neointimal mass in this model may be termed *migratory/*

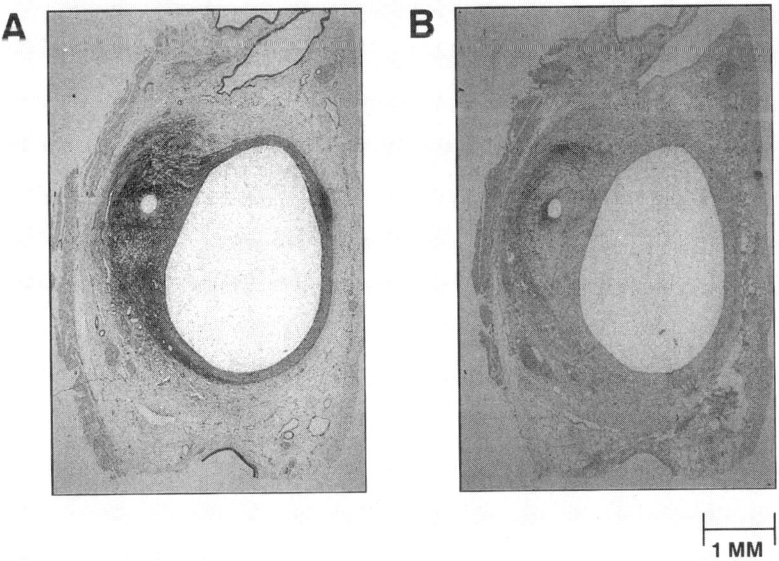

Figure 3 Histological sections were prepared for immunohistochemistry 28 days after deploying a platinum single strut stent in the porcine LAD. Smooth muscle alpha-actin-like immunoreactivity was apparent throughout the media and neointima (A). At 28 days, PCNA-like immunoreactivity was localized sparsely throughout the neointima (B).

synthetic and is thought to include luminal migration of synthetic smooth muscle cells, which expand the lesion by producing extracellular matrix. At 4 weeks the neointima is composed primarily of smooth muscle cells and matrix (Fig. 3A). In this regard, the neointimal lesion in the porcine model and the human condition appear to have a similar proportion of cells to matrix (12).

One potential component of the lesion unique to stent models of restenosis is the chronic inflammation associated with a foreign body reaction. The materials used for stents in this model, i.e., stainless steel, tantalum, and platinum, are generally thought to be biologically inert. The initial studies by Schwartz et al. (12) report only a minimal amount of chronic inflammation, which was judged to be an insignificant factor in lesion development. However, in a later study by Karas et al. (15), it was noted that most of the tantalum stent struts were surrounded by inflammatory infiltrates composed of lymphocytes, eosinophils, histiocytes (macrophages), and occasional multinucleated giant cells. We have made similar observations when using platinum stents. One common feature in all of these studies was that the inflammatory reaction surrounding stent struts occurred only following deep vascular injury involving the adventitia. This inflammatory reaction was often associated with thickening of the adventitia (Fig. 1). Chronic inflammatory reactions have been observed following deep balloon overinflation injury in the pig and in some atherosclerotic/postangioplasty human coronary artery specimens (13). Thus, it appears that deep vascular injury, unlike intimal or medial damage, activates histiocytes and undifferentiated mesenchymal cells in the adventitia.

IV. CONCLUSION

Coronary artery restenosis in the pig represents an important model for understanding the vascular response to injury (24,25). The lesions produced in this model closely resemble human coronary restenotic vessels produced by balloon angioplasty or stent procedures. The major clinical problems associated with these procedures, thrombosis and intimal hyperplasia, are also important processes in the development of restenotic lesions in the porcine model. In addition, the predictable relationship between coronary injury and neointimal response in the porcine model make it attractive for evaluating approaches to limit restenosis. Thus, the challenge is to identify and regulate important restenotic mechanisms in the pig model that will have the hope of direct application to the treatment of human coronary restenosis.

REFERENCES

1. Lee KT. Swine as animal models in cardiovascular research. In: Swine in Biomedical Research, Vol. 3, 1986:1481–1496.
2. Hughes HC. Swine in cardiovascular research. Lab Animal Sci 1986; 36:348–350.
3. Horneffer PJ, Gott VL, Gardner TJ. Swine as a cardiac surgical model. In: Swine in Biomedical Research, Vol. 1.
4. Smith GS, Smith JL, Mameesh MS, et al. Hypertension and cardiovascular abnormalities in starved-refed swine. J Nutr 1964; 82:172–182.
5. Mahley RW, Weisgraber KH. An electrophoretic method for the quantitative isolation of human and swine plasma lipoproteins. Biochemistry 1974; 13:1964–1969.
6. Folts JD, Rowe GG. Acute thrombus formation in stenosed pig coronary arteries, causing sudden death by ventricular fibrillation. Circulation 1983; 68(suppl III):264.
7. Leach CM, Thorburn GD. A comparative study of collagen-induced throm-

boxane release from platelets of different species: implications for human atherosclerosis models. Prostaglandins 1982; 24:47–59.
8. Jokinen MP, Clarkson TB, Prichard PW. Recent advances in molecular pathology: animal models in atherosclerosis research. Exp Mol Pathol 1985; 42:1–28.
9. Getty R. Gross and microscopic occurrence and distribution of spontaneous atherosclerosis in the arteries of swine. In: Comparative Atherosclerosis. Roberts and Straus eds. New York: Harper & Row, 1965:11–20.
10. Zugibe FT. Atherosclerosis in the miniature pig. In: Comparative Atherosclerosis. Roberts and Straus eds. New York: Harper & Row, 1965:37–42.
11. Rodgers GP, Minor ST, Robinson K, et al. Adjuvant therapy for intracoronary stents: investigations in atherosclerotic swine. Circulation 1990; 82(2):560–569.
12. Schwartz RS, Murphy JG, Edwards WD, et al. Restenosis after balloon angioplasty: A practical proliferative model in porcine coronary arteries. Circulation 1990; 82(6):2190–2200.
13. Virmani R, Farb A, Burke AP. Coronary angioplasty from the perspective of atherosclerotic plaque: morphologic predictors of immediate success and restenosis. Am Heart J 1994; 127:163–179.
14. Schwartz RS, Huber KC, Murph JG, Edwards WD, Camrud AR, Vlietstra RE, Holmes DR. Restenosis and the proportional neointimal response to coronary artery injury: results in a porcine model. J Am Coll Cardiol 1992; 19:267–274.
15. Karas SP, Gravanis MB, Santoian EC, Robinson KA, Anderberg KA, King SB. Coronary intimal proliferation after balloon injury and stenting in swine: an animal model of restenosis. JACC 1992; 20(2):467–474.
16. Steele PM, Chesebro JH, Stanson, AW, et al. Balloon angioplasty: natural history of the pathophysiological response to injury in a pig model. Circ Res 1985; 57:105–112.
17. Humphrey WR, Simmons CA, Toombs, CF and Shebuski RJ. Induction of neointimal hyperplasia by coronary angioplasty balloon overinflation: comparison of feeder pigs to Yucatan minipigs. Am Heart J 1994; 127:20–31.
18. Buchwald AB, Unterberg C, Nebendahl K, Grone HJ, Wiegand V. Low-molecular-weight heparin reduces neointimal proliferation after coronary stent implantation in hypercholesterolemic minipigs. Circulation 1992; 86:531–537.
19. Grinstead WC, Rodger GP, Mazure W. French BA, Cromeens D, Van Pelt C, West SM, Raizner AE. Comparison of three porcine restenosis models: the relative importance of hypercholesterolemia, endothelial abrasion, and stenting. Coronary Artery Dis 1994; 5:425–434.
20. Schwartz RS, Edwards WD, Bailey KR, Camrud AR, Jorgenson MA, Holmes DR Jr. Differential neointimal response to coronary artery injury in pigs and dogs: implications for restenosis models. Arterioscler Thromb 1994; 14:395–400.
21. Schwartz SM, deBois D, Obrien ERM. The intima. Circ Res 1995; 77:445–465.
22. White CJ, Ramee SR, Banks AK, Mesa JE, Chokshi S, Isner JM. A new

balloon-expandable tantalum coil stent: angiographic patency and histologic findings in an atherogenic serine model. JACC 1992; 19(4):870–876.
23. Carter AJ, Laird JR, Farb A, Kufs W, Wortham DC, Virmani R. Morphologic characteristics of lesion formation and time course of smooth muscle cell proliferation in a porcine proliferative restenosis model. JACC 1994; 24(5):1398–1405.
24. Schwartz RS, Holmes DR. Pigs, dogs, baboons and man: lessons for stenting from animal studies. J Interven Cardiol 1994; 7:355-368.
25. Schwartz RS, Edwards WD, Huber KC, Antoniades LC, Bailey KR, Camrud AR, Jorgenson MA, Holmes DR. Coronary restenosis: prospects for solution and new perspectives from a porcine model. Mayo Clin Proc 1993; 68:54–62.

15

The Pharmacology of Restenosis in Experimental Animals

Stephen A. Douglas
SmithKline Beecham Pharmaceuticals, King of Prussia, Pennsylvania

I. INTRODUCTION

Advanced coronary and peripheral atherosclerosis (leading to myocardial infarction and cerebrovascular disease) is the primary cause of death in the United States, Europe, and Japan. The nonsurgical treatment of occlusive peripheral (femoral) artery disease was first described by Dotter and Judkins in 1964 and was subsequently adapted over a decade later by Grüntzig for percutaneous transluminal coronary angioplasty (PTCA) (1,2). Subsequently, PTCA has become an increasingly popular alternative to coronary artery bypass surgery for the treatment of angina and myocardinal infarction and can now be used in high-risk patients to treat complex lesions with multiple foci in both proximal and distal coronary artery segments. Nevertheless, although procedural advances (in both medical therapy and equipment, e.g., atherectomy catheters, excimer lasers, rotablators, stents, etc.) have led to a high primary success rate and low incidence of acute complications ($<5\%$), the long-term efficacy of PTCA is still limited by restenosis: vascular reocclusion, usually defined angiographically as a $>50\%$ loss of the initial gain in minimal luminal diameter, typically occurs within 1–3 months of surgery. Only 60% of patients who achieve a successful PTCA go on to experience a long-term, event-free outcome. Although cardiologists have almost two decades worth of experience in performing PTCA, the development of pharmacological adjuncts to coronary angioplasty has met with marginal success. As such, restenosis still constitutes a major unmet clinical need in modern interventional cardiology. This chapter describes the use of animal models of restenosis and reviews the various therapeutic approaches that have been adopted in the quest to develop drugs to inhibit vascular reocclusion. Prior to describing the pharmacological agents that have been developed, however, it is first necessary to describe the basic pathology that underlies the phenomenon of restenosis and how well, or poorly, such animal models relate to this clinical process.

II. BASIC PATHOPHYSIOLOGY OF RESTENOSIS

Angiogenesis/vasculogenesis are usually processes associated with embryonic development. However, geometric and structural vascular remodeling are dynamic processes evident throughout life. The intrinsic capacity of a blood vessel to sense changes in its physical (transluminal pressure, shear, flow rate, compliance, reactivity) and chemical (accumulation of metabolites) environment endows the circulatory system with the ability to adapt to the long-term metabolic requirements of the organs it perfuses. Ion channels and cytoskeletal components, such as those present in endothelial cells, sense a wide range of physicochemical changes such as fluctuations in shear stress, a variable that can range from <1 to >100 dynes cm^{-2} at the carotid sinus bulb and iliac bifurcations/flow dividers, respectively. Normally, structural adaptation is under strict control, a sensitive balance existing between the actions of numerous growth factors, chemoattractants, and proteases. However, a disturbance in this status quo can result in chronic pathophysiological remodeling such as is seen in hypertension, diabetes, atherosclerosis, and restenosis. In order to understand the pharmacological approaches employed to attenuate restenosis, it is necessary to have a rudimentary understanding of the processes leading to luminal narrowing. Essentially, four principal cellular events occur following vascular trauma: (a) thrombosis, (b) cellular proliferation, (c) cellular migration and infiltration, and (d) matrix production (Table 1). Although the relative importance of each of these four basic processes is intrinsically interdependent, it varies within individuals and from species to species. Nevertheless, it is these four processes that offer the potential for pharmacological intervention. Virtually all mechanistic studies have been performed using animal models of restenosis. This chapter will describe the various models that have been employed (Sec. III) along with how these models have been used to assess the efficacy of potential pharmacological adjuncts to PTCA (Sec. IV). The relevance of these models to the clinical setting will also be addressed (Sec. V) along with the challenges that lie

Table 1 Atherosclerosis and the Pathogenesis of Restenosis: Sites for Pharmacological Intervention

DEVELOPMENT OF PRIMARY ATHEROSCLEROTIC LESIONS (decades)

(i) T-lymphocytes and lipid rich macrophages aggregate within intima of blood vessel to form fatty streak.
(ii) Intimal cells undergo clonal expansion, releasing growth factors/cytokines thereby stimulating further proliferation of resident cells (macrophages and smooth muscle cells) to form intermediate lesion.
(iii) Cells elaborate matrix rich in elastic fibers, collagen and proteoglycans.
(iv) Further accumulation of free and unesterified cholesterol occurs within the vessel wall.
(v) Lesion becomes increasingly fibrous, maturing into the advanced or complex lesion.
(vi) Dense connective tissue cap forms over embedded smooth muscle cells, lipid core and necrotic debris.
(vii) Plaque matures, lumen caliber is reduced thereby compromising coronary blood flow.
(viii) Process manifests itself as angina when myocardial oxygen supply no longer meets demand.
(ix) Plaque may rupture resulting in thrombus or microemboli formation, myocardial infarction or sudden death.
(x) PTCA performed to restore coronary blood flow (alternative to coronary artery bypass graft).

⇓
⇓
⇓

A. THROMBOSIS (within minutes - hours after PTCA)

(i) Vessel is stretched during balloon dilation resulting in endothelial denudation/disruption.
(ii) Plaque splitting/rupturing occurs, especially at the shoulder region.
(iii) Thrombogenic subendothelial matrix exposed to lumen contents.
(iv) Platelet aggregation and degranulation occurs.
(v) Intramural microthrombi form and fibrin deposition evident.

⇓

B. CELLULAR PROLIFERATION AND MIGRATION (within hours - days after PTCA)

(i) Smooth muscle cell proliferation is an essential step in process of restenosis.
(ii) Migration is believed to be important but may not be essential since cells are resident in intima at time of angioplasty. Both proteoglycan and musculoelastic layers of tunica intima contain resident smooth muscle cells. Nonfibrous proteoglycan layer contains "synthetic" and "contractile" phenotypes of α-actin positive smooth muscle cells (cells are not oriented in layers as in the media), isolated T-lymphocytes, macrophages and mast cells. Collagen rich musculoelastic layer is a more abundant source of smooth muscle cells.

⇓

C. MATRIX ELABORATION AND MATURATION (within weeks - months after PTCA)

(i) Cells resorb intramural thrombi and undergo further rounds of proliferation as lesion begins to adopt a more fibroproliferative character.
(ii) Smooth muscle cells elaborate large amounts of extracellular matrix, primarily proteoglycan rich.
(iii) Matrix composition changes as chondroitin/dextran sulfate replaced by large amounts of collagen.
(iv) Scar contraction occurs and smooth muscle cell apoptosis may become more prevalent.

⇓
⇓
⇓

CLINICAL OUTCOME (within months after PTCA)

(i) Primary PTCA is successful in >60% of the subjects who have a successful acute outcome.
(ii) Where restenosis occurs, narrowing rarely exceeds that originally observed. Even when restenosis can be detected (angiography/ultrasound), patient may be asymptomatic with good prognosis.
(iii) However, restenosis for many patients leads to recurrent angina and occasionally myocardial infarction.
(iv) Repeat PTCA can be performed (although this is a known clinical risk factor for restenosis)
(v) Alternatively, patient may become a candidate for coronary artery bypass grafting.

ahead as to how these animal models should be used to assess pharmacological efficacy and to identify novel targets suitable for pharmacological manipulation (Sec. VI).

III. ANIMAL MODELS OF RESTENOSIS

Traditionally, animal models are the cornerstone of strategies aimed at developing treatments for clinical conditions and for understanding basic pathophysiological mechanisms. In this respect, restenosis is no exception, and numerous models have been developed and utilized in an attempt to develop a pharmacological adjunct to PTCA. Both mechanical and chemical stimuli have been used to produce fibroproliferative lesions in a wide variety of blood vessels form several different species (Table 2), the most frequently studied species being rats, rabbits, and pigs (although dogs and nonhuman primates are becoming increasingly popular). The severity of mechanical injury varies greatly from a mild mechanical stimulus (introduction of a nylon filament within the vessel lumen) to severe trauma (external mechanical crushing of the artery), and differences in the underlying pathologies mean that each model is best suited to studying a particular aspect of restenosis. With respect to clinical restenosis, the relevance and the advantages and disadvantages of each particular model are discussed (Table 3).

Table 2 Types of Models Used to Study Neointima Formation

SPECIES	TYPES OF ARTERY	TYPES OF STIMULI
Baboon	Abdominal aorta	Air desiccation
Dog	Central ear artery	Allograft transplantation
Guinea-pig	Common carotid artery	Balloon denudation
Mouse	Coronary (LAD, LCX, RCA)	Balloon inflation
Pig	Femoral artery	Chemical irritants (lathycrinic acid)
Rabbit	Iliac artery	Compression/crush injury
Rat	Renal artery	Extravascular polyethylene cuffs
	Subclavian artery	Electrical stimulation
		Focal hypoxia (ligation of vasa vasorum)
		Nylon loop insertion
		Oversize biocompatible (e.g. tantalum) stents
		Polymer anastomosis

LAD, left anterior descending coronary artery (CA); LCX, left circumflex CA; RCA, right CA.

Table 3 Comparison of Archetypal Animal Models

SPECIES	RAT	RABBIT	PIG	DOG	BABOON
A. TYPES OF INJURY FREQUENTLY STUDIED					
Balloon denudation	+++++	++++	+	+	+
Balloon inflation	+	++	+++++	+	++++
Polyethylene cuff	++	+++	+	+	+
Crush injury	+	++	+	++++	+
Luminal air desiccation	++	++	+	+	+
Oversized biocompatable stents	+	++	+++++	+	++++
B. TYPES OF VESSEL COMMONLY STUDIED					
Abdominal aorta	+++	++++	+	+	+
Central ear artery	+	++	+	+	+
Common carotid artery	+++++	+++++	++	++	++
Coronary artery	+	+	+++++	+++++	+++++
Femoral artery	+++	++++	++	++	++
Iliac artery	+++	+++	+	+	+
Subclavian artery	+	++	+	+	+
C. TYPICAL CHARACTERISTICS DEEMED TO BE DESIRABLE IN A MODEL					
Historical pharmacological/histopathological database	+++++	++++	+++	+	+
Technical ease	+++++	++++	++	++	+
Inexpensive	+++++	++++	++	+++	+
Well characterized/available reagents (*e.g.* antibodies)	+++++	++++	+++	++	+
Genetic manipulation (knockout, transfection)	+++++	++	+++++	+	+
Small quantities of investigational drugs required	+++++	+++	+	++	+
Multivessel lesions routinely produced	++	++++	+++	+	+++
Intima typically present in normal vessels	+	++++	+++++	+++++	+++++
Angiographically defined lumen compromise	+	++	+++++	+++++	+++++
Elastic or muscular arteries typically studied	+	++	+++++	+++++	++++
Internal elastic lamina disruption necessary	+	+++	+++++	+++++	+++++
Injury of preexisting primary lesions studied	++	+++++	+	+	+
Hypercholesterolemia readily induced (dietary, familial)	+	+++++	++	++	++
Thrombotic component involved	+	++	+++++	+++	++++
Migratory component	+++++	+++	++	++	++
Proliferative component important	+++++	+++	++	++	++

+, least practical, frequently used, desirable, or important; "+++++," most practical, frequently used, desirable, or important.

A. Rat Models of Restenosis

The rat common carotid artery angioplasty model involves the induction of a fibroproliferative lesion within a long unbranched segment of artery using a 2F embolectomy catheter (3). Essentially, following denudation of the endothelium, a hyperplastic neointimal response to injury is induced following the repeated withdrawal of an inflated balloon catheter. Unlike many species, simple denudation of the endothelium alone is sufficient to induce lesion formation in pigs, dogs, and, in all probability, humans (discrete rupturing of the internal elastic lamina is a prerequisite). Since this model was one of the first described and is not a technically challenging model, it has become the most extensively utilized. Subsequently our knowledge of the underlying pathophysiological mechanisms of lesion formation in this model and the efficacy of numerous pharmacological interventions is the most extensive. As a consequence, numerous investigational tools and molecular markers have been identified and characterized and are available for use in this model. In addition, being a relatively small animal, very small amounts of potentially scarce and/or expensive test compound are required for initial pilot studies. Therefore, despite numerous disadvantages, the rate model is likely to remain in the armory of the investigative scientists for some time to come.

However, the rat is far from a perfect species. Although the rat's size gives it distinct advantages over larger animals (ease of handling, expense of husbandry, compound supply, etc.), its small body may constitute a distinct, albeit subtle, disadvantage. Dynamic vessel wall shear stress is an important determinant of the remodeling process, since shear stress is determined by blood viscosity, velocity (both similar between species), and vessel radius. It is not surprising, therefore, that the typical stress experienced by the aortic wall of an adult rat (55 dynes cm^{-2}) is an order of magnitude greater than that experienced by a 70 kg human. Furthermore, the carotid artery of the rat is an elastic vessel, unlike the human coronary circulation, which is composed of muscular arteries. Thus, this model does not accurately reproduce the vasomotor components observed clinically. These differences are less evident in larger species such as dogs and pigs.

Classically, the response to injury in this model is referred to as the "three-wave paradigm" whereby endothelial denudation produces medial smooth muscle cell proliferation (peaking 3 days after injury), smooth muscle cell migration (from the media to the subendothelial/intimal border 4 days following injury), and, finally, intimal proliferation coincidental with matrix synthesis (resulting in neointima formation, peaking 1–2 weeks after injury). As such, the rat carotid artery model is an ideal model for studying the efficacy of antiproliferative agents. However, there are major differences between the mechanisms occurring in this animal model and pathophysiological mechanisms that underlie clinical restenosis.

Since the rat carotid artery contains no intima prior to injury, the migration of smooth muscle cells from the media to the intima is a critical step in lesion formation. In contrast, the human coronary artery contains a preexistent intima, rich in cellular material (Table 1). Indeed, the lesion formed in the rat is essentially a smooth muscle cell–rich lesion: unlike the human restenotic lesion, T-lymphocytes, macrophages, and mast cells, although not absent, are relatively scarce. Although smooth muscle cell replication is important in lesion formation in humans, it is probably fair to say that this phenomenon is more important in the rat.

Furthermore, unlike porcine, canine, and nonhuman primate models, angioplasty-induced platelet adherence, intramural microthrombi formation, and fibrin deposition are relatively unimportant processes in the rat. This is in contrast to the profound activation of the coagulation system that occurs in humans after PTCA.

PTCA is performed by simply expanding an inflatable balloon catheter against a primary atherosclerotic plaque or secondary restenotic lesions—no "rubbing" of the vessel is performed. However, in the rat model mechanical trauma is induced by rubbing the luminal surface of an normal vessel where no atherosclerosis is evident. Indeed, unlike rabbits, rats are notoriously resistant to dietary manipulation of their serum lipid levels and rarely develop primary atherosclerotic lesions.

The response to injury is usually assessed in rats using histological endpoints (image analysis) or surrogate biochemical markers ([^{3}H]thymidine labeling, PCNA staining). This is in contrast to clinical restenosis, which is usually defined as angiographically determined luminal narrowing. However, current technology means that the rat is too small to facilitate clear angiographic resolution of lesion formation. Indeed, relative to other species, lumen patency is infrequently compromised in the rat. Hopefully, technological advances in the use of angiography, intravascular ultrasound, or magnetic resonance imaging will mean that noninvasive analytical techniques will become amenable to use in small animal species such as the rat.

B. Rabbit Models of Restenosis

Along with the rat, rabbits have been used extensively for developing experimental restenosis models (4). As with the rat, the popularity of rabbit models reflects the relative ease with which they can be studied and the fact that it is also a relatively inexpensive model. However, several important differences exist between these two species. Unlike rats, hypercholesterolemia can be induced readily in rabbits using either modified diets or strains of rabbits with a genetic predisposition to developing hypercholesterolemia (WHHL rabbits). Although the lipid profiles obtained in rabbits bear little relationship to those seen in humans, reproducible foam cell–rich lesions, detectable by angiography, can be induced. Although these lesions are distinct from those usually observed clinically (ulceration and mural thrombus formation are rare and lesions tend to be concentric), the development of these models has meant that, in contrast to the rat, angioplasty (both balloon-rubbing and -dilation) can be performed on diseased vessels containing a preexistent intima. Indeed, a technique of "double-ballooning" has also been utilized whereby a normal vessel undergoes angioplasty, the animal is allowed to recover from surgery, and then approximately 6 weeks later the same site is ballooned a second time.

C. Porcine Models of Restenosis

The use of porcine models of restenosis is becoming increasingly popular (5). The types of lesions seen in the coronary circulation of both minipigs and domestic swine, usually induced by balloon dilation or the implantation of biocompatible metallic stents, most closely mimic those seen in humans in terms of their anatomy, pathology, morphology, and histology. Immediately following the rupturing of the internal elastic lamina, extensive intramural microthrombi are evident (due to the pig's intrinsically low fibrinolytic capacity). These fibrin-rich thrombi are resolved as the lesion becomes colonized by α-actin–imunopositive cells (smooth muscle cells) and leukocytes (T-lymphocytes, monocytes, and macrophages). Proliferation is also accompanied by significant matrix deposition. However, the expense of these animals and the strain that they can place on experimental compound supply means that they are probably best suited for late-stage compound evaluation of candidate molecules, which have been identified as efficacious in smaller models such as the rat or rabbit.

D. Canine Models of Restenosis

Dogs, a species notoriously resistant to the formation of neointimal lesions following balloon angioplasty, have long been regarded as unsuitable for the investigation of pharmacological adjuncts to restenosis. Even more so than in the pig and the baboon, the integrity of the internal elastic lamina is the primary determinant of the remodeling response to injury, and, as such, very poor neointimal responses have been observed in dogs in response to standard balloon injury. Recently, a canine model of neointimal injury has been described where lesions are induced in the canine coronary circulation using a crush-type mechanical injury, similar to that used in the rabbit central ear artery model (6). However, this model differs from the rabbit model in that the myocardium must first be "preconditioned" (thereby facilitating collateralization) by exposing it to a period of ischemia prior to crush injury. Significant smooth muscle cell proliferation and fibrin deposition occurs in this model, and the high thrombolytic capacity of this species may make it of significant utility to investigators. As is the case in the pig, substantial neovascularization of the lesion also occurs as the lesion matures.

E. Baboon Models of Restenosis

The excessive cost of using nonhuman primates (e.g., baboons) in preclinical animal modeling has made their use in basic science inhibitory. However, these types of models are becoming increasingly popular as the existing models fail to act as faithful predictors of therapeutic efficacy in the clinic (Sec. V). Since the anatomy, morphology, and histology of the lesions observed in nonhuman primates most closely mimics that of the human, such animals are likely to become pivotal in the quest to increase our understanding of the basic pathophysiological mechanisms that underlie restenosis.

F. Mouse Models of Restenosis

The relatively small size of mice has made this species somewhat unattractive since injury is produced using intravascular techniques. However, the mouse may become an increasingly useful species to the investigative scientist since it is the species of choice for genetic manipulation: the identification of molecular targets involved in the pathobiology of restenosis (Sec. VI) will undoubtedly increase the use of transgenic and knockout technology.

IV. PHARMACOLOGY OF PUTATIVE MEDIATORS OF RESTENOSIS

Restenosis is the result of four basic cellular events that occur following vascular trauma. As such, thrombosis, cellular proliferation and migration and matrix production constitute prime targets for pharmacological intervention. These discrete processes are mediated by a variety of molecules (Table 4), many of which have complex, multiple actions (TGF-β, for example, both promotes and inhibits cellular proliferation in vitro in addition to inducing chemokinesis and matrix elaboration). This chapter describes the pharmacology of those factors considered as playing major pathogenic roles in the pathogenesis of restenosis, with a focus being placed on those studied most extensively in animal models.

A. Vasoactive Factors

In addition to playing a pivotal role in the control of vascular smooth muscle tone, many vasodilator (adenosine, nitric oxide, PGI_2/E_2) and vasoconstrictor (angiotensin II, endothelin-1, catecholamines, 5-hydroxytryptamine, TXA_2) hormones have profound actions on the growth characteristics of the vasculature. As such, not only have these factors been implicated in the acute vasospastic episodes that occur as a result of PTCA, they may also play a significant role in the chronic remodeling processes that occur subsequent to coronary angioplasty.

1. Angiotensin II

Production of angiotensin II (AII), a vasoactive octapeptide formed from an inactive decapeptide angiotensin I following the renin-induced cleavage of angiotensinogen, is under the direct control of the dipeptidyl carboxypeptidase angiotensin converting enzyme (ACE). The development of ACE inhibitors (captopril, enalapril, cilazapril; Table 5) has delineated the role of AII in the pathogenesis of experimental and clinical restenosis. Recent advances have also included the development of AII receptor

Table 4 Endogenous Factors Identified as Putative Modulators of Restenosis

Vascular tone	Cellular growth	Matrix production	Coagulation	Cellular migration
Vasoconstrictors	**Mitogens**	**Degradadtion inhibitors**	**Procoagulants**	**Chemoattractants**
ET-1	a/bFGF	PAI-1	PAI-1	EGF
TXA_2	PDGF	Antiplasmin		IGF-1
5-HT	TGF-α/β	TIMPs		PDGF
AII	EGF	Nexin		TGF-β
NE	IGF-1			LTB_4
PDGF	IL-1β			Fibronectin
EGF	IL-6			MG-CSF
	TNF-α			VEGF
	Thrombin			bFGF
	Nicotine			MCP-1
	OxLDL			OxLDL
	5-HT			Osteopontin
	AII			
	ET-1			
	NE			
	Vasopressin			
	LTB_4			
	SP			
	TXA_2			
	Thrombospondin			
	GM-CSF			
	Osteopontin			
	VEGF			
Vasodilators	**Cytostatic factors**	**Degradadtion stimulators**	**Anticoagulants**	**Antimigratory factors**
NO	NO	tPA	Heparin	Heparin
PGI_2	PGI_2	Plasmin	tPA	Osteonectin
PGE_2	PGE_2	Collagenase	Urokinase	
ANF	ANF	Stromelysin	NO	
SP	Heparin	Elastase	PGI_2	
LTB_4	Fibronectin	Endoglycosidase		
Adenosine	TGF-β	Hyaluronidase		
	IFN-γ	Heparinase		

ET-1 endothelin-1; TXA_2, thromboxane A_2; 5-HT, serotonin; AII, angiotensin II; NE, norepinephrine; PDGF, platelet-derived growth factor; EGF, epidermal growth factor; NO, nitric oxide; PGI_2, prostacyclin; PGE_2, prostaglandin E_2, ANF, atrial natriuretic factor; SP, substance P; LTB_4, leukotriene B_4; PAI-1, plasminogen activator inhibitor-1; tPA, tissue plasminogen activator; TIMPS, tissue inhibitors of matrix metalloproteinases; TGF-α/β, transforming growth factor-α/β; a/bFGF, acidic/basic fibroblast growth factor; IL-1β, interleukin-1β; IL-6, interleukin-6; IGF-1, insulin-like growth factor-1; TNF-α, tissue necrosis factor-α; OxLDL, oxidized low density lipoprotein; GM-CSF, colony stimulating factor; VEGF, vascular endothelial growth factor; IFN-γ, interferon-γ; MCP-1, monocyte chemotactic protein-1.

antagonists selective for both the AT_1- (DuP 753, CV11974, SR 47436) and the AT_2-receptor subtype. Stimulation of the AT_1-receptor is associated with vascular smooth muscle cell contraction, sympathetic nervous system activation, and aldosterone release (little is known about the function of

Table 5 Vasculoprotective Agents That Interfere with Vasoconstrictor and Vasodilator Factors

Target	Pharmacological agents
angiotensin II	ACE inhibitors (captopril, enalapril, cilazapril, quinapril, benazapril, lisinopril, perindopril, trandolopril, fosinopril, ramipril) AT_1-receptor selective antagonists (DuP-753, CV11974, SR 47436)
Ca^{2+}	Ca^{2+} antagonists (verapamil, SIM 6080, nifedipine, nisoldipine, nicardipine, nimodipine, nilvadipine, amlodipine, diltiazem, clentiazem, lanthanum, Ro 40-5967, flunarizine)
catecholamines	α/β-adrenoceptor antagonists (labetalol), α_1/β-adrenoceptor antagonists (carvedilol), α-selective antagonists (bunazosine), α_1-selective antagonists (urapidil, prazosin), β-selective antagonists (propranolol)
cyclic nucleotides	Non-hydrolysable cyclic nucleotides (8-bromo-cAMP, 8-bromo-cGMP) Adenylate/guanylate cyclase stimulants (forskolin, L-arginine/nitric oxide) Adenosine and A2-selective analogs (octynyladenosine, ethylcarboxamidoadenosine, phenylisopropyladenosine) Antiplatelet agents (dipyridamole, AH-P719) PDE inhibitors (isobutylmethylxanthine, cilostazol, SCH48936, SCH47687) Pertussis toxin Nitric oxide donors (sodium nitroprusside, glceryl trinitrate, SIN-1, SNAP, isosorbide dinitrate, SPM-5185) NOS inhibitors (N^{ω}-nitro-L-arginine, N^{ω}-nitro-L-arginine methyl ester)
endothelin-1	Dual $ET_{A/B}$ receptor antagonists (SB 209670, Ro 46-2005, TAK-044) and ET_A-selective receptor antagonists (BMS 182874, FR 139317)
5-hydroxytryptamine	$5\text{-}HT_2$-selective receptor antagonists (ketanserin, naftidrofuryl, methiotepine, ICS-205-930, LY215840) 5-HT-uptake inhibitors (fluoxetine)

the AT_2 receptor, although it has been linked to collagen synthesis in cultured fibroblasts). More importantly, the AT_1-receptor mediates peptide-induced hyperplasia in cultured human vascular smooth muscle cells via intracellular tyrosine phosphorylation and activation of the MAP kinase cascade. In addition, AII stimulates the release of "classical" growth factors (e.g., PDGF, bFGF, ET-1, IGF-1) with which it can synergize to function as a comitogen (7–9). Although the role of AII as a direct mitogen has been questioned (since AII induces the formation of polyploidal cell populations and hypertrophy at lower concentrations than those required for hyperplasia), ACE inhibitors are probably the most widely studied class of inhibitors in the restenosis field, both experimentally and in the clinic (see Sec. V).

Infusion of exogenous AII increases the neointimal smooth muscle labeling index in both normal rat carotid arteries and those injured using a balloon catheter (10). ACE inhibitors are vasculoprotective in a diverse range of animal models of restenosis (including the rat, rabbit, guinea pig, and, to a modest degree, pig) as a result of inhibition of smooth muscle cell proliferation and migration (11–14). Since ACE is also involved in the catabolism of bradykinin (an endothelium-dependent vasodilator peptide), inhibitors of this enzyme may possess an indirect vasculoprotective mechanism, enhancing the release of the cytostatic free radical nitric oxide from the endothelium (see below). Paradoxically, however, the bradykinin antagonist Hoe-140 potentiates the protective actions of rampril. In contrast to AT_2-selective antagonists (PD 123177, CPG 422112A), AT_1-selective antagonists (DuP-753, CV11974) are also efficacious in the rat and the rabbit (12,15). Collectively these data strongly suggest a role for AII in the pathogenesis of restenosis.

2. Calcium Antagonists

The divalent calcium cation (Ca^{2+}) is an important intracellular second messenger molecule, playing a seminal role in the regulation of several fundamental cellular processes (membrane depolarization, smooth muscle contraction, control of enzyme activity). Sustained increases in cytosolic free Ca^{2+} are almost exclusively dependent upon the activation of voltage-dependent (L-type) channels located in the cell membrane, and, therefore, these channels represent attractive targets for pharmacological intervention. Ca^{2+} channel blockers (phenylalkylamines, dihydropyridines, and benzothiazepines; Table 5) are used extensively in cardiovascular medicine to treat angina, stroke, hypertension, and supraventricular arrhythmias. The experimental use of these antagonists has led to the proposition that Ca^{2+} channel activation is critical in the transition of quiescent smooth muscle cells to those undergoing active proliferation. As such, Ca^{2+} channel activation controls replication "activation," and the ability to attenuate proliferation is lost once a population of cells has begun to undergo proliferation (16). Although verapamil is inactive in the rat, significant inhibition of neointima formation has been reported with Ro 40–5967 and clentiazem (TA-3090) in rat and rabbit angioplasty models (17,18). Interestingly, lanthanum can displace Ca^{2+} binding in vascular smooth muscle cell cultures and is also vasculoprotective in an experimental angioplasty model (19). However, the clinical relevance of these vasculoprotective effects is unclear since typically they occur at concentrations that exceed those routinely obtained in patients. Indeed, diltiazem, nifedipine, and verapamil have failed to demonstrate clinical efficacy. Although meta-analysis of several small randomized clinical trials shows a very modest reduction in the rate of angiographically defined restenosis, a significant positive effect awaits confirmation in a large randomized, double-blind, placebo-controlled study (20). Nevertheless, whether or not such studies are performed, many patients will continue to receive Ca^{2+} antagonists due to their inherent vasodilator activity: since many candidate PTCA patients suffer from angina, Ca^{2+} antagonists (along with β-blockers and nitrates) are routinely administered (to increase myocardial blood flow/reduce oxygen demand and oppose acute coronary artery vasospasm such as is seen following PTCA).

3. Catecholamines

The catecholamines norepinephrine and epinephrine, synthesized within the adrenal medulla and postganglionic sympathetic neurons, exhibit diverse biological functions including the control of vascular tone and structure. Both α- and β-adrenoceptors (epinephrine-, norepinephrine, phenylephrine-, and isoproteranol-induced) mediate rat and bovine smooth muscle cell mitogenesis (21–24). These responses are sensitive to blockade of either α-(nonselective, bunazocine; α_1-selective, prazosin) or β-(propranolol) adrenoceptors, or both (labetolol), although this response is subject to phenotype modulation (butoxamine-sensitive α_2-adrenoceptor activation inhibits cellular growth in cultured cells of high passage number). Exogenous epinephrine administration augments DNA synthesis in vivo, whereas surgical and chemical sympathectomy (superior cervical ganglion ablation, 6-hydroxydopamine administration) have the opposing effect (25–27). This led to the investigation of the vasculoprotective activities of numerous adrenoceptor antagonists. Indeed, α_1-adrenoceptor antagonism (urapidil, prazosin) attenuates lesion formation in the rat (28). The renal-sparing vasodilator carvedilol is an α_1- and β-adrenoceptor antagonist (with weak affinity for Ca^{2+} channels) used in the management of hypertension and CHF. This agent potently inhibits norepinephrine-induced rat and human smooth muscle cell proliferation, with cells derived from restenotic lesions appearing to be particularly sensitive, and inhibits neointima formation by >80% in the rat carotid artery model (29,30). On first appearances this might indicate a significant role for catecholamines in the pathogenesis of lesion formation, at least in the experimental animal. However, the vasculoprotective mechanism of carvedilol may be unrelated to an interaction with adrenoceptors since this compound (a) inhibits the mitogenic actions of a diverse group of pharmacologically distinct growth factors (including serum), (b) attenuates cellular migration, and (c) opposes free radical generation (29). Indeed, adrenoceptor antagonists have failed to exhibit efficacy in the clinic, but, as with Ca^{2+} antagonists and nitrate vasodilators, their administration to PTCA patients, at least acutely, will undoubtedly be continued for the treatment of angina pectoris, acute vasospasm, and/or hypertension.

4. *Cyclic Nucleotides*

Intracellular levels of the nucleotide second messengers cyclic adenosine monophosphate (cAMP) and cyclic guanosine monophosphate (cGMP) control the growth characteristics of cultured vascular smooth muscle cells (31). In vitro, these actions can be mimicked by nonhydrolyzable analogs (8-bromo-cAMP and -cGMP; Table 5), factors that suppress neointima formation in human saphenous vein organ cultures (32). Intracellular cyclic nucleotide levels can also be elevated by directly stimulating adenylate or guanylate cyclase (e.g., forskolin). Indeed, numerous agents can activate these intracellular signaling pathways, thereby attenuating the mitogenic properties of a diverse range of pharmacologically unrelated smooth muscle mitogens. Such factors include adenosine and its analogs, phosphodiesterase inhibitors, dipyridamole, and nitric oxide.

Adenosine. The cAMP metabolite adenosine is a potent vasodilator, particularly within the coronary circulation where the adenosine A_2 receptor mediates adenylate cyclase activation. Adenosine and its ethylcarboxamido and phenylisopropyl analogs attenuate PDGF-induced smooth muscle proliferation. Since intracoronary adenosine levels are depressed following PTCA, A_2-selective spasmolytic agonists have been proposed as adjuncts to restenosis. Although the ability of such compounds to reduce clinical restenosis awaits investigation, 2-octynyladenosine (YT-146) attenuates neointima formation in the rat photochemical injury femoral artery model (33,34).

Dipyridamole. The conversion of cAMP/cGMP to adenosine/guanosine is controlled by intracellular phosphodiesterases (PDE). Inhibition of platelet and smooth muscle PDE activity elevates intracellular cAMP. Although the antiplatelet agent dipyridamole (and its analog AH-P719) possesses multiple actions (stimulating PGI_2 production, attenuating adenosine uptake), its ability to inhibit cultured smooth muscle proliferation is directly related to smooth muscle PDE inhibition. Indeed, numerous other smooth muscle/platelet PDE inhibitors have been identified (cilostazol, isobutylmethylxanthine, SCH48936). Such compounds oppose vasospasm, platelet aggregation, and cellular proliferation and, along with dipyridamole, suppress neointima formation in the rat, dog, and baboon vascular injury models and human saphenous vein organ culture (32,35). However, despite these positive findings, dipyridamole was reported to increase intimal smooth muscle cell number in cholesterol-fed rabbits and did not attenuate lesion size in either rabbit aortic balloon or pig coronary stent models (36–38). Indeed, dipyridamole has failed to exhibit efficacy in the clinic (39).

EDRF/Nitric Oxide. The endothelium-derived relaxing factor nitric oxide ($NO^{\cdot}$) is formed, along with L-citrulline, from L-arginine under the influence of a family of $NO^{\cdot}$ synthase isozymes. Both $NO^{\cdot}$ and the nitrate vasodilators sodium nitroprusside, SNAP, and isosorbide dinitrate attenuate agonist-induced DNA synthesis in cultured smooth muscle cells by elevating intracellular cGMP levels subsequent to soluble guanylate cyclase activation. Administration of L-arginine attenuates neointima formation in a rabbit aortic balloon model via a mechanism that can be reversed by coadministration of the $NO^{\cdot}$ synthase inhibitor N^{ω}-nitro-L-arginine (40). In accord, the $NO^{\cdot}$ donor SPM-5185 inhibits neointimal injury in the rat as does Sendai virus/liposome-mediated transfer of the gene encoding endothelial cell NOS (41,42).

5. *Endothelin-1*

Endothelin(ET)-1, an endothelium-derived 21-amino-acid residue peptide, is the most potent mammalian vasoconstrictor known. ET-1, formed under the action of a novel metalloprotease, ET-converting enzyme-1 (ECE-1), mediates its biological actions through two distinct receptor subtypes, the ET_A and the ET_B receptors. ET-1 is a potent vascular smooth muscle mitogen, a response mediated by either the ET_A or the ET_B receptor (43,44). In addition, ET-1 induces the release of several distinct growth factors/chemokines (e.g., PDGF, EGF, bFGF) with which it synergizes to function as a comitogen within the vasculature. ET-1 also facilitates cellular migration and matrix production (e.g., collagen), either directly or via the synthesis and/or release of secondary mediators (TGF-β, ICAM-1, TNF-α, MCP-1, IL-1β, IL-6, and IL-8).

In addition to being elevated within the vessel wall during the development of primary atherosclerotic lesions, plasma ET-1 levels are elevated as a consequence of PTCA, both acutely (as a result of endothelial cell destruction) and chronically (due to de novo peptide synthesis) (45–47). Furthermore, neointima formation (in rat balloon angioplasty or cardiac allograft transplantation models) is associated with elevated levels of ET-1 mRNA and ET-like immunoreactivity (48,49). In addition, mRNAs for ECE-1 and both ET_A and ET_B receptors are also enhanced in the rat carotid artery after balloon angioplasty, and both acute and chronic administration of synthetic ET-1 augment the degree of neointimal injury observed. However, a definitive role for endogenous ET-1 in the pathogenesis has only recently been established with the availability of potent receptor antagonists (50–52). Dual $ET_{A/B}$ receptor antagonists such as SB 209670, Ro 46–2005, and TAK-044 reduce lesion formation in the rat carotid and rabbit iliac artery models (50,53,54). Since the ET_A-selective antagonist BQ-123, a cyclic pentapeptide, does not share this action in these species, it was postulated that ET_B receptor activation played a pivotal role in lesion formation (55,56). Indeed, a "non-ET_B" receptor (BQ-123-insensitive) has been identified in the rabbit neointima (57). Whether this receptor is a novel receptor subtype or a "BQ-123-insensitive ET_A" receptor remains to be clarified since other ET_A-selective antagonists (BMS 182874, FR 139317) have demonstrated efficacy in the rat and rabbit carotid and iliac arteries and aorta (54,58,59). Since ET_A antagonists reduce fatty-streak formation in hypercholesterolemic hamsters, these effects warrant further investigation in additional restenosis models (60).

6. *Serotonin (5-Hydroxytryptamine)*

The biogenic amine serotonin, or 5-hydroxytryptamine (5-HT), is involved in the control of a variety of biological processes including hemostasis, neurotransmission, and gastric function. Circulating 5-HT is stored almost exclusively in platelets (although the endothelium serves as an important secondary source; 61). When vascular trauma occurs, such as is seen following PTCA, platelets aggregate and adhere to the site of injury, after which they degranulate, releasing potent vasoconstrictors including 5-HT. 5-HT further interacts with platelet 5-HT_2 receptors to stimulate additional aggregation/degranulation, thereby amplifying this "response to injury" by promoting the secondary release of additional vasoconstrictors, mitogens/chemokines with which it can synergize (ADP, TXA_2, PDGF). These actions are normally abrogated by a functional endothelium, which either catabolizes 5-HT or releases vasodilator/antiggregatory factors (5-HT_1–like receptor-mediated release of $NO^{\bullet}$ and PGI_2). However, where the endothelium is damaged or dysfunctional, such as at primary atherosclerotic lesions or sites of vascular trauma seen after balloon angioplasty, 5-HT gains access to the underlying smooth muscle where its contractile/mitogenic actions occur functionally unopposed. In addition to inducing vasoconstriction, 5-HT_2 receptors mediate smooth muscle proliferation, leading investigators to study the role of 5-HT in the pathogenesis of restenosis using 5-HT_2 receptor antagonists (ketanserin, naftidrofuryl) and 5-HT uptake inhibitors (fluoxetine; 62,63). Furthermore, 5-HT is a potent chemokine for T-lymphocytes and smooth muscle cells (a response sensitive to 5-HT_2 antagonists; ketanserin, methiotepine, ICS-205–930), and, thus, 5-HT may recruit inflammatory cells to the site of injury either directly or indirectly (through the release of a novel 15 kDa T-lymphocyte–selective chemokine/mitogen factor from the endothelium; 64–66). However, although ketanserin reduces myointimal hyperplasia in the rabbit vein graft model, the novel 5-HT_2 receptor antagonist LY215840 is not vasculoprotective in the rat carotid artery model (67,68). Indeed, a recent randomized, double-blind, placebo-controlled trial (PARK) reported that ketanserin did not attenuate overall clinical outcome or restenosis rate (69).

B. Coagulation and Inflammation

In addition to acute vasospasm, vascular trauma induces platelet adherence and degranulation and initiates the activation of the coagulation cascade resulting in thrombus formation, putatively a critical step in the pathogenesis of neointima formation. As such, numerous agents that interfere with these processes have been assessed as adjuncts to PTCA.

1. Eicosanoids

Since the identification in the 1930s of a vasoactive, lipid-soluble substance by von Euler (erroneously thought to be synthesized by the prostate), the eicosanoid family is now known to contain some 90 distinct lipid mediators derived from arachidonic acid which play a critical role in the control of vascular smooth muscle tone and structure. Arachidonic acid, derived from long-chain fatty acids via the action of phospholipase A_2, can be metabolized in platelets, endothelial cells, and smooth muscle cells to several different vasoactive eicosanoids as a consequence of the action of two principal enzymes: cyclooxygenase (producing PGG_2 and PGH_2, which are further metabolized to either the prostaglandins or the thromboxanes) and lipoxygenase (producing the leukotrienes via a 5-hydroperoxy-arachidonic acid intermediate). These factors have an extremely diverse range of effects on vascular tone, platelet aggregation, cellular proliferation, and migration and, as such, have become the focus of interest as targets in the quest to develop pharmacological adjuncts to PTCA (Table 6; 70,71).

Prostaglandins. Prostaglandin synthesis and release is stimulated by a wide variety of both mechanical and chemical stimuli (e.g., 5-HT, PDGF, AII, and IL-1β). Prostacyclin (PGI_2), PGE_1, and PGE_2, metabolites of the enzyme cyclooxygenase, exert a wide range of biological actions including vasodilation and inhibition of platelet aggregation (even stimulating dysaggregation). Along with the spasmogenic cyclooxygenase product $PGF_{2\alpha}$, these factors inhibit smooth muscle proliferation in vitro. Although PGI_2 and PGE_2 are potent antiaggregatory/antimitogenic factors, they are notoriously labile molecules with extremely short biological half-lives, a characteristic of arachidonate metabolites. This has led to the development of several stable analogs such as the PGI_2 analogs epoprostenol, iloprost, carbacyclin, and ciprostene, which potently attenuate serum-induced human smooth muscle proliferation by stimulating adenylate cyclase (see above). Although acute administration of PGI_2 analogs is insufficient to

Table 6 Agents That Modulate Coagulation and Inflammatory Processes

Target	Pharmacological agents
phospholipase A_2	natural and synthetic corticosteroids (hydrocortisone, corticosterone, methylprednisolone, prednisolone, dexamethasone)
PGI_2	PGI_2 mimetics (epoprostenol, iloprost, carbacyclin, ciprostene)
TXA_2	TXA_2 mimetics (U46619, 9,11-epithio-11,12-methano TXA_2) TXA_2 synthase inhibitors (dazoxiben, CV-4151, CGS 13080, nafagrel [DP-1904], 5-(3-pyridinylmethyl)benzofuran-2-carboxylate, ridogrel [R-68060], furegrelate [U63557A]) TXA_2 receptor antagonists (vapiprost [GR-32191], sulotroban [BM-13177], ridogrel [R-68060], SQ-28668, SQ-29548)
cyclooxygenase	cyclooxygenase inhibitors (aspirin, flurbiprofen, ibuprofen, indomethacin, sulfinpyrazone)
lipoxygenase	5-lipoxygenase inhibitors (nordihydroguiaretic acid [NDGA], caffeic acid)
platelet	platelet stabilizers (dipyridamole, ticlodipine, U-53,059)
heparin	low molecular weight heparin (LMWH) derivatives and heparin-mimetics (GMI-077, CY-216, enoxaparin, tedelparin, β-cyclodextrin tetradecasulfate)
vitamin K	vitamin K inhibitor (coumadin [warfarin sodium])
integrins	$GPII_b/III_a$ antibodies (c7E3), $\alpha_v\beta_3$ integrin antibodies (LM609), RGD/KGD-containing peptides (barbourin, SB-1, SB-6, echistatin, G4120, GpenGRGDSPCA),
thrombin/related factors	thrombin mimetics (SFLLRN-containing peptides) endogenous thrombin inhibitors (antithrombin III and α_1-antitrypsin) mono- and polyclonal thrombin antibodies dual thrombin catalytic/exosite inhibitors (hirudin, hirugen, hirulog) thrombin inhibitors (PPACK [D-Phe-L-propyl-L-Argchloromethylketone], argatroban [argipidine]) factor Xa inhibitors (antistatin [ATS], tick anticoagulant peptide [TAP])
cytokines	immunosuppressants (cyclosporin A) and corticosteroids (see phospholipase A_2)

attenuate restenosis in animal models, chronic administration of a irreversible inhibitor of cyclooxygenase, aspirin, is vasculoprotective in rat and rabbit angioplasty models (72,73). However, since both $PGI_2/PGE_{1/2}$ (antiaggregatory, antimitogenic, vasodilator factors) and TXA_2/TXB_2 (proaggregatory, mitogenic, vasoconstrictor factors; see below) are products of cyclooxygenase, it is not surprising that cyclooxygenase inhibition (with aspirin, flurbiprofen, ibuprofen, indomethacin, sulfinpyrazone) has generally failed to alter neointima formation in rat, rabbit, and dog models (presumably because this therapy blocks both the synthesis of the proaggregatory factors in platelets [TXA_2] and antiaggregatory factors in the endothelium [PGI_2]) (74–77).

Thromboxanes. In contrast to PGI_2/PGE_2, TXA_2 and its stable analogs (U46619 and epithiomethano-TXA_2 analog) are potent smooth muscle mitogens and vasoconstrictors which promote platelet aggregation. Since cyclooxygenase inhibitors block the production of both PGI_2 (antiproliferative) and TXA_2 (mitogenic), efforts have focused on developing selective TXA_2 receptor antagonists (vapiprost, sulotroban, SQ-28668, SQ-29548) and inhibitors of TXA_2 synthase (dazoxiben, CV-4151, CGS 13080, nafagrel, pyridinylmethyl-benzofuran-2-carboxylate, furegrelate), the enzyme specifically responsible for TXA_2 production. In addition, combined TXA_2 receptor antagonist/synthase inhibitors (ridogrel) have also been reported. However, although such compounds have been reported to inhibit platelet deposition and mural thrombus formation in several animal models (and may, therefore, be useful in attenuating the incidence of acute complications following PTCA), they have generally failed to attenuate both experimental and clinical restenosis (e.g., the CARPORT trials) (78,79).

Leukotrienes. Collectively, the leukotrienes are potent vasoconstrictors, mitogens, and chemoattractants (inducing leukocyte aggregation and adherence to the endothelium), responses mediated via distinct membrane-bound receptors. The leukotrienes LTB_4 and the sulfidopeptide analogs LTC_4, LTD_4, and LTE_4 are active metabolic products of 5-lipoxygenase (71). Inhibition of this enzyme with nordihydroguiaretic acid or caffeic acid inhibits human umbilical artery smooth muscle proliferation, but, as such, leukotriene inhibitors and antagonists have received relatively little attention as antirestenosis agents.

2. *Cytokines and Inflammatory Mediators*

The role of cytokines as inflammatory mediators has received widespread attention leading to the proposal of a cascade model for restenosis where mechanical trauma induces the expression of a diverse range of cytokines leading to a complex tissue injury response involving smooth muscle cells and leukocytes resident within the vessel wall. Various cytokines synergize and initiate a wound-healing process, acting as both autocrine and paracrine factors promoting monocyte/macrophage and T-lymphocyte proliferation, chemokinesis, and migration to the site of injury. As such, these cytokines represent novel targets for pharmacological intervention.

Glucocorticoids. Hypothalamic and anterior pituitary hormones (corticotrophin and CRF) control the release of corticosteroids from the adrenal cortex. Both natural and synthetic corticosteroids (hydrocortisone, corticosterone, methylprednisolone, prednisolone, hydrocortisone, dexamethasone) inhibit smooth muscle cell proliferation, T-lymphocyte migration and proliferation, and matrix production (80–82). Indeed, both prednisolone and dexamethasone attenuate neointima formation in rat and rabbit carotid, femoral, and central ear artery models (although hypophysectomy does not enhance neointima formation following vascular injury, nor does local delivery of dexamethasone prevent myointimal proliferation in the pig carotid stent model; 83–87).

Glucocorticoids have complex mechanisms of action, their anti-inflammatory effects being derived largely from their ability to induce lipocortin-1 expression (a 37 kDa member of the annexin superfamily of calcium-binding proteins that inhibits phospholipase A_2). Inhibition of PLA_2 prevents the metabolism of cellular phospholipids to platelet-activating factor (PAF) and arachidonic acid, and, hence, corticosteroids reduce eicosanoid production (an effect synergistic with more recent reports where attenuated cyclooxygenase mRNA production has been observed).

In addition, glucocorticoids are potent inhibitors of cytokine expression, and, as such, they modulate the expression of numerous immunomodulators including IL-1β, IFN-γ, TNF-α, and MCP-1 by altering nuclear transcription (88). Binding to a specific extracellular globulin results in delivery of the glucocorticoid to the cells cytoplasm where, following displacement of heat shock protein 90 (hsp90), it binds to its type I or type II receptor. The resultant homo- and heterodimeric complexes translocate to the nucleus where, upon binding to specific glucocorticoid response elements within the genomic DNA, gene transcription is either inhibited or upregulated. The specifics of this interaction are unclear, but altered transcription may be due to interference with AP-1 (c-*jun*:c-*fos* dimers) or nuclear factor κB (p65 subunit of NF-κB) binding. However, although cytokines are believed to play a critical role in the process of restenosis and, as such, they make an attractive target for pharmacological intervention, it should be noted that acute administration of methylprednisolone does not reduce the frequency of restenosis following PTCA (89,90).

Cyclosporin A. Cyclosporin A, an immunosuppressive agent used clinically to reduce the incidence of tissue rejection following organ transplantation, has been investigated as an adjunct to PTCA. Although the data is conflicting, cyclosporin A has been reported to inhibit cultured smooth muscle cell proliferation and prevent neointima formation in the rat, but not the rabbit carotid artery model (91–93).

3. *Antiplatelet Agents*

In addition to specific inhibitors of eicosanoid synthesis or function, a diverse collection of compounds has been described which attenuate platelet function via distinct mechanisms. Many of these loosely defined "antiplatelet agents" are described elsewhere (nonsteroidal anti–inflammatory agents such as aspirin, dipyridamole, 5-HT antagonists, PDGF inhibitors). However, one antiplatelet agent warrants comment, namely, ticlodipine. This factor inhibits platelet aggregation/degranulation via an unknown mechanism but may relate to this compound's ability to stabilize platelet membranes in vitro, thus interfering with integrin receptor interactions. However, although ticlodipine reduces neointima formation induced in the rabbit by balloon injury (but not crush injury), this compound has no effect on late clinical events (TACT trial; 77,94,95).

4. Heparinoids

Vascular trauma, such as is seen after PTCA, exposes the subendothelial matrix to the circulating contents of the vascular lumen resulting in activation of the extrinsic/intrinsic coagulation cascade. In order to minimize platelet aggregation, formation of emboli and intramural thrombi, large doses of heparin are routinely used during interventional procedures such as PTCA. Heparin, a ubiquitous and heterologous group (2–40 kDa) of glycosaminoglycans, and related molecules such as heparan sulfate are found within the extracellular matrix of blood vessels where they reversibly bind anticoagulant factors such as antithrombin III and prevent thrombin formation. Both the anticoagulant and nonanticoagulant fractions [low molecular weight heparin (LMWH)] of heparin and heparin mimetics (β-cyclodextrin tetradecasulfate) decrease smooth muscle cell proliferation and migration in vitro via a poorly understood mechanism, possibly an indirect result of an ability of heparin to scavenge cationic proteins (but certainly unrelated to any proteolytic interaction with thrombin; 96–98). Numerous factors with diverse functions are "heparin-binding proteins," including chemokines (PF-4, IL-8, RANTES, MCP-1), matrix proteins (laminin, thrombospondin, collagen, fibronectin, vitronectin) growth factors (a/bFGF and its receptor, PDGF, TGF-β, VEGF), and enzymes (SOD, elastase, cathepsin G; 98). An interaction with one of more of these proteins undoubtedly underlies the cytostatic actions of heparin and related glycosaminoglycans. Despite demonstrating vasculoprotective effects in rat and rabbit models of restenosis, heparin administration has failed to reduce clinical restenosis (99,100). Table 6 shows several LMWH derivatives (developed since they have a reduced bleeding liability) and heparin-mimetics (GMI-077, CY-216, enoxaparin, tedelparin, cyclodextrin) that decrease platelet/fibrin deposition and neointima formation in rabbit aorta and iliac, femoral, and carotid artery balloon injury models and pig stent models (96, 101–103). However, as with heparin, LMWH have produced disappointing clinical results (as reported in the ERA study; 104,105). As an alternative to heparin, oral anticoagulation can be readily obtained using coumadin, or warfarin sodium, an agent that attenuates neointima formation in the rat (although its propensity for untoward drug interactions makes it an unattractive clinical adjunct) (74).

5. *Glycoprotein II_b/III_a and Related Integrins*

Integrins, the family of cell surface receptors that mediate extracellular matrix and cell-cell adhesion, are involved in the regulation of many cellular functions (hemostasis, embryogenesis, tumor cell growth/metastasis, apoptosis, inflammation, bone resorption). More than 20 different integrins have bene identified to date, all of which are composed of α and β transmembrane subunits (16 α and 8 β subunits of 95–200 kDa) that heterodimerize to produce distinct receptors that bind specific ligands.

Glycoprotein (GP) II_b/III_a is an surface integrin complex normally restricted in its expression to platelets (and the megakaryocytes from which they are derived). Upon activation, the GP II_b/III_a complex functions as a receptor for fibrinogen and other ligands (including von Willebrand factor, fibronectin, vitronectin) and, as such, constitutes a common pathway by which platelet aggregation is initiated. Therefore, this integrin constitutes a major target for the development of both antithrombotic agents and, consequently, adjuncts to PTCA (106).

Dysintegrins, a family of highly homologous cysteine-rich polypeptides (snake venoms constituents, fibrinogen, fibronectin, von Willebrand factor, collagen) also competitively inhibit integrin-ligand binding at this platelet receptor. These polypeptides contain the arginine–glycine–aspartic acid (RGD) consensus sequence, the "integrin recognition sequence." In addition to RGD peptides, dysintegrin polypeptides containing the lysine–glycine–aspartic acid (KGD) recognition sequence, such as barbourin, can also bind to the $GPII_b/III_a$ receptor. The antithrombotic effects of chimeric monoclonal antibodies to GP II_b/III_a have been demonstrated in dogs and baboons using the chimeric human-murine c7E3 F(ab')2 fragment (107). However, although c7E3 reduces the incidence of postprocedural ischemic complications following angioplasty in high-risk patients, a significant antirestenotic effect remains to be established in a general population of patients undergoing PTCA (108,109). The medical community awaits with anticipation reports describing the efficacy of specific peptidic and nonpeptidic GP II_b/III_a receptor antagonists in experimental and, hopefully, clinical studies (SK&F 107260, SK&F 106760, SB 207448, DMP728).

In addition to the GP II_b/III_a receptor, the use of numerous RDG-containing peptides and related antibodies (SB-1, SB-6, echistatin, G4120, GpenGRGDSPCA, LM609) has led to the suggestion that, by facilitating smooth muscle cell migration, the vitronectin integrin receptor, $\alpha_v\beta_3$ is involved in the pathogenesis of restenosis. Indeed, $\alpha_v\beta_3$ inhibitors attenuate myointimal hyperplasia in hamsters and rabbits (110–112). However, since both normal and diseased (primary atherosclerotic and secondary restenotic plaques) human conduit arteries contain resident intimal smooth muscle cells, $\alpha_v\beta_3$ antagonists require evaluation in animal models (pig or baboon) where the general vascular anatomy/histopathology more closely resembles that of the human, i.e., smooth muscle migration may not be prerequisite in the pathogenesis of clinical restenosis.

6. Thrombin, Hirudin, and Related Inhibitors

Thrombosis is hypothesized as playing a central role in the pathogenesis of restenosis after angioplasty. Central to thrombus formation is thrombin (factor IIa), a coagulation factor derived from prothrombin under the actions of factors V and Xa. This serine protease is responsible for the cleavage of fibrinogen to fibrin prior to clot formation and for the activation of several other distinct coagulation factors (V, VIII, and XIII). Thrombin stimulates platelet activation, smooth muscle, monocyte, and neutrophil proliferation and migration/chemotaxis, and the release of secondary vasoactive/prothrombotic factors (e.g., ET-1). Thrombin receptors are activated following an interaction between the receptor anion binding exosite and a 6 amino acid consensus sequence (SFLLRN) present within thrombin (the "tethered" ligand). Several distinct intracellular signaling pathways are activated including adenylate cyclase and, more importantly, tyrosine kinase pathways.

Physiologically, thrombin is inactivated by several distinct factors including antithrombin III and α_1-antitrypsin. Pharmacologically, however, thrombin inhibition has been achieved using factors that interfere with the catalytic and/or substrate recognition site of thrombin (Table 6). Hirudin, a 65 amino acid polypeptide isolated from the leech hirudis medicinalis, is a specific thrombin inhibitor that inhibits the cleavage of fibrinogen to fibrin by binding to both the active catalytic site (fibrinogen-binding site) and the substrate- recognition site (exosite) of thrombin. Hirudin reduces angiographically defined restenosis in rabbit aorta and femoral artery and pig coronary artery balloon-injury models, an action shared by both hirugen and hirulog (peptidomimetics that also interact with the thrombin- binding domains; 113,119). The alternative thrombin activator inhibitors PPACK (D-Phe-L-propyl-L-Arg-chloromethylketone) and argatroban (argipidine—a synthetic piperidinecarboxylate peptide derivative) also bind to the active site of thrombin and attenuate neointima formation in the rabbit (113,114). Antistatin (ATS, originally derived from the Mexican leech) and tick anticoagulant peptide (TAP) are long- and short-acting factor Xa inhibitors, respectively. These anticoagulant peptides also modulate the vascular remodeling process since both reduce neointima formation observed 4 weeks after balloon injury in atherosclerotic rabbit femoral arteries (115).

However, despite promising results obtained in experimental animal models (where neointima formation has been effectively attenuated) and positive effects on the acute clinical events associated with PTCA, anticoagulant factors have, in general, been reported to have little effect on the process of clinical restenosis.

C. Growth Factors and Cytostatic Agents

As described above, smooth muscle replication plays a pivotal role in experimental intimal hyperplasia and in clinical restenosis. As such, interfering with the cellular processes that control cellular replication has attracted much interest in the quest to develop pharmacological adjuncts to angioplasty.

1. Growth Factors

Although not all growth factors have been implicated in the pathogenesis of restenosis [vascular endothelial growth factor (VEGF) attenuates neointima formation in the rat by selectively facilitating endothelial regeneration], many such molecules are believed to promote lesion formation following vascular trauma and, as such, represent putative targets for pharmacological manipulation (116). However, in addition to proliferation, many growth factors also facilitate other cellular processes in vitro, e.g., directed migration or matrix deposition (Table 4). Thus, many factors classically considered as "mitogens" actually promote neointima formation via an integrated mechanism that is far more complex than their "growth factor" name implies. The purpose of this section, however, is to focus on describing the pharmacology of the five most extensively studied growth factors implicated in the pathogenesis of restenosis (PDGF, TGF-β, EGF, FGF, and IGF-I; Table 7).

Platelet-Derived Growth Factor. PDGF, a 30 kDa polypeptide, is synthesized in a wide variety of cells including platelets, smooth muscle and endothelial cells, and macrophages. PDGF exists in three possible dimeric forms (PDGF-A/A, -A/B, and -B/B), which are potent inducers of mitogenesis (predominantly the A chain homodimer) and chemotaxis/cellular migration (predominantly the B-chain homodimer or the heterodimer). Enhanced expression of mRNA and protein encoding both PDGF-A and -B chains and its high-affinity cell surface receptor occurs after vascular trauma in the rat, rabbit, and baboon, both acutely (prior to neointima formation) and several weeks after injury (in neointimal smooth muscle cells and macrophages; 117–121). Infusion of PDGF-BB induces a 20-fold increase in angioplasty-induced intimal thickening and smooth muscle migration in the rat, whereas a specific PDGF antibody reduces lesion formation in athymic nude rats (122,123). The triazolopyrimidine derivative trapidil exhibits specific affinity for PDGF

Table 7 Agents That Modulate Growth Factor Function and Cellular Replication

Target	Pharmacological agents
PDGF	receptor antagonists (trapidil [triazolopyrimidine], SCH 13929) tyrosine kinase inhibitors (genistein, tyrophostins[AG1295, AG1296, RG-50872]) PDGF receptor antibodies
TGF-β	polyanionic coagulant (heparin) and non-coagulant (fucoidan, polyinosinate) binding factors
EGF	EGF receptor antibodies receptor antagonists (SCH 13929) chimeric fusion proteins (αPE4EKDEL, DAB389, TGFαPE40)
FGF	bFGF antibodies chimeric fusion proteins (aFGF-PE) adenovirus-mediated transfection of secretable form of aFGF
IGF-I	somatostatin analogs (angiopeptin [BIM23014C], BIM23034, ocreotide and lanreotide) IGF-I receptor antibodies
dihydrofolate reductase	inhibitors (methotrexate)
antimetabolites	purine analogs (cytarabine, azathioprine)
topoisomerase II	inhibitors (etoposide, doxorubicin)
microtubules	inhibitors (colchicine, vincristine)
rentinoblastoma gene	adenovirus-mediated transfection of a nonphosphorylatable, constitutively active form of Rb gene product
DNA	alkylating agents (mitomycin C) photodynamically activated antineoplastic agents (8-methoxypsoralen)

receptors (124). Alternatively, since the PDGF receptor possesses intrinsic tyrosine kinase activity, the biological effects of PDGF are attenuated by genistein or tyrophostin (AG1295, AG1296, RG-50872) exposure (125,126). Trapidil attenuates neointima formation in rat and rabbit models, as does SCH 13929, a novel PDGF receptor antagonist (127–129). However, such inhibition may not be due to an antiproliferative mechanism of action. Although a potent mitogen in vitro, the principal biological role of PDGF in vivo is that of a chemokine facilitating smooth muscle, monocyte, neutrophil, and T-lymphocyte migration to the site of vascular injury (bFGF has been proposed as being the primary in vivo smooth muscle mitogen; 123,130). Most importantly, however, recent clinical studies, including the randomized, double-blind STARC trial, report that trapidil reduces the incidence of restenosis (in addition to improving overall clinical outcome; 131,132).

Transforming Growth Factor-β. The five members of the TGF-β family of polypeptides are prototypical multifunctional cytokines with actions in a broad spectrum of cells. Mitogenesis represents only one of their many diverse functions. For example, TGF-β promotes cellular migration and enhances extracellular matrix/integrin expression, a consequence of enhanced protein synthesis (collagen, fibronectin, vitronectin, osteopontin, tenascin and proteoglycan expression) and protease inhibition (stromelysin, collagenase). These actions are, however, complex and dependent upon cellular phenotype and culture conditions: as with many heparin-binding growth factors and cytokines (FGF, PDGF, VEGF, IL-8, MCP-1), such actions are modulated in vitro by a variety of cell culture variables ranging from seeding density, passage number, and cellular phenotype to variations in the extent of growth factor binding to extracellular matrix glycosaminoglycans such as heparin.

Vascular trauma results in enhanced expression of TGF-β (mRNA and protein) in rat femoral and carotid arteries, a response that occurs prior to neointima formation suggesting a pivotal role in stimulating cellular migration (117,122,133,134). However, enhanced expression persists for several weeks implicating this factor in additional, chronic processes such as proliferation and matrix elaboration (122,135). Indeed, direct gene transfer of a TGF-β_1 expression plasmid into porcine arteries results in pronounced matrix production (procollagen, collagen, proteoglycans) accompanied by intimal and medial hyperplasia (although proliferation was less pronounced than that observed using the PDGF-B gene; 136). Similarly, exogenous TGF-β_1 administration also promotes neointima formation in the rat (137). Since TFG-β is also known to bind to several discrete polyanionic coagulant (heparin) an non coagulant (fucoidan, polyinosinate) substrates, these substances can also be used to attenuate intimal hyperplasia (138). However, a detailed investigation of the pathophysiological role of endogenous TGF-β production is currently hampered by the relative lack of specific pharmacological tools.

Epidermal Growth Factor. Both epidermal growth factor (EGF) and transforming growth factor-α (TGF-α) bind to the extracelluar N-terminal domain of the EGF receptor glycoprotein. Ligand binding and subsequent receptor dimerization result in activation of the receptor's intracellular tyrosine kinase domain, which, in turn, leads to phosphorylation of specific protein substrates that function as intracellular second messengers. EGF receptor expression is associated with primary atherosclerotic plaques (139). Unfortunately, although EGF receptor antibodies are available, investigation of the role of EGF in the control of the vascular remodeling process has been severely hampered by the relative lack of selective pharmacological tools. Although the PDGF antagonist SCH 13929 also exhibits significant affinity for EGF receptor, this secondary action is not thought to contribute to its vasculoprotective efficacy in the rat (129). Recently, however, chimeric fusion proteins specifically designed to recognize the EGF receptor have been described (αPE4EKDEL, DAB389, TGFαPE40) (140–142). These chimeric molecules are genetically engineered to combine an EGF receptor consensus sequence (TGF-α or heparinlike EGF-binding protein) with a cytotoxic element that preferentially targets rapidly proliferating cells including smooth muscle cells (protein synthesis inhibitors such as Pseudomonas exotoxin or diphtheria toxin). The utility and in vivo efficacy of these chimeric fusion proteins await evaluation in animal models of restenosis.

Fibroblast Growth Factor. The FGFs comprise a family of nine structurally related heparin-binding polypeptides, including the prototypical growth factors acidic FGF-1 (aFGF) and basic FGF-2 (bFGF; 143). Both aFGF and bFGF exert a wide range of biological actions in various tissues, and, as their name implies, these proteins are potent mitogens, inducing fibroblast, smooth muscle, and endothelial cell proliferation, differentiation, in addition to migration. Administration of bFGF enhances the degree of angioplasty-induced smooth muscle proliferation in the rat, an effect more profound than that observed with PDGF or TGF-β, indicating that bFGF is the principal mitogen that controls smooth muscle replication in vivo (PDGF/TGF-β controlling subsequent migration and matrix elaboration; 123,130,144,145). Indeed, bFGF antibodies significantly reduce smooth muscle replication and neointima formation in the rat (145). In addition to direct type I FGF receptor-mediated mitogenesis, FGFs act as comitogens and facilitate the production of other growth factors, including AII (146,147). The introduction of a eukaryotic expression vector encoding a secreted form of aFGF (aFGF and bFGF do not contain signal sequences) promotes intimal hyperplasia and neocapillary formation in pig arteries (148). Although few pharmacological tools are available, chimeric fusion proteins for the FGF receptor have been expressed in and await evaluation in restenosis models (149).

Insulin-like Growth Factor-1 and Somatostatin. Insulin-like growth factors (namely, IGF-I and -II), ubiquitous single-chain polypeptides, are found in the circulation in the form of a stable ternary complex involving specific IGF-binding proteins and an acid-labile glycoprotein subunit. In addition to modulating numerous metabolic processes, IGFs play a seminal role in the control of cellular proliferation and differentiation in numerous tissues ranging from bone to the cardiovascular system. Although encoded by a single copy gene, regulation of IGF-1 mRNA transcription is complex and under the influence of numerous factors, the most notable of which is growth hormone (GH). The tetradecapeptide somatostatin and several stable synthetic analogs including the cyclic octapeptide antiopetpin, BIM23034, ocreotide and lanreotide inhibit GH release from the pituitary. These factors modulate many of the biological actions of IGF-I in a complex manner via both direct and indirect mechanisms (altered GH release, smooth muscle adenylate cyclase activity, immediate early gene expression). Angioplasty increases IGF-I mRNA and protein expression in the rat (although the IGF-I receptor may compensate for this response by downregulating), and angiopeptin inhibits neointima formation in rats, rabbits, and pigs after both angioplasty and cardiac transplantation (150–159). IGF-I is associated with smooth muscle cells present in primary atherosclerotic and restenotic human coronary artery plaques. However, whereas Grant et al. (160) reported that somatostatin analogs attenuated IGF-1-induced human smooth muscle proliferation but not migration, Bornfeldt et al. (161) found that IGF-I was only a weak mitogen but a potent chemokine (an action blocked by a specific antibody to the IGF-I receptor). Irrespective of these conflicting observations, however, angiopeptin does not reduce the incidence of angiographically defined restenosis in the clinic (162).

2. *Antineoplastic Agents*

Numerous laboratory techniques, including standard histobiochemical assays ([^{3}H]thymidine incorporation, 5-BrDU- and PCNA-labeling) and in vivo gene transfer studies (e.g. overexpression of nonphosphorylatable form of the retinoblastoma gene product), demonstrate that aberrant smooth muscle proliferation is a hallmark of experimental restenosis (163). Although the clinical significance of this event has been questioned (since PCNA staining varies enormously in clinical specimens), mathematical considerations show that even a very subtle increase in the smooth muscle replication rate can drastically alter vascular smooth muscle cell mass over a period of several months. This fact alone has led numerous investigators to assess the utility of standard chemotherapeutic agents as adjuncts to angioplasty.

Several antineoplastic agents routinely used to inhibit malignant cancer cell growth attenuate human vascular smooth muscle cell proliferation in vitro (Table 7; 164–166). Such agents exhibit diverse mechanisms of action: dihydrofolate reductase inhibitors (methotrexate), antimetabolites (cytarabine, azathioprine), topoisomerase II inhibitors (etoposide, doxorubicin), inhibitors of microtubule function (colchicine, vincristine, taxol), alkylating agents (mitomycin C), and agents with less well-defined mechanisms (8-methoxypsoralen, an agent reported to form DNA adducts and interfere with EGF receptor function upon photodynamic activation). As with most chemotherapeutic strategies, the low therapeutic index of these drugs is a potential concern to the cardiologist: although chronic high-dose colchicine administration attenuates neointima formation in rabbits (causing metaphase arrest by blocking microtubule formation), it is unclear whether a comparable dosage regimen could be tolerated by humans without causing excessive damage to other cells undergoing rapid cell division (bone marrow, gastrointestinal and reproductive tracts; 167). The problem of systemic cytotoxicity may be overcome, to some extent, by local intramural drug administration (using porous balloon catheters or polymer coated stents) and may not even be an issue with some drugs, such as taxol, which inhibits neointima formation the rat at plasma concentrations 100-fold lower than those routinely used by oncologists (168). However, several antineoplastic agents (methotrexate, azathioprine, doxorubicin) have failed to demonstrate efficacy in rabbit and pig angioplasty models, and colchicine does not reduce the incidence of clinical restenosis following PTCA (169–173).

D. Agents That Modulate with Lipid Biochemistry

Hypercholesterolemia is a recognized risk factor for the development of atherosclerosis and advanced coronary artery disease. In addition, however, it is also recognized as a risk factor for vascular reocclusion following PTCA. As such, many investigators have studied the effects of drugs that alter lipid metabolism in the pathogenesis of restenosis (Table 8).

Table 8 Vasculoprotective Agents That Interfere with Lipid Biochemistry

Target	Pharmacological agents
HMG CoA reductase	HMG CoA reductase inhibitors (lovastatin, pravastatin, simvastatin, fluvastatin, mevinolin, compactin, fenofibric acid, γ-tocotrienol, perillyl alcohol, geraniol and d-limonene)
Dietary lipids	ω3-polyunsaturated fatty acids (eicosapentanoic acid [EPA], docosahexanoic acid [DHA])
Free radicals	antioxidants (probucol, vitamin C [ascorbic acid], vitamin E [α-tocopherol])

1. HMG CoA Reductase Inhibitors

The enzyme responsible for the production of mevalonic acid, 3-hydroxy-3-methylglutaryl coenzyme A (HMG CoA) reductase, is the rate-limiting enzyme in cholesterol synthesis. In addition to the widely prescribed hypocholesterolemic statins)lovastatin, pravastatin, simvastatin, and fluvastatin), this enzyme can be inhibited by numerous other agents including mevinolin, compacting, fenofibric acid, and additional isoprenoids. However, the HMG CoA reductase inhibitor lovastatin induces G_1 phase cell cycle arrest via a mechanism unrelated to any hypolipidemic action or inhibition of sterol synthesis (e.g., reducing the posttranslational prenylation of proteins, such as nuclear lamins, required for DNA synthesis). Indeed, serum-induced smooth muscle proliferation is attenuated by lovastatin, fluvastatin, and fenofibrate via a mechanism reversed by mevalonate but not squalene or cholesterol) (174–176). Administration of HMG CoA reductase inhibitors blocks intimal hyperplasia in rats and rabbits (177,178). However, despite promising preliminary data, chronic high-dose lovastatin administration does not attenuate the incidence of clinical restenosis (the FLARE trial with fluvastatin is currently ongoing) (179,180). The efficacy of HMG CoA reductase inhibitors may be augmented by combining them with LDL-aphersis, a technique that lowers plasma lipoprotein (a) and LDL levels using dextran sulfate–cellulose columns (L-ART trial) (181).

2. Fish Oils and ω3-Fatty Acids

The low incidence of coronary artery disease observed in Eskimos is attributed to a diet rich in salt water fish, an excellent source of ω3-polyunsaturated fatty acids [eicosapentanoic acid, (EPA), docosahexanoic acid (DHA)]. Although their precise mechanism(s) of action are poorly understood (inducing complex changes in plasma lipid levels, fibrinogen production, etc.), fish oils are vasculoprotective in rabbit and nonhuman primate restenosis models and clearly alter the relative production of vasoconstrictor and vasodilator eicosanoids within the vasculature (favoring PGI_2 production, thereby enhancing platelet dysaggregation, etc.; 182). Meta-analysis of several randomized clinical trials suggests that fish oils may reduce the rate of restenosis. However, many of these trials are seriously flawed since (a) they were conducted on small patient populations, (b) they were not blinded, (c) patient compliance was low (low tolerance to the taste and gastrointestinal effects associated with fish oils), and (d) restenosis was both poorly defined and measured indirectly (e.g., stress tests). Indeed, doubt surrounding the therapeutic efficacy of fish oils has recently arisen after two large randomized, double-blind, placebo-controlled clinical trials reported that EPA administration failed to alter the incidence of angiographically defined restenosis following PTCA (183,184).

3. *Antioxidants*

The aberrant generation of oxygen-derived free radicals can lead to excessive peroxidation of plasma lipoproteins, producing high circulating and tissue levels of oxidized low-density lipoprotein (ox-LDL), a recognized risk factor for atherosclerosis and restenosis. Uptake and accumulation of ox-LDL by macrophages/foam cells and smooth muscle cells stimulates the production of numerous cytokines and growth factors. Thus, due to their ability to scavenge free radicals, antioxidant agents have been investigated as potential therapeutic adjuncts to PTCA. Administration of probucol, vitamin C (ascorbic acid), or vitamin E (α-tocopherol) improves endothelial cell function, prevents mitogen-induced (ox-LDL, PDGF, or serum) smooth muscle proliferation, and attenuates neointima formation in atherosclerotic rabbits and cholesterol-fed rats and pigs (an antioxidant mechanism may also underlie the vasculoprotective actions of the β-blocker carvedilol; 185–191). Indeed, it has been claimed that probucol prevents restenosis following PTCA in a small clinical study whereas a similar double-blind, placebo-controlled trial failed to find a significant effect with α-tocopherol (192,193). Thus, the efficacy of antioxidant therapy, therefore, warrants further clinical investigation.

V. THE PREDICTIVITY OF ANIMAL MODELS OF RESTENOSIS

The list of compounds that have demonstrated efficacy in laboratory animal models but have failed to reduce clinical restenosis is extensive, including Ca^{2+} channel-, adrenoceptor-, 5-HT-antagonists, antiplatelet agents, anticoagulants, anti-inflammatory agents, hypolipidemic drugs, and antioxidants. An inability to identify efficacious clinical adjuncts to PTCA has led investigators to question the validity and predictability of standard animal models of restenosis, most notably the rat carotid artery model (although this probably reflects the fact that this model is the most extensively studied, as much as anything). To this end, serious attempts have been made to improve the predictability of this, and other, animal models (Table 9). This lack of animal model predictability is exemplified by the ACE inhibitors, probably the most extensively studied group of agents to date. ACE inhibitors are, along with AT_1-antagonists, clearly vasculoprotective in small animal models (rat, rabbit, guinea pig) and, to a modest degree, in pigs, However, randomized, double-blind, placebo-controlled clinical trials show that ACE inhibitors, even in high doses, do not improve the incidence of restenosis following PTCA (cilazapril, enalapril, fosinopril; MERCATOR and MARCATOR trials; 194–196).

Table 9 Increasing the Predictivity of Restenosis Models

APPROACH	TYPICAL DRAWBACK	AIM
Muscular arteries	The rat carotid artery is an elastic vessel lacking the structural and functional (e.g. vasomotion) characteristics of a coronary artery.	To use coronary arteries (and other vessels) of rabbits and pigs which, like human coronary arteries, are muscular vessels.
Branch points and bifurcations	Typically, traumatic injury of the rat carotid artery is performed using long, straight unbranched portions of concentric artery.	To employ tortuous, eccentric coronary arteries that are amenable to injury at the site of flow dividers.
Vessels dimensions	The hemodynamic characteristics of the arteries of small animals, especially rats, experience shear stresses which far exceed those observed clinically.	To use coronary vessels of pigs where the shear stresses experienced by the vessel wall more closely mimic those observed in patients.
Primary and secondary lesions: atherosclerosis and lipidemia	Many angioplasty models involve injuring naive/normal vessels with no preexisting lesion. Experimental angioplasty (e.g. rat carotid artery, a species resistant to experimental hyperlipidemia) is performed in the absence of atheroma.	To use techniques such as double balloon injury where trauma can be induced in vessels with preexisting, cellular/matrix rich lesions. In addition, angioplasty can be performed in vessels where primary atherosclerotic lesions have been induced (dietary manipulation, genetic strains of rabbit/pig).
Microthrombi	Unlike the clinical situation, platelet deposition and subsequent thrombotic events play a relatively unimportant role in neointima formation in the rat.	Models should be studied where coagulation cascades and mural microthrombi play a significant role in the pathogenesis of lesion formation (i.e. dogs, pigs and nonhuman primates).
Presence of intima: migration	The rat carotid artery contains no intima other than a single layer of squamous endothelial cells, hence no subendothelial intimal cells are present. Therefore, neointima formation is dependent upon the infiltration/migration of cells *e.g.* smooth muscle cells.	To use conduit vessels of rabbits and larger species which contain a substantial intima, rich in cellular and matrix components. Therefore, the proliferation of resident cells can make a significant contribution to lesion formation.
Mode of injury	Balloon -induced endothelial denudation (rubbing) or extravascular trauma (crush injury) are considered to be severe forms of vascular trauma.	Coronary artery balloon inflation (no intentional rubbing) or stent implantation in rabbits or larger species may mimic clinical procedures more closely.
Endpoints	Injury is analyzed by quantitative morphometry (vessel cross section) or a surrogate markers of injury is used (platelet deposition, proliferation index)	Analysis of lesion formation by angiography, intravascular ultrasound or MRI.
Time course	Typically, the degree of lesion is assessed at 2 weeks after injury in the rat carotid artery	Injury assessed after lesion has had a chance to mature, allowing matrix maturation, scar contraction to occur (>4 weeks)
Dosage regimens of investigational drug	The doses of investigational drugs employed in animal models are frequently excessive (>10 mg kg^{-1}) and multiple daily dosing regimens are employed (drugs are frequently administered continuously).	The dose of drug and the plasma levels obtained should reflect its pharmacology, both its pharmacodynamic and clinical pharmacokinetic profile. The effect of acute and chronic drug administration should be investigated.
Concomitant therapy	Investigators rarely study drug interactions and synergism with other drugs.	Clinically, patients are usually already receiving vasodilator therapy (Ca^{2+} antagonists, β-blockers, nitrates) and anticoagulant therapy. Drugs of interest should be shown to be efficacious when coadministered with the types of drugs described.

With hindsight, it is now clear why the rat carotid artery model was a poor predictor of the clinical efficacy of these agents. In this model, medial smooth muscle migration is an essential step in neointimal lesion formation, i.e., neointima formation is dependent on cellular migration, a process readily blocked by ACE inhibitors. However, in humans lesion formation is less dependent on the migration of medial smooth muscle cells to the site of injury since the intima of primary atherosclerotic lesions already contains resident cells (Table 1). Indeed, several investigators reported that cilazapril, enalapril, and DuP-753 did not inhibit lesion formation in rabbit, pig, and baboon vessels, which possess an intrinsic tunica intima replete with resident cells (Table 10).

However, this does not necessarily mean that larger animal models make better animal models, and their reliability must also challenged: ACE inhibition or AT_1-receptor antagonism produces significant vasculoprotective effects in a pig coronary stent model but does not inhibit angioplasty-induced lesion formation in pig or rabbit carotid and femoral arteries (Table 10; 14,194,195,197–200). Indeed, this lack of predictability is not limited to ACE inhibitors, nor is it limited to pigs: angiopeptin, ω3-fatty acids, and dipyridamole all reduce lesion formation in pig and baboon models yet fail to inhibit clinical restenosis (35,39,158,162,182,184). Thus, although pigs and nonhuman primates are becoming increasingly popular animals for the investigation of adjunct therapies, currently no one animal model has been shown satisfactorily to be entirely predictive of the human condition. Although these models are certainly promising, producing lesions that appear to more closely mimic those observed in humans, they have not yet been extensively studied.

The "inconsistent" predictability of the most commonly used restenosis animal models has led to the development of every more costly and complex models in larger species where the anatomical, pathological, and procedural aspects of clinical restenosis are more closely mimicked. However, such models are not amenable to large-scale, rapid, easy screening of pharmacological agents. As a consequence, many research groups are adopting a process whereby initial screening of compounds of interest is performed using several different cells-based in vitro assays of proliferation, migration, matrix production, etc. Once candidate molecules have been identified, they can be studied extensively in small animals such as the rat and rabbit prior to selecting the most promising compounds for study in larger models such as the pig and, ultimately, baboon (Table 11). This lack of predictability underscores a fundamental lack of understanding of the basic molecular mechanisms that control vascular reocclusion in the clinic.

Table 10 Vasculoprotective Efficacy of Angiotensin Inhibitors in Animal Models: Predictivity of Clinical Restenosis

SPECIES	COMPOUND	DOSE	COMMENTS
POSITIVE EXPERIMENTAL STUDIES			
ACE INHIBITORS			
Rat	Cilazapril	10 mg kg^{-1} day^{-1}	Significant inhibition of neointima formation in carotid artery 2 weeks after balloon injury
Rabbit	Perindopril	2 mg kg^{-1} day^{-1}	Significant inhibition of neointima formation in carotid artery 2 weeks after balloon injury
Guinea-pig	Cilazapril	30 mg day^{-1}	Significant inhibition of neointima formation in femoral artery 3 weeks after photochemical injury
Pig	Trandolapril	10 mg day^{-1}	Significant inhibition of neointimal thickness per unit injury induced by oversized stent
AT_1-ANTAGONISTS			
Rat	DuP-753	12.5 mg day^{-1}	Significant inhibition of neointima formation in carotid artery 2 weeks after balloon injury
Rabbit	DuP-753	1 mg day^{-1}	Significant inhibition of neointima formation in carotid artery 2 weeks after balloon injury
NEGATIVE EXPERIMENTAL STUDIES			
ACE INHIBITORS			
Pig	Cilazapril	20 mg kg^{-1} day^{-1}	No significant inhibition of neointima formation in carotid artery 4 weeks after balloon injury
Baboon	Cilazapril	20 mg kg^{-1} day^{-1}	No significant inhibition of neointima formation in femoral artery 3 months after balloon injury
AT_1-ANTAGONISTS			
Rabbit	DuP-753	50 mg day^{-1}	No significant inhibition of minimum luminal diameter in carotid artery 4 weeks after balloon injury
CLINICAL STUDIES			
ACE INHIBITORS			
	Cilazapril	10 mg day^{-1} for 6 months	Randomized, double-blind, placebo-controlled study (n=595) where low dose ACE inhibition does not attenuate angiographically-defined (minimum luminal diameter) restenosis or alter clinical outcome.
	Cilazapril	20 mg day^{-1} for 6 months	Randomized, double-blind, placebo-controlled study (n=1436) where high dose ACE inhibition does not attenuate angiographically-defined (minimum luminal diameter) restenosis or alter clinical outcome.
	Fosinopril	40 mg day^{-1} for 6 months	Randomized, double-blind, placebo-controlled study (n=304) where ACE inhibition does not attenuate angiographically-defined (minimum luminal diameter) restenosis or alter clinical outcome.
	Enalapril	10 mg day^{-1} for 6 months	Randomized study (n=304) where ACE inhibition does not attenuate angiographically-defined (minimum luminal diameter) restenosis.

Table 11 Hypothetical Screen to Identify Candidates for Entrance into Clinical Restenosis Trials

1° *IN VITRO* ASSAYS
Examine rat, rabbit or porcine cells Study smooth muscle cells, endothelial cells, macrophages, T-lymphocytes and platelets in cell-based assays of proliferation (cell number, [^{3}H]thymidine incorporation, protein synthesis, FACS analysis), migration (Boyden chamber assay), matrix production (matrix synthesis, collagenase inhibition) and platelet function (collagen-induced aggregation) Study cells derived from peripheral (e.g aortic smooth muscle) and coronary vessels Assess efficacy in neonatal/contractile or adult/synthetic smooth muscle cell phenotype (isolate by proteolytic digestion or explant, early [≤P5] and late passage [≥P10] cells) Stimulate cells with both appropriate receptor specific agonist and also examine inhibition of serum-induced responses

⇓

2° *IN VITRO* ASSAYS
Perform above assays in cells derived from human coronary vessels Examine antagonist/inhibitor in human artery organ culture (study interaction between multiple cell types)

⇓

1° *IN VIVO* SCREEN: RAT MODELS
Use histological endpoints in common carotid artery model Perform dose-ranging studies Examine acute (2 weeks after angioplasty) and mature/chronic (1-3 monthsafter angioplasty) lesions Establish effect on antagonist-induced inhibition of neointima formation without prophylactic treatment, or following withdrawl of drug after acute dosage perod Study effect of coadministration of other drugs used as standard clinical adjuncts to PTCA (Ca^{2+} channel blockers, anticoagulants, β-blockers, aspirin) Examine multiple lesion formation in additional blood vessels (aorta, iliac or femoral arteries)

⇓

2° *IN VIVO* SCREEN: INTERMEDIATE ANIMAL MODELS
Use "double-balloon" rabbit models where pre-existing lesion can be injured Introduce lipid component to rabbit models - familial hypercholesterolemia, high cholesterol diet Preliminary study of thrombotic components in canine model Use "nonhistological" endpoints - angiography, MRI

⇓

3° *IN VIVO* SCREEN: PIG AND NON-HUMAN PRIMATE MODELS
Aiming to simulate procedural techniques/molecular and cellular mechanisms/anatomical aspects to those encountered during clinical PTCA using both pig and baboon Examine lesions in coronary vasculature Balloon inflation (or stent implacement) rather than balloon "rubbing"

VI. FUTURE DIRECTIONS

An alternative approach to enhancing the predictability of restenosis models would be to better understand the intracellular events that occur following vascular trauma, particularly at the molecular level. Hopefully, this can be accomplished by combining recent interventional developments (e.g., there use of directional atherectomy to harvest samples from human lesions) with advances made in the fields of molecular biology (e.g., differential display).

A. Molecular Mechanisms of Restenosis: Application of Differential Display

Traditionally, differentially expressed mRNAs have been identified using techniques such as subtractive hybridization. However, such techniques are time consuming and are restrictive where tissue specimens are small and/or scarce since they require the generation of large quantities of purified poly(A^+) mRNA for cDNA library construction. However, the recent development of differential display reverse transcription polymerase chain reaction (DD-RT-PCR) and the related RNA arbitrary primed PCR (RAP-PCR) have overcome these limitations (since they are PCR based, small quantities of total cellular RNA can be used to rapidly generate large quantities of cDNA; 201,202). DD-RT-PCR has identified several genes that are selectively expressed in cancer, diabetes, and embryogenesis (203). This technique is based upon the isolation of undergraded mRNA, which is reverse transcribed to a corresponding subset of single-stranded cDNAs using oligo(dT) primers (where the final 3'-nucleotide is either G, A, or C), which anneal to the mRNAs 3'poly(A^+) tail. An initial round of PCR amplification is performed using an arbitrary anchor primer, which anneals to the cDNA at some point downstream of the 5'-poly(T^+) tail. Additional PCR is performed, after which the amplified products are separated and displayed on a denaturing polyacrylamide gel. Once identified, a differentially expressed cDNA can be recovered from the gel, reamplified, cloned, and sequenced.

DD-RT-PCR has been used to identify novel mRNA transcripts in rats, the expression of which is selectively associated with the neointima that forms as a result of either balloon angioplasty or cardiac allograft transplant rejection. Specifically, cDNA transcripts have been differentially displayed that have identifiable homologies to mRNA's encoding proteins associated with cell replication (14–3-3γ, a member of a family of proteins that may control Ras/Raf coupling during mitosis, and P1-protein, a polypeptide involved in DNA replication) and cell-cell interactions (galactose/N-acetylgalactosamine macrophage lectin) (204–206). The combination of this technology with the collection of human tissue biopsies may greatly aid our understanding of the molecular mechanisms and mediators of restenosis following PTCA.

B. Inhibition of Molecular Targets

Along with standard cDNA library screening, subtractive hybridization techniques, major advances in the field of recombinant DNA technology, and the use of molecular biological techniques such as DD-RT-PCR will aid greatly in the quest to identify gene products controlling the pathogenesis of restenosis. However, alone, these techniques can do no more than identify mRNAs whose altered expression is associated with an aberrant cellular process. They cannot, for example, establish a direct cause-and-effect relationship between altered mRNA expression (which may occur indirectly or may not translate to a change in protein expression) and restenosis. In order to identify a direct link between a functional response and induced/suppressed gene expression, investigators must assess the effect of selectively modulating the expression of such genes in angioplasty models using emerging molecular technologies such as antisense therapy and gene transfer.

1. Antisense Technology

Gene expression can be selectively attenuated by administration of oligonucleotides, short antisense sequences complementary to a portion of a target mRNA. Oligonucleotides bind to a target transcript and form a duplex, thereby inhibiting mRNA translation (oligonucleotides that target DNA transcription can also be used). Antisense oligonucleotides are usually introduced into a host cell using liposome carriers, pluronic gels, or electroporation (occasionally direct injection is used). Since these short nucleotide polymers are subject to rapid intracellular degradation by RNAses, synthetic oligonucleotides with modified sugar-phosphate backbones have been developed to increase oligonucleotide stability [e.g., phosphorothioates, peptidic oligonucleotides (PNAs)]. Alternative modifications include the introduction of the catalytic domain of the hammerhead-ribozyme. These oligonucleotides not only bind to a target mRNA, they also promote its enzymatic cleavage. Experimental restenosis has been attenuated by extra- and intraluminal delivery of antisense oligonucleotides directed against immediate early genes (c-myb and c-myc), although inhibition may involve a nonantisense mechanism (207–210). Immediate early genes have been popular targets for antisense oligonucleotide therapy due to the relatively labile nature of these oligonucleotide molecules. The short biological half life of these molecules may explain why some investigators have failed to block neointima formation in vivo using c-myb antisense oligonucleotides (211). For this reason, gene therapy may make a more practical approach to the utilization of molecular medicine.

2. *Gene Therapy*

Rather than simply using exogenous "naked" DNA/RNA, the aim of gene therapy is to facilitate the stable in situ overexpression of an antisense (or sense) RNA. This is achieved by efficiently introducing (transfecting) foreign DNA into a somatic target cell, such as a smooth muscle or endothelial cell, using viral transfer (replication-defective retroviral vectors and amphotrophic adenoviruses, e.g., Sendai virus– or adenovirus-mediated transfection). The successful transfection of rat carotid and porcine femoral arteries with eukaryotic expression vectors encoding several distinct genes has helped confirm a role (both positive and negative) for their protein products in the genesis of experimental restenosis, e.g., endothelial NOS, inactive retinoblastoma gene product, PDGF-B, TGF-β1, aFGF (42,136,148,163). Similar effects have been achieved by targeting cyclin B1 and CDC2 kinase or by transfecting arteries with thymidine kinase (an enzyme that activates the nucleoside analog prodrug, ganciclovir, thereby facilitating cytotoxicity within a specific region of the artery; 212,213). Although atherosclerosis may significantly reduce the efficiency of viral transfection, the development of specialized catheters (double-tipped balloons, porous Wilensky balloons) suggests that gene therapy may provide an novel approach to standard pharmacological intervention in the treatment of vascular disorders such as restenosis in the future. Even if clinical variables limit the routine use of gene therapy, this technique will help in identifying critical molecular targets suitable for conventional pharmacotherapy.

VII. SUMMARY

Almost two decades after the first PTCA was performed, restenosis still constitutes the major unmet clinical obstacle in modern interventional cardiology. The identification of clinical candidates has been based, primarily, on data obtained in animal models of restenosis and has met with frustrating results. However, the failure to identify efficacious agents cannot alone be accounted for by poor experimental design (e.g., experimental dosage regimens of drug that have little clinical relevance). Instead, these shortfalls underline the paucity of knowledge concerning the precise cellular and molecular mechanisms that drive clinical restenosis. An inability to identify relevant mechanism has led to an obvious inability to design animal models that faithfully reproduce them. In addition, the mechanisms that have evolved to control vascular remodeling contain a tremendous degree of intrinsic redundancy, i.e., restenosis is controlled by several distinct growth factors and chemokines. Understanding how such factors interact may help identify common mechanistic pathways/processes amenable to pharmacological manipulation. Hopefully, the advances currently being made in molecular medicine, coupled with procedural advances, will help identify such processes in humans and aid the development of efficacious therapeutic adjuncts to PTCA.

ACKNOWLEDGMENTS

The author would like to express his sincere gratitude to Ms. Elisabeth A. Minthorn, Department of Drug Metabolism and Pharmacokinetics, SmithKline Beecham Pharmaceuticals, for her help and support during the preparation of this manuscript.

REFERENCES

1. Dotter CT, Judkins MP. Transluminal treatment of atherosclerotic obstruction: description of a new technique and preliminary report of its application. Circulation 1964; 30:654.
2. Grüntzig A. A transluminal dilatation of coronary artery stenosis. Lancet 1978; 1:263.
3. Clowes AW, Reidy MA, Clowes MM. Kinetics of cellular proliferation after arterial injury. I: smooth muscle growth in the absence of endothelium. Lab Invest 1983; 49:327–333.
4. Block PC, Baughman KL, Pasternak RC, Fallon JT. Transluminal angioplasty: correlation of morphologic and angiographic findings in an experimental model. Circulation 1980; 61:778–785.
5. Schwartz RS, Huber KC, Murphy JG, Edwards WD, Camrud AR, Vlietstra RE, Holmes DR. Restenosis and the proportional response to coronary artery injury: results in a porcine model. J Am Coll Cardiol 1992; 19:267–274.
6. Scheinowitz M, Shou M, Banai S, Gertz SD, Lazarus DF, Unger EF. Neointimal proliferation in canine coronary arteries: a model of restenosis permitting local and continuous drug delivery. Lab Invest 1994; 71:813–819.
7. Dzau VJ. Vascular renin-angiotensin system and vascular protection. J Cardiovasc Pharmacol 1993; 22(suppl 5):S1-S9.
8. Huckle WR, Earp HS. Regulation of cell proliferation and growth by angiotensin II. Prog Growth Factor Res 1994; 5:177–194.
9. Sung CP, Arleth AJ, Storer BL, Ohlstein EH. Angiotensin type 1 receptors

mediate smooth muscle proliferation and endothelin biosynthesis in rat vascular smooth muscle. J Pharmacol Exp Ther 1994; 271:429–437.

10. Daemon MJAP, Lombardi DM, Bosman FT, Schwartz SM. Angiotensin II induces smooth muscle proliferation in the normal and injured rat arterial wall. Circ Res 1991; 68:450–456.
11. Powell JS, Clozel JP, Müller RKM, Kuhn H, Hefti F, Hosang M, Baumgartner HR. Inhibitors of angiotensin-converting enzyme prevent myointimal proliferation after vascular injury. Science 1989; 245:186–188.
12. Janiak P, Libert O, Vilaine JP. The role of the renin-angiotensin system in neointima formation after injury in rabbits. Hypertension 1994; 24:671–678.
13. Hirata Y, Umemura K, Kondoh K, Uematsu T, Nakashima M. Experimental intimal thickening studies using the photochemically induced thrombosis model in the guinea-pig femoral artery. Atherosclerosis 1994; 107:117–124.
14. Huber KC, Schwartz RS, Edwards WD, Camrud AR, Bailey KR, Jorgenson MA, Holmes DR Jr. Effects of angiotensin converting enzyme inhibition on neointimal proliferation in a porcine coronary injury model. Am Heart J 1993; 125:695–701.
15. Taguchi J, Abe J, Ohno M, Schwartz SM, Kurokawa K. Topical application of AT_1 receptor antagonists prevents medial and neointimal proliferation after balloon injury. Blood Pressure 1994; 5:S38-S42.
16. Munro E, Patel M, Chan P, Betteridge L, Gallagher K, Schachter M, Wolfe J, Sever P. Effect of calcium channel blockers on the growth of human vascular smooth muscle cells derived from saphenous vein and vascular graft stenosis. J Cardiovasc Pharmacol 1994; 23:779–784.
17. Powell JS, Muller RK, Rouge M, Kuhn H, Hefti F, Baumgartner HR. The proliferative response to vascular injury is suppressed by angiotensin-converting enzyme inhibition. J Cardiovasc Pharmacol 1990; 16(suppl 4):S42-S49.
18. Saso Y, Ohtani A, Odawara A, Iwasaki H, Takashima K, Morita T. Inhibitory effect of clentiazem (TA-3090), a new calcium antagonist, on balloon catheter-induced intimal thickening of rabbit aorta. Cardiovasc Drug Ther 1993; 7:257–264.
19. Jackson CL, Bush RC, Bowyer DE. Inhibitory effect of calcium antagonists on balloon catheter-induced arterial smooth muscle cell proliferation and lesion size. Atherosclerosis 1988; 69:115–122.
20. Hillegass WB, Ohman EM, Leimberger JD, Califf RM. A meta-analysis of randomized trials of calcium antagonists to reduce restenosis after coronary angioplasty. Am J Cardiol 1994; 73:835-839.
21. Kuriyama S, Nakamura K, Kaguchi Y, Kimura M, Tamura H, Tamai K, Hashimoto T, Miyahara T. The effects of vasoactive agents on the proliferation of vascular smooth muscle cells grown in vitro. J Hypertension 1988; 6(suppl 4):S154-S156.
22. Blaes N, Boissel JP. Growth-stimulating effect of catecholamines on rat smooth muscle cells in culture. J Cell Physiol 1983; 116:167–172.

23. Bell L, Madri JA. Effect of platelet factors on migration of cultured bovine aortic endothelial and smooth muscle cells. Circ Res 1989; 65:1057–1065.
24. Nakaki T, Nakayama M, Yamamoto S, Kato R. α_1-Adrenergic stimulation and β_2-adrenergic inhibition of DNA synthesis in vascular smooth muscle cells. Mol Pharmacol 1990; 37:30–36.
25. Cavellero C, Di Tondo U, Mingazzini PL, Pesando PC, Spagnoli LG. Cell proliferation in the atherosclerotic lesions of cholesterol fed rabbits. Atherosclerosis 1973; 17:49–62.
26. Bevan RD. Effect of sympathetic denervation on smooth muscle cell proliferation in the growing rabbit ear artery. Circ Res 1975; 37:14–19.
27. Fronek K, Bloor CM, Amiel D, Chvapil M. Effect of long-term sympathectomy on the arterial wall in rabbits and rats. Exp Mol Pathol 1978; 28:279–289.
28. Fingerle J, Sanders KH, Fotev Z. Alpha 1-receptor antagonists urapidil and prazosin inhibit neointima formation in the rat carotid artery induced by balloon catheter injury. Basic Res Cardiol 1991; 86(suppl 1):75–81.
29. Ohlstein EH, Douglas SA, Sung CP, Yue TL, Louden C, Arleth A, Poste G, Ruffolo RR Jr, Feuerstein GZ. Carvedilol, a cardiovascular drug, prevents smooth muscle cell proliferation, migration and neointimal formation following vascular injury. Proc Natl Acad Sci USA 1993; 90:6189–6193.
30. Patel MK, Chan P, Betteridge LJ, Schachter M, Sever PS. Inhibition of human smooth muscle cell proliferation by the novel multiple-action antihypertensive agent carvedilol. J Cardiovasc Pharmacol 1995; 25:652–657.
31. Bennett MR, Littlewood TD, Hancock DC, Evan GI, Newby AC. Down-regulation of the c-myc proto-oncogene in inhibition of vascular smooth muscle cell proliferation: a signal for growth arrest. Biochem J 1994; 302:701–708.
32. Soyombo AA, Angelini GD, Newby AC. Neointima formation is promoted by surgical preparation and inhibited by cyclic nucleotides in human saphenous vein organ cultures. J Thoracic Cardiovasc Surg 1995; 109:2–12.
33. Guieu R, Paganelli F, Sampieri F, Bechis G, Levy S, Rochat H. The use of HPLC to evaluate the variations of blood coronary adenosine levels during percutaneous transluminal angioplasty. Clin Chim Acta 1994; 230:63–68.
34. Takiguchi Y, Nagano M, Ikeda Y, Nakashima M. Early administration of YT-146, an adenosine A2 receptor agonist, inhibits neointimal thickening after rat femoral artery endothelium injury. Eur J Pharmacol 1995; 281:205–207.
35. Harker LA, Ross R, Slichter SJ, Scott CR. Homocysteine-induced atherosclerosis: the role of endothelial cell injury and platelet response in its genesis. J Clin Invest 1976; 58:731–741.
36. Bomberger RA, Wilburn J, dePalma RG. Aspirin and dipyridamole increase intimal thickening after injury. Surg Forum 1983; 34:475–477.
37. Koster JK, Tryka AF, H'Doubler P, Collins JJ. The effect of low dose aspirin and dipyridamole upon atherosclerosis in the rabbit. Artery 1981; 9:405–413.
38. Rogers GP, Minor ST, Robinson K, Cromeens D, Woolbert SC, Stephens LC, Guyton JR, Wright K, Roubin GS, Raizner AE. Adjuvant therapy for in-

tracoronary stents: investigations in atherosclerotic swine. Circulation 1990; 82:560–569.
39. Schwartz L, Bourassa MG, Lesperance J. Aldridge HE, Kazim F. Aspirin and dipyridamole in the prevention of restenosis after percutaneous transluminal coronary angioplasty. N Engl J Med 1988; 318:1714–1719.
40. McNamara DB, Bedi B, Aurora H, Tena L, Ignarro LJ, Kadowitz PJ, Akers DL. L-Arginine inhibits balloon catheter-induced intimal hyperplasia. Biochem Biophys Res Commun 1993; 193:291–296.
41. Guo JP, Milhoan KA, Tuan JS, Lefer AM. Beneficial effect of SPM-5185, a cysteine-containing nitric oxide donor, in rat carotid artery intimal injury. Circ Res 1994; 75:77–84.
42. Von der Leyen HE, Gibbons GH, Morishita R, Lewis NP, Zhang L, Nakajima M, Kaneda Y, Cooke JP, Dzau VJ. Gene therapy inhibiting neointimal vascular lesion: in vivo transfer of endothelial cell nitric oxide synthase gene. Proc Natl Acad Sci USA 1995; 92:1137-1141.
43. Ohlstein EH, Douglas SA. Endothelin modulates vascular smooth muscle structure and vasomotion: implications in cardiovascular pathology. Drug Dev Res 1993; 29:108–128.
44. Ohlstein EH, Douglas SA, Brooks D, Hay DWP, Feuerstein GZ, Ruffolo RR Jr. Functions mediated by peripheral endothelin receptors. In: Ruffolo RR Jr., ed. Endothelin Receptors: from the Gene to the Human. Boca Raton, FL: CRC Press, 1995:109–185.
45. Lerman A, Edwards BS, Hallett JW, Heublein DM, Sandberg SM, Burnett JC Jr. Circulating and tissue endothelin immunoreactivity in advanced atherosclerosis. N Engl J Med 1991; 325:997–1001.
46. Malatino LS, Grassi R, Stancanelli B, Polizzi G, Leonardi C, Tamburino C, Tamburino G. Release of immunoreactive endothelin from the heart during percutaneous transluminal coronary angioplasty. Am Heart J 1993; 126:700–702.
47. Tahara A, Kohno M, Yanagi S, Itagane H, Toda I, Akioka K, Teragaki M, Yasuda M, Takeuchi K, Takeda T. Circulating immunoreactive endothelin in patients undergoing percutaneous transluminal coronary angioplasty. Metabolism 1992; 40:1235–1237.
48. Wang X, Douglas SA, Feuerstein GZ, Ohlstein EH. Temporal expression of ECE-1, ET-1, ET-3, ET_A and ET_B receptor mRNAs after balloon angioplasty in the rat. J Cardiovasc Pharmacol 1995; 26(suppl 3):S22-S25.
49. Watschinger B, Sayegh MH, Hancock WW, Russell ME. Up-regulation of endothelin-1 mRNA and peptide expression in rat cardiac allografts with rejection and atherosclerosis. Am J Pathol 1995; 146:1065–1072.
50. Douglas SA, Vickery-Clark LM, Storer BL, Hart T, Louden C, Elliott JD, Ohlstein EH. A role for endogenous endothelin-1 in neointima formation following rat carotid artery balloon angioplasty: antiproliferative effects of the non-peptide endothelin receptor antagonist SB 209670. Circ Res 1994; 75:190-197.
51. Trachtenberg JD, Sun S, Choi ET, Callow AD, Ryan US. Effect of

endothelin-1 infusion on the development of intimal hyperplasia after balloon catheter injury. J Cardiovasc Pharmacol 1993; 22(suppl 8):S355-S359.
52. Douglas SA, Meek TD, Ohlstein EH. Novel receptor antagonists welcome a new era in endothelin biology. Trends Pharmacol Sci 1994; 15:313–316.
53. Tsujino M, Hirata Y, Eguchi S, Watanabe T, Chatani F, Marumo F. Nonselective ET_A/ET_B receptor antagonist blocks proliferation of rat vascular smooth muscle cells after balloon angioplasty. Life Sci 1995; 56:449–454.
54. Hele D J, Birrell M, Bush RC, Flynn DA, Brown T J, Roach AG. Selective ET_A and mixed ET_A/ET_B receptor antagonists inhibit balloon catheter-induced smooth muscle cell proliferation in the rat thoracic aorta. Br J Pharmacol 1994; 114:P199.
55. Douglas SA, Vickery-Clark LM, Louden C, Ohlstein EH. Selective ETA receptor antagonism with BQ-123 is insufficient to inhibit angioplasty induced neointima formation in the rat. Cardiovasc Res 1995; 29:641–646.
56. Azuma H, Hamasaki H, Niimi Y, Terada T, Matsubara O. Role of endothelin-1 in neointima formation after endothelial removal in rabbit carotid arteries. Am J Physiol 1994; 267:H2259-H2267.
57. Azuma H, Hamasaki H, Sato J, Isotani E, Obayashi S, Matsubara O. Different localization of ET_A and ET_B receptors in the hyperplastic vascular wall. J Cardiovasc Pharmacol 1995; 25:802–809.
58. Moreland S, Jenkins-West T, Valentine M, Ferrer P. BMS-182874 inhibits intimal lesion formation in balloon-injured rat carotid arteries. J Cardiovasc Pharmacol. In press.
59. Wessale J, Adler A, Novosad E, Burke S, Dayton B, Opgenorth T. Endothelin antagonism reduces neointima formed following balloon injury in the rabbit. J Cardiovasc Pharmacol. In press.
60. Kowala MC, Rose PM, Stein PD, Goller N, Recce R, Beyer S, Valentine M, Barton D, Durham SK. Selective blockade of the endothelin subtype A receptor decreases early atherosclerosis in hamsters fed cholesterol. Am J Pathol 1995; 146:819–826.
61. Loesch A, Bodin P, Burnstock G. Colocalization of endothelin vasopressin and serotonin in cultured endothelial cells of rabbit aorta. Peptides 1991; 12:1095–1103.
62. Bodin P, Travo P. Effects of naftidrofuryl on the contraction and proliferation of cultured myocytes evoked by serotonin. J Cardiovasc Pharmacol 1990; 16(suppl 3):S25-S28.
63. Sigal SL, Gellman J, Anderson GM, True LD, Chen Q, Tselentakis MJ, Ling FS, Ezekowitz MD. Potentiation of the vasospastic response to angioplasty by pretreatment with fluoxetine. A study in the atherosclerotic rabbit. Arterioscl Throm 1993, 13:907–914.
64. Bell L, Madri JA. Effect of platelet factors on migration of cultured bovine aortic endothelial and smooth muscle cells. Circ Res 1989; 65:1057–1065.
65. Bondesson L, Nordlind K, Liden S, Sundstrom E. Inhibiting effects of serotonin antagonists on the migration of mononuclear leukocytes. Immunopharmacol Immunotoxicol 1993; 15:243–250.

66. Katz MF, Farber HW, Dodds-Stitt Z, Cruikshank WW, Beer DJ. Secretion of a novel T-lymphocyte cytokine possessing both chemotactic and growth factor activity by serotonin-stimulated human aortic endothelial cells. Exp Cell Res 1994; 212:113–119.
67. Massey MF, Davies MG, Svendsen E, Klyachkin ML, Schwartz LB, Barber L, McCann RL, Hagen PO. Reduction of experimental vein graft intimal hyperplasia by ketanserin. J Surg Res 1993; 54:530–538.
68. Kauffman RF, Bean JS, Bloomquist WE, Cohen ML. Vascular serotonin 5-HT_2 receptor blockade by LY215840: lack of effect upon neointima formation in balloon-injured rat carotid arteries. J Pharmacol Exp Ther 1993; 266:450–455.
69. Serruys PW, Klein W, Tijssen JP, Rutsch W, Heyndrickx GR, Emanuelsson H, Ball SG, Decoster O, Schroeder E, Liberman H. Evaluation of ketanserin in the prevention of restenosis after percutaneous transluminal coronary angioplasty. A multicenter randomized double-blind placebo-controlled trial. Circulation 1993; 88:1588–1601.
70. Fletcher JR. Eicosanoids. Critical agents in the physiological process and cellular injury. Arch Surg 1993; 128:1192–1196.
71. Vane JR, Botting RM. Pharmacodynamic profile of prostacyclin. Am J Cardiol 1995; 75:3A-10A.
72. Hehrlein C, Svenson RH, McKusik AP, Chuang CH, Tuntelder JR, Tatsis GP, Littmann L, Thompson M. Thermal laser arterial injury and prostacyclin administration in dogs: thrombotic and hyperplastic consequences. J Cardiovasc Surg 1992; 33:366–371.
73. Völker W, Faber V. Aspirin reduces the growth of medial and neointimal thickenings in balloon-injured rat carotid arteries. Stroke 1990; 21(suppl IV):44–45.
74. August D, Tilson MD. Modification of myointimal response to arterial injury: effects of aspirin and warfarin. Surg Forum 1980; 31:337–338.
75. Clowes AW, Karnovsky MJ. Failure of certain antiplatelet drugs to affect myointimal thickening following arterial endothelial injury in the rat. Lab Invest 1977; 36:452–464.
76. Bush HL, Jakubowski JA, Sentissi JM, Curl GR, Hayes JA, Deykin D. Neointimal hyperplasia occurring after carotid endarterectomy in a canine model: effect of endothelial seeding vs. perioperative aspirin. J Vasc Surg 1987; 5:118–125.
77. Ingerman-Wojenski CM, Silver MJ. Model system to study the interaction of platelets with damaged arterial wall. II: inhibition of smooth muscle cell proliferation by dipyridamole and AH-P719. Exp Mol Pathol 1988; 48:116–134.
78. Serruys PW, Rutsch W, Heyndrickx GR, Danchin N, Mast EG, Wijns W, Rensing BJ, Vos J, Stibbe J. Prevention of restenosis after percutaneous transluminal coronary angioplasty with thromboxane A_2-receptor blockade: a randomized, double-blind, placebo-controlled trial. Coronary artery restenosis prevention on repeated thromboxane-antagonism study (CARPORT). Circulation 1991; 84:1568–1580.

79. Hattori R, Kodama K, Takatsu F, Yui Y, Kawai C. Randomized trial of a selective inhibitor of thromboxane A_2 synthase, (E)-7-phenyl 7-(3-pyridyl)-6-heptenoic acid (CV-4151), for prevention of restenosis after coronary angioplasty. Jpn Circ J 1991; 55:324–329.
80. Longenecker JP, Kilty LA, Johnson LK. Glucocorticoid influence on growth of vascular wall cells in culture. J Cell Physiol 1982; 113:197–202.
81. Longenecker JP, Kilty LA, Johnson LK. Glucocorticoid inhibition of vascular smooth muscle cell proliferation: influence of homologous extracellular matrix and serum mitogens. J Cell Biol 1984; 98:534–540.
82. Voisard R, Seitzer U, Baur R, Dartsch PC, Osterhues H, Hoher M, Hombach V. Corticosteroid agents inhibit proliferation of smooth muscle cells from human atherosclerotic arteries in vitro. Int J Cardiol 1994; 43:257–267.
83. Hirosumi J, Nomoto A, Ohkubo Y, Sekiguchi C, Mutoh S, Yamaguchi I, Aoki H. Inflammatory response in cuff-induced atherosclerosis in rabbits. Atherosclerosis 1987; 64:243–254.
84. Chervu A, Moore WS, Quinones-Baldrich WJ, Henderson T. Efficacy of corticosteroids in suppression of intimal hyperplasia. J Vasc Surg 1989; 10:129–134.
85. Colburn MD, Moore WS, Galebert HA, Quinones-Baldrich WJ. Dose responsive suppression of myointimal hyperplasia by dexamethasone. J Vasc Surg 1992; 15:510–518.
86. Villa AE, Guzman LA, Chen W, Golomb G, Levy RJ, Topol EJ. Local delivery of dexamethasone for prevention of neointimal proliferation in a rat model of balloon angioplasty. J Clin Invest 1994; 93:1243–1249.
87. Muller DW, Golomb G, Gordon G, Levy RJ. Site-specific dexamethasone delivery for the prevention of neointimal thickening after vascular stent implantation. Coronary Artery Dis 1994; 5:435-442.
88. Wilckens T. Glucocorticoids and immune function: physiological relevance and pathogenic potential of hormonal dysfunction. Trends Pharmacol Sci 1995; 16:193–197.
89. Libby P, Schwartz D, Brogi E, Tanaka H, Clinton SK. A cascade model for restenosis. A special case of atherosclerosis progression. Circulation 1992; 86(suppl 6):III47-III52.
90. Stone GW, Rutherford BD, McConahay DR, Johnson WL, Giorgi LV, Ligon RW, Hartzler GO. A randomized trial of corticosteroids for the prevention of restenosis in 102 patients undergoing repeat coronary angioplasty. Cath Cardiovasc Dis 1989; 18:227–231.
91. McKenney PA, Currier JW, Haudenschild LL, Heyman D, Faxon DP. Cyclosporin A does not inhibit restenosis in experimental angioplasty. Circulation 1991; 84(suppl II):70.
92. Jonasson L, Holm J, Hansson GK. Cyclosporin A inhibits smooth muscle proliferation in the vascular response to injury. Proc Natl Acad Sci USA 1988; 85:2303–2306.
93. Ferns G, Reidy MA, Ross R. Vascular effects of cyclosporin A in vivo and in vitro. Am J Pathol 1990; 137:403–413.

94. Reece AH, Walton PL. Inhibition of intimal proliferation of rabbit aorta by ticlodipine. Thromb Haemost 1979; 42:367.
95. Bertrand ME, Allain H, LaBlanche JM. Results of a randomized trial of ticlodipine versus placebo for prevention of acute closure and restenosis after coronary angioplasty (PTCA): the TACT study. Circulation 1990; III:190.
96. Herrmann HC, Okada SS, Hozakowska E, Le Veen RF, Golden MA, Tomaszewski JE, Weisz PB, Barnathan ES. Inhibition of smooth muscle cell proliferation and experimental angioplasty restenosis by beta-cyclodextrin tetradecasulfate. Arteriosc1 Thromb 1993; 13:924–931.
97. Letourneur D, Logeart D, Avramoglou T, Jozefonvicz J. Antiproliferative capacity of synthetic dextrans on smooth muscle cell growth: the model of derivatized dextrans as heparin-like polymers. J Biomat Sci 1993; 4:431–444.
98. Tyrrell DJ, Kilfeather S, Page CP. Therapeutic uses of heparin beyond its traditional role as an anticoagulant. Trends Pharmacol Sci 1995; 16:198–204.
99. Clowes AW, Karnovsky MJ. Suppression by heparin of smooth muscle proliferation in injured arteries. Nature 1977; 265:625-626.
100. Berk BC, Gordon JB, Alexander RW. Pharmacological roles of heparin and glucocorticoids to prevent restenosis after coronary angioplasty. J Am Coll Cardiol 1991, 17:111B-117B.
101. Currier JW, Pow TK, Haudenschild CC, Minihan AC, Faxon DP. Low molecular weight heparin (Enoxaparin) reduces restenosis after iliac angioplasty in the hypercholesterolemic rabbit. J Am Coll Cardiol 1991; 17:118B-125B.
102. Oberhoff M, Hanke H, Hassenstein S, Hanke S, Kamenz J. Inhibition of smooth muscle proliferation after experimental balloon angioplasty: comparison of LMWH and unfractionated heparin. Circulation 1991; 84:II80.
103. Unterberg C, Buchwald AB, Nebendahl K, Wiegand V. Low molecular weight heparin reduces intimal proliferation after coronary stenting. J Am Coll Cardiol 1992; 19:291A.
104. More RS, Brack MJ, Gershlick AC. Heparin after angioplasty: an unresolved issue? Eur Heart J 1993; 14:1543–1547.
105. Faxon DP, Spiro T, Minor S, Douglas J, Cote G. Enoxaparin, a low molecular weight heparin in the prevention of restenosis after angioplasty: result of a double-blind randomized trial. J Am Coll Cardiol 1991; 19:258A.
106. Lefkovits J, Plow EF, Topol EJ. Platelet glycoprotein IIb/IIIa receptors in cardiovascular medicine. N Engl J Med 1995; 332:1553–1559.
107. Bates ER, McGillem MJ, Mickelson JK, Pitt B, Mancini GB. A monoclonal antibody against the platelet glycoprotein IIb/IIIa receptor complex prevents platelet aggregation and thrombosis in a canine model of coronary angioplasty. Circulation 1991; 84:2463-2469.
108. Use of monoclonal antibody directed against the platelet glycoprotein IIb/IIIa receptor in high-risk coronary angioplasty. The EPIC investigation. N Engl J Med 1994; 330:956–961.
109. Topol EJ, Califf RM, Weisman HF, Ellis SG, Tcheng JE, Worley S, Ivanhoe R, George BS, Fintel D, Weston M. Randomized trial of coronary interven-

tion with antibody against platelet IIb/IIIa integrin for reduction of clinical restenosis: results at six months. The EPIC Investigators. Lancet 1994; 343:881–886.
110. Matsuno H, Stassen JM, Vermylen J, Deckmyn H. Inhibition of integrin function by a cyclic RGD-containing peptide prevents neointima formation. Circulation 1994; 90:2203–2206.
111. Choi ET, Engel L, Callow AD, Sun S, Trachtenberg J, Santoro S, Ryan U. Inhibition of neointimal hyperplasia by blocking alpha V beta 3 integrin with a small peptide antagonist GpenGRGDSPCA. J Vasc Surg 1994; 19:125–134.
112. Imura Y, Stassen JM, Vreys I, Ledaffre E, Gold HK, Collen D. Synergistic antithrombotic properties of G4120, a RGD-containing synthetic peptide, and argatroban, a synthetic thrombin inhibitor, in a hamster femoral vein platelet-rich thrombus model. Thromb Haemostas 1992; 68:336–340.
113. Walters TK, Gorog DA, Wood RF. Thrombin generation following arterial injury is a critical initiating event in the pathogenesis of the proliferative stages of the atherosclerotic process. J Vasc Res 1994; 31:173–177.
114. Sarembock IJ, Gertz SD, Gimple LW, Owen RM, Powers ER, Roberts WC. Effectiveness of recombinant desulphatohirudin in reducing restenosis after balloon angioplasty of atherosclerotic femoral arteries in rabbits. Circulation 1991; 84:232–243.
115. Ragosta M, Gimple LW, Gertz SD, Dunwiddie CT, Vlasuk GP, Haber HL, Powers ER, Roberts WC, Sarembock IJ. Specific factor Xa inhibition reduces restenosis after balloon angioplasty of atherosclerotic femoral arteries in rabbits. Circulation 1994; 89:1262–1271.
116. Asahara T, Bauters C, Pastore C, Kearney M, Rossow S, Bunting S, Ferrara N, Symes JF, Isner JM. Local delivery of vascular endothelial growth factor accelerates reendothelialization and attenuates intimal hyperplasia in balloon-injured rat carotid artery. Circulation 1995; 91:2793–2801.
117. Hoch JR, Stark VK, Turnipseed WD. The temporal relationship between the development of vein graft intimal hyperplasia and growth factor gene expression. J Vasc Surg 1995; 22:51–58.
118. Lindner V, Giachelli CM, Schwartz SM, Reidy MA. A subpopulation of smooth muscle cells in injured rat arteries express platelet-derived growth factor-B chain mRNA. Circ Res 1995; 76:951–957.
119. Bilder GE, Kasiewski CJ, Costello RJ, Hodge TG, Perrone MH. Electrode cuff-induced changes in DNA and PDGF gene expression in the rat carotid artery. Atherosclerosis 1993; 100:103–112.
120. Kraiss LW, Raines EW, Wilcox JN, Seifert RA, Barrett TB, Kirkman TR, Hart CE, Bowen-Pope DF, Ross R, Clowes AW. Regional expression of the platelet-derived growth factor and its receptors in a primate graft model of vessel wall assembly. J Clin Invest 1993; 92:338–348.
121. Marmur JD, Poon M, Rossikhina M, Taubman MB. Induction of PDGF-responsive genes in vascular smooth muscle. Implications for the early response to vessel injury. Circulation 1992; 86(suppl 6):III53-III60.
122. Majesky MW, Giachelli CM, Reidy MA, Schwartz SM. Rat carotid neointimal

smooth muscle cells reexpress a developmentally regulated mRNA phenotype during repair of arterial injury. Circ Res 1992; 71:759–768.
123. Ferns GA, Raines EW, Sprugel KH, Montani AS, Reidy MA, Ross R. Inhibition of neointimal smooth muscle accumulation after angioplasty by an antibody to PDGF. Science 1991; 253:1129–1132.
124. Munro E, Patel M, Chan P, Betteridge L, Gallagher K, Schachter M, Wolfe J, Sever P. Growth inhibition of human vascular smooth muscle cells by fenofibrate: a possible therapy for restenosis. Cardiovasc Res 1994; 28:615–620.
125. Kovalenko M, Gazit A, Bohmer A, Rorsman C, Ronnstrand L, Heldin CH, Waltenberger J, Bohmer FD, Levitzki A. Selective platelet-derived growth factor receptor kinase blockers reverse sis-transformation. Cancer Res 1994; 54:6106–6114.
126. Cosigny PM, Barry JJ, Vitali NJ. Local delivery of an antiproliferative drug with use of hydrogel-coated angioplasty balloons. J Vasc Int Radiol 1994; 5:553–560.
127. Tiell ML, Sussman H, Gordon PB, Saunders RN. Suppression of fibroblast proliferation in vitro and of myointimal hyperplasia in vivo by triazolopyrimidine. Artery 1983; 12:33–50.
128. Liu MW, Roubin GS, Robinson KA, Black AJ, Hearn JA, Siegel RJ, King SB III. Trapidil in preventing restenosis after balloon angioplasty in the atherosclerotic rabbit. Circulation 1990; 81:1089–1093.
129. Mullins DE, Hamud F, Reim R, Davis HR. Inhibition of PDGF receptor binding and PDGF-stimulated biological activity in vitro and of intimal lesion formation in vivo by 2-bromomethyl-5-chlorobenzene sulfonylphthalimide. Arteroscl Thromb 1994; 14:1047-1055.
130. Jawien A, Bowen-Pope DF, Lindner V, Schwartz SM, Clowes AW. Platelet-derived growth factor promotes smooth muscle migration and intimal thickening in a rat model of balloon angioplasty. J Clin Invest 1992; 89:507–511.
131. Okamoto S, Inden M, Setsuda M, Konishi T, Nakano T. Effects of trapidil (triazolopyrimidine), a platelet-derived growth factor antagonist, in preventing restenosis after percutaneous transluminal coronary angioplasty. Am Heart J 1992; 123:1439–1444.
132. Maresta A, Balducelli M, Cantini L, Casari A, Chioin R, Fabbri M, Fontanelli A, Monici Preti PA, Repetto S, De Servi S. Trapidil (triazolopyrimidine), a platelet-derived growth factor antagonist, reduces restenosis after percutaneous transluminal coronary angioplasty. Results of the randomized, double-blind STARC study: studio trapidil versus aspirin nella restenosis coronarica. Circulation 1994; 90:2710–2715.
133. Hancock WW, Adams DH, Wyner LR, Sayegh MH, Karnovsky MJ. CD4+ mononuclear cells induce cytokine expression, vascular smooth muscle cell proliferation, and arterial occlusion after endothelial cell injury. Am J Pathol 1994; 145:1008–1014.
134. Brown SL, Lundgren CH, Nordt T, Fujii S. Stimulation of migration of

human aortic smooth muscle cells by vitronectin: implications for atherosclerosis. Cardiovasc Res 1994; 28:1815-1820.
135. Li Z, Alavi MZ, Moore S. The proliferation of neointimal smooth muscle cells cultured from rabbit aortic explants 15 weeks after de-endothelialization by a balloon catheter. Int J Exp Pathol 1994; 75:169–177.
136. Nabel EG, Shum L, Pompili VJ, Yang ZY, San H, Shu HB, Liptay S, Gold L, Gordon D, Derynck R. Direct transfer of transforming growth factor beta 1 gene into arteries stimulates fibrocellular hyperplasia. Proc Natl Acad Sci USA 1993; 90:10759-10763.
137. Majesky MW, Lindner V, Twardzik DR, Schwartz SM, Reidy MA. Production of transforming growth factor beta 1 during repair of arterial injury. J Clin Invest 1991; 88:904–910.
138. McCaffrey TA, Falcone DJ, Borth W, Brayton CF, Weksler BB. Fucoidan is a non-coagulant inhibitor of intimal hyperplasia. Biochem Biophys Res Commun 1992; 184:773–781.
139. Bauriedel G, Heidemann P, Klingel K, Windstetter U, Hofling B, Kandolf R. In situ detection of EGF receptor mRNA in arteriosclerotic lesions in man: implications for the proliferative activity of smooth muscle cells. Z Kardiol 1992; 81:519–524.
140. Epstein SE, Siegall, Biro S, Fu, YM, Fitzgerald D, Pastan I. Cytotoxic effects of a recombinant chimeric toxin on rapidly proliferating vascular smooth muscle cells. Circulation 1991; 84:778–787.
141. Pickering JG, Bacha PA, Weir L, Jekanowski J, Nichols JC, Isner JM. Prevention of smooth muscle outgrowth from human atherosclerotic plaque by a recombinant cytotoxin specific for the epidermal growth factor receptor. J Clin Invest 1993; 91:724–729.
142. Fu, YM, Mesri EA, Yu ZX, Kreitman RJ, Pastan I, Epstein SE. Cytotoxic effects of vascular smooth muscles of the chimeric toxin, heparin binding TGF alpha-Pseudomonas exotoxin. Cardiovasc Res 1993; 27:1691–1697.
143. Friesel RE, Maciag T. Molecular mechanisms of angiogenesis: fibroblast growth factor signal transduction. FASEB J 1995; 9:919-925.
144. Reidy MA, Jackson CL. Factors controlling growth of arterial cells following injury. Toxicol Pathol 1990; 18:547–553.
145. Lindner V, Majack RA, Reidy MA. Basic FGF stimulates endothelial regrowth and proliferation in denuded arteries. J Clin Invest 1990; 85:2004–2008.
146. Xin X, Johnson AD, Scott-Burden T, Engler D, Casscells W. The predominant form of fibroblast growth factor receptor expressed by proliferating human arterial smooth muscle cells in culture is type I. Biochem Biophys Res Commun 1994; 204:557–564.
147. Fishel RS, Thourani V, Eisenberg SJ, Shai SY, Corson MA, Nabel EG, Bernstein KE, Berk BC. Fibroblast growth factor stimulates angiotensin converting enzyme expression in vascular smooth muscle cells. Possible mediator of the response to vascular injury. J Clin Invest 1995; 95:377–387.

148. Nabel EG, Yang ZY, Plautz G, Forough R, Zhan X, Haudenschild CC, Maciag T, Nabel GJ. Recombinant fibroblast growth factor-1 promotes intimal hyperplasia and angiogenesis in arteries in vivo. Nature 1993; 362:844–846.
149. Siegall CB, Epstein S, Spier E, Hla T, Forough R, Maciag T, Fitzgerald DJ, Pastan I. Cytotoxic activity of chimeric proteins composed of acidic fibroblast growth factor and Pseudomonas exotoxin on a variety of cell types. FASEB J 1991; 5:2843–2849.
150. Khorsandi MJ, Fagin JA, Giannella-Neto D, Fortester JS, Cercek B. Regulation of insulin-like growth factor-I and its receptor in rat aorta after balloon denudation. Evidence for local bioactivity. J Clin Invest 1992; 90: 1926–1931.
151. Mooradian DL, Fernandes B, Diglio CA, Lester BR. Angiopeptin (BIM23014C) inhibits vascular smooth muscle cell migration in vitro through G-protein-mediated pathway and is associated with inhibition of adenylyl cyclase and cAMP accumulation. J Cardiovasc Pharmacol 1995; 25:611–618.
152. Bauters C, Van Belle E, Wernert N, Delcayre C, Thomas F, Dupuis B, Lablanche JM, Bertrand ME, Swynghedauw B. Angiopeptin inhibits oncogene induction in rabbit aorta after balloon denudation. Circulation 1994; 89:2327–2331.
153. Foegh ML, Asotra S, Conte JV, Howell M, Kagan E, Verma F, Ramwell PW. Early inhibition of myointimal proliferation by angiopeptin after balloon catheter injury in the rabbit. J Vasc Surg 1994; 19:1084–1091.
154. Lundergan CF, Foegh ML, Vargas R, Eufemio M, Bormes GW, Kot PA, Ramwell PW. Inhibition of myointimal proliferation of the rat carotid artery by the peptides, angiopeptin and BIM 23034. Atherosclerosis 1989; 80:49–55.
155. Asotra S, Foegh ML, Conte JV, Cai BR, Ramwell PW. Inhibition of 3H-thymidine incorporation by angiopeptin in the aorta of rabbits after balloon angioplasty. Transplant Proc 1989; 21:3695–3696.
156. Howell M, Adams MM, Wolfe MS, Foegh M, Ramwell PW. Angiopeptin inhibition of myointimal hyperplasia after balloon angioplasty in large arteries in hypercholesterolaemic rabbits. Clin Sci 1993; 85:183–188.
157. Howell M, Orskov H, Frystyk J, Flyvbjerg A, Gronbaek H, Foegh M. Lanreotide, a somatostatin analogue, reduces insulin-like growth factor I accumulation in proliferating aortic tissue in rabbits. A preliminary study. Eur J Endocrinol 1994; 130:422–425.
158. Santoian ED, Schneider JE, Gravanis MB, Foegh M, Tarazona N, Cipolla GD, King SB III. Angiopeptin inhibits intimal hyperplasia after angioplasty in porcine coronary arteries. Circulation 1993; 88:11–14.
159. Mennander A, Raisanen A, Paavonen T, Hayry P. Chronic rejection in the rat allograft. V: Mechanism of the angiopeptin (BIM23014C) effect on the generation of allograft atherosclerosis. Transplantation 1993; 55:124–128.
160. Grant MB, Wargovich TJ, Ellis EA, Caballero S, Mansour M, Pepine CJ. Localization of insulin-like growth factor I and inhibition of coronary smooth

muscle growth by somatostatin analogues in human coronary smooth muscle cells. A potential treatment for restenosis. Circulation 1994; 89:1511–1517.
161. Bornfeldt KE, Raines EW, Nakano T, Graves LM, Krebs EG, Ross R. Insulin-like growth factor-I and platelet-derived growth factor-BB induce directed migration of human arterial smooth muscle cells via signaling pathways that are distinct from those of proliferation. J Clin Invest 1994; 93:1266–1274.
162. Emanuelsson H, Beatt KJ, Bagger JP, Balcon R, Heikkila J, Piessens J, Schaeffer M, Suryapranata H, Foegh M. Long term effects of angiopeptin treatment in coronary angioplasty. Reduction of clinical events but not angiographic restenosis. European angiopeptin study group. Circulation 1995; 91:1689–1696.
163. Chang MW, Barr E, Seltzer J, Jiang YQ, Nabel GJ, Nabel EG, Parmacek MS, Leiden JM. Cytostatic gene therapy for vasculoproliferative disorders with a constitutively active form of the retinoblastoma gene product. Science 1995; 267:518–522.
164. Bauriedel G, Heimerl J, Beinert T, Welsch U, Hofling B. Colchicine antagonizes the activity of human smooth muscle cells cultivated from arteriosclerotic lesions after atherectomy. Cornonary Artery Dis 1994; 5:531–539.
165. Tanaka K, Honda M, Kuramochi T, Morioka S. Prominent inhibitory effects of tranilast on migration and proliferation of and collagen synthesis by vascular smooth muscle cells. Atherosclerosis 1994; 107:179–185.
166. Voisard R, Dartsch PC, Seitzer U, Hannekum A, Roth D, Kochs M, Hombach V. The in-vitro effect of antineoplastic agents on proliferative activity and cytoskeletal components of plaque-derived smooth-muscle cells from human coronary arteries. Cornonary Artery Dis 1993; 4:935–942.
167. Curtier JW, Pow TK, Minihan AC, Haudenschild CC, Faxon DP. Colchicine inhibits restenosis after iliac angioplasty in the atherosclerotic rabbit. Circulation 1989; 80(suppl 2):1166.
168. Sollott SJ, Cheng L, Pauly RR, Jenkins GM, Monticone RE, Kuzuya M, Froehlich Crow MT, Lakatta EG, Rowinsky EK. Taxol inhibits neointimal smooth muscle cell accumulation after angioplasty in the rat. J Clin Invest 1995; 95:1869–1876.
169. Murphy JG, Schwartz RS, Edwards WD, Camrud AR, Ko J. Methotrexate and azathioprine fail to inhibit porcine coronary restenosis. Circulation 1990; 82 (suppl 2):II429.
170. Curtier JW, Kalan JM, Franklin SM, Mejias Y, Cody C. Effects of local infusion of doxorubicin or saline on restenosis following angioplasty in atherosclerotic rabbits. Restenosis Summit 1992; IV:A9.
171. Cox DA, Anderson PG, Roubin GS, Chou CY, Agrawal SK. Local delivery of heparin and methotrexate fails to inhibit in vivo smooth muscle proliferation. Circulation 1991; 84(suppl 2):II71.
172. Mullet DW, Topol EJ, Abrams GD, Gallagher KP, Ellis SG. Intramural methotrexate therapy for the prevention of the neointimal thickening after balloon angioplasty. J Am Coll Cardiol 1992; 20:460–466.

173. O'Keefe JH Jr, McCallister BD, Bateman TM, Kuhnlein DL, Ligon RW, Hartzler GO. Ineffectiveness of colchicine for the prevention of restenosis after coronary angioplasty. J Am Coll Cardiol 1992; 19:1597–1600.
174. Pascal M, Sepulchre C, Chazan JB, Majoie B. Evidence for the inhibition of platelet-derived growth factor induced rat smooth muscle cells DNA synthesis by fenofibric acid at the G_0/G_1 cell cycle level. Life Sci 1983; 33:925-933.
175. Munro E, Patel M, Chan P, Betteridge L, Clunn G, Gallagher K, Hughes A, Schachter M, Wolfe J, Sever P. Inhibition of human vascular smooth muscle cell proliferation by lovastatin: the role of isoprenoid intermediates of cholesterol synthesis. Eur J Clin Invest 1994; 24:766–772.
176. Rogler G, Lacknet KJ, Schmitz G. Effects of fluvastatin on growth of porcine and human vascular smooth muscle cells in vitro. Am J Cardiol 1995; 76:114A-116A.
177. Gellman J, Ezekowitz MD, Sarembock IJ, Azrin MA, Nochomowitz LE, Lerner E, Haudenschild CC. Effect of lovastatin on intimal hyperplasia after balloon angioplasty: a study in an atherosclerotic hypercholesterolemic rabbit. J Am Coll Cardiol 1991; 17:251–259.
178. Wolda SL, Glomset JA. Evidence for modification of lamin B by a product of mevalonic acid. J Biol Chem 1988; 263:5997–6000.
179. Sahni R, Maniet AR, Voci G, Banka VS. Prevention of restenosis by lovastatin after successful coronary angioplasty. Am Heart J 1991; 121:1600–1608.
180. Weintraub WS, Boccuzzi S J, Klein JL, Kosinski AS, King SB III, Ivanhoe R, Cedarholm JC, Stillabower ME, Talley JD, DeMaio SJ. Lack of effect of lovastatin on restenosis after coronary angioplasty. Lovastatin restenosis trial study group. N Engl J Med 1994; 331:1331–1337.
181. Yamaguchi H, Lee YJ, Daida H, Yokoi H, Miyano H, Kanoh T, Ishiwata S, Kato K, Nishikawa H, Takatsu F. Effectiveness of LDL-apheresis in preventing restenosis after percutaneous transluminal coronary angioplasty (PTCA): LDL-apheresis angioplasty restenosis trial (L-ART). Chem Phys Lipids 1994; 67:399–403.
182. Harker LA, Kelly AB, Hanson SR, Krupski W, Bass A, Osterud B, Fitzgerald GA, Goodnight SH, Connor WE. Interruption of vascular thrombus formation and vascular lesion formation by dietary n-3 fatty acids in fish oil in nonhuman primates. Circulation 1993; 87:1017–1029.
183. Franzen D, Schannwell M, Oette K, Hopp HW. A prospective, randomized and double-blind trial on the effect of fish oil on the incidence of restenosis following PTCA. Cath Cardiovasc Diag 1993; 28:301–310.
184. Leaf A, Jorgensen MB, Jacobs AK, Cote G, Schoenfeld DA, Scheer J, Weiner BH, Slack JD, Kellet MA, Raizner AE. Do fish oils prevent restenosis after coronary angioplasty. Circulation 1994; 90:2248–2257.
185. Ferns GA, Forster L, Stewant-Lee A, Konneh M, Nourooz-Zadeh J, Anggard EE. Probucol inhibits neointimal thickening and macrophage accumulation after balloon injury in the cholesterol-fed rabbit. Proc Natl Acad Sci USA 1992; 89:11312–11316.
186. Schneider JE, Berk BC, Gravanis MB, Santoian EC, Cipolla GD, Tarazona

N, Lassegue B, King SB III. Probucol decreases neointimal formation in a swine model of coronary artery balloon injury. A possible role for antioxidants in restenosis. Circulation 1993; 88:628–637.
187. Baumann DS, Doblas M, Schonfeld G, Sicard GA, Daugherty A. Probucol reduces the cellularity of aortic intimal thickening at anastomotic regions adjacent to prosthetic grafts in cholesterol-fed rabbits. Arterioscl Thromb 1994; 14:162–167.
188. Nunes GL, Sgoutas DS, Redden RA, Sigman SR, Gravanis MB, King SB III, Berk BC. Combination of vitamins C and E alters the response to coronary balloon injury in the pig. Arterioscl Thromb Vasc Biol 1995; 15:156–165.
189. Lafont AM, Chai YC, Cornhill JF, Whitlow PL, Howe PH, Chisholm GM. Effect of alpha-tocopherol on restenosis after angioplasty in a model of experimental atherosclerosis. J Clin Invest 1995; 95:1018–1025.
190. Konneh MK, Rutherford C, Li SR, Anggard EE, Ferns GA. Vitamin E inhibits the intimal response to balloon catheter injury in the carotid artery of the cholesterol-fed rat. Atherosclerosis 1995; 113:29–39.
191. Yue TL, Wang X, Gu JL, Ruffolo RR Jr, Feuerstein GZ. Carvedilol, a new vasodilating beta-adrenoceptor blocker, inhibits oxidation of low-density lipoproteins by vascular smooth muscle cells and prevents leukocyte adhesion to smooth muscle cells. J Pharmacol Exp Ther 1995; 273:1442–1449.
192. Setsuda M, Inden M, Hiraoka N, Okamoto S, Tanaka H, Okinaka T, Nishimura Y, Okano H, Kouji T, Konishi T. Probucol therapy in the prevention of restenosis after successful percutaneous transluminal coronary angioplasty. Clin Ther 1993; 15:374–382.
193. DeMaio SJ, King SB III, Lembo NJ, Roubin GS, Hearn JA, Bhagavan HN, Sgoutas DS. Vitamin E supplementation, plasma lipids and the incidence of restenosis after percutaneous transluminal coronary angioplasty (PTCA). J Am Coll Nutr 1992; 11:68–73.
194. Faxon DP. Effect of high dose angiotensin-converting enzyme inhibition on restenosis: final results of the MARCATOR study, a multicenter, double-blind, placebo-controlled trial of cilazapril. J Am Coll Cardiol 1995; 25:362–369.
195. Desmet W, Vrolix M, De Schreerder I, Van Lierde J, Willems JL, Piessens J. Angiotensin-converting enzyme inhibition with fosinopril sodium in the prevention of restenosis after coronary angioplasty. Circulation 1994; 89:385–392.
196. Kaul U, Chandra S, Bahl VK, Sharma S, Wasir HS. Enalapril for prevention of restenosis after coronary angioplasty. Indian Heart J 1993; 45:469–473.
197. Lam JY, Lacoste L, Bourassa MG. Cilazapril and early atherosclerotic changes after balloon injury of carotid arteries. Circulation 1992; 85:1542–1547.
198. Hanson SR, Powell JS, Dodson T, Lumsden A, Kelly AB, Anderson JS, Clowes AW, Harker LA. Effects of angiotensin converting enzyme inhibition with cilazapril on intimal hyperplasia in injured arteries and vascular grafts in the baboon. Hypertension 1991; 18(suppl 4):II70-II76.
199. Aberg G, Ferrer P. Effects of captopril on atherosclerosis in cynamologous monkeys. J Cardiovasc Pharmacol 1990; 15(suppl 5):S65-S72.

200. Chobanian AV, Haudenschild C, Nickerson C, Drago R. Antiatherogenic effect of captopril in the Watanabe heritable hyperlipidemic rabbit. Hypertension 1990; 15:327–331.
201. Liang P, Pardee AB. Differential display of eukaryotic messenger RNA by means of the polymerase chain reaction. Science 1992; 257:967–971.
202. Welsh T, Chada K, Dalal SS, Chang R, Ralph D, McClelland MM. Arbitrary primed PCR fingerprinting of RNA. Nucl Acids Res 1992; 20:4965–4970.
203. Liang P, Pardee AB. Recent advances in differential display. Curr Opin Immunol 1995; 7:274–280.
204. Russell M, Utans U, Wallace AF, Liang P, Arceci MJ, Karnowsky MJ, Wyner LR, Yamashita Y, Tarn C. Identification and upregulation of galactose/N-acetylgalactosamine macrophage lectin in rat cardiac allografts with atherosclerosis. J Clin Invest 1994; 94:722–730.
205. Autieri MV, Feuerstein GZ, Yue TL, Ohlstein EH, Douglas SA. Use of differential display to identify differentially expressed mRNAs induced by rat carotid artery balloon angioplasty. Lab Invest 1995; 72:656–661.
206. Utans U, Liang P, Wyner LR, Karnowsky MJ, Russell M. Chronic cardiac rejection: identification of five upregulated genes in transplanted hearts by differential mRNA display. Proc Natl Acad Sci USA 1994; 91:6463–6467.
207. Simons M, Edelman ER, De Keyser JL, Langer R, Rosenberg RD. Antisense c-myb oligonucleotides inhibit intimal arterial smooth muscle accumulation in vivo. Nature 1992; 359:67–70.
208. Burgess TL, Fisher EF, Ross SL, Bready JV, Qian YX, Bayewitch LA, Cohen AM, Herrera CJ, Hu SS, Kramer TB. The antiproliferative activity of c-myb and c-myc antisense oligonucleotides in smooth muscle cells is caused by a nonantisense mechanism. Proc Natl Acad Sci USA 1995; 92:4051–4055.
209. Villa AE, Guzman LA, Poptic EJ, Labhasetwar V, D'Souza S, Farrell CL, Plow EF, Levy RJ, Di Corleto PE, Topol EJ. Effects of antisense c-myb oligonucleotides on vascular smooth muscle cell proliferation and response to vessel wall injury. Circ Res 1995; 76:505–513.
210. Morishita R, Gibbons GH, Kaneda Y, Ogihara T, Dzau VJ. Pharmacokinetics of antisense oligodeoxyribonucleotides (cyclin B1 and CDC 2 kinase) in the vessel wall in vivo: enhanced therapeutic utility for restenosis of HVJ-liposome delivery. Gene 1994; 149:13-19.
211. Shi Y, Fard A, Galeo A, Hutchinson HG, Vermani P, Dodge GR, Hall DJ, Shaheen F, Zalewski A. Transcatheter delivery of c-myc antisense oligomers redues neointimal formation in a porcine model of coronary artery balloon injury. Circulation 1994; 90:944–951.
212. Bennett MR, Anglin S, McEwan JR, Jagoe R, Newby AC, Evan GI. Inhibition of vascular smooth muscle cell proliferation in vitro and in vivo by c-myc antisense oligodeoxynucleotides. J Clin Invest 1994; 93:820–828.
213. Guzman RJ, Hirschowitz EA, Brody SL, Crystal RG, Epstein SE, Finkel T. In vivo suppression of injury-induced vascular smooth muscle accumulation using adenovirus mediated transfer of the herpes simplex virus thymidine kinase gene. Proc Natl Acad Sci USA 1994; 91:10732–10736.

16

Clinical Determinants of Restenosis

H. Vernon Anderson
University of Texas Health Science Center, Houston, Texas

Coronary angioplasty is a useful and effective method of revascularization for many patients with atherosclerotic coronary artery disease. Initially it was developed only for patients with single, discrete lesions in the proximal portion of one major coronary artery. Success rates were quite good, with 90–95% of lesions being adequately reduced. The general overall success of angioplasty naturally led to expansion beyond its original "borders." The past decade has witnessed dramatic growth in the number of procedures, as well as development of several additional complementary techniques. Newly acquired experiences of aggressive young operators fueled a heady and appropriate optimism. Many more patients than the originally envisioned groups are able to be successfully treated now, including patients with complex multivessel disease, severely diseased saphenous vein grafts, chronic totally occluded coronary arteries, and impaired left ventricular function. Success rates have remained high in spite of more difficult situations. The changes have come about because of tremendous advances in equipment design, angioplasty techniques, and adjunctive antithrombotic therapies. These advances have helped to support hemodynamically precarious patients and attenuate the risk of vessel thrombosis, thereby reducing immediate risk of interventions.

While immediate success rates of angioplasty are gratifyingly high, one of the problems with angioplasty as a therapeutic modality is the fact that the treated lesion or lesions may recur ("restenosis"). Approximately 25–50% of first-time angioplasty procedures will have to be repeated within 6 months to a year, and another 10% or so of treated patients will have to have coronary bypass surgery performed, all because restenosis has occurred (1–4). While the advances in equipment design, techniques, and adjunctive pharmacological agents have made angioplasty far safer and more immediately effective over the past 18 years, the daunting challenge of restenosis has not yet been surmounted (5).

I. RECOGNITION OF RESTENOSIS

Although the immediate thrombotic risk of vessel closure with angioplasty was understood from the outset, restenosis was not initially foreseen. It was only after the first few years of clinical experience that the phenomenon was appreciated (1). Early efforts recognized that in order to understand the clinical ramifications of restenosis, large clinical datasets and multivariate analyses would be needed (6–8). More than a decade of clinical research work has now been spent trying to identify and understand factors associated with restenosis and to possibly reduce the incidence of restenosis by employing various therapies. A literature review (9) evaluated 212 published reports—the equivalent of the appearance of almost two publications per month for 10 years. Despite the time and energy (and money) spent on restenosis, the problem is nearly as great as ever. Only recently has it appeared possible that, with proper application of intracoronary stents, restenosis could be attenuated significantly.

II. DEFINING RESTENOSIS

Since coronary arterial lesions are identified and treated with the use of angiography, one would hope that an angiographic definition of restenosis exists. In fact, at least six different angiographic definitions of restenosis have been used commonly in various studies (Table 1). The existence of so many definitions of restenosis has at times led to confusion, and it has hampered investigations in this field (10). The lack of a uniform angiographic definition of restenosis is a major limitation to studies of the problem and presents quite a challenge when attempting to apply basic biological principles to clinical observations. The fact that investigators use a single definition for their own group comparisons and, as a result, their studies are at least internally consistent is helpful. Problems arise when attempting to compare and contrast different studies. Additional difficulties arise with the (not infrequent) discordance between angiography and

Table 1 Commonly Used Arteriographic Definitions of Restenosis After Coronary Angioplasty

1. An increase of ≥30% from immediate postangioplasty diameter stenosis to follow-up stenosis (NHLBI-1).
2. An initial diameter stenosis <50% after angioplasty, increasing to ≥70% at follow-up angiography (NHLBI-2).
3. An increase in diameter stenosis at follow-up angiography to within 10% of the preangioplasty value (NHLBI-3).
4. A loss of ≥50% of the initial diameter stenosis gain achieved by angioplasty, from immediate postangioplasty to follow-up angiography (NHLBI-4).
5. A postangioplasty diameter stenosis <50% increasing to >50% at follow-up angiography.
6. A decrease in the minimal luminal diameter at the lesion of >0.72 mm from immediate postangioplasty to follow-up angiography.

NHLBI, National Heart, Lung, and Blood Institute Percutaneous Transluminal Coronary Angioplasty Registry.

clinical status. Occasionally, patients will undergo angiography at some point after angioplasty and be found to have measurable lesions that fit the angiographic criteria for recurrence, and yet these patients will be asymptomatic and/or have exercise tests indicating absence of ischemia. They likely would not have been recatheterized on clinical grounds alone. On the other hand, a few patients will have recurrence of their symptoms, along with exercise tests indicating ischemia, and yet on angiography be found to have lesions that do not qualify as measurable restenosis. It is clear then that restenosis is neither a purely clinical nor a purely angiographic phenomenon.

III. DETECTING RESTENOSIS

Angioplasty was first proposed as a treatment for the symptoms of angina pectoris that accompany significant coronary disease. It is remarkably successful in this. Thus it is natural for clinicians to be on the lookout for symptoms and attribute a great deal of meaning to their presence or absence. As mentioned above, symptom status by itself has been found to be a useful but imperfect clinical indicator for restenosis (1–4,6–8). In general, symptoms recur more frequently than significant coronary lesions do. In a recent review of a number of large trials, Califf and colleagues (7) noted that by angiographic criteria restenosis had occurred in 37% of all patients. Yet fully 56% of all patients were symptomatic at their follow-up contact. It has been estimated from a number of comprehensive surveys that about one third of patients with symptom recurrence will actually be free from restenosis. On the other hand, approximately 15% of patients without any symptoms will in fact have restenosis by angiographic criteria ("silent restenosis").

Treadmill exercise tests have long been employed to evaluate possible ischemia in both symptomatic as well as asymptomatic persons (11–16). As a diagnostic maneuver for helping detect restenosis after angioplasty, they have been found to be wanting. There are a number of confounding factors that probably influence this. These include the use of angioplasty in patients with multivessel disease or previous infarction, where positive or negative exercise tests may be difficult to interpret. Also, problems with inadequate levels of stress, and the coexistence of conditions such as left ventricular hypertrophy or conduction defects, as well as the use of medications such as beta adrenergic blocking agents or calcium channel antagonists, can all influence test results and cloud interpretation.

In contrast to the limited value of plain treadmill exercise testing in restenosis detection, exercise thallium or sestamibi perfusion imaging considerably improves the value of stress testing (17–22). This includes both the positive value for detecting presence of restenosis as well as the negative value for detecting absence of restenosis (the two are not symmetrical). From a practical standpoint, a negative exercise perfusion scintigram in an asymptomatic patient, with an acceptable level of stress, performed more than 4 months after angioplasty has a better than 90% predictive value for absence of restenosis. While not applicable to all patients undergoing coronary angioplasty, the strategy of 4- to 6-month noninvasive testing using scintigraphy can be applied to many of them.

IV. CLINICAL CORRELATES OF RESTENOSIS

Many clinical studies have been performed to identify correlates of restenosis (or lack of restenosis, taking the opposite view) (23–30). Traditionally, they have been divided into three different categories of variables: clinical patient-related factors, coronary lesion–related factors, and angioplasty procedure–related factors. The concept has been put forward that categorization like this allows the clinician to form risk estimates sequentially at each step in the treatment process. Obviously these factors are interrelated. Clinicians choose to perform angioplasty on some patients and not on others based upon an evaluation of the patient and the lesion or lesions. Many of the technical details of angioplasty, including balloon choice and positioning, inflation times, and a myriad of other procedural items, are based upon clinical judgments that take into account patients and lesions. Therefore, dividing a continuum of interrelated factors into categories is at best somewhat arbitrary.

Table 2 Patient-Related Factors Associated with Restenosis After Coronary Angioplasty

Older age (>65 years)
Male gender
Unstable angina prior to initial procedure
Continued smoking after procedure
Diabetes[a]
Hypertension[a]

[a]Noted as a weak correlate only in some studies.

V. PATIENT-RELATED FACTORS

A number of specific patient-related variables appear to be associated with increased risks of restenosis. These include older age, male gender, unstable angina prior to angioplasty, and continued smoking after angioplasty (Table 2). Diabetes mellitus and hypertension have been associated with restenosis in some large studies but not in others. It is interesting that several other factors known to be involved in development or progression of coronary disease have not been shown to be associated with restenosis, or appear to have much weaker associations. These include a family history of coronary disease and hypercholesterolemia. It is possible that intensive treatment of diabetes, hypertension, and elevated cholesterol may serve to blunt the contribution these conditions might make to restenosis.

VI. LESION-RELATED FACTORS

These include multilesion and multivessel angioplasty procedures, very severe ("tight") lesions, ostial lesions, longer lesions (>15 mm), total occlusions, and lesions located either in the proximal portion of a vessel, the left anterior descending artery, or a saphenous vein graft (Table 3). The issue of recurrences in patients with multiple lesions requires elaboration. If more than one lesion is treated with angioplasty, then multiple combinations of recurrences are theoretically possible. For example, with two lesions, Lesion A and Lesion B, it is possible for A to recur but not B, for B to recur but not A, and for both lesions or neither lesion to recur. Thus with two lesions there are four possibilities, three of which include a recurrence of some sort. With more than two lesions there are even more possibilities. Mathematically it would appear that if restenosis were an independent lesion-related process, each lesion with its own probability of recurrence, then with three or four lesions treated, a recurrence would be virtually guaranteed. This scenario has not been found to be the case (31).

Table 3 Lesion-Related Factors Associated with Restenosis After Coronary Angioplasty

Multivessel disease
Multilesion treatment
Severe lesions (DS > 90%)
Ostial lesions
Long lesions (>15 mm)
Total occlusions
Proximal vessel location
LAD location
Vein graft location

DS, diameter stenosis; LAD, left anterior descending artery.

Restenosis appears in some sense to be a "systemic" process, and multiple lesions do not behave entirely independently, although multiple lesion angioplasty is associated with somewhat increased recurrence rates over single lesion treatment. The biological reasons underlying the increased recurrence rates for the factors listed in Table 3 are not known.

VII. PROCEDURE-RELATED FACTORS

The only procedure-related factor that has emerged as a correlate of recurrence is higher post angioplasty residual stenosis (e.g., a "suboptimal result." Many other procedure-related factors, such as number of balloon inflations, duration of balloon inflations, balloon pressures, type of balloon material used, etc., have not been found to be consistently related to higher risk for restenosis and may in fact be related more to inability to achieve a good result, which may then be related indirectly to restenosis. The ability of intracoronary stents to reduce restenosis rates is very likely related to the ability to achieve excellent initial results, thereby obtaining large residual diameters at the conclusion of the procedures.

One other procedure-related factor that has received a great deal of attention has been tear or dissection of the treated coronary artery. While dissection can be angiographically dramatic at times and increases the risk of abrupt closure, often necessitating deployment of a stent, it does not by itself appear to increase the risk of subsequent restenosis (32–34). The important element with dissection may be that a successful initial result was achieved, with low residual stenosis values and good flow, and not the presence or absence of dissection per se.

VIII. LIMITATIONS OF CLINICAL RESTENOSIS STUDIES

Clinical restenosis studies have suffered to various degrees from methodological problems. Many studies are quite small, having followed fewer than 100 patients after successful angioplasty. Many have enrolled or followed heterogeneous patient groups. The timing and method of follow-up for restenosis studies has been quite varied. Some follow-up intervals have been as short as 3 months, while others have been 6–12 months or longer. Ideally, a restenosis study should have 100% angiographic follow-up. This is rare or impossible for social, technical, and financial reasons. In a comprehensive review of clinical restenosis studies (9), only 4 out of 31 carefully screened reports had 100% angiographic follow-up, although 6 others had greater than 90% angiographic follow-up. Weintraub and colleagues (25) have demonstrated that clinically important variables are skewed between the patient group with angiography and the group without angiography, creating biases. Kuntz and colleagues (26) and Califf and colleagues (30) have demonstrated that observed restenosis rates in one population could vary quite markedly, depending only upon the mix of patients included when follow-up angiography is less than complete. Indeed, many restenosis studies have relied on retrospective reviews of patients who happened to undergo coronary arteriography at some point after a successful angioplasty procedure. Often this angiogram may have been initiated because the patient had return of symptoms, or an exercise text was performed and the results were either indicative of ischemia or indeterminate. Therefore, selection bias in choosing patients for follow-up angiography can cloud the interpretation of restenosis studies.

The final and major problem with clinical correlative restenosis studies is the fact that they can be misleading if applied too readily to patient care. All patients undergoing coronary angioplasty must have some follow-up evaluation. No constellation of variables has yet been found that indicates complete freedom from restenosis. Conversely, no group of variables has been identified that will make restenosis absolutely certain. The majority of patients have mixtures of variables that are both favorable and unfavorable toward restenosis. In one sense, then, restenosis variable definition is irrelevant because it will not help with individual patient care. Identifying these variables may be useful from a research standpoint, especially because it can help keep therapeutic trials balanced. From a very practical standpoint, it is only the anatomical location of the lesion that is paramount: patients who have important coronary disease are always at risk for recurrence or progression of their important disease.

IX. CONCLUSIONS

Restenosis remains an important issue in use of angioplasty as a treatment for coronary disease. Its importance is mostly economic, inasmuch as the major costs are not measured in terms of lives lost or infarctions treated, but in terms of the expense required to follow, test, and retreat these patients. Prevention of restenosis after angioplasty does not appear imminent at present, even though stents hold promise for reducing restenosis rates somewhat. Any advances are eagerly awaited and could radically alter expectations with this beautiful technique.

REFERENCES

1. Gruentzig AR, King SB, Schlumpf M, Siegenthaler W. Long-term follow-up after percutaneous transluminal coronary angioplasty. The early Zurich experience. N Engl J Med 1987; 316:1127–1132.
2. Fanelli C. Aronoff R. Restenosis following coronary angioplasty. Am Heart J 1990; 119:357–368.
3. Nobuyoshi M. Kimura T, Nosaka H, Mioka S, Ueno K, Yokoi H. Hamasaki N, Horiuchi H, Ohishi H. Restenosis after successful percutaneous transluminal coronary angioplasty: serial angiographic follow-up of 229 patients. J Am Coll Cardiol 1988; 12:616–623.
4. Serruys PW, Luijten HE, Beatt KH, Geuskens, R, de Feyter PJ, van den Brand M, Reiber JHC, ten Katen JH, van Es GA, Hugenholtz PG. Incidence of restenosis after successful coronary angioplasty: a time-related phenomenon. Circulation 1988; 77:361–371.
5. Hermans WRM, Rensing BJ, Strauss BH, Serruys PW. Prevention of restenosis after percutaneous transluminal coronary angioplasty: the search for a "magic bullet." Am Heart J 1991; 122:171–187.
6. Holmes DR, Vlietrstra RE, Smith HC, Vetrovec GW, Kent KM, Cowley MJ, Faxon DP, Gruentzig AR, Kelsey SF, Detre KM, Van Raden M, Mock MB. Restenosis after percutaneous transluminal coronary angioplasty (PTCA): a report from the PTCA registry of the National Heart, Lung, and Blood Institute. Am J Cardiol 1984; 53:77C-81C.
7. Califf Rm, Ohman EM, Frid DJ, Fortin DF, Mark DB, Hlatky MA, Herndon JE, Bengtson JR. Restenosis; the clinical issues. In: Topol EJ, ed. Textbook of Interventional Cardiology. Philadelphia: W.B. Saunders, 1990:363–394.
8. Hirshfeld JW, Schwartz JS, Jugo R, MacDonald RG, Goldberg S, Savage MP, Bass TA, Vetrovec G, Cowley M, Taussig AS, Whitworth HB, Margolis JR, Hill JA, Pepine CJ. Restenosis after coronary angioplasty: a multivariant statistical model to relate lesion and procedural variables to restenosis. J Am Coll Cardiol 1991; 18:647-656.
9. Bobbio M, Detrano R, Colombo A, Lehmann KG, Park JB. Restenosis rate after percutaneous transluminal coronary angioplasty: a literature overview. J Invas Cardiol 1991; 3:214-224.

10. Serruys PW, Rensing BJ, Hermans WRM, Beatt KJ. Definition of restenosis after percutaneous transluminal coronary angioplasty: a quickly evolving concept. J Intervent Cardiol 1991; 4:265–276.
11. El-Tamimi H, Davies GJ, Sritara P, Hackett D, Crea F, Maseri A. Inappropriate construction of small coronary vessels as a possible cause of a positive exercise test early after successful coronary angioplasty. Circulation 1991; 84:2307–2312.
12. Kipfer PH, Hess OM, Gaglione A, Krayenbuehl HP. Exercise-induced ST-segment depression after successful PTCA: incomplete revascularization or altered coronary vasomotor tone? Coronary Artery Dis 1991; 2:595–604.
13. El-Tamimi H, Davies GJ, Hackett D, Fragasso G, Crea F, Maseri A. Very early prediction of restenosis after successful coronary angioplasty: anatomical and functional assessment. J Am Coll Cardiol 1990; 15:259–264.
14. Ernst SMPG Hillebrand FA, Klein B, Ascoop CA, van Tellingen C, Plokker HWM. The value of exercise tests in the follow-up of patients who underwent transluminal coronary angioplasty. Int J Cardiol 1985; 7:267–279.
15. Rosing DR, van Raden MJ, Mincemoyer RM, Bonow RO, Bourassa MG, David PR, Ewels CJ, Detre KM, Kent KM. Exercise, electrocardiographic and functional responses after percutaneous transluminal coronary angioplasty. Am J Cardiol 1984; 53:36C-41C.
16. Honan MB, Bengtson JR, Pryor DB, Rendall DS, Stack RS, Hinohara T, Skelton TN, Califf RM, Hlatky MA, Mark DB. Exercise treadmill testing is a poor predictor of anatomic restenosis after angioplasty for acute myocardial infarction. Circulation 1989; 80:1585–1594.
17. Hecht HS, Shaw RE, Bruce TR, Ryan C, Stertzer SH, Myler RK. Usefulness of tomographic thallium-201 imaging for detection of restenosis after percutaneous transluminal coronary angioplasty. Am J Cardiol 1990; 66:1314–1318.
18. Manyari DE, Knudtson M, Kloiber R, Roth D. Sequential thallium-201 myocardial perfusion studies after successful percutaneous transluminal coronary angioplasty: delayed resolution of exercise-induced scintigraphic abnormalities. Circulation 1988; 77:86–95.
19. Wijns W, Serruys PW, Reiber JHC, de Feyter PJ, van den Brand M, Simoons ML, Hugenholtz, PG, Tijssen JGP. Early detection of restenosis after successful percutaneous transluminal coronary angioplasty by exercise-redistribution thallium scintigraphy. Am J Cardiol 1985; 55:357–361.
20. Wijns W, Serruys PW, Simoons ML, van den Brand M, de Feyter PJ, Reiber JH, Hugenholtz PG. Predictive value of early maximal exercise test and thallium scintigraphy after successful percutaneous transluminal angioplasty. Br Heart J 1985; 53:194–200.
21. Scholl JM, Chaitman BR, David PR, Dupras G, Brevers G, Val PG, Crepeau J, Lesperance J, Bourassa MG. Exercise electrocardiography and myocardial scintigraphy in the serial evaluation of the results of percutaneous transluminal coronary angioplasty. Circulation 1982; 66:380–390.
22. Hardoff R, Shefer A, Gips S, Merdler A, Flugelman MY, Halon DA, Lewis

BS. Predicting late restenosis after coronary angioplasty by very early (12 to 24 h) thallium-201 scintigraphy: implications with regard to mechanisms of late coronary restenosis. J Am Coll Cardiol 1990; 15:1486–1492.
23. Renkin J, Melin J, Robert A, Richelle F, Bachy JL, Col J, Detry JMR, Wijns W. Detection of restenosis after successful coronary angioplasty: improved clinical decision making with use of a logistic model combining procedural and follow-up variables. J Am Coll Cardiol 1990; 1333–1340.
24. Weintraub WS, Kosinski AS, Brown CL, King SB. Can restenosis after coronary angioplasty be predicted from clinical variables? J Am Coll Cardiol 1993; 21:6–14.
25. Weintraub WS, Ghazzal ZMB, Douglas JS, Liberman HA, Morris DC, Cohen CL, King SB. Long-term clinical follow-up in patients with angiographic restudy after successful angioplasty. Circulation 1993; 87:831–840.
26. Kuntz RE, Keaney KM, Senerchia C, Baim DS. A predictive method for estimating the late angiographic results of coronary intervention despite incomplete ascertainment. Circulation 1993; 87:815–830.
27. Rensing BJ, Hermans WRM, Vos J, Tijssen JGP, Rutch W, Danchin N, Heyndrickx GR, Mast EG, Wijns W, Serruys PW. Luminal narrowing after percutaneous transluminal coronary angioplasty. Circulation 1993; 88:975–985.
28. Mick MJ, Piedmonte MR, Arnold AM, Simpfendorfer C. Risk stratification for long-term outcome after elective coronary angioplasty: a multivariate analysis of 5,000 patients. J Am Coll Cardiol 1994; 24:74–84.
29. Melkert R, Violaris AG, Serruys PW. Luminal narrowing after percutaneous transluminal coronary angioplasty: a multivariate analysis of clinical, procedural and lesion related factors affecting long-term angiographic outcome in the PARK study. J Invas Cardiol 1994; 6:160–171.
30. Califf RM, Fortin DF, Frid DJ, Harlan WR, Ohman EM, Bengtson JR, Nelson CL, Tcheng JE, Mark DB, Stack RS. Restenosis after coronary angioplasty: an overview. J Am Coll Cardiol 1991; 17:2B-13B.
31. Gibson CM, Kuntz RE, Nobuyoshi M, Rosner B, Baim DS. Lesion-to-lesion independence of restenosis after treatment by conventional angioplasty, stenting, or directional atherectomy. Circulation 1993; 87:1123–1129.
32. Leimgrumber PP, Roubin GS, Anderson HV, Bredlau CE, Whitworth HB, Douglas JS, King SB, Gruentzig AR. Influence of intimal dissection on restenosis after successful coronary angioplasty. Circulation 1985; 72:530–535.
33. Matthews BJ, Ewels CJ, Kent KM. Coronary dissection: a predictor of restenosis? Am Heart J 1988; 115:547–554.
34. Hermans WRM, Rensing BJ, Foley DP, Deckers JW, Rutsch W, Emanuelsson H, Danchin N, Wijns W, Chappuis F, Serruys PW. Therapeutic dissection after successful coronary balloon angioplasty: no influence on restenosis or on clinical outcome in 693 patients. J Am Coll Cardiol 1992; 20:767–780.

17

Clinical Trials of Restenosis

David Eccleston and Eric J. Topol
Cleveland Clinic Foundation, Cleveland, Ohio

I. INTRODUCTION

Although advances in technology since the inception of percutaneous transluminal coronary angioplasty (PTCA) in 1977 have radically expanded its role, deficiencies in our understanding of basic processes have restricted our ability to impact upon the problem of restenosis. In 1991, over 350,000 coronary angioplasty procedures were performed in the United States, increasing to approximately 410,000 per year in 1994 (1,2). With an average cost of $16,000 per procedure to third-party payers in 1991, this accounted for approximately $5.6 billion in initial hospitalization costs (1). Within 6 months of initial PTCA there is a 30–40% incidence of restenosis, leading approximately 20–25% of patients to undergo repeat angioplasty, and 5–8% to receive coronary bypass surgery for symptomatic restenosis. In addition to patients suffering the burden of recurrent symptoms and repeat procedures, the cost of these repeat revascularization procedures is estimated to be as high as $2.0 billion per year (1). A reduction of restenosis rates from 33 to 25% might save as much as $750 million annually (3). This chapter will outline the critical methodological issues and potential pitfalls in performing clinical trials of agents to prevent restenosis, review current study results, and examine key concepts for future clinical trials.

II. PATHOBIOLOGY OF THE ARTERIAL RESPONSE TO INJURY AND RESTENOSIS: THERAPEUTIC TARGETS AND AGENTS

The contemporary view of the vascular response to injury is of a multifactorial cascade of events commencing with exposure of subintimal components of the vessel wall with resultant platelet deposition, thrombus formation, and the release of growth factors from platelets, circulating monocytes, macrophages, endothelium, and smooth muscle cells (4). These mitogens stimulate the transformation of medial smooth muscle cells from a resting contractile state to a synthetic phenotype and promote their proliferation and migration to the intima. Subsequently, synthesis and secretion of extracellular connective tissue matrix occurs leading to progressive luminal narrowing (5–7). However, the dominant role of the proliferative response in restenosis has recently been challenged. Other mechanisms such as early elastic recoil, organization of mural thrombus, subintimal hemorrhage, and unfavorable vascular remodeling responses lend impetus to the restenotic process, which is complete by 3–6 months. Of particular note, recent intravascular ultrasound studies suggest that after all percutaneous interventions except stenting, mechanisms such as recoil and remodeling may predominate (5–11). Evidence exists that the ability of devices such as directional atherectomy and stents to provide a larger lumen at 6 months than conventional balloon angioplasty appears more related to their ability to achieve a larger acute gain than to any reduction in late loss, as late loss for both devices may actually be greater than twice that seen with balloon angioplasty (12). Intravascular ultrasound studies suggest that late loss is not associated with significant intimal thickening in approximately 70% of cases after balloon angioplasty (13–16). However, serial ultrasound studies fail to show evidence of chronic Palmaz-Schatz stent recoil, suggesting that restenosis in stents is primarily due to neointimal proliferation (17). Intimal hyperplasia and matrix secretion are the principal mechanisms of restenosis in animal models, and to date research has largely focused on attenuation of the proliferative response to vascular injury. The responses to injury are mediated and amplified by multiple and redundant pathways, and it is likely that the optimal therapeutic approach would arrest the process at an early stage prior to amplification or inhibit a final common pathway. This cascade of events can be conceptually divided into early, middle, and late phases.

A. The Early Phase

After local injury platelets adhere to the arterial wall and leukocytes migrate into the thrombus (Fig. 1). Following increased surface expression of

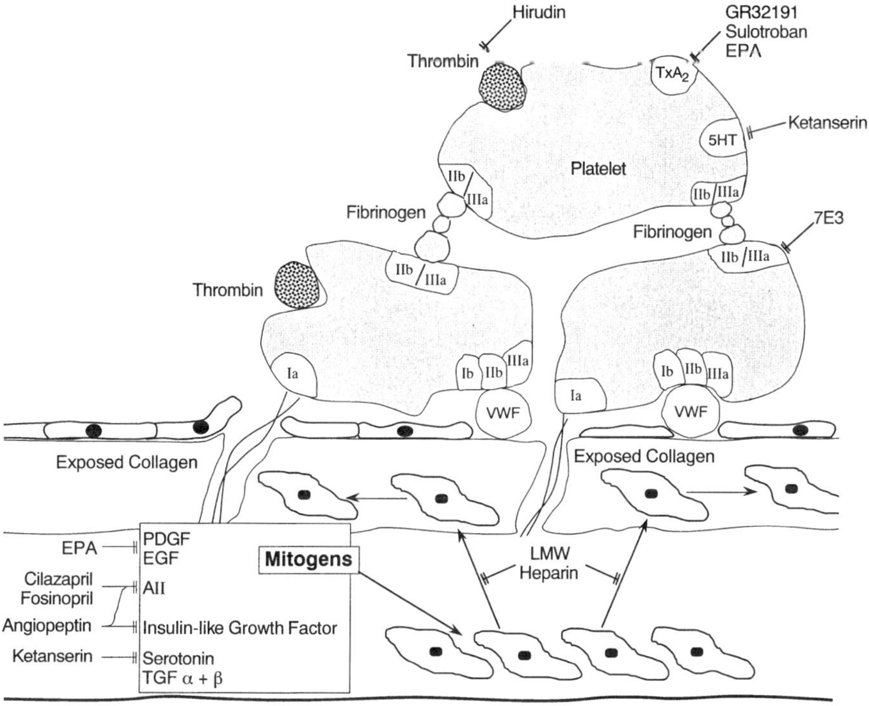

Figure 1 Interactive biological processes resulting in restenosis after coronary angioplasty. Platelet adhesion and aggregation are mediated by platelet glycoprotein receptors Ia, Ib, and IIb/IIIa, which bind to collagen; von Willebrand factor (vWF); and fibrinogen. As a result of arterial injury and platelet aggregation, a variety of mitogen factors are released including platelet-derived growth factor (PDGF), epidermal growth factor (FGF), angiotensin II (A II), and transforming growth factor (TGF). A variety of potential inhibitors may block platelet aggregation, smooth muscle cell proliferation, and growth factor release. EPA, eicosapentanoic acid; 7E3, murine monoclonal antibody to glycoprotein IIb/IIIa receptor; TxA_2 thromboxane A_2; 5HT, serotonin; LMW, low molecular weight. Reprinted with permission from the American Heart Association. Circulation 1991;84:1426–1436.

the glycoprotein integrin IIb/IIIa, platelet aggregation is stimulated, with fibrinogen serving as the key ligand. The importance of platelets in the restenotic process is emphasized by the reduction in late revascularization events following angioplasty after blockade of the platelet glycoprotein IIb/IIIa receptor (10). As well as their role in the formation of mural thrombus, platelets may promote restenosis by initiation of the coagulation cascade with generation of thrombin and by enhancing cellular proliferation and migration via the action of platelet derived growth factor (10). The amount of intramural and intraluminal thrombus is injury dependent (18). Thrombus consists mainly of platelets, white cells, and fibrin and acts as a reservoir of mitogenic substances, influencing the proliferative response of the arterial wall. Thrombus constituents other than platelets may also be mechanistically responsible for cellular migration, smooth muscle cell proliferation, and the development of neointima. Thrombin is central to thrombus development; after activation by either the intrinsic or extrinsic systems and Factor X_a, thrombin cleaves fibrinogen to fibrin. In addition, it activates platelets, stimulates plasma proteins (factors V, VIII, and XIII, proteins C and S), activates white cells, stimulates endothelial cells to release endothelin and tissue factor, and both has a mitotic effect on and stimulates growth factor release from smooth muscle cells (SMC) (19). Thrombin has also been shown to stimulate the production of plasminogen activator inhibitor (PAI-1) by SMC in a dose-dependent manner, thereby promoting continued thrombosis (20).

The mechanical injury itself triggers growth factor expression by the endothelium, SMC, and circulating platelets and monocytes (21). Targets for intervention thus include the GP Ib and GP IIb/IIIa integrins, which mediate adhesion and aggregation, amplification factors such as cyclooxygenase, and coagulation factors such as Xa and thrombin. Aspirin, thromboxane inhibitors, ticlopidine, and heparin have been ineffective in limiting restenosis (6,22), and the direct thrombin inhibitor hirudin has not yielded salutary results (4,23).

B. Middle and Late Phases

The middle phase is characterized by complex interactions between growth factors, second messengers, and gene regulatory proteins resulting in phenotypic change from a quiescent state, characterized by a differentiated contractile phenotype, to a proliferative state and proliferation of SMC (24). By about 48 h after injury in humans, SMC begin to proliferate and then migrate to the injured area. Experimental use of antimitotic and antiproliferative agents has been uniformly unsuccessful, however, even when prolonged high tissue concentrations of drug have been demonstrated (25). Local application of antisense oligonucleotides to the proto-oncogenes *c-myb* (26) and *c-myc* (27) have reduced myointimal proliferation in animal models, and other potential targets include heparin-binding growth factors such as basic fibroblast growth factor (28). Recently, local delivery of vascular endothelial growth factor (VEGF) was shown to speed reendothelialization and reduce neointimal thickening after injury in a rat model (29). Gene transfer may be accomplished by direct application of single genes, by the use of biological carrier systems (vectors), or by local delivery of genetically modified endothelial cells. Gene therapy may modify the vascular injury response at multiple sites; delivery of genetically modified cells may facilitate reendothelialization of the target site and simultaneously deliver biologically active products. Cell-based techniques using harvested endothelial cells which are transfected in cell culture and reintroduced percutaneously have achieved successful colonization of the endothelium (25). However, the impracticality and logistic drawbacks of this process, which requires many weeks, have seen the emergence of direct in situ gene-transfer techniques, which are more likely to be clinically applicable. Several gene-transfer systems have been investigated using balloon catheters coupled with various biological carriers. Gene transfer can be accomplished using plasmid DNA containing the therapeutic gene (lipofection) or by retroviral and adenoviral vectors containing therapeutic genes introduced into a modified viral genome "crippled" by deletion of endogenous genes, rendering virions incapable of infection or replication. Viral vectors offer greater transfer efficiency than plasmids, probably because of binding and internalization by specific cellular receptors. Although progress in this field has been rapid, vectors and delivery systems are still in evolution, and issues of safety and transfer efficiency must be addressed before gene therapy enters the clinical arena for prevention of restenosis.

Late phase events (weeks to months) include the generation of proteoglycan matrix, which comprises the bulk of mature restenotic tissue, and vascular remodeling. SMCs invade the intimal area and the local thrombus where they proliferate and enter a secretory phase within 7 days after injury. Transforming growth factor-β (TGF-β) regulates their production of large amounts of extracellular matrix, rich in chondroitin sulfate and dermatan sulfate, replacing fibronectin as the predominant extracellular matrix material. Both chondroitin sulfate and dermatan sulfate promote further SMC migration and proliferation. Heparin sulfate stimulates the proteoglycan production of secretory SMCs. Extracellular matrix production continues for up to 20–25 weeks, during which time the proteoglycan matrix is gradually replaced by collagen and elastin, and the synthetic SMCs become quiescent mesenchymal cells. Reendothelialization from adjacent cells completes the healing process; the resulting neointima is mostly composed of fibrotic extracellular matrix material with only an estimated 10% of cellular constituents, as derived from human coronary atherectomy specimens.

While these concepts of the pathobiology of restenosis are almost certainly incomplete, coronary stenting limits recoil and remodeling and has provided the first clinically efficacious approach to this process (30–32).

However, these promising results pertain to a highly select group of patients with single-vessel, single-stent disease; the role of stenting in restenotic lesions, small vessels, and long lesions requiring multiple stents remains to be clarified. Biological therapies may be developed that are even more successful through impacting on all aspects of the arterial response to injury, yet remain cost-effective. The optimal approach to the problem of restenosis will likely involve combining mechanical and biological approaches.

III. DEFINITIONS OF RESTENOSIS FOR CLINICAL TRIALS

There is much debate among investigators regarding the most appropriate definition of restenosis, especially as to whether restenosis is best defined angiographically, functionally, or clinically. However, the utility of interventions should be defined in a way that provides the most prognostic information about the patient's overall clinical outcome.

A. Angiographic Definitions

Angiographic definitions of restenosis have been the most controversial. First, the severity of the angiographic obstruction must be measured. Second, the angiographic parameters or thresholds that provide the most information about the biology or clinical consequences of restenosis must be determined.

Several reports illustrate the difficulties of using visual methods of assessment, with significant overestimation (15–20%) of lesion severity compared with quantitative methods, further obscuring the likelihood of detecting real changes in vessels undergoing angioplasty (3). These reports also suggest that visual assessment is highly inaccurate in the midrange of diameter stensosis estimates (25–75%). The conventional approach to determining procedural success or failure has depended on precision in this range. While the use of core laboratory systems and automated edge detection algorithms to quantify the severity of coronary lesions remains the "gold standard" in the research arena, issues such as variability in quantitative measurements between different systems need to be resolved before they can be recommended for routine clinical use. This arises from operator-dependent factors such as the technical quality of the angiogram, angiographic projection, lesion and frame selection, the presence of radiolucency or dissection, and catheter characteristics.

At a pathophysiological level, restenosis is not a binary phenomenon. Rather, virtually all patients have some degree of lumen renarrowing at late follow-up compared to the initial angiographic result after PTCA, and this process follows a near Gaussian distribution (33). Thus, any angiographic threshold for classifying restenosis is largely arbitrary, and to be useful it needs to be correlated with functional significance or clinical outcome. However, while a continuous measure of the degree of luminal obstruction may give greater statistical power for detecting prognostic and treatment effects in clinical trials and observational studies, for clinical decision making a classification of restenosis as present or absent is more relevant. Thus, in a study evaluating the best clinical treatment for restenosis, development of a 40% diameter stenosis would not be a meaningful adverse outcome, because such lesions are most frequently associated with a benign prognosis.

The process of angiographic restenosis has further been separated into "acute gain," "late loss," and "net gain." Acute gain refers to the change in luminal area from before PTCA to immediately after. This measure provides useful information about the initial impact of one device versus another. In a nonrandomized series, Kuntz et al. have demonstrated significant differences in the acute gain achieved by intracoronary stent versus balloon angioplasty versus laser angioplasty (34). In the Coronary Angioplasty Versus Excisional Atherectomy Trial (CAVEAT) and the Canadian Coronary Atherectomy Trial (CCAT), directional atherectomy produced a significantly greater acute gain than balloon angioplasty (35,36). Late loss refers to the reduction in luminal diameter between the postangioplasty result and the follow-up angiogram. This measurement presumably documents the neointimal hyperplastic response and elastic recoil and vascular remodeling. Isolating the neointimal proliferative response may help determine risk factors or interventions that may modulate the biology of restenosis. Net gain represents the difference between acute gain and late loss.

Given our failure to develop effective therapies to reduce late loss by modulating the neointimal proliferative response, considerable attention has been focused on the role of acute gain in minimizing restenosis. Although one 2444-patient study suggested that the magnitude of acute gain is not related to subsequent late loss of arterial area, this was limited by a 52% angiographic follow-up rate, raising concerns about withdrawal bias (37). Most studies suggest a strong link between the amount of acute gain and subsequent late loss (8). Kuntz et al. have found that acute gain is the best predictor of subsequent restenosis regardless of the interventional device used to obtain this gain (34). However, the quest for an angiographically or ultrasound-guided normal final result, with the possibility of reducing restenosis rates, may have to be tempered at least in the case of balloon angioplasty by an increased risk of periprocedural complications (35).

Standardization of angiographic measurements is necessary to permit comparisons between trials and allow for generalizability of trial results to the wider clinical setting. Ideally, baseline, early postprocedural (yielding the acute gain) and 24-h angiograms (to characterize the degree of elastic recoil) are preferable (38). Follow-up at 6 months after the procedure, when the remodeling process will be completed, provides the critical comparative measure (determining long-term success or failure and calculation of late loss and net gain). However, basing a definition of restenosis solely on differences in percentage stenosis may lead to underestimation of the true change in stenosis severity, as the reference diameter often undergoes changes similar in size to changes in the minimal luminal diameter (MLD). It is also essential to decide which angiographic view will be utilized for measurement of the residual percentage stenosis, as restenosis rates reported from the worst view (as in CAVEAT) will be higher (by 10% or more) than those determined from an average of all views (as in most trials). These problems can be avoided by reporting absolute measurements, either MLD (mm) or cross-sectional area (mm^2), in addition to percentage diameter stenosis, to describe changes in vessel dimensions, in addition to reporting the luminal diameter of the reference segment of the vessel.

Another area that warrants investigation is whether angiographic criteria alone are adequate for declaring procedural success or whether it will be useful to demonstrate reversal of ischemia or other metabolic abnormalities by such techniques as thallium-201 scintigraphic studies, positron emission tomography, or Doppler-flow guidewires. As an alternative, measurement of translesional pressure gradients has been found to have an excellent correlation with visual estimates of stenosis severity (39) and may be useful as an adjunct to angiography to determine procedural success. The role of early remodeling of the vessel, including elastic recoil, incorporation of thrombus into the lesion, and resolution of intimal flaps, may be critical in these abnormal functional studies.

B. Clinical Definitions

In the past, clinical outcomes after PTCA were largely not used to define restenosis due to the number of patients required to detect a difference reliably. However, as restenosis trials have increased in size, it has become possible to examine the occurrence of clinical events such as death, nonfatal myocardial infarction, and the need for repeat percutaneous revascularization or coronary artery bypass grafting (CABG). Two clinical trials of antiplatelet agents (GRASP, M-HEART-II) with a negative angiographic outcome yet a reduction in clinical events among the patients receiving active therapy suggest that the net clinical benefit of some agents is not accounted for by angiographic outcomes alone (40,41). Conversely,

CAVEAT demonstrated a reduction in angiographic restenosis but a higher clinical event rate with atherectomy (35). Thus, clinical events after PTCA are a better primary endpoint to measure than angiographic restenosis to define the clinical value of post-PTCA therapies.

Despite reported anatomical restenosis rates of 40–50% in most trials, there is a need for repeat revascularization in only 20–30% of patients. This apparent discrepancy has arisen from the use of binary restenosis definitions of greater than 50% residual stenosis. Many cases classified as restenosis have been in the 50–70% diameter stenosis range, where generally a clinician would avoid further invasive strategies. In CAVEAT, although the binary restenosis rates were different between directional atherectomy and balloon angioplasty, neither severe restenosis nor rates of repeat revascularization procedures were different between the two groups (35). For this reason, the restenosis data should be displayed as a cumulative distribution function when comparative restenosis rates are reported.

In undertaking clinical trials, several important statistical issues must be considered. Random error, due to sampling variation, is influenced by the variance and size of the sample population. Two types of error may result from sampling variation. The first, leading to a false-positive study, rejects the null hypothesis when it is actually true (type I). A type I error may be produced when multiple statistical comparisons are made during the analysis phase of a study, since any association found may be entirely due to chance. This may be minimized by limiting comparisons to one for every 10 endpoints (the "rule of 10s"), adjusting the *p*-value required for significance (Bonferroni correction) or validating the study results in another, entirely independent sample ("bootstrapping") (31). Studies of restenosis often include sample sizes that are inadequate for a particular outcome, leading to the incorrect conclusion of a negative study (type II error). A study should have a sample size sufficient to reduce the probability of a type II error to less than 20% for the smallest clinically meaningful benefit. In over 60 reported randomized trials of therapies for restenosis, only 5 had sample sizes sufficient to be 80% confident that a clinically meaningful therapeutic benefit was not missed (42).

One other important factor to consider is withdrawal bias, where patients who do not have symptoms, and who presumably have lower rates of restenosis, are less likely to return for a follow-up restudy. Patients who die, and who presumably have higher restenosis rates, are unable to return, thus the true restenosis rate may be under- or overestimated if angiographic follow-up is significantly incomplete. With a less than 90% follow-up rate, the statistical basis for inference based on randomization is suspect and the generalizability of the results to other populations of patients is questionable. One method shown to better estimate the true restenosis rate is to classify patients by symptoms; then knowing the restenosis rates in the patients in each symptom class (asymptomatic, atypical, or typical symptoms) who undergo repeat angiography, as well as the proportion of patients in each symptom class who do not undergo follow-up angiography, a better estimate of the "true" restenosis rate should be possible for the patients being studied (43).

In principal, clinical trials assessing therapies for restenosis should measure clinical outcomes (death, myocardial infarction, repeat revascularization procedures, symptomatic angina, and recurrence of ischemia as documented by functional testing for provocable ischemia) as the primary endpoint, while retaining the ability to assess the angiographic outcomes in a predefined subset of patients. The degree of stenosis before treatment, immediately after treatment, and at long-term follow-up should be ascertained, and the difference between the immediate and long-term results should be quantified to estimate the overall restenosis effect. This measure ideally should be adjusted for changes occurring in the normal or reference portions of the vessel.

IV. PREDICTORS OF RESTENOSIS

Diabetes and unstable angina have been the only two consistent patient-related variables associated with an increased risk of restenosis. These relationships were initially suggested by the NHLBI Registry; subsequent studies suggest a doubling of relative risk of restenosis in diabetics compared with nondiabetics (3). Carrozza and others have documented that late loss of initial luminal gain after coronary stenting is substantially greater in patients with insulin-dependent diabetes (44). When unstable angina is defined as new-onset angina (<2 months), recent-onset angina (<6 months), or increased frequency or severity of angina, the relative risk of restenosis appears to be 1.2–1.7 times higher than in patients with chronic stable symptoms (3). Morphological features including stenosis location, baseline percentage diameter stenosis, stenosis length, adjacent artery diameter, and postangioplasty stenosis severity have been found to be independent predictors of restenosis in both univariate and multivariate analyses (45).

V. CLINICAL TRIALS

A. Strategies to Prevent Restenosis

Initial attempts to deal with the problem of restenosis focused predominantly upon mechanical strategies and systemic drug therapy. Despite 15 years of technological progress, utilization of new devices such as atherectomy or laser to "debulk" lesions had, until recently, generally resulted in restenosis rates that were unchanged from the first series reported by Gruentzig et al. (46). In the recent Benestent and STRESS trials, elective coronary stenting was associated with a moderate reduction in restenosis rates (22 and 32% angiographic restenosis at 6 months), however, these results pertain to a select patient group with de novo lesions (30,47). Even with high-pressure deployment techniques, stenting is associated with a small but significant risk of subacute thrombosis, vascular and bleeding complications, and considerable cost. In addition, ultrasound studies now suggest that late lumen loss is accentuated in patients with stents, predominantly due to excessive neointimal proliferation. The early results of treatment for in-stent restenosis by balloon angioplasty or further stent deployment are disappointing, with subsequent restenosis rates of 30–40%. Use of multiple and especially overlapping stents has been associated with restenosis rates of up to 64% (48), and preliminary data suggest that stenting of restenotic lesions leads to restenosis rates as high as 40% (49). Clearly, these patients are not optimally treated by current mechanical approaches alone, prompting the exploration of adjunctive pharmacological therapies.

Pharmacological therapy, however, has thus far largely fallen short of its potential for preventing restenosis. Despite considerable evidence from in vitro and animal models that numerous pharmacological agents are efficacious in reducing neointimal hyperplasia, in clinical trials these agents have failed to attenuate the restenotic process and have nearly been abandoned (50). This may reflect interspecies differences in the biology of restenosis, or the etiological significance of causative factors other than neointima formation (51). However, this failure to reproduce clinically the positive results observed in animal experiments may simply reflect patients' inability to tolerate the high systemic drug concentrations required to achieve therapeutic levels for sufficient time at the target site. For example, while both the low molecular weight heparin enoxaparin (5 mg/kg/day) and the angiotensin-converting enzyme inhibitor cilazapril (5–10 mg/kg/day) attenuated neointimal proliferation in animal systems, they failed to reduce restenosis in humans possibly because the doses used (40 and 2–20 mg/day, respectively) were an order of magnitude smaller (52,53). A widespread occurrence of similar results with systemic therapies has necessitated a shift in the focus of therapeutic agents for the prevention of restenosis to local or site-specific delivery.

B. Pharmacological Trials

Most pharmacological trials have examined whether systemically administered pharmacological agents reduce the risk of angiographic restenosis

(54–56). Over 20 different agents have been tested to date, yet until the EPIC trial none had demonstrated effectiveness (57). Agents used can be grouped according to their hypothesized pathophysiological targets as platelet antagonists, anticoagulants or antiproliferative agents. In Tables 1 and 2, data from randomized trials are pooled using broad pharmacological groups. An overview of this nature should be interpreted cautiously as there may be publication bias, with some negative trials not reported and others presented only in abstract form. Nevertheless, meta-analysis suggests that some interesting features are emerging.

1. Platelet Antagonists

Platelet adhesion and activation are fundamental steps in vascular healing during the first few days after angioplasty. Several trials have tested platelet antagonists such as aspirin, ticlopidine, thromboxane A_2 inhibitors, and prostacyclin analogs such as ciprostene. A meta-analysis of 573 patients from trials of various aspirin dosages showed no significant reduction in angiographic restenosis (odds ratio, 0.81; 95% C.I. 0.7–1.4), although immediate postangioplasty acute closure was reduced (3). Similarly, dipyridamole and ticlopidine do not have any beneficial effect on restenosis (3, 58–60).

Thromboxane A_2 is a potent vasoconstrictor and promotes platelet aggregation. Three large randomized studies (GRASP, M-HEART II, and CARPORT) examining thromboxane A_2 inhibition all showed a failure of these agents to reduce angiographic restenosis either individually or in combination (22,40,41).

CARPORT (Coronary Artery Restenosis Prevention on Repeated Thromboxane Antagonism) (22). Vapiprost (GR32191B) is a novel thromboxane A_2 receptor blocker. In this multicenter European trial, 697 patients were randomized to oral vapiprost 80 mg before angioplasty and 80 mg/day for 6 months or 250 mg of i.v. aspirin before angioplasty and then placebo for 6 months in a double-blind fashion. Eighty-nine percent of patients had follow-up quantitative angiography at 6 months. Restenosis was defined as loss of $\geqslant$ 0.72 mm of MLD. Intention-to-treat analysis did not show any reduction in restenosis rate (21% in treatment group vs. 19% in placebo group) or in the incidence of ranked clinical events including death, CABG, re-PTCA, and nonfatal MI. The trial concluded that long-term thromboxane A_2–receptor blockade with vapiprost is not beneficial in reducing restenosis.

GRASP (Glaxo Restenosis and Symptom Project) (40). This U.S. trial also evaluated vapiprost (GR32191B). A total of 1192 patients were randomized to one of the three arms consisting of 325 mg of aspirin the day before angioplasty and placebo; thereafter, 80 mg of vapiprost prior to

Table 1 Meta-Analysis of Clinical Trials of Restenosis: Antiplatelet and Anticoagulant Agents

Study		N	% Angio. follow-up	Agent and dose	Definition of restenosis	Restenosis rate		Odds ratio (95% C.I.)
						Drug	Control	
Aspirin vs. placebo								
Schwartz	(1988)	376	66	ASA 990/dipyr 225 mg	>50% stenosis	38%	39%	1.0 (0.7–1.3)
White	(1987)	157	71	ASA 650/dipyr 225 mg	>70% stenosis	18%	20%	0.9 (0.4–1.9)
Finci	(1988)	40	73	ASA 100 mg	>50% stenosis	33%	14%	2.3 (0.5–10.1)
Cheseboro	(1989)	207	83	ASA 975/dipyr 225 mg	Δ MLD (mm)	1.33	1.34	p = ns
Bove	(1992)	755	55	ASA 325 mg	Δ MLD (mm)	1.59	1.43	p = ns
High vs. low-dose aspirin								
Dyckmans	(1988)	203	42	ASA 1500/320 mg	>50% stenosis	38%	39%	1.0 (0.7–1.3)
Mufson	(1988)	453	37	ASA 1500/80 mg	>50% stenosis	51%	47%	1.1 (0.7–1.6)
Schanzenbacher	(1988)	79	100	ASA 1000/100 mg	Clin. events 6 m	21%	17%	1.2 (0.5–2.9)
Kadel	(1990)	188	92	ASA 1400/350 mg	N/A	31%	21%	1.5 (0.9–2.5)
Total		923	55					1.3 (0.8–1.8)
Ticlopidine vs. placebo								
White	(1987)	157	76	Ticlopidine 750 mg	>70% stenosis	29%	20%	1.6 (0.7–3.6)
Bertrand	(1990)	266	92	Ticlopidine 200 mg	Loss>50 % gain	50%	41%	1.1 (0.7–1.9)
Kitazume	(1988)	189	100	Ticlopidine 200 mg	>50% stenosis	27%	38%	0.5 (0.3–1.2)
Total		612	90					1.0 (0.7–1.4)
Thromboxane A_2 blocker vs. placebo								
Yabe	(1989)	33	100	TxA_2 synthesis inhibitor 600 mg (DP-1904)	Loss>50% gain	22%	53%	0.4 (0.0–1.4)
Serruys	(1991)	697	89	TxA_2 receptor blocker 80 mg Vapiprost	Loss≥0.72 mm	21%	19%	1.1 (0.8–1.6)
Feldman	(1992)	1192	94	TxA_2 receptor blocker 40–80 mg Vapiprost	>70% stenosis	28%	31%	0.9 (0.7–1.2)
Total		1673	92					0.9 (0.6–1.3)
Bove	(1992)	755	55	TxA_2 receptor blocker Sulotroban 3200 mg	Δ MLD (mm)	1.43	1.43	p = ns

Table 1 Continued

Study		N	% Angio. follow-up	Agent and dose	Definition of restenosis	Restenosis rate		Odds ratio (95% C.I.)
						Drug	Control	
Prostacyclin analogs vs. placebo								
Raizner	(1988)	311	80	Ciprostene 120 ng/kg/min	>50% stenosis	41%	53%	0.8 (0.6–1.0)
Knudtson	(1990)	270	93	Prostacyclin 5 ng/kg/min	>50% stenosis	27%	32%	0.8 (0.5–1.4)
Gershlick	(1990)	132	80	Prostacyclin 4 ng/kg/min	Loss>50% gain	31%	34%	0.9 (0.2–4.3)
Total		693	83					0.7 (0.5–1.0)
Anticoagulants vs. placebo								
Ellis	(1989)	416	61	Heparin≤24 h, target PTT	>50% stenosis	41%	37%	1.1 (1.0–1.2)
Lehmann	(1991)	30	77	Heparin 10,000 U/day	>50% stenosis	82%	33%	2.5 (0.1–6.4)
Thornton	(1984)	248	72	Coumadin, target PT	Loss>50% gain	27%	36%	0.7 (0.4–1.1)
Urban	(1988)	110	77	Coumadin, target INR	>50% stenosis	29%	37%	0.7 (0.3–1.6)
Faxon	(1994)	458	86	Enoxaparin 40 mg	Loss>50% gain	52%	51%	1.0 (0.7–1.5)
Cairns	(1994)	814	97	Enoxaparin 30 mg	Loss>50% gain	47%	47%	1.0 (0.7–1.4)
Serruys	(1995)	1141	100	Hirudin 40 mg vs heparin	Clin. events 6 m	37%	33%	0.8 (0.6–1.1)
Glycoprotein IIb/IIIa inhibitors vs. placebo								
Topol (EPIC)	(1994)	2099	100	c7E3 bolus/12 h infusion	Clin. events 6 m	27%	35%	0.7 (0.5–0.9)
EPILOG	(1995)	1500	100	c7E3 bolus/infusion + low/standard-dose heparin	Clin. events 30 d	2.6%	8.1%	0.3 (0.2–0.6)
Tcheng	(1995)	150	100	Integrelin bolus/infusion	Clin. events 6 m	4.1%	12.2%	0.3 (0.1–1.6)
Lincoff	(1995)	918	100	Integrelin bolus/infusion	>50% stenosis	47%	52%	0.9 (0.6–1.2)

MLD = minimal luminal diameter; clin. events 6 m = clinical events at 6-month follow-up; 30 d = 30-day follow-up; ns = not statistically significant; Δ = change.

Table 2 Meta-Analysis of Clinical Trials of Restenosis: Other Pharmacological Agents

Study		N	% Angio. follow-up	Agent and dose	Definition of restenosis	Restenosis rate		Odds ratio (95% C.I.)
						Drug	Control	
Calcium antagonists vs. placebo								
Corcos	(1985)	92	100	Diltiazem 270 mg	>70% stenosis	15%	22%	0.7 (0.2–2.3)
O'Keefe	(1991)	201	60	Diltiazem 240 mg	>70% stenosis	36%	32%	1.1 (0.5–2.2)
Whitworth	(1986)	241	82	Nifedipine 40 mg	>50% stenosis	28%	30%	0.9 (0.3–3.6)
Hoberg	(1990)	196	88	Verapamil 480 mg	Loss>50% gain	43%	63%	0.7 (0.5–0.9)
Unverdorben	(1993)	189	90	Diltiazem 180 mg	>50% stenosis	21%	38%	0.6 (0.3–1.1)
Total		919	82					0.7 (0.5–0.9)
Steroids vs. placebo								
Rose	(1987)	66	88	48 mg Prednisone	>50% stenosis	33%	33%	1.0 (0.4–1.4)
Stone	(1989)	102	53	60 mg Prednisone	>50% stenosis	59%	56%	1.1 (0.5–1.5)
Pepine	(1990)	722	71	1 g Methylprednisone	>50% stenosis	43%	43%	1.0 (0.8–1.2)
Total		890	70					1.0 (0.8–1.2)
ACE inhibitors vs. placebo								
Serruys	(1992)	693	86	Cilazapril 10 mg	Loss>50% gain	37%	39%	0.9 (0.9–1.1)
Faxon	(1995)	1436	75	Cilazapril 2–20 mg	>50% stenosis	37%	33%	1.2 (0.9–1.5)
Desmet	(1994)	336	90	Fosinopril 40 mg	Loss>50% gain	46%	41%	1.2 (0.8–1.9)
Total		2465	80					1.0 (0.9–1.2)
Fish oil (EPA/DHA) vs. placebo								
Slack	(1987)	162	85	7.4 g	Clin events 6 m	16%	33%	0.5 (0.2–1.0)
Reis	(1989)	186	30	6.0 g	>70% stenosis	34%	23%	1.5 (0.9–2.5)
Milner	(1989)	194	100	4.5 g	Clin. events 6 m	22%	35%	0.6 (0.4–1.0)
Dehmer	(1988)	82	100	3.2 g	>50% stenosis	19%	46%	0.4 (0.2–0.8)
Grigg	(1989)	108	91	3.0 g	Loss>50% gain	34%	33%	1.0 (0.6–1.8)
Cheng	(1990)	50	86	3.0 g	>50% stenosis	20%	34%	0.6 (0.1–2.7)

Table 2 Continued

Study		N	% Angio. follow-up	Agent and dose	Definition of restenosis	Restenosis rate		Odds ratio (95% C.I.)
						Drug	Control	
Nye	(1990)	69	100	4.0 g	>50% stenosis	11%	30%	0.4 (0.1–0.2)
Franzen	(1990)	200	65	3.2 g	>50% stenosis	37%	33%	1.1 (0.5–2.4)
Bairati	(1992)	205	60	4.5 g	>50% stenosis	31%	48%	0.5 (0.2–1.0)
Leaf	(1994)	551	93	6.9 g	>50% stenosis	52%	46%	1.3 (0.9–1.9)
Cairns	(1994)	814	97	5.4 g	Loss>50% gain	38%	37%	1.0 (0.8–1.5)
Total		2621	81					0.9 (0.7–1.0)
PDGF antagonist vs. placebo								
Nishikawa	(1992)	160	85	Trapidil 600 mg	Loss>50% gain	20%	38%	0.4 (0.2–0.9)
Okamoto	(1992)	97	74	Trapidil 600 mg	Loss>50% gain	19%	42%	0.3 (0.1–1.0)
Maresta	(1992)	305	83	Trapidil 300 mg	Loss>50% gain	24%	40%	0.5 (0.3–0.8)
Total		562	82					0.4 (0.3–0.7)
Serotonin antagonist vs. placebo								
Klein	(1989)	43	100	Ketanserin 80 mg	>50% stenosis	33%	29%	1.2 (0.3–4.3)
Heik	(1992)	97	89	Ketanserin 80/40 mg	>50% stenosis	22%	38%	0.5 (0.2–1.2)
Serruys	(1993)	658	90	Ketanserin 80 mg	Δ MLD (mm)	0.27	0.24	p = ns
Lovastatin vs. placebo								
Sahni	(1991)	157	50	20/40 mg	>50% stenosis	14%	38%	0.3 (0.1–0.7)
Weintraub	(1994)	404	92	80 mg	>50% stenosis	44%	46%	0.9 (0.6–1.4)
Tanajura	(1995)	150	84	40 mg	>50% stenosis	38%	45%	0.7 (0.3–1.4)
Angiopeptin vs. placebo								
Kent	(1993)	1246	87	190/750/3000 μg	>50% stenosis	37%	39%	0.9 (0.7–1.2)
Eriksen	(1993)	112	82	750 μg	>50% stenosis	7.5%	38%	0.2 (0.1–0.6)

Abbreviations as for Table 1.

angioplasty followed by 40 or 80 mg/day for 6 months. Restenosis was defined as change in MLD of ≥ 0.72 mm by quantitative angiography at 6 months. The restenosis rate was 39% in the treatment group and 35% in the control group, indicating no reduction in restenosis with vapiprost treatment.

M-Heart II (Multi-Hospital Eastern Atlantic Restenosis Trial-2) (61). Sulotroban (BM-13177), a sulfonamide, is a specific thromboxane A_2 receptor antagonist. In this multicenter trial, 755 patients were randomized to receive 800 mg qid of oral Sulotroban, or 325 mg/day of aspirin or placebo for 6 months in a double-blind fashion. Restenosis was defined as > 0.72-mm change in MLD by quantitative angiography at 6 months; 55% of patients had angiographic follow-up. Clinical events were also assessed. There was no significant reduction in angiographic restenosis among these three groups. Change in MLD was 1.43 mm in the treatment and control groups. However, the aspirin group had fewer adverse ischemic clinical events. It was concluded that neither selective thromboxane A_2 receptor blockage with sulotroban nor nonselective thromboxane A_2 inhibition with aspirin affects restenosis.

2. *Anticoagulants*

The use of anticoagulants such as heparin or low molecular weight heparin (LMWH) has been evaulated in a series of clinical trials. In addition to its antithrombotic effects, heparin has been shown to inhibit the proliferation and migration of vascular SMCs in animal studies. Although a retrospective subgroup analysis by Hirshfeld et al. (45) showed a reduction in angiographic restenosis, this was not confirmed in two other larger studies (3,62). Heparin does significantly decrease acute complications like abrupt closure. Unfortunately, to date there have been no adequate trials of intravenous heparin for several (5–7) days and in a large enough patient population. Low molecular weight heparins have weaker anti-IIa and greater anti-Xa and antiproliferative properties. These are discussed below.

Two small randomized trials have evaluated long-term anticoagulation with warfarin and found no reduction in restenosis (63,64). These studies have been inadequate so far to refute or document a therapeutic benefit.

Low Molecular Weight Heparins. Heparin is a mixture of glycosaminoglycans with a wide range of molecular weights and can be fractionated into its anticoagulant and nonanticoagulant components. The low molecular weight nonanticoagulant fragments have antiproliferative properties (65).These fragments, in addition to scavenging cationic growth factors like fibroblast growth factor (FGF) and platelet-derived growth factor (PDGF), are internalized by SMCs and prevent cell division by S-phase inhibition (66). These heparin fragments have weaker anti-IIa and greater anti-Xa activity and cause much less systemic anticoagulation and spontaneous bleeding. In animal models, heparin reduces SMC proliferation and migration, albeit only when administered within 3 days of vascular injury (66–68), and low molecular weight heparin has been demonstrated to reduce restenosis after angioplasty (69).

ERA Trial (Enoxaparin Restenosis After Angioplasty). Enoxaparin is a LMWH fragment which has been shown to inhibit restenosis in the hyperlipidemic rabbit model. In this multicenter trial, 459 patients were randomized to receive either 40 mg/day of Enoxaparin or placebo subcutaneously in a double-blind fashion for 1 month. Restenosis was defined as loss of $>$ 50% of initial gain at quantitative angiographic follow-up at 6 months. Eighty-six percent of the patients had follow-up angiography. No reduction in clinical events or restenosis rate was noted with Enoxaparin therapy (52 vs. 51% with placebo), although the dose and the route of administration may have been inadequate (53).

EMPAR Trial (Enoxaparin Max EPA for Prevention of Angioplasty Restenosis). In this multicenter Canadian trial, 800 patients were randomized in a two-by-two factorial design to receive either 30 mg bid of Enoxaparin subcutaneously for 6 weeks starting 2 h after sheath removal, 5.4 g/day of eicosapentanoic acid (EPA) for 4 months starting 7 days prior to angioplasty, both treatments, or placebo (70). Endpoints were restenosis (defined as $\geqslant$ 50% loss of initial gain at 6-month follow-up angiography) and clinical events (periprocedural complications and recurrent ischemia). No reduction in restenosis rates was seen for enoxaparin compared with placebo (47 vs. 47%, $p = 1.0$), or for MaxEPA compared with placebo (47 vs. 46%, $p = 1.0$).

FACT. Preliminary results from this study randomizing 354 patients to nadroparin or placebo also failed to show any benefit with LMWH in terms of clinical or angiographic outcomes at 6 months (71). The failure of heparin to prevent restenosis in humans despite clear benefits in animal systems may relate to species specificity, where the effect of heparin on promoters of migration and proliferation of SMCs, such as basic FGF and PDGF, is relatively weak in primates (72).

3. Antiproliferative Agents

Several antiproliferative agents targeting smooth muscle cell migration and proliferation have been evaluated, including glucocorticoids, colchicine, angiotensin-converting enzyme (ACE) inhibitors, and trapidil. Glucocorticoids have multiple effects but may inhibit inflammatory cell function, altering the production of smooth muscle cell mitogens. While animal studies have shown reduced smooth muscle cell proliferation with glucocorticoids, three human trials using regimens associated with low risk for systemic toxicity in 890 patients have shown no reduction in restenosis rates (3,73–75). This may be due to the fact that the animal study used sustained local steroid delivery, whereas the clinical trials employed only oral pulse dose therapy.

Colchicine. Colchicine is a plant alkaloid that exerts its antiproliferative effects by causing metaphase arrest of the cell cycle by interfering with intracellular microtubular functions and cell secretory functions. High-dose colchicine was shown to reduce restenosis in the rabbit model (76), however, no benefit was seen in two randomized placebo-controlled clinical trials (77,78). Thus, it can be inferred that systemically administered colchicine is unlikely to be effective in restenosis prevention.

ACE Inhibitors. There is evidence from cell culture and animal studies to suggest that angiotensin II is either a mitogen or a co-mitogen to SMCs. Although one review suggested that patients on ACE inhibitors had significantly less restenosis, in a small nonrandomized study, enalapril as a part of a multidrug regimen did not reduce restenosis (79,80). Two large clinical studies (MERCATOR and MARCATOR), with over 2129 patients combined, examining cilazapril (a third-generation ACE inhibitor) failed to show any impact on restenosis rates (52,81).

In the MERCATOR Trial (Multicenter European Research trial with Cilazapril after Angioplasty to prevent Transluminal coronary Obstruction and Restenosis), 735 patients were randomized in a double-blind fashion to 2.5 mg of cilazapril on the day of angioplasty followed by 5 mg bid for 6 months or matched placebo. All patients received aspirin for 6 months. With 81% quantitative angiographic follow-up at 6 months, neither restenosis (defined as loss of > 50% of initial gain, 37 vs. 39%) nor the incidence of clinical events including death, nonfatal MI, and coronary revascularization differed between the cilazapril group and controls.

The companion North American MARCATOR Trial (Multicenter American Research trial with Cilazapril after Angioplasty to prevent Transluminal coronary Obstruction and Restenosis) was designed to evaluate different doses of cilazapril after 5 mg bid did not reduce restenosis in MERCATOR. Patients (n = 1436) were randomized to placebo plus aspirin or to 2.5, 5, or 10 mg bid of oral cilazapril plus aspirin for 24 weeks. Restenosis (using MERCATOR criteria) was 46% in the cilazapril group and 41% in controls; there was no difference in clinical events between the groups.

A further study using fosinopril, a novel phosphinic acid–containing ACE inhibitor, was commenced prior to the release of these trial results (82). Patients received either fosinopril or matched placebo 10 mg more than 18 h prior to PTCA, 20 mg more than 4 h prior to PTCA, and 40 mg daily thereafter for 6 months. This trial was stopped after 509 patients were randomized once the negative results of the MERCATOR trial became available, and the interim analysis for the first 100 patients showed no benefit from fosinopril therapy. Of the 509 patients randomized, 173 patients (86 fosinopril, 87 control) were excluded from the study early due to an unsuccessful PTCA or symptomatic hypotension from study medication, leaving 153 in the fosinopril group and 151 in the placebo group eligible for final analysis. No significant difference in restenosis rates (45.7% in fosinopril vs. 40.7% in placebo) or in the incidence of ranked clinical events, such as death, MI, repeat revascularization, and recurrent ischemic events, was noted between the groups. Thus, the available data from three large trials do not indicate a useful role for ACE inhibition in the prevention of restenosis.

PDGF Antagonists. Trapidil (triazolopyrimidine) is chemically related to dipyridamole and is a competitive antagonist of the PDGF receptor. In cell culture studies this agent is shown to inhibit PDGF-induced proliferation, and in the rabbit model it significantly reduced neointimal hyperplasia (83). In two recent small but randomized clinical trials trapidil therapy reduced the restenosis rate (84,85). This finding was confirmed in a larger cohort. In the 305-patient, multicenter STARC (Studio Trapidil vs. ASA nella Restenosi Coronarica) trial, patients were randomized to trapidil 100 mg tid or aspirin 100 mg tid orally in a double-blind fashion (86). With 83% follow-up, restenosis (defined as loss of $> 50\%$ of initial gain at 6-month angiography) was reduced with trapidil compared to aspirin (24.2 vs. 39.7%, $p = 0.01$). Further study in large-scale trials is needed to determine whether there is a clinical role for trapidil.

Angiopeptin. Several growth factors are identified as important mediators of SMC proliferation, including insulin-like growth factor 1 (IGF-1), whose effects are potentiated by PDGF. Angiopeptin, a cyclic octapeptide analog of somatostatin, prevents an increase in IGF-1 in the vascular wall after balloon injury and alters its responsiveness to PDGF (87,88). It has been shown to reduce intimal hyperplasia after balloon injury in several different animal models (89–91).

A multicenter U.S. trial (92) tested the efficacy of three different doses of subcutaneous angiopeptin (190, 750, and 3000 mg/day) for the prevention of restenosis. Cumulatively, 1246 patients were randomized to placebo or one of the three subcutaneous doses of angiopeptin, begun 2 h prior to angioplasty and continued twice daily for 10 days. Angiographic follow-up was 87% complete. Using a dichotomous definition, restenosis rates (36.5 vs. 38.6%) and clinical event rates did not differ between treatments. This may have been due to a suboptimal daily dosing regime or to inadequate periprocedural drug levels. The Scandinavian Angiopeptin Pilot Study randomized 112 patients in a double-blind fashion to either 750 g/day of subcutaneous angiopeptin as a continuous infusion or matched placebo for 6–24 h before and 4 days after angioplasty (93). With 82% of patients returning for 6-month angiographic follow-up, the restenosis rate was 7.5% in the angiopeptin group compared with 37.8% in the placebo group, suggesting that angiopeptin at more appropriate doses may significantly reduce restenosis.

However, even with similar high doses and prolonged drug delivery, this promising finding was not confirmed by a recent 553-patient randomized multicenter European study (94). Using the same dosing regimen as the Scandinavian Pilot study, angiopeptin decreased clinical events at 12-month follow-up from 36.4% with placebo to 28.4% in angiopeptin-treated patients ($p = 0.046$), principally due to a decrease in the rate of repeat angioplasty procedures (20.7 vs. 14.7%). However, with 92% angiographic follow-up, there was no difference in restenosis rate (36 vs. 37%, $p = 0.85$). It remains to be demonstrated that angiopeptin, even when given for several days, is an effective antirestenosis strategy, although one study has shown a clinical benefit.

Nonsteroidal Anti-inflammatory Agents. Ebselen, a synthetic selenium-containing heterocyclic agent with anti-inflammatory and antioxidant properties, was recently tested in a small Japanese randomized trial (95). A total of 79 patients were randomized to treatment with either 200 mg twice a day of oral ebselen ($n = 29$), or placebo ($n = 50$), initiated 3 days prior to angioplasty and continued for 3 months. Restenosis was defined as loss of $> 50\%$ of initial luminal gain by quantitative angiography at 3-month follow-up. Restenosis was significantly reduced in the ebselen compared to the placebo group (18.6 vs. 38.2%, $p < 0.05$). These results clearly need to be confirmed by a larger study.

4. *Vasodilators*

Serotonin Antagonists. Serotonin is released at the injury site by platelet degranulation. It causes vasoconstriction, promotes platelet activation, and is mitogenic to SMCs. Ketanserin is a specific S_2 receptor antagonist (96). While one small study of ketanserin showed a clinical benefit with a reduction in abrupt closure (97), the double-blind multicenter PARK (Post-Angioplasty Restenosis Ketanserin) trial ($n = 658$) demonstrated no angiographic or clinical benefit from ketanserin 40 mg bid for 6 months compared to placebo (96).

Calcium Channel Blockers. From a pooled analysis it has been suggested that calcium channel antagonists may decrease restenosis by reducing coronary vasospasm (56). They have been studied in 919 patients; two randomized trials evaluating diltiazem (3,98) and one evaluating nifedipine (99) did not show a beneficial effect, although there was a trend towards an angiographic reduction in restenosis when all studies were combined (3,98–101). However, the potential toxicity of these agents and the lack of any definitive data make this trend suspect. Further large studies are required to confirm that these observations are not due to reporting bias.

Prostanoids. Prostacyclin is a vasodilator and antiaggregatory agent which may have an antirestenotic effect. In one trial with ciprostene (a prostacyclin analog), Raizner and coworkers reported on 311 patients randomized to placebo or preangioplasty intracoronary ciprostene followed by 2 days of intravenous infusion (102). There was a trend towards a reduction in visual angiographic restenosis rates in the ciprostene group compared to controls (41 vs. 53%, $p = 0.058$). Twenty-three percent of the treatment patients experienced death, nonfatal myocardial infarction, repeat PTCA, or CABG during 6 months of follow-up compared to 38% in the placebo group ($p = 0.004$). Reanalysis using QCA of 68% of the films showed a significant reduction in restenosis in ciprostene group (0.24 mm less late loss, $p = 0.034$). Additionally, when data from a 321-patient European companion trial were pooled, a 35% reduction in clinical events at 6 months was seen ($p = 0.001$). These encouraging results suggest that this class of agents needs further investigation in a large prospective clinical study.

5. *Lipid-Altering Agents*

Although the association between hyperlipidemia and restenosis is not as clear as that with atherosclerosis (103), reducing low-density lipoprotein (LDL) cholesterol levels decreases platelet aggregability (104), and lipid-altering agents may inhibit SMC proliferation. Lovastatin, an HMG-Co-A reductase inhibitor, has been shown to reduce neointimal hyperplasia in animal models (105). Elevated serum lipoprotein has been shown to be a risk factor for clinical recurrence after PTCA (106). Thus, lipid metabolism and lipoproteins have attracted interest in the search to prevent restenosis. Although there are conflicting data, some studies have suggested that alterations in lipid profile may have a favorable effect on restenosis. In a randomized, placebo-controlled trial, lovastatin was shown to significantly reduce restenosis; however, the trial was hampered by inadequate angiographic follow-up (107). In a small nonrandomized trial aggressive lipid lowering with lovastatin and colestipol did not lower restenosis compared to historical controls (3).

Further, in a large randomized multicenter study, the 404 patient Lovastatin Restenosis Trial (LRT), high-dose lovastatin with pretreatment was ineffective in decreasing restenosis after angioplasty (108). In 203 patients with total cholesterol levels of 180–300 mg/dl randomized to 40 mg bid of lovastatin started 7–10 days prior to angioplasty, restenosis was not reduced despite a 40% reduction in LDL levels compared to a matched group given placebo ($n = 201$). This finding was repeated in a 150-patient randomized trial of lovastatin 20 mg bid started either 3–10 days before or at the time of PTCA, with no reduction in restenosis compared to placebo (38 vs. 45%, p = ns) (109).

The omega-3 fatty acids may favorably influence restenosis by altering synthesis of arachidonic acid and thromboxane production (from TXA_2 and PGI_2 to TXA_3 and PGI_3, thus providing a less pro-aggregatory and vasoreactive milieu), altering lipid metabolism, and reducing various smooth muscle cell mitogens. To date nine clinical trials with fish oils rich in omega-3 fatty acids have been performed to examine whether this substance can reduce restenosis (110–118). The dose of fish oil varied between 2.5 and 6.0 g per dose. Although the results from individual small clinical trials have been conflicting, a meta-analysis of the combined trials in 1358 patients shows a 39% (95% C.I. 19–54) reduction of a mixture of clinical and angiographic endpoints for restenosis (3,119). Two large randomized trials were conducted in an attempt to confirm these findings.

The FORT (Fish Oil Restenosis Trial) study is a 551-patient multicenter, double-blind, placebo-controlled trial evaluating the efficacy of 10 g/day omega-3 fatty acids for 6 months after adequate pretreatment in preventing restenosis. Using a primary endpoint of angiographic restenosis at 6 months, there was no benefit associated with use of fish oils (120). The EMPAR trial (previously described) is a large Canadian fish oil trial in which 814 patients were randomized in a two-by-two factorial design to receive either 30 mg twice daily of enoxaparin subcutaneously for 6 weeks starting 2 h after sheath removal, 5.4 g/day of eicosapentanoic acid (EPA) for 4 months starting 7 days prior to angioplasty, both treatments, or placebo. No reduction in restenosis rates (defined as $\geqslant$ 50% loss of initial gain at 6-month follow-up angiography) or clinical events (periprocedural complications and recurrent ischemia) was seen in any treatment group when compared to placebo. Despite the trend towards benefit seen in the meta-analysis of earlier trials, from the large-scale FORT and EMPAR data it appears that there is no role for fish oils in the prevention of restenosis.

In summary, as of 1994 no systemic pharmacological agent had been shown conclusively to produce a clinically worthwhile reduction in restenosis after PTCA. Although these data rest on clinical trials with the previously described weaknesses, some agents (ketanserin, thromboxane A_2 antagonists, cilazapril, calcium channel blockers, fish oils, lipid-modifying drugs, and glucocorticoids) can likely be rejected as systemic monotherapy to prevent angiographic restenosis. While many of these agents are active in vitro or in animal studies against components of the restenotic process, their failure in clinical trials likely relates to maximum tolerable systemic doses in humans, the shortcomings of animal models to mimic human pathology, and the complexity of the vascular healing response. Other agents such as prostacyclin analogs and trapidil have shown some promise and deserve further study.

C. Recent Pharmacological Studies

1. Platelet Glycoprotein IIb/IIIa Antagonists

EPIC Trial (Evaluation of c7E3 for the Prevention of Ischemic Complications). Since the platelet glycoprotein IIb/IIIa integrin is the final common pathway for platelet aggregation, it was postulated that blocking this receptor with a chimeric monoclonal antibody Fab (c7E3) fragment would result in a reduction of restenosis. This, however, does not prevent platelet adhesion with a monolayer formation at the site of injury. A total of 2099 high-risk patients were randomized to receive c7E3 bolus pre-PTCA then a 12-h infusion (n = 708), c7E3 bolus only (n = 695), or placebo (n = 696), in a double-blind fashion, in addition to aspirin and heparin (121). Over a 6-month follow-up period, the composite endpoint of ischemic events (death, MI, and the need for repeat revascularization) was used as clinical evidence of restenosis. A significant 26% reduction of the composite endpoint was seen at 6-month follow-up, mostly due to a reduction in the need for repeat procedures, in the bolus and infusion of c7E3 group, likely due to less restenosis (57). No beneficial effect was noted in the bolus-only or placebo groups. Although bleeding complications were increased with c7E3, this was mainly in patients who were older, female, given higher doses of heparin per kg body mass (larger dose or lower weight), and in those with prolonged procedures and delayed sheath removal (122). These findings suggest that more specific antiplatelet therapy with c7E3 bolus and infusion may be beneficial in reducing restenosis and improving clinical outcome and that bleeding complications may potentially be decreased with a reduction in heparin dosing.

EPILOG. The EPILOG (Evaluation of PTCA to Improve Long-term Outcome by c7E3 GP IIb/IIIa receptor blockade) trial was planned as a 5000 patient multicenter, randomized, placebo-controlled study to assess the potential benefit of the GP IIb/IIIa integrin blocker c7E3 with low (70 U/kg) or standard dose heparin in elective coronary intervention, in terms of clinical events at 30 days. However, the trial was halted at 3000 patients enrolled after an interim analysis of data from the first 1500 patients revealed a highly significant 68% reduction in the incidence of the 30-day composite of death and acute myocardial infarction from 8.1% in controls to 2.6% in the c7E3/low-dose heparin group ($p < 0.0001$). Bleeding complications were not increased in the c7E3 groups. As a result, the trial has been restructured to include a 1000-patient stent substudy and an angiographic follow-up arm to determine the effect of c7E3 on restenosis, which should provide important data on a representative sample of the combined cohort of approximately 4000 patients at the trial's conclusion (123).

IMPACT + IMPACT-II. The IMPACT (Integrelin to Minimize Platelet Aggregation and prevent Coronary Thrombosis) study was the first clinical trial during coronary angioplasty of the synthetic cyclic heptapeptide integrelin, a peptide with high specificity and affinity for the GP IIb/IIIa integrin, as well as the first trial of a GP IIb/IIIa antagonist during elective PTCA (124). In this phase II trial, 150 patients were randomized to placebo, or a 90 μg/kg bolus of integrelin prior to PTCA followed by a 1.0 μg/kg-min infusion for 4 or 12 h. Although the bolus + infusion of Integrelin resulted in an 86% inhibition of platelet aggregation, there was only a trend towards reduced clinical events in the Integrelin compared to placebo groups (12.2 vs. 4.1%, $p = 0.13$). There was no increase in bleeding complications with Integrelin, provisionally supporting its safety in this setting. This led to a further examination of the role of integrelin in the phase III IMPACT-II trial.

IMPACT-II was a multicenter double-blind, placebo-controlled study of 4010 low- or high-risk patients undergoing coronary intervention randomized to 135 mg/kg bolus of Integrelin followed by either a 0.75 μg/kg-min infusion ($n = 1335$) or a 0.5 μg/kg-min infusion ($n = 1348$) for 24 h, or placebo ($n = 1327$). There was a nonsignificant trend towards a reduction in the composite clinical endpoint (death, MI, and need for urgent intervention) at 30 days with Integrelin compared to placebo (9.5 vs. 11.4%, $p = 0.07$) (125). However, there was no evidence of reduction in restenosis rates in the angiographic substudy ($n = 918$), either in terms of minimal luminal diameter (1.20 vs. 1.33 mm, $p =$ ns) or dichotomous restenosis rate (52 vs. 47%, $p =$ ns) at 6-month follow-up (126). There was no increase in bleeding complications in either Integrelin group compared to controls. A dose response was not observed in the study, probably due to the fact that plasma drug levels were similar between the two Integrelin groups for the first 12 h of the study. The lack of clear clinical benefit in this study may have been due to inadequate drug dosing. Low-risk patients seemed to derive greater benefit compared to placebo in terms of the composite clinical endpoint (8.6 vs. 11.6%, $p = 0.02$) than those in the high-risk group (10.9 vs. 11.5%, $p = 0.7$). High-risk patients, defined as those presenting with unstable angina or acute myocardial infarction, have in other studies been shown to have enhanced platelet activation, requiring greater plasma concentrations of Integrelin to achieve similar suppression of platelet activation. Thus, the role of Integrelin needs to be clarified by studies using higher bolus or infusion doses in high-risk patients.

Alternatively, direct thrombin inhibitors like the prototypic agent hirudin may be useful. In the HELVETICA [Hirudin in a European triaL Versus heparin in The prevention of restenosIs after ptCA) trial, 1141 patients were randomized to receive intravenous heparin for 24 h or subcutaneous hirudin for 3 days either with or without an initial intravenous bolus of hirudin (127). Although there was a reduction in cardiac events in the first 96 h in the hirudin group, by 7 months there was no difference in clinical events or angiographic restenosis rates between the strategies. These results may relate to inadequate drug doses, as markers of thrombosis (prothrombin fragments F1+2) were not reduced by hirudin therapy, or perhaps to an insufficient duration of drug effect. Similarly, a trial of a hirudin analog, hirulog, during high-risk coronary angioplasty found no benefit compared to heparin in terms of 30-day or 6-month ischemic events (128).

2. *Antisense Oligonucleotides*

With the hypothesis that the failure of several antiproliferative agents to impact upon restenosis may be due to the amplification and redundancy present in the process of protein signaling and production, attempts were made to block gene expression in the cell nucleus. Antisense oligonucleotides, by acting at the initial stage of protein regulation, may be more effective even in very small doses if present during a critical interval after arterial injury (129,130). Several antisense oligonucleotides directed at the proto-oncogenes *c-myb* (26) and *c-myc* (131), proliferating cell nuclear antigen, and cell cycle regulatory genes such as cdc2-kinase and cdk2-kinase (132,133) have reduced neointimal hyperplasia in the balloon-injured rat carotid model. This technology is limited, however, by low rates of cellular uptake and concerns regarding the tissue specificity of these agents and some conflicting results, which may be related to the problem of satisfactory drug delivery and efficacy (134). A pilot study demonstrated the preliminary safety of intracoronary delivery of *c-myc* antisense oligonucleotides (135); a large clinical trial will be required to fully assess the role and safety of this approach.

D. Trials of Mechanical Therapies for Restenosis

Multiple new technologies have been developed in an effort to reduce angiographic restenosis. The goals of these new devices are to safely provide better acute gains (a bigger lumen), either by debulking or by scaffolding with stenting, and to prevent late loss, and thus potentially lower restenosis rates, as well as to broaden the spectrum of lesions safely amenable to angioplasty. Several important clinical trials have examined these issues (Table 3).

1. Autoperfusion Devices

Studies in an animal model have shown prolonged, slow balloon inflation to be associated with less restenosis. This finding suggested that either mechanical approaches such as retroperfusion or pretreatment with beta-blockers, nitrates, or oxygenated fluorocarbons may permit prolonged inflations that could reduce restenosis. Autoperfusion devices permit significantly extended balloon inflations, and a pilot study of 67 patients with 90% angiographic follow-up found a somewhat lower restenosis rate than that observed with standard angioplasty (3). A multicenter randomized trial of 1-min versus 15-min inflations found no significant improvement in clinical outcome or long-term restenosis despite a modest improvement in initial gain with longer inflations (136). Thus, at present perfusion balloon catheters, although useful in treating complex lesions and for "bail-out" in dissection or abrupt closure, have no role in the prevention of restenosis.

2. Atherectomy

This procedure is a potentially important approach to restenosis because it physically removes the atherosclerotic plaque, often leaving a normal or nearly normal lumen as visualized angiographically at the completion of the interventional procedure. Intravascular ultrasound (IVUS) usually demonstrates significant residual stenosis, however, as well as diffuse disease in the adjacent "normal" segment.

CAVEAT I and II (Coronary Angioplasty Versus Excisional Atherectomy Trials). CAVEAT was a multicenter trial of 1012 patients with de novo native coronary lesions randomized to either atherectomy ($n = 512$) or balloon angioplasty ($n = 500$) (35). Endpoints were clinical outcomes and restenosis (defined as $\geqslant$ 50% stenosis at 6 months) determined from baseline and 6-month follow-up angiograms, which were quantitatively analyzed by an independent and blinded core laboratory. All procedures were performed by experienced operators, and all patients received aspirin and a calcium channel blocker for at least a month and heparin peri-procedurally. Angiographic follow-up was 90% complete. Overall, restenosis rates, using worst-view analysis, did not differ significantly between the atherectomy and balloon angioplasty groups (50 vs. 57%, $p = 0.06$); however, in a subgroup of patients with proximal LAD lesions, restenosis rates were lower with atherectomy than with balloon angioplasty (51 vs. 63%, $p =$

Table 3 Meta-Analysis of Clinical Trials of Restenosis: Device Trials

Study		N	% Angio. follow-up	Device/ technique	Definition of restenosis	Restenosis rate (%) Device	Control	Odds ratio (95% C.I.)
Autoperfusion devices								
Ohman	(1994)	478	77	1 vs. 15 min inflation	>50% stenosis	44	44	1.0 (0.7–1.4)
Directional atherectomy vs. balloon angioplasty								
Topol	(1993)	1012	90	DCA:<20% residual	>50% stenosis	50	57	0.8 (0.6–1.0)
Adelman	(1993)	274	97	Standard DCA	>50% stenosis	46	43	1.1 (0.7–1.8)
Holmes	(1995)	305	80	DCA:<20% residual	>50% stenosis	46	51	0.8 (0.5–1.3)
Total		1591	89					0.8 (0.7–1.0)
Primary stent vs. balloon angioplasty								
Serruys	(1994)	520	90	PS stent, ASA Coumadin	>50% stenosis	22	32	0.6 (0.4–0.9)
Fischman	(1994)	410	91	PS stent, ASA Coumadin	>50% stenosis	32	41	0.6 (0.4–1.0)
Total		930	91					0.6 (0.5–0.8)
Excimer laser vs. balloon angioplasty								
Appelman	(1996)	308	92	Laser ± balloon	>50% stenosis	52	41	1.5 (0.9–2.5)

DCA = directional coronary atherectomy; PS = Palmaz-Schatz coronary stent.

0.04). Compared with balloon angioplasty, atherectomy had a higher initial procedural success (89 vs. 80%, $p < 0.001$), larger initial luminal dimension (1.05 vs. 0.86 mm, $p < 0.001$), but more early complications (11 vs. 5% $p < 0.001$) and higher probability of death or MI within 6 months (8.6 vs. 4.6%, $p = 0.007$). With atherectomy, there was no clinical benefit noted after 6 months of follow-up. One-year follow-up data from this trial showed that the modest reduction in angiographic restenosis with atherectomy did not result in a lower rate of repeat procedures, and the difference in death and nonfatal MI between groups persisted (137). Criticisms of this study included the fact that the mean postprocedural stenosis, as determined by core laboratory analysis, was 29% in the atherectomy group, which may have been inadequate to reduce the incidence of restenosis and clinical events. However, in two large randomized trials of stenting compared with balloon angioplasty (STRESS, Benestent), restenosis rates were reduced in stent patients although their mean postprocedural stenosis of 21% was only slightly lower than that achieved in CAVEAT (32,138). The CAVEAT trial did suggest that with both directional atherectomy and balloon angioplasty, the larger the initial lumen, the lower the rate of subsequent restenosis. This trial validated the concept of debulking with atherectomy to reduce angiographic restenosis, but the effect was too modest and the complications too great for widespread adoption of this technology to impact on clinical restenosis.

CAVEAT II compared the outcomes of 305 patients with de novo vein bypass graft stenoses randomized to either directional atherectomy or angioplasty (139). Although initial angiographic success (89% vs. 79%, $p < 0.02$) and luminal gain (1.45 vs. 1.12 mm, $p < 0.001$) were greater with atherectomy than balloon angioplasty, there was an increase in distal embolization (13.4 vs. 5.1%, $p = 0.012$) and more non–Q-wave myocardial infarctions in the atherectomy patients (16.1 vs. 9.6%, $p = 0.09$). Also, there was no difference in 6-month restenosis rates (45.6 vs. 50.5%, $p = 0.49$), although primary atherectomy patients tended to require less target lesion revascularization (18.6 vs. 26.2%, $p = 0.09$).

CCAT (Canadian Coronary Atherectomy Trial). CCAT was a multicenter trial of 274 patients with de novo proximal LAD lesions randomized to undergo either atherectomy ($n = 138$) or balloon angioplasty ($n = 136$) (36). The primary endpoint was restenosis, defined as > 50% stenosis, assessed by quantitative angiography at 6 months. Of the eligible patients, 97% had angiographic follow-up. Compared with balloon angioplasty, atherectomy led to a higher initial procedural success rate (94% vs. 88%, $p = 0.061$), larger initial luminal dimension (1.45 ± 0.47 vs. 1.16 ± 0.44 mm, $p < 0.001$) and larger late loss (0.79 ± 0.61 vs. 0.47 ± 0.64 mm, $p < 0.001$), however, restenosis rates were not significantly different between the two groups (46 vs. 43%, $p = 0.71$). The frequency of major in-hospital complications or clinical outcomes at 6 months did not differ between the groups. The conclusion that atherectomy did not result in better late angiographic or clinical outcomes than balloon angioplasty in patients with elective revascularization of de novo coronary lesions is concordant with the overall findings of CAVEAT.

The final results of further trials, including BOAT (Balloon vs. Optimal Atherectomy Trial) and OARS (Optimal Atherectomy Restenosis Study), studies investigating more aggressive intravascular ultrasound-guided atherectomy that may safely allow greater plaque removal and improved acute and long-term results, are pending. OARS, a 200-patient multicenter registry, was designed to assess the impact of using IVUS-guided "optimal" directional atherectomy to achieve a residual stenosis of less than 10% by visual estimate. Initial results revealed a higher procedural success rate (98 vs. 88%) and an improved final result compared to CAVEAT in terms of residual stenosis (7 vs. 29%). While cognizant that different revascularization goals and different angiographic core laboratories were utilized in these two studies, it is noteworthy that there were fewer adverse outcomes in OARS than CAVEAT in terms of composite clinical events (death, MI, and target lesion revascularization—23.7 vs. 36.5%) and the target lesion revascularization rate (19 vs. 26.5%) at 12 months, and the angiographic restenosis rate at 6 months (29.6 vs. 50.0%), with angiographic follow-up 81% complete (140). These results lend support to the concept of debulking with atherectomy to reduce angiographic restenosis. The initial phase of the 1000-patient, 37-site BOAT comparing "optimal" atherectomy (target of a final stenosis < 20% by quantitative angiography) with balloon angioplasty was recently completed. Overall, the procedural angiographic goal was achieved in 68% of the atherectomy group, compared with only 23% of the PTCA group, with the acute results of atherectomy superior to those from balloon angioplasty both in terms of residual diameter stenosis (14.6 vs. 29.2%, $p < 0.001$) and minimal luminal diameter (2.82 ± 0.54 vs. 2.31 ± 0.48 mm, $p < 0.001$). The 6-month follow-up results should help to clarify the role of DCA for the prevention of restenosis.

3. *Coronary Stent Implantation*

Coronary stents also produce a widely patent artery immediately following the interventional procedure. Unfortunately, preliminary data indicated a substantial restenosis rate with all available stents, although restenosis was diminished when the final stent diameter was greater than 3.2 mm and when a single stent, as opposed to multiple stents, was deployed. Careful evaluation and IVUS studies are consistent with the concept that stent implantation can eliminate elastic recoil, so that even with the same degree of intimal proliferation, the lumen can remain widely patent after stent implantation. This early experience was substantially impacted by two large randomized studies.

Benestent Trial (Belgian-Netherlands Stent Trial). In this multicenter European trial, 520 patients with stable angina and de novo native coronary lesions were randomized to Palmaz-Schatz stent implantation or balloon angioplasty (32). Primary success was achieved in 93% of stent (n = 262) patients and 89% of the PTCA (n = 258) group. The primary clinical endpoint, a composite of death, cerebrovascular accident, MI, or the need for a repeat revascularization procedure at 7 months, was reduced by 32% in the stent compared to balloon angioplasty group (20 vs. 30%, $p = 0.02$), mainly due to a reduced need for repeat PTCA. Although the primary angiographic endpoint of minimal luminal diameter at follow-up did not differ between stent and balloon angioplasty groups (1.82 ± 0.64 vs. 1.73 ± 0.55 mm, $p = 0.09$), using a dichotomous definition, the rate of restenosis was reduced from 32 to 22% in stent patients at 6-month quantitative angiography ($p = 0.02$). However, vascular complications and the need for transfusion were higher in the stent group (13.5 vs. 3.1%, $p < 0.001$), in association with a markedly longer mean hospital stay (8.5 vs. 3.1 days, $p < 0.001$). Thus, clinical and angiographic outcomes were better at 7-month follow-up in patients who received a stent rather than standard angioplasty, at the cost of significantly more vascular complications and a longer hospital stay.

STRESS (STent REStenosis Study) Trial. This multicenter trial compared Palmaz-Schatz stenting with balloon angioplasty in > 3.0 mm native vessel de novo lesions. A total of 410 patients were randomized to stent (n = 207) or balloon angioplasty (n = 203) (138). Stent patients had a higher rate of procedural success (96.1 vs. 89.6, $p = 0.011$), a larger initial lumen increase (1.72 vs. 1.23 mm, $p < 0.001$), and a larger final luminal diameter (2.49 vs. 1.99 mm, $p < 0.001$). At 6 months, minimal luminal diameter (1.74 vs. 1.56, mm $p = .007$) was higher and dichotomous restenosis rate was lower (31.6 vs. 42.1%, $p = 0.046$) in the stent group; however, the composite clinical endpoint of death, MI, coronary bypass surgery, or need for repeat angioplasty was not significantly different between groups (19.5 vs. 23.8%, $p = 0.16$). There was a trend for reduced need for target lesion revascularization in the stent group (10.2 vs. 15.4%, $p = 0.06$). Bleeding and vascular complications were similar in the two groups (7.3 vs. 4.0%, $p = 0.14$); however, length of stay was increased in the stent group (5.8 vs. 2.8 days, $p < 0.001$). The results of this trial confirm the benefits of stent deployment in elective intervention on de novo coronary stenoses found in the Benestent trial.

Recently, Colombo and coworkers combined high-pressure balloon inflation with IVUS guidance to optimize stent deployment and thereby reduce the need for anticoagulation with its negative sequelae (141). Patients were treated with aspirin and ticlopidine alone, resulting in a low incidence of bleeding complications. Despite this, there was a low subacute thrombosis rate (0.3%) and only a 17.6% rate of ischemic events (death, MI, or target lesion revascularization) at 6 months. These findings are supported by a recent trial in which patients randomized to ticlopidine for one month plus short-term aspirin ($n = 123$) after IVUS-guided stenting had a lower incidence of subacute thrombosis (0.8 vs. 2.9%, $p = 0.2$) than those given aspirin alone ($n = 103$) and tended to have fewer major clinical events (0.8 vs. 3.9%, $p = 0.1$) at 30 days (142). Several studies are in progress to attempt to confirm these promising results.

The predominant mechanism for restenosis in stents appears to be intimal proliferation, rather than the recoil seen with other interventional devices (12,143). This finding has led to trials of antiproliferative agents during coronary stenting. In the Benestent II pilot study, stents with a covalently bonded heparin coating were deployed in four groups of patients ($n = 207$) with aspirin, warfarin, and decreasing doses of heparin, or aspirin and ticlopidine alone. Angiographic restenosis occurred in 13% of patients at 6 months (compared to 22% in Benestent) in association with a significant decrease in the incidence of the major complications of stent deployment from that noted in the original Benestent trial (144). Subacute thrombosis decreased from 3.5 to 0% ($p = 0.005$), suggesting that the sustained local action of the stent heparin may have played a significant role, while avoiding systemic side effects, as the incidence of vascular surgery fell from 9.7 to 2.8% ($p < 0.005$) and blood transfusion rates fell from 3.9 to 1.0% ($p = 0.07$). These findings are being further examined in the large multicenter Benestent II trial comparing balloon angioplasty with heparin-coated stents and reduced anticoagulation. With 400 patients enrolled to date, there have been no subacute stent thromboses in this study.

4. *Excimer Laser Coronary Angioplasty*

The excimer laser (ELCA) system exhibits favorable characteristics for ablation of atherosclerotic tissue compared to other laser devices, because of its small penetration depth and the induction of limited damage to the vascular wall (145,146). Several nonrandomized series have suggested a benefit for ELCA compared with balloon angioplasty for complex lesions, in terms of improved primary success rates and reduced procedural complications (147,148). However, the first randomized trial comparing ELCA (n

= 151) with PTCA (n = 157) found no difference in either restenosis rates (51.6 vs. 41.3%, p = 0.13) or the composite clinical endpoint (death, MI, coronary bypass grafting, or repeat angioplasty—33.1 vs. 29.9%, p = 0.55) between the two treatments at 6 months (149).

5. *Endovascular Irradiation*

Gamma radiation limits cell proliferation by inhibiting cell division and reducing the number of stem cells. Recently, low-dose gamma radiation was shown to inhibit neointimal growth and prevent restenosis after balloon angioplasty in rabbit iliac and both balloon-injured and stented porcine coronary models (150–154). Although promising in these animal systems, the potential risks of this therapy require careful consideration before it reaches the clinical arena. A pilot study of coronary stenting followed by catheter delivery of intracoronary ^{192}Iridium seeds, releasing 800 cGy locally, is in progress with 10 patients treated without complication to date (155).

VI. CARDINAL CONCEPTS FOR FUTURE TRIALS

A. Trial Design: Clinical vs. Angiographic Endpoints

Angiographic endpoints have so far been considered the "gold standard" for measuring restenosis rates. Caveats with using angiographic endpoints alone include inadequate restudy rates with inherent withdrawal and selection bias, nonuniform definitions of angiographic restenosis, interobserver variability, the expense involved, patient discomfort, and poor correlation between angiographic restenosis and clinical outcomes, which may have limited the generalizability of many trials to the clinical setting (3,156). Although angiography has been refined by the use of computerized quantitative techniques and endpoints such as minimal luminal diameter, acute gain, and late loss to assess the extent and mechanisms of restenosis, it provides only a two-dimensional outline of the vessel lumen, without precise information regarding the vessel wall and lesion itself. Intravascular ultrasound may provide important additional information to assist in our interpreting trial results to draw clinically relevant conclusions. Alternately, future restenosis trials should utilize clinical outcomes as primary endpoints. Utilizing a composite clinical endpoint will increase discriminating power in determining the overall therapeutic profile of an agent. Califf and coworkers proposed one such weighted index including the clinical outcomes of death, nonfatal MI or stroke, repeat elective and emergent revascularizations (angioplasty or CABG) for documented restenosis at the site of initial intervention, positive exercise stress test, recurrence of symptoms, and angiographic-only restenosis (54). Clinically relevant angiographic restenosis that requires repeat revascularization is considered the critical outcome since death and infarction are extremely uncommon in the first 6 months after successful angioplasty.

Also, future clinical trials should ideally use a factorial design combining multiple, simultaneous treatment approaches and multiple-dose regimens. This will permit evaluation of the benefit of individual, additive, and synergistic effects of each approach in a cost-effective manner. Evaluation of any agent in restenosis trials should ideally follow a multistage approach. After efficacy is established in cell culture and in vitro studies, the agent should be tested in at least two animal species. If this preclinical testing shows effectiveness and a small phase I pilot study establishes safety, a small-scale clinical trial with 6-month angiographic and "soft clinical" endpoints can be carried out. Such phase II and III trials will require 350–500 patients. Particular attention needs to be turned towards the appropriate dosing strategy of the drug and ideally achieving a dose-response effect. If benefit is noted, a large clinical trial with 2000–4000 patients (adequate to detect 25–30% reduction in endpoints) can be performed to study the effect on hard clinical endpoints such as death, MI, and need for repeat percutaneous or surgical revascularization. This large trial should include a systematic, predefined angiographic substudy with 250–300 patients per treatment group to assess angiographic outcomes and their correlation with clinical outcomes. In such a way, clinically meaningful trials of restenosis will be accomplished.

B. Local Drug Delivery Systems

Although in cardiology several systemic therapies such as thrombolysis for myocardial infarction and IIb/IIIa inhibitors in high-risk coronary angioplasty have been extremely effective, benefit has been achieved at the cost of significant side effects. Use of a bolus and 12-h infusion of the glycoprotein IIb/IIIa inhibitor c7E3 in the EPIC study reduced ischemic complications by 23% at 6 months; however, this was at the expense of major bleeding complications unrelated to bypass surgery in 10.6% and blood product transfusions in 16.8% (10).

The major advantage that local drug delivery may provide is the ability to achieve high and in some cases sustained local concentrations of drug without requiring the large systemic doses needed to obtain similar local concentrations. High local drug concentrations can be attained even when agents are rapidly metabolized or have short half-lives when administered systemically. Second, delivering drug to the treatment site while avoiding significant systemic delivery will minimize systemic toxicity or side effects.

Arterial injury after angioplasty produces a localized response, thus ideally therapies for the prevention of restenosis should only act at the injury site. Several systems have been developed for local drug and genetic material delivery to the angioplasty site (4). The Wolinsky balloon with multiple microscopic pores has been documented to deliver marker agents and genetic material into the arterial walls of animals by hydrostatic pressure. Polymer-coated balloons such as the Hydrogel catheter have also successfully delivered marker agents into the arterial wall. Polymer intracoronary stents with drug-delivery capabilities are also under development. Even if devices such as porous balloons can deliver drug locally with minimal additional arterial wall injury, their use may be limited by the rapidity with which infused drug leaches out from the delivery site. Almost all previous studies show a marked reduction in local drug levels within hours of infusion, which may be the reason for poor results to date (157). However, local delivery systems have the potential to establish and maintain local drug action, either by preventing its efflux from the arterial wall or by using vehicles or agents that have a prolonged duration of action. Sustained release may be essential to influence the vascular healing process, which occurs over a period of weeks, and to achieve passivation of the injury site and to favorably influence the processes of reendothelialization and restenosis.

C. Nitric Oxide Regulation

Nitric oxide (NO), or endothelium-derived relaxing factor (EDRF), has been shown to inhibit platelet aggregation (158), leukocyte adhesion, and smooth muscle cell migration and proliferation (159). NO production is reduced following endothelial injury due to downregulation of the inducible NO synthetase (iNOS) found on SMCs and macrophages by factors such as PDGF and IGF-1 (160–162). In an elegant gene-transfer study, transfection of balloon-injured rat carotid arteries with endothelial cell NOS (ec-NOS) without NOS-specific regulatory sites or controls increased NO production and inhibited neointimal formation by 70% compared to controls (163). Coating stents with an NO donor reduces their thrombogenicity (164); administration of an NO donor, S-nitrosoglutathione, has been shown to inhibit platelet expression of P-selectin and the GP IIb/IIIa integrin following PTCA in a small preliminary clinical study (165).

D. Arterial Reendothelialization

Previously, the goal of antirestenosis therapies has been to modulate the response of the smooth muscle cell to arterial injury, however, recent data support the potential value of attempting to rapidly restore normal endothelial integrity and function. In addition to its properties as a physical barrier, the endothelium has a central role in the modulation of growth factor signals and the process of vascular remodeling. Vascular endothelial growth factor (VEGF) is unique among angiogenic growth factors by virtue of the fact that its high-affinity binding sites (*Flt-1* and *Flk-1/KDR*) are present solely on endothelial cells (166–168). Consequently, the effects of VEGF are limited to endothelial cells (169). Using a local delivery system, a 30-min infusion of VEGF has been demonstrated to accelerate reendothelialization and reduce neointimal hyperplasia by 34% in a rat carotid balloon injury model (29). However, VEGF may, in addition to promoting neovascularization, produce increased endothelial permeability, leading to extravasation of humoral factors such as fibrinogen and thrombin, which may lead to a local inflammatory response. These and other concerns must be answered before VEGF can reach clinical trials (170).

E. Apoptosis

Apoptosis, or programmed cell death, is an important regulator of cell populations in normal tissues (171). Isner and coworkers demonstrated that foci of apoptosis were present in 86% of tissue specimens obtained during directional atherectomy for restenosis compared to 29% of de novo lesions (172). Apoptosis was limited to hypercellular tissue and comprised less than 2% of total cell numbers. It has been proposed that restenosis may be impeded by facilitating apoptosis within the SMC population in the treated arterial segment, possibly by gene transfection.

VII. CONCLUSIONS

Despite rapid advances in molecular biology and in our understanding of the complex process of restenosis after PTCA, modulating this response for net therapeutic benefit remains one of the greatest challenges to interventional cardiology research. Unsuccessful clinical trials of agents shown to prevent restenosis in animal models highlight the importance of issues such as achieving adequate site-specific drug doses for sufficient time, species specificity of many signal pathways and cellular systems, and the limitations of conducting adequate clinical trials using only angiographic endpoints. The primary endpoints of restenosis trials should shift from exclusively angiographic to prioritize clinical outcomes such as death, nonfatal myocardial infarction, and subsequent revascularization rates, as well as utilizing new imaging modalities such as intravascular ultrasound. This will require larger trials with simplified designs while specifying angiographic and IVUS substudies for pathophysiological information. The reduction in clinical adverse events documented in several randomized trials despite no angiographic benefit validates the concept of studying the net clinical effect of an intervention.

The effectiveness of new therapies including potent antiplatelet agents and stenting to reduce restenosis, along with improved comprehension of the restenosis paradigm, has renewed the potential to remove the major limitation of coronary angioplasty. Other developing areas for future trials include sophisticated site-specific approaches such as bioerodable stents, local drug-delivery systems, and genetic therapies that may improve the therapeutic index of treatments to modify luminal renarrowing and vessel repair after angioplasty. The continued appeal of angioplasty as an alternative or adjunct to medical therapy and bypass surgery will rely on our ability to understand and control the restenotic process in a cost-effective manner.

REFERENCES

1. Topol E, Ellis S, Cosgrove D, Bates E, Muller D, Schork N, et al. Analysis of coronary angioplasty practice in the United States with an insurance-claims data base. Circulation 1993; 87:1489–1497.
2. USCI Division of CR Bard, Inc. Industry Assessment 1994. Internal publication.
3. Hillegass WB, Ohman EM, Califf RM. Restenosis: the clinical issues. In: Topol EJ, ed. Textbook of Interventional Cardiology. 2nd ed. Philadelphia: WB Saunders, 1994:415–435.
4. Lincoff AM, Topol EJ, Ellis SG. Local drug delivery for the prevention of restenosis. Fact, fancy, and future. Circulation 1994; 90:2070–2084.
5. Schwartz R, Holmes Jr D, Topol E. The restenosis paradigm revisited: an alternative proposal for cellular mechanisms. J Am Coll Cardiol 1992; 20:1284–1293.
6. Muller DWM, Ellis SG, Topol EJ. Experimental models of coronary artery restenosis. J Am Coll Cardiol 1992; 19 (2):418–432.
7. Strauss BH, Chisholm RJ, Keeley FW, Gotlieb AI, Logan RA, Armstrong PW. Extracellular matrix remodeling after balloon angioplasty injury in a rabbit model of restenosis. Circ Res 1994; 75:650–658.
8. Serruys PW, Luijten HE, Beatt KJ, Geuskens R, de Feyter PJ, van den Brand M, et al. Incidence of restenosis after successful coronary angioplasty: a time-related phenomenon. Circulation 1988; 77:361–371.
9. Healy B. Women's health, public welfare (editorial). JAMA 1991; 266(4):566–568.
10. Glagov S. Intimal hyperplasia, vascular modeling, and the restenosis problem. Circulation 1994; 89:2888–2891.
11. Nobuyoshi M, Kimura T, Nosaka H, Mioka S, Ueno K, Yokoi H, et al. Restenosis after successful percutaneous transluminal coronary angioplasty:

serial angiographic follow-up of 229 patients. J Am Coll Cardiol 1988; 12:616–623.
12. Kuntz R, Baim D. Defining coronary restenosis. Newer clinical and angiographic paradigms. Circulation 1993; 88:1310–1323.
13. Tenaglia A, Buller C, Kisslo K, Stack R, Davidson C. Mechanisms of balloon angioplasty and directional coronary atherectomy as assessed by intracoronary ultrasound. J Am Coll Cardiol 1992; 20:685–691.
14. Isner JM. Vascular remodeling: Honey, I think I shrunk the artery. Circulation 1994; 89:2937–2942.
15. Currier JW, Faxon DP. Restenosis after percutaneous transluminal coronary angioplasty: Have we been aiming at the wrong target? J Am Coll Cardiol 1995; 25:516–520.
16. Losordo D, Rosenfield K, Pieczek A, Baker K, Harding M, Isner J. How does angioplasty work? Serial analysis of human iliac arteries using intravascular ultrasound. Circulation 1992; 86:1845–1858.
17. Painter JA, Mintz GS, Wong SC, Popma JJ, Pichard AD, Kent KM, et al. Serial intravascular ultrasound studies fail to show evidence of chronic Palmaz-Schatz stent recoil. Am J Cardiol 1995; 75:398–400.
18. Beatt KJ, Serruys PW, Luijten HE, Rensing BJ, Suryapranata H, de Feyter P, et al. Restenosis after coronary angioplasty: the paradox of increased lumen diameter and restenosis. J Am Coll Cardiol 1992; 19:258–266.
19. Fuster V, Ik-Kyung J. Role of platelet-inhibitor agents in coronary artery disease. In: Topol E, ed. Textbook of Interventional Cardiology. 2d ed. Philadelphia: WB Saunders, 1994:3–22.
20. Noda-Heiny H, Fujii S, Sobel B. Induction of vascular smooth muscle cell expression of plasminogen activator inhibitor-1 by thrombin. Circ Res 1993; 72:36–43.
21. Majesky MW, Lindner V, Twardzik DR, Schwarts SM, Reidy MA. Production of transforming growth factor B1 during repair of arterial injury. J Clin Invest 1991; 88:904–910.
22. Serruys PW, Rutsch W, Heyndrickx GR, Danchin N, Mast EG, Wijns W, et al. Prevention of restenosis after percutaneous transluminal coronary angioplasty with thromboxane A_2-receptor blockade—a randomized, double-blind, placebo-controlled trial. Circulation 1991; 84:1568–1580.
23. Sarembock IJ, Gertz D, Gimple LW, Owen RM, Powers ER, Roberts WC. Effectiveness of recombinant desulphatohirudin in reducing restenosis after balloon angioplasty of atherosclerotic femoral arteries in rabbits. Circulation 1991; 84(1):232–243.
24. Casscells W. Migration of smooth muscle and endothelial cells. Critical events in restenosis. Circulation 1993; 86:723–729.
25. Muller D. Site-specific therapy for the prevention of restenosis. In: Topol E, ed. Textbook of Interventional Cardiology. 2d ed. Philadelphia: WB Saunders, 1994: 436–448.
26. Simons M, Edelman E, DeKeyser J-L, Langer R, Rosenberg R. Antisense c-myb oligonucleotides inhibit intimal arterial smooth muscle cell accumulation in vivo. Nature 1992; 359:67–70.

27. Shi Y, Fard A, Galeo A, Hutchinson H, Vermani P, Dodge G, et al. Transcatheter delivery of c-myc antisense oligomers reduces neointimal formation in a porcine model of coronary artery balloon injury. Circulation 1994; 90:944–951.
28. Lindner V, Reidy MA. Proliferation of smooth muscle cells after vascular injury is inhibited by an antibody against basic fibroblast growth factor. Proc Natl Acad Sci 1991; 88:3739–3743.
29. Asahara T, Bauters C, Pastore C, Kearney M, Rossow S, Bunting S, et al. Local delivery of vascular endothelial growth factor accelerates reendothelialization and attenuates intimal hyperplasia in balloon-injured rat carotid artery. Circulation 1995; 91:2793–2801.
30. Fischman D, Leon M, Baim D, Schatz R, Savage M, Penn I, et al. A randomized comparison of coronary-stent placement and balloon angioplasty in the treatment of coronary artery disease. N Engl J Med 1994; 331:496–501.
31. DiSciascio G, Cowley MJ, Vetrovec GW, Kelly KM, Lewis SA. Triple vessel coronary angioplasty: acute outcome and long-term results. J Am Coll Cardiol 1988; 12:42–48.
32. Serruys PW, de Jaegere P, Kiemeneij F, Macaya C, Rutsch W, Heyndrickx G, et al. A comparison of balloon-expandable stent implantation with balloon angioplasty in patients with coronary artery disease. N Engl J Med 1994; 331:489–495.
33. Rensing B, Hermans W, Deckers J, de Feyter P, Tijssen J, Serruys P. Lumen narrowing after percutaneous transluminal coronary balloon angioplasty follows a near Gaussian distribution: a quantitative angiographic study in 1,445 successfully dilated lesions. J Am Coll Cardiol 1992; 19:939–945.
34. Kuntz R, Gibson C, Nobuyoshi M, Baim D. Generalized model of restenosis after conventional balloon angioplasty, stenting and directional atherectomy. J Am Coll Cardiol 1993; 21:15–25.
35. Topol E, Leya F, Pinkerton C, Whitlow P, Hofling B, Simonton C, et al. A comparison of directional atherectomy with coronary angioplasty in patients with coronary artery disease, N Engl J Med 1993; 329:221–227.
36. Adelman A, Cohen E, Kimball B, Bonan R, Ricci D, Webb J, et al. A comparison of directional atherectomy with balloon angioplasty for lesions of the left anterior descending coronary artery. N Engl J Med 1993; 329:228–233.
37. Liu MW, Roubin GS, King SB. Does an optimal luminal result after PTCA reduce restenosis? Circulation 1989; 80:II-63.
38. Rensing BJ, Hermans WRM, Beatt KJ, Laarman GJ, Suryapranata H, van den Brand M, et al. Quantitative angiographic assessment of elastic recoil after percutaneous transluminal coronary angioplasty. Am J Cardiol 1990; 66:1039–1044.
39. Anderson HV, Roubin GS, Leimgruber PP, Cox WR, Douglas JSJ, King SBI, et al. Measurement of transstenotic pressure gradient during percutaneous transluminal coronary angioplasty. Circulation 1986; 73:1223–1230.
40. Feldman RL, Bengston JR, Pryor DB, Zimmerman MB. The GRASP study: use of a thromboxane A2 receptor blocker to reduce adverse clinical events after coronary angioplasty. J Am Coll Cardiol 1992; 19:259A.

41. Savage MP, Goldberg S, MacDonald RG, Bass TA, Margolis JR, Whitworth HB, et al. Multi-Hospital Eastern Atlantic Restenosis Trial II: a placebo controlled trial of thromboxane blockade in the prevention of restenosis following coronary angioplasty. Am Heart J 1991; 122:1239–1244.
42. Hillegas WB, Ohman EM. What have we learned from randomized trials of restenosis? Choices Cardiol 1993; 7:164–167.
43. Kuntz R, Keaney K, Senerchia C, Baim D. A predictive method for estimating the late angiographic results of coronary intervention despite incomplete ascertainment. Circulation 1993; 87:815–830.
44. Carrozza J, Kuntz R, Fischman R, Baim D. Restenosis after arterial injury caused by coronary stenting in patients with diabetes mellitus. Ann Intern Med 1993; 118:344–350.
45. Hirshfeld JW Jr, Schwartz JS, Jugo R, MacDonald RG, Goldberg S, Savage MP, et al. Restenosis after coronary angioplasty: a multivariate statistical model to relate lesion and procedure variables to restenosis. J Am Coll Cardiol 1991; 18(3):647–656.
46. Gruentzig AR, King SBI, Schlumpf M, Siegenthaler W. Long-term follow-up after percutaneous transluminal coronary angioplasty: the early Zurich experience. N Engl J Med 1987; 316:1127–1132.
47. Gal D, Rongione AJ, Slovenkai GA, DeJesus ST, Lucas A, Fields CD, et al. Atherosclerotic Yucatan microswine: an animal model with high-grade, fibrocalcific, nonfatty lesions suitable for testing catheter-based interventions. Am Heart J 1990; 119:291–300.
48. Ellis S, Savage M, Fischman D, Baim D, Leon M, Goldberg S, et al. Restenosis after placement of Palmaz-Schatz stents in native coronary arteries: initial results of a multicenter experience. Circulation 1992; 86:1836–1844.
49. Nunes GL, Hanson SR, King Sr, Sahatjian RA, Scott NA. Local delivery of a synthetic antithrombin with a hydrogel-coated angioplasty balloon catheter inhibits platelet-dependent thrombosis. J Am Coll Cardiol 1994; 23(7):1578–83.
50. Tanguay JF, Zidar JP, Phillips HR, Stack RS. Current status of biodegradable stents. Cardiol Clin 1994; 12:699–713.
51. Nunes GL, Hanson SR, King SB, Sahatjian RA, Scott NA. Local delivery of a synthetic antithrombin with a hydrogel-coated angioplasty balloon catheter inhibits platelet-dependent thrombosis. J Am Coll Cardiol 1994; 23:1578–1583.
52. The Multicenter European Research Trial with Cilazapril After Angioplasty to Prevent Transluminal Coronary Obstruction and Restenosis (MERCATOR) Study Group. Does the new angiotensin converting enzyme inhibitor cilazapril prevent restenosis after percutaneous transluminal coronary angioplasty? Results of the MERCATOR Study. Circulation 1992; 86:100–110.
53. Faxon D, Spiro T, Minor S, Cote G, Douglas J, Gottlieb R, et al. Low molecular weight heparin in the prevention of restenosis after angioplasty. Results of enoxaparin restenosis (ERA) trial. Circulation 1994; 90:908–914.
54. Califf RM, Fortin DF, Frid DJ, Harlan WR, Ohman EM, Bengtson JR, et al.

Restenosis after coronary angioplasty: an overview. J Am Coll Cardiol 1991; 17:2B–13D.
55. Popma JJ, Califf RM, Topol EJ. Clinical trials of restenosis after coronary angioplasty. Circulation 1991; 84(3):1426–1436.
56. Hillegass WB, Ohman EM, Leimberger JD, Califf RM. A meta-analysis of randomized trials of calcium antagonists to reduce restenosis after coronary angioplasty. Am J Cardiol 1994; 73:835–839.
57. Topol EJ, Califf RM, Weisman HF, et al. Randomized trial of coronary intervention with antibody against platelet IIb/IIIa integrin for reduction of clinical restenosis: results at six months. Lancet 1994; 343:881–886.
58. Schwartz L, Bourassa MG, Lesperance J, Aldridge HE, Kazim F, Salvatori VA, et al. Aspirin and dipyridamole in the prevention of restenosis after percutaneous transluminal coronary angioplasty. N Engl J Med 1988; 318:1714–1719.
59. Schwartz L, Lesperance J, Bourassa MG, Eastwood C, Kazim F, Arafah M, et al. The role of antiplatelet agents in modifying the extent of restenosis following percutaneous transluminal coronary angioplasty. Am Heart J 1990; 119:232–236.
60. Kitaz H, Kubo I, Iwama T, Ageishi Y, Suzuki Au. Combined use of aspirin, ticlopidine and nicorandil prevented restenosis after coronary angioplasty (abstr). Circulation 1988; 78:II–633.
61. Bove A, Savage M, Deutsch E, R M, Bass T, Vetrovec G, et al. Effects of selective and non-selective thromboxane A_2 blockage on restenosis after PTCA: M-HEART-II (abstr). J Am Coll Cardiol 1992; 19:259A.
62. Ellis SG, Roubin GS, Wilentz J, Douglas JS, King SB. Effect of 18- to 24-hour heparin administration for prevention of restenosis after complicated coronary angioplasty. Am Heart J 1989; 117:777–782.
63. Thornton MA, Gruentzig AR, Hollman J, King III SB, Douglas JS. Coumadin and aspirin in prevention of recurrence after transluminal coronary angioplasty: a randomized study. Circulation 1984; 69:721–727.
64. Urban P, Buller N, Fox F, Shapiro L, Bayliss J, Richards A. Lack of effect of warfarin on the restenosis rate or on clinical outcome after balloon coronary angioplasty. Br Heart J 1988; 60:485–488.
65. Hanke H, Oberhoff M, Hanke S, Hassenstein S, Kamenz J, Schmid KM, et al. Inhibition of cellular proliferation after experimental balloon angioplasty by low-molecular-weight heparin. Circulation 1992; 85:1548–1556.
66. Reilly CF, Fritze LMS, Rosenberg RD. Heparin inhibition of smooth muscle cell proliferation: a cellular site of action. J Cell Physiol 1986; 129:11–19.
67. Guyton JR, Rosenberg RD, Clowes AW, Karnovsky MJ. Inhibition of rat arterial smooth muscle cell proliferation by heparin: in vivo studies with anticoagulant and non-anticoagulant heparin. Circ Res 1980; 46:625–634.
68. Dryiski M, Mikat E, Bjornsson TD. Inhibition of intimal hyperplasia after arterial injury by heparins and heparinoids. J Vasc Surgery 1988; 8:623–633.
69. Currier JW, Pow TK, Haudenschild CC, Minihan AC, Faxon DP. Low molecu-

lar weight heparin (Enoxaparin) reduces restenosis after iliac angioplasty in the hypercholesterolemic rabbit. J Am Coll Cardiol 1991; 17:118B–125B.
70. Cairns J, Gill J. Morton B, Roberts R, Gent M, Hirsh J, et al. Enoxaparin and MaxEPA for the prevention of angioplasty restenosis (EMPAR) (abstr). Circulation 1994; 90:I–651.
71. LaBlanche J-M. Low molecular weight heparin in the prevention of restenosis after coronary angioplasty. Results of the FACT study (abstr). J Am Coll Cardiol 1995; 25:226A.
72. Geary RL, Koyama N, Wang TW, Vergel S, Clowes AW. Failure of heparin to inhibit intimal hyperplasia in injured baboon arteries. The role of heparin-sensitive and -insensitive pathways in the stimulation of smooth muscle cell migration and proliferation. Circulation 1995; 91:2972–2781.
73. Villa A, Guzman L, Chen W, Golomb G, Levy R, Topol E. Local delivery of dexamethasone for prevention of neointimal proliferation in a rat model of balloon angioplasty. J Clin Invest 1994; 93:1243–1249.
74. Pepine CJ, Hirshfeld JW, MacDonald RG, Henderson MA, Bass TA, Goldberg S, et al. A controlled trial of corticosteroids to prevent restenosis after coronary angioplasty. Circulation 1990; 81:1753–1761.
75. Stone GW, Rutherford BD, McConahay DR, Johnson WL, Giorgi LV, Ligon RW, et al. A randomized trial of corticosteroids for the prevention of restenosis in 102 patients undergoing repeat coronary angioplasty. Cathet Cardiovasc Diagn 1989; 18:227–231.
76. Muller DWM, Ellis SG, Topol EJ. Colchicine and antineoplastic therapy for the prevention of restenosis after percutaneous coronary interventions. J Am Coll Cardiol 1991; 17:126B–131B.
77. O'Keefe JHJ, McCallister BD, Bateman TM, Kuhnlein DL, Ligon RW, Hartzler GO. Ineffectiveness of colchicine for the prevention of restenosis after coronary angioplasty. J Am Coll Cardiol 1992; 19:1597–1600.
78. Grines CL, Rizik D, Levine A, et al. Colchicine angioplasty restenosis trial (CART) (abstr). Circulation 1991; 84:II–365.
79. Freed M, Safian M, Safian R, et al. An intensive poly-pharmaceutical approach to the prevention of restenosis: the Mevacor, ACE-inhibitor, Colchicine (BIG-MAC) pilot trial (abstr). Circulation 1993; 21:33A.
80. Brozovich FV, Morganroth J, Gottlieb NB, Gottlieb RS. Effect of angiotensin converting enzyme inhibition on the incidence of restenosis after percutaneous transluminal coronary angioplasty. Cathet Cardiovasc Diagn 1991; 23:236–267.
81. Marquis J-F, Schwartz L, Aldridge H, Majid P, Henderson M, Matushinsky E. Acute coronary artery occlusion during percutaneous transluminal coronary angioplasty treated by redilation of the occluded segment. J Am Coll Cardiol 1984; 4:1268–1271.
82. Desnet W, Vrolix M, De Scheerder I, Van Lierde J, Willems J, Piessens J. Angiotensin-converting enzyme inhibition with fosinopril sodium in the prevention of restenosis after coronary angioplasty. Circulation 1994; 89:385–392.
83. Liu MW, Roubin GS, Robinson KA, et al. Trapidil in preventing restenosis

after balloon angioplasty in the atherosclerotic rabbit. Circulation 1990; 81:1089–1093.
84. Nishikawa H, Ono N, Motoyasu M, et al. Preventive effects of trapidil (PDGF antagonist) on restenosis after PTCA (abstr). Circulation 1992; 86:1–53.
85. Okamoto S, Inden M, Setsuda M, Konishi T, Nakano T. Effects of trapidil (triazolopyrimidine), a platelet-derived growth factor antagonist, in preventing restenosis after percutaneous transluminal coronary angioplasty. Am Heart J 1992; 123:1439–1444.
86. Maresta A, Balducelli M, Cantini L, et al. Trapidil (triazolopyrimidine), a platelet-derived growth factor antagonist, reduces restenosis after percutaneous transluminal coronary angioplasty. Results of the randomized, double-blind STARC study. Studio Trapidil versus Aspirin nella Restenosi Coronarica. Circulation 1994; 90:2710–2715.
87. Grant MB, Wargovich TJ, Ellis EA, Caballero S, Mansour M, Pepine CJ. Localization of insulin-like growth factor I and inhibition of coronary smooth muscle cell growth by somatostatin analogues in human coronary smooth muscle cells: A potential treatment for restenosis? Circulation 1994; 89:1511–1517.
88. Howell M, Orskov H, Frystyk F, Flybjerg A, Gronback H, Foegh M. Lanreotide, a somatostatin analogue, reduces insulin-like growth factor-1 accumulation in proliferating aortic tissue in rabbits in vitro. Eur J Endocrinol 1994; 130:422–425.
89. Lundergan CF, Foegh ML, Ramwell PW. Peptide inhibition of myointimal proliferation by angiopeptin, a somatostatin analogue. J Am Coll Cardiol 1991; 17:132B–136B.
90. Santoian E, Schneider J, Gravanis M, Foegh M, Tarazona N, Cipolla G, et al. Angiopeptin inhibits intimal hyperplasia after angioplasty in porcine coronary arteries. Circulation 1993; 88:11–14.
91. Foegh ML, Asotra S, Conte JV, et al. Early inhibition of myointimal proliferation by angiopeptin after balloon catheter injury in the rabbit. J Vasc Surg 1994; 19:1084–1091.
92. Kent KM, Williams DO, Cassagneau B, et al. Double blind, controlled trial of the effect of angiopeptin on coronary restenosis following balloon angioplasty (abstr). Circulation 1993; 88:1–506.
93. Eriksen U. Amtorp, Bagger J, et al. Randomized double-blind Scandinavian trial of angiopeptin versus placebo for the prevention of clinical events and restenosis after coronary balloon angioplasty. Am Heart J 1995; 130:1–8.
94. Emanuelsson H, Beatt KJ, Bagger J-P, Balcon R, Heikkila J, Piessens J, et al. Long-term effects of angiopeptin treatment in coronary angioplasty: reduction of clinical events but not angiographic restenosis. Circulation 1995; 91:1689–1696.
95. Hirayama A, Nanto S, Ohara T, et al. Preventive effect on restenosis after PTCA by ebselen: a newly synthesized anti-inflammation agent (abstr). J Am Coll Cardiol 1992; 19:259A.
96. Serruys P, Klein W, Tijssen J. Rutsch W, Heyndrickx G, Emanuelsson H, et al. Evaluation of ketanserin in the prevention of restenosis after percutaneous

transluminal coronary angioplasty. A multicenter randomized double-blind placebo-controlled trial. Circulation 1993; 88:1588–1601.
97. Klein W, Brandt D, Eber B, Dusleag J. Prävention der frühen Restenosierung nach perkutaner transluminaler Koronarangioplastie mit Serotonin-Antagonisten. Cor Vasa 1988; 5/6(234–237).
98. O'Keefe JH, Giorgi LV, Hartzler GO, Good TH, Ligon RW, Webb DL, et al. Effects of diltiazem on complications and restenosis after coronary angioplasty. Am J Cardiol 1991; 67:373–376.
99. Whitworth HB, Roubin GS, Hollman J, Meier B, Leimgruber PP, Douglas Jr JS, et al. Effect of nifedipine on recurrent stenosis after percutaneous transluminal coronary angioplasty. J Am Coll Cardiol 1986; 8:1271–1276.
100. Corcos T, David PR, Val PG, Renkin J, Dangiosse V, Rapold HG, et al. Failure of diltiazem to prevent restenosis after percutaneous transluminal coronary angioplasty. Am Heart J 1985; 109:926–931.
101. Hoberg E, Dietz R, Frees U, Katus H, Rauch B, Schomig A, et al. Verapamil treatment after coronary angioplasty in patients at high risk of recurrent stenosis. Br Heart J 1994; 71:254–260.
102. Raizner A, Hollman J, Abukhalil J, Demke D, for the Cioprostene Investigators. Ciprostene for restenosis revisited: Quantitative analysis of angiograms (abstr). J Am Coll Cardiol 1993; 21:321A.
103. Meier B. "Occlusion angioplasty" light at the end of the tunnel or dead end. Circulation 1992; 85:1214–1216.
104. Carvalho A, Colman R, Lees R. Platelet function in hyperlipidemia. N Engl J Med 1974; 290:434–438.
105. Gellman J, Ezekowitz MD, Sarembock IJ, Azrin MA, Nochomowitz LE, Lerner E, et al. Effect of lovastatin on intimal hyperplasia after balloon angioplasty: a study in an atherosclerotic hypercholesterolemic rabbit. J Am Coll Cardiol 1991; 17:251–259.
106. Kaltenbach M, Beyer J, Walter S, Klepzig H, Schmidts L. Prolonged application of pressure in transluminal coronary angioplasty. Cathet Cardiovasc Diagn 1984; 10:213–219.
107. Sahni R, Maniet AR, Voci G, Banka VS. Prevention of restenosis by lovastatin after successful coronary angioplasty. Am Heart J 1991; 121:1600–1608.
108. Feldman RC. Transcatheter aspiration of a thrombus in an aortocoronary saphenous vein graft. Am J Cardiol 1987; 60:379–380.
109. Tanajura L, Cano M, Nunes G, Pinto I, Chaves A, Cenemero M, et al. A propsoective randomized trial of lovastatin for prevention of coronary restenosis (abstr). Circulation 1995; 92:I–345.
110. Slack JD, Pinkerton CA, Van Tassel J, et al. Can oral fish oil supplement minimize restenosis after percutaneous transluminal coronary angioplasty? (abstr). J Am Coll Cardiol 1987; 9:64A.
111. Dehmer GJ, Popma JJ, van den Berg EK, Eichhorn EJ, Prewitt JB, Campbell WB, et al. Reduction in the rate of early stenosis after coronary angioplasty by a diet supplemented with n-3 fatty acids. N Engl J Med 1988; 319:733–740.

112. Milner MR, Gallino RA, Leffingwell A, Pichard AD, Brooks-Robinson S, Rosenberg J, et al. Usefulness of fish oil supplements in preventing clinical evidence of restenosis after percutaneous transluminal coronary angioplasty. Am J Cardiol 1989; 64:294–299.
113. Nye ER, Ablett MS, Robertson MC, et al. Effect of eicosapentaenoic acid on restenosis rate, clinical course and blood lipids in patients after percutaneous transluminal coronary angioplasty. Aust N Z J Med 1990; 20:549–552.
114. Bairati I, Roy L, Meyer F. Double-blind, randomized, controlled trial of fish oil supplements in prevention of recurrence of stenosis after coronary angioplasty. Circulation 1992; 85:950–956.
115. Grigg LE, Kay TWH, Valentine PA, Larkins R, Flower DJ, Manolas EG, et al. Determinants of restenosis and lack of effect of dietary supplementation with eicosapentaenoic acid on the incidence of coronary artery stenosis after angioplasty. J Am Coll Cardiol 1989; 13:665–672.
116. Reis GJ, Sipperly ME, McCabe CH, Sacks FM, Boucher TM, Silverman DI, et al. Randomized trial of fish oil for prevention of restenosis after coronary angioplasty. Lancet 1989; II:177–181.
117. Cheng A, Bustami M, Norell MS, et al. The effect of omega-3 fatty acids on restenosis after coronary angioplasty. Eur Heart J 1990; 11(suppl):368.
118. Franzen D, Schannwell M, Oette K, Hopp H. A prospective, randomized, and double-blind trial on the effect of fish oil on the incidence of restenosis following PTCA. Cathet Cardiovasc Diagn 1993; 28:301–310.
119. Gapinski J, VanRuiswyk J, Heudebert F, Schectman G. Preventing restenosis with fish oils following coronary angioplasty. Arch Intern Med 1993; 153:1595–1601.
120. Leaf A, Jorgensen MB, Jacobs AK, Cote G, Schoenfeld DA, Scheer J, et al. Do fish oils prevent restenosis after coronary angioplasty? Circulation 1994; 90:2248–2257.
121. The EPIC Investigators. Use of a monoclonal antibody directed against the platelet glycoprotein IIb/IIIa receptor in high-risk coronary angioplasty. N Engl J Med 1994; 330:956–961.
122. Aguirre F, Topol E, Ferguson J, et al. Bleeding complications with the chimeric antibody to platelet glycoprotein IIb/IIIa in patients undergoing percutaneous coronary intervention. Circulation 1995; 91:2882–2890.
123. Topol EJ. Important protocol change as a result of data and safety monitoring committee interim analysis. Clinical Event Committee Communication, 1995.
124. Tcheng JE, Harrington RA, Kottke-Marchant K, Kleiman NS, Ellis SG, Kereiakes DJ, et al. Multicenter, randomized, double-blind placebo-controlled trial of the platelet integrin glycoprotein IIb/IIIa blocker integrelin in elective coronary intervention. Circulation 1995; 91:2151–2157.
125. Tcheng JE, Lincoff Am, Sigmon KN, Kitt MM, Califf RM, Topol EJ. Platelet glycoprotein IIb/IIIa inhibition with integrelin during percutaneous coronary intervention (abstr). Circulation 1995; 92:I–543.
126. Lincoff AM, Tcheng JE, Ellis SG, Moliterno DJ, Kitt MM, Debowey D, et al. Randomized trial of platelet glycoprotein IIb/IIIa inhibition with integrelin for

prevention of restenosis following coronary intervention: the IMPACT II angiographic substudy (abstr). Circulation 1995; 92:I–607.
127. Serruys PW, Herrman JPR, Simon R, Rutsch W, Bode C, Laarman GJ, et al. A comparison of hirudin with heparin in the prevention of restenosis after coronary angioplasty. N Engl J Med 1995; 333:757–763.
128. Bittl JA, Strony J, Brinker JA, et al. Treatment with bivalirudin (hirulog) as compared with heparin during coronary angioplasty for unstable or post-infarction angina. N Engl J Med 1994; 333:764–769.
129. Epstein S, Speir E, Finkel T. Do antisense approaches to the problem of restenosis make sense? Circulation 1993; 88:1351–1353.
130. Epstein SE, Speir E, Unger EF, Guzman RJ, Finkel T. The basis of molecular strategies for treating coronary restenosis after angioplasty. J Am Coll Cardiol 1994; 23:1278–1288.
131. Bennett M, Anglin S, McEwan J, Jagoe R, Newby A, Evan G. Inhibition of vascular smooth muscle cell proliferation in vitro and in vivo by C-myc antisense oligodeoxynucleotides. J Clin Invest 1994; 93:820–828.
132. Morishita R, Gibbons G, Ellison K, Nakajima M, Zhang L, Kaneda Y, et al. Single intraluminal delivery of antisense cdc2 kinase and proliferating-cell nuclear antigen oligonucleotides results in chronic inhibition of neointimal hyperplasia. Proc Natl Acad Sci USA 1993; 90:8474–8478.
133. Morishita R, Gibbons GH, Ellison KE, Jakajima M, von dr Leyen H, Zhang L, et al. Intimal hyperplasia after vascular injury is inhibited by antisense cdk2 kinase oligonucleotides. J Clin Invest 1994; 93:1458–1464.
134. Ivanhoe RJ, Weintraub WS, Douglas JSJ, Lembo NJ, Furman M, Gershony G, et al. Percutaneous transluminal coronary angioplasty of chronic total occlusions. Primary success, restenosis, and long-term clinical follow-up. Circulation 1992; 85:106–115.
135. Villa AE, Guzman LA, Poptic EJ, Labhasetwar V, D'Souza S, Farrell CL, et al. Effects of antisense c-myb oligonucleotides on vascular smooth muscle cell proliferation and response to vessel wall injury. Circ Res 1995; 76:505–513.
136. Ohman E, Marquis J, Ricci D, Brown R, Knudtson M, Kereiakes D, et al. A randomized comparison of the effects of gradual prolonged versus standard primary balloon inflation on early and late outcome. Results of a multicenter clinical trial. Circulation 1994; 89:1118–1125.
137. Elliott JM, Berdan LG, Holmes DR, Isner JM, King SB, Keeler GP, et al. One-year follow-up in the coronary angioplasty versus excisional atherectomy trial (CAVEAT I). Circulation 1995; 91:2158–2166.
138. Fischman DL, Leon MB, Baim DS, Schatz RA, Savage MP, Penn I, et al. A randomized comparison of stent placement and balloon angioplasty in the treatment of coronary artery disease. N Engl J Med 1994; 331:496–501.
139. Holmes DR, Topol EJ, Califf RM, Berdan LG, Leya F, Berger PB, et al. A multicenter, randomized trial of coronary angioplasty versus directional atherectomy for patients with saphenous vein bypass graft lesions. Circulation 1995; 91:1966–1974.
140. Simonton CA, Leon MB, Kuntz RE, Popma JJ, Hinohara T, Bersin RM, et

al. Acute and late clinical and angiographic results of directional atherectomy in the Optimal Atherectomy Restenosis Study (OARS) (abstr). Circulation 1995; 92:I–545.

141. Colombo A, Hall P, Nakamura S, Almagor Y, Maiello L, Martini G, et al. Intracoronary stenting without anticoagulation accomplished with intravascular ultrasound guidance. Circulation 1995; 91:1676–1688.
142. Hall P, Nakamura S, Maiello L, Itoh A, Blengino S, Martini G, et al. A randomized comparison of combined ticlopidine and aspirin therapy versus aspirin alone after successful intravascular ultrasound-guided stent implantation. Circulation 1996; 93:215–222.
143. Trivedi A, Voci G, Banka VS. Coronary angioplasty of septal perforator. Am Heart J 1988; 115:466–468.
144. Serruys P, on behalf of the Benestent Study Group BENESTENT-II pilot study: 6-month follow-up of phase 1, 2 and 3 (abstr). Circulation 1995; 92:I–542.
145. Grundfest WS, Litvack F, Forrester J. Laser angioplasty. Coron Artery Dis 1990; 1:430–437.
146. Isner J, Rosenfield K, Losordo DW. Excimer laser atherectomy. The greening of sisyphus. Circulation 1990; 81:2018–2021.
147. Bittl J, Sanborn T, Tcheng J, Siegel R, Ellis S, for the percutaneous excimer laser coronary angioplasty registry. Clinical success, complications and restenosis rates with excimer laser coronary angioplasty. Am J Cardiol 1992; 70:1533–1539.
148. Litvack F, Eigler N, Margolis J, Rothbaum D, Bresnahan J, Holmes D, et al. Percutaneous excimer laser coronary angioplasty: results in the first consecutive 3,000 patients. J Am Coll Cardiol 1994; 23:323–329.
149. Appelman Y, Plek J, Strikwerda S, Tijsson J, de Feyter P, David G, et al. Randomized trial of excimer laser angioplasty versus balloon angioplasty for treatment of obstructive coronary artery disease. Lancet 1996; 347:79–84.
150. Weidermann JG, Marboe C, Amols H, Schwartz A, Weinberger J. Intracoronary irradiation markedly reduces restenosis after balloon angioplasty in a porcine model. J Am Coll Cardiol 1994; 23:1491–1498.
151. Waksman R, Robinson KA, Crocker IR, Gravanis MB, Cipolla GD, King SB. Endovascular low-dose irradiation inhibits neointima formation after coronary artery balloon injury in swine. Circulation 1995; 91:1533–1539.
152. Waksman R, Robinson KA, Crocker IR, Gravanis MB, Palmer SJ, Wang C, et al. Intracoronary radiation before stent implantation inhibits neointima formation in stented porcine coronary arteries. Circulation 1995; 92:1383–1386.
153. Hehrlein C, Gollan C, Donges K, Metz J, Riessen R, Fehsenfeld P, et al. Low-dose radioactive endovascular stents prevent smooth muscle cell proliferation and neointimal hyperplasia in rabbits. Circulation 1995; 92:1570–1575.
154. Wiedermann JG, Marboe C, Amols H, Schwartz A, Weinberger J. Intracoronary irradiation markedly reduces neointimal proliferation after balloon angioplasty in swine: persistent benefit at 6-month follow-up. J Am Coll Cardiol 1995; 25:1451–1456.

155. Teirstein P, Massulo V, Jani S, Russo R, Schatz R, Steuterman S, et al. Catheter-based radiation therapy to inhibit restenosis following coronary stenting. Circulation 1995; 92:I–543.
156. Topol EJ, Nissen SE. Our preoccupation with coronary luminology: the dissociation between clinical and angiographic findings in ischemic heart disease. Circulation 1995; 92:2333–2342.
157. Fernandez-Ortiz A, Meyer BJ, Mailhac A, Falk E, Badimon L, Fallon JT, et al. A new approach for local intravascular drug delivery: iontophoretic balloon. Circulation 1994; 89:1518–1522.
158. Radomski M, Palmer R, Moncada S. An L-arginine/nitric oxide pathway present in human platelets regulates aggregation. Proc Natl Acad Sci USA 1990; 87:5193–5197.
159. Garg U, Hassid A. Nitric oxide generating vasodilators and 8-bromo-cyclic guanosine monophosphate inhibit mitogenesis and proliferation of cultured rat vascular smooth muscle cells. J Clin Invest 1989; 83:1774–1777.
160. Scott-Burden T, Schini V, Elizondo E, Junquero D, Vanhoutte P. Platelet-derived growth factor suppresses and fibroblast growth factor enances cytokine-induced production of nitric oxide by cultured smooth muscle cells: effects on cell proliferation. Circ Res 1992; 71:1088–1100.
161. Schini VB, Catovsky S, Schray-Utz B, Busse R, Vanhoutte PM. Insulin-like growth factor I inhibits induction of nitric oxide synthase in vascular smooth muscle cells. Circ Res 1994; 74:24–32.
162. Schini-Kerth VB, Fiblthaler B, Andersen TT, Fenton JW, Vanhoutte PM, Busse R. Thrombin prevents the expression of inducible nitric oxide synthase in vascular smooth muscle cells by a proteolytically-activated thrombin receptor. Thromb Haemost 1995; 74:980–986.
163. von der Leyen HE, Gibbons GH, Morishita R, Lewis NP, Zhang L, Nakajima M, et al. Gene therapy inhibiting neointimal vascular lesion: in vivo transfer of endothelial cell nitric oxide synthase gene. Proc Natl Acad Sci USA 1995; 92:1137–1141.
164. Folts J, Maalej N, Keaney JJ, Loscalzo J. Coating Palmaz-Schatz stents with a unique NO donor renders them much less thrombogenic when placed in pig carotid arteries (abstr). Circulation 1995; 92:I–670.
165. Langford E, Brown A, Wainwright R, et al. Inhibition of platelet activity by S-nitrosoglutathione during coronary angioplasty. Lancet 1994; 344:1458–1460.
166. De Vries C, Escobedo JA, Ueno H, Houck K, Ferrara N, Williams LT.The fms-like tyrosine kinase, a receptor for vascular endothelial growth factor. Science 1992; 255:989–991.
167. Millauer B, Wizigmann-Voos S, Snurch H, Martinez R, Moller N, Risau W, et al. High affinity VEGF binding and developmental expression suggest *Flk-1* as a major regulator of vasculogenesis and angiogenesis. Cell 1993; 72:835–846.
168. Terman B, Dougher-Vermozen M, Carrion M, Dimitrov D, Armellino D, Gospodarowicz D, et al. Identification of the KDR tyrosine kinase as a receptor for vascular endothelial growth factor. Biochem Biophys Res Commun 1992; 187:1579–1586.

169. Ferrara N, Henzel W. Pituitary follicular cells secrete a novel heparin-binding growth factor specific for vascular endothelial cells. Biochem Biophys Res Commun 1989; 161:851–855.
170. Casscells W. Growth factor therapies for vascular injury and ischemia. Circulation 1995; 91:2699–2702.
171. Kerr J Shrinkage necrosis: a distinct mode of cell death. J Pathol 1971; 105:13–21.
172. Isner J, Kearney M, Bortman S, Passeri J. Apoptosis in human atherosclerosis and restenosis. Circulation 1995; 91:2703–2711.

18

The Clinical Approach to Prevention of Restenosis: What Has Been Done and Where Do We Go from Here?

Diane K. Jorkasky and Bernard E. Ilson
SmithKline Beecham Pharmaceuticals and University of Pennsylvania, Philadelphia, Pennsylvania

Coronary artery disease is a common cause of cardiovascular morbidity and mortality in modern western societies. Percutaneous transluminal coronary angioplasty (PTCA) is a safe, cost-effective, and efficacious therapy for clinically significant coronary artery disease. Primary success rates for PTCA are in the range of 90–95%, and the complication rate is relatively low (4–5%) (1). However, the cost-effectiveness and efficacy of PTCA in the long term have been limited by restenosis of successfully dilated coronary vessels. Restenosis complicates 30–50% of all initially successful PTCA procedures, usually within the first 6 months after PTCA (2). Restenosis may be effectively treated by repeat angioplasty; however, repeat PTCA entails additional cost, and the redilated lesions are more prone to the development of restenosis than naive lesions. Various pharmacological therapies for the prevention of restenosis following successful PTCA have been tried, and the clinical trials of these therapies will be discussed in this chapter. In addition, some perspectives will be given on future clinical trials and therapeutic strategies.

I. DEFINITION

Any discussion of restenosis following successful PTCA must begin with an agreement on a definition of restenosis. However, a uniform definition of restenosis is currently lacking. Restenosis may be defined on the basis of coronary angiographic criteria (for example, loss of >50% of the improvement at PTCA), evidence of myocardial ischemia (such as an abnormal exercise test or thallium perfusion scan), or clinical syndromes (recurrence of angina). This issue is reviewed in greater detail in the discussion of the evaluation of clinical trials data. Restenosis must be distinguished from the outcome of unsuccessful PTCA procedures. In general, if ischemic episodes recur very early following PTCA (within several days to weeks), it is more likely the result of a technical problem that occurred at angioplasty (inadequate dilation, dissection, etc.) than of the proliferative lesion characteristic of restenosis. Restenosis generally occurs 3–6 months following successful PTCA (3).

II. PATHOLOGY

The pathophysiology of restenosis following successful PTCA is very complex. It is likely that restenosis following successful PTCA is a different process than atherosclerosis. Primary atherosclerotic plaque contains a complex mixture of smooth muscle cells, fibrous tissue, and cholesterol. Restenotic lesions are much more fibrous in nature with few cholesterol pools. The fibrous nature of the restenotic plaque may protect it against rupture, which may explain the rarity of recurrent infarction as a presenting manifestation of restenosis because myocardial infarction is generally believed to result from fissuring of an atherosclerotic plaque in an area overlying a lipid pool (4). Restenosis is most likely part of the normal healing process in response to arterial injury. During angioplasty, there is mechanical injury of the coronary artery. The muscularis of the artery is interrupted, and there is separation of the vascular layers and dissection. Platelets and thrombin interact with the injured vessel wall, followed by the elaboration of various biologically active mediators (TGF-β, PDGF, etc.). Subsequent to the initial phase, there is activation and replication of medial smooth muscle cells, followed by their migration into the subintima. Finally, there is autoreplication of smooth muscle cells that have migrated into the intima, followed by remodeling of the blood vessel with modulation of the extracellular matrix. Smooth muscle cell migration and proliferation and excessive matrix formation are characteristic of the restenosis lesion. Factors such as residual volume of plaque and elastic recoil of the dilated artery are thought to relate primarily to technical aspects of the initial PTCA procedure.

It should be noted that proliferative plaque phenomena are also present in some naturally occurring atherosclerotic lesions. Similar proliferative lesions have been found in patients who have had coronary artery bypass graft (CABG) surgery and in patients who present with unstable angina or myocardial infarction who have never had angioplasty or coronary artery surgery. It is thought that these patients have had plaques that ruptured spontaneously, resulting in severe damage to the vessel wall. The subsequent proliferation occurs as a result of intrinsic damage to the plaque that occurs in ordinary life. Plaque rupture and hemorrhage disrupts the plaque, and then the plaque responds with proliferation as part of the normal healing process (3).

III. INTERPRETATION OF CLINICAL TRIALS OF PHARMACOLOGICAL THERAPY

A number of variables have made the interpretation of clinical trials difficult; these include the lack of stratification of patients based on their risk factors for restenosis and the manner in which angiographic and clinical data have been evaluated. Clinical trials have also been limited by inadequate drug therapy and study design flaws.

A. Risk Factors for Restenosis

Risk stratification should be considered when analyzing the results of PTCA clinical trials. Individual patients may respond differently following successful PTCA depending on a number of factors. For example, patients who are at high risk for restenosis may not respond to preventive therapy regardless of which therapy is chosen. On the other hand, patients who are at low risk for restenosis may do well without any preventive treatment (3). Risk factors for restenosis include lesion-related and procedure-related factors (1,4,5). Lesion characteristics such as stenosis location (left anterior descending coronary artery, bend points, vein graft, or prior angioplasty), pre-PTCA percent stenosis, stenosis length, and the presence of multiple lesions in a single vessel tend to correlate with an increased risk for restenosis. Postangioplasty stenosis severity, pressure gradient across the dilated lesion, and the presence or absence of dissection are procedure-related factors which may influence risk for restenosis.

Patient-related risk factors such as unstable angina, diabetes mellitus, smoking, male sex, absence of a prior myocardial infarction, hyperlipidemia, and fibrinolytic system variables have been investigated. Some authors have found that diabetes mellitus and unstable angina pectoris confer an increased risk for restenosis (4,6); however, no patient-related factors have been consistently associated with the risk of restenosis. Risk factors for atherosclerosis and restenosis appear to be different, lending further evidence to the notion that restenosis is distinct from primary atherosclerosis.

B. Data Evaluation

One of the problems with interpreting the results of clinical trials of restenosis prevention is that "restenosis" has been defined in a number of different ways, and these definitions are not consistent. Restenosis has been defined based on clinical endpoints such as patient symptoms (angina) or evidence of myocardial ischemia on exercise testing. Clinical endpoints, however, may underestimate restenosis by as much as 30% (2). Only 60–70% of patients with recurrent angina have angiographic evidence of clinically significant restenosis. On the other hand, approximately 10–20% of those patients without recurrent angina have restenosis on angiography (4,5). In addition, antianginal drug therapy may affect symptomatology.

Definitions of restenosis based on coronary angiography have not been consistent from one clnical trial to another. Angiographic criteria for restenosis have been defined as >50% stenosis, immediate post-PTCA diameter of <50% increasing to >70% at follow-up, an increase in stenosis severity to within 10% or less than the predilation diameter stenosis at follow-up, loss of 50% of the gain in luminal diameter achieved at PTCA, decrease in minimal luminal diameter of >0.72 mm with respect to the post-PTCA angiogram, and other assessments of minimal luminal diameter (relative gain, relative loss, and net gain index) (7,8). Objective quantification of angioplasty results is an important aspect of angiographic definitions of restenosis. Visual estimation of stenosis severity with or without caliper measurements of percent diameter stenosis are subject to bias, inaccuracy, and variability between observers. Noncritical stenoses tend to be overestimated and critical stenoses underestimated (9). Caliper measurements also have poor overall reproducibility. Automated quantitative angiography using videodensitometry or an automated edge-tracing device has been suggested as an objective measure of anatomic restenosis (4,5,8).

Many studies have used follow-up angiographic data to define restenosis as a discrete, binary event (i.e., present or absent, based on an arbitrarily defined cutoff value). Alternatively, continuous measurements of the absolute change in vessel dimensions have been proposed as a more sensitive method of comparing different groups of patients and different therapies (4,8). Restenosis is a continuous, time-related event, which occurs to some extent in all patients. Continuous measurements of minimal luminal diameter over time may be more reflective of the biological process that can lead to restenosis rather than discrete angiographic endpoints. It has been suggested that clinical outcome measures must be integrated with the measurement of absolute and relative changes in the dimensions of the vessel lumen (4). Another problem with follow-up coronary angiography as an endpoint for restenosis clinical trials is the failure of 100% compliance to repeat coronary angiography. Studies with 70–90% follow-up probably allow for reasonable estimates of restenosis rates. In many studies, the timing of repeat coronary arteriography has been dictated by symptom status. Patients with recurrent chest pain have proceeded to repeat angiography earlier than asymptomatic patients. This has introduced a bias favoring restenosis since patients who have recurrence of angina are more likely to have restenosis (50–76%) than asymptomatic patients (4–17%) (4,5). In addition, patients who are asymptomatic are less likely to agree to have repeat coronary angiography performed. It is important to know, therefore, the proportion of patients without follow-up angiography in each symptom class (asymptomatic, atypical, or typical symptoms) and the restenosis rates in the patients undergoing repeat angiography in each class in order to obtain a better estimate of the true restenosis rate for the patients under study (4).

C. Inadequate Drug Therapy, Study Design Flaws

Many of the trials have utilized drug regimens that may have been inadequate. For example, two large studies of the angiotensin converting enzyme inhibitor cilazapril used a dose of cilazapril 7–10 times lower than the minimally effective dose in experimental studies in animal models (2). Many of the treatment regimens were not started prior to PTCA. The process leading to restenosis likely begins immediately upon vessel dilatation/injury, and, therefore, treatment strategies aimed at the earliest events (i.e., platelet activation) should be initiated well before PTCA. Adequate assessments of the proposed mechanism of action of drugs has not taken place in the clinical trials. For example, in many of the trials of antiplatelet therapies, assessments of platelet function (platelet aggregation, bleeding times) have not been performed in the patients undergoing PTCA. Some of the trials have suffered from an inadequate sample size or poor angiographic or clinical follow-up. Some of these trials with small sample size or inadequate follow-up have demonstrated positive results which have created a false impression of therapeutic benefit.

IV. THERAPEUTIC STRATEGIES

Since restenosis following successful PTCA is a multifactorial process, therapeutic strategies for the prevention of restenosis have been directed against a host of potential mediators and mechanisms. These therapies may be divided, for purposes of discussion, into six broad categories: antiplatelet therapies, anticoagulant therapies, lipid-lowering therapies, and therapies aimed at inhibition of cellular proliferation, inflammation, or coronary vasospasm. Clinical trials of each of these therapeutic strategies will be discussed. All of the clinical trials included in this review had a follow-up period for their patients of at least 3–6 months post-PTCA.

A. Antiplatelet Therapies

Antiplatelet therapies (Table 1) cover a broad range of pharmacological agents and treatment strategies.

1. Aspirin

Aspirin has been the cornerstone of this approach, and it has been extensively evaluated in a number of clinical trials of restenosis prevention. Aspirin has often been used as "conventional" therapy in clinical trials of other therapies aimed at preventing restenosis. Aspirin doses have ranged from 80 to 1500 mg/day and have been evaluated alone and in combination with dipyridamole and other drugs. All of the studies that were reviewed started their patients on aspirin therapy at least 1 day prior to PTCA and continued treatment through to follow-up. None of the studies reported on assessment of platelet function (platelet aggregation or bleeding times) either before or after aspirin therapy was begun. Placebo-controlled trials of aspirin alone (10,11) or aspirin in combination with dipyridamole (12,13) have generally shown no significant effect on restenosis rates or minimum luminal diameter. Taylor et al. (11), however, did find fewer restenotic lesions in the aspirin-treated group (25%) compared to the placebo-treated group (38%) ($p < 0.025$), and aspirin-treated lesions had lost 16% of lumen compared to 22% loss of lumen in placebo-treated lesions ($p < 0.01$). It should be noted that there were more left anterior descending lesions in the placebo group, and these lesions had a higher recurrence rate than other lesions. High-dose aspirin regimens have shown no benefit compared to low-dose regimens (14–16), although it has been noted that more side effects have been associated with high-dose regimens (15). In a randomized, double-blind, placebo-controlled study of ticlopidine (an inhibitor of ADP-induced platelet aggregation) vs. aspirin/dipyridamole, there was no benefit of either regimen compared to placebo (17). In a nonrandomized, uncontrolled study of aspirin vs. aspirin/ticlopidine vs. aspirin/ticlopidine/nicorandil, there was a significant effect of the addition of nicorandil (a potassium channel activator) in reducing restenosis rates compared to the regimens without nicorandil. All patients were treated with an unspecified calcium channel blocker as part of the standard therapy in this study (18).

Table 1 Antiplatelet Therapies

Study	Patients (n)	Study design	Therapy	Endpoint	Follow-up (%)	Results[a]	p
Aspirin							
Finci (10)	40	R, PC	ASA 100 mg/day; or placebo	Angio	73	33% ASA 14% placebo	NS
Taylor (11)	216	R, PC	ASA 100 mg/day; or placebo	Angio	98	35% ASA vs. 43% placebo (patients); 25% ASA vs. 38% placebo (lesions)	NS $p > 0.025$
Schwartz (12)	376	R, DB, PC	ASA 330 mg tid +dipyridamole 75 mg tid; or placebo	Angio	66	37.7% ASA/dip 38.6% placebo	NS
Chesebro (13)	207	R, DB, PC	ASA 975 mg/day +dipyridamole 225 mg/day; or placebo	Angio	83	Minimum luminal diameter: −0.15 mm ASA/dip −0.18 mm placebo	NS
Mufson (14)	495	R	ASA 80 mg/day (LD); or ASA 1500 mg/day (HD)	Angio	37	47% LD 51% HD	NS
Dykmans (15)	203	R	ASA 320 mg/day (LD); or ASA 1500 mg/day (HD)	Angio	42	31% LD 21%HD	—
Schanzenbacher (16)	79	—	ASA 100 mg qd; or ASA 1000 mg qd	Angio, ETT	100	18% LD 21% HD	NS
White (17)	236	R, DB, PC	ticlopidine 250 mg tid; or ASA 325 mg bid +dipyridamole 75 mg tid; or placebo	Angio	75	39% ticlopidine 33% ASA + dip 25% placebo	NS vs. placebo NS vs. placebo
Kitazume (18)	309	—	ASA 300 mg/day; or ASA 300 mg/day +ticlopidine 200 mg/day;	Angio	96	37.8% ASA ($n = 82$)	$p = 0.002$ ASA + tpd +nrd vs. ASA

Table 1 Continued

Study	Patients (n)	Study design	Therapy	Endpoint	Follow-up (%)	Results[a]	p
			or ASA 300 mg/day +ticlopidine 200 mg/day +nicorandil 30 mg/day			26.5% ASA + tpd ($n = 107$) 16.3% ASA + tpd + nrd ($n = 108$)	$p = 0.04$ ASA + tpd + nrd vs. ASA + tpd $p = 0.07$ ASA + tpd vs. ASA
Prostacyclin (PGI_2)							
Gershlick (19)	135	R, DB, PC	PGI_2 4 ng/kg/min iv × 36 h or placebo	Angio	93	29.2% PGI_2 38.3% placebo	NS
Knudtson (20)	270	R, PC	PGI_2 5–8 ng/kg/min × 48 h; or placebo	Angio	93	27% PGI_2 32% placebo	NS
Thromboxane-A_2 antagonists							
Hattori (21)	105	R, DB, PC	CV-4151 200 mg/day ($n = 58$); or placebo ($n = 27$)	Angio	81	38.3% CV-4151 31.4% placebo	NS
Feldman (22) (GRASP)	1089	R, DB, PC	GR32191 20 mg bid; or GR32191 40 mg bid; or placebo	Angio, clinical events	86	Clinical event rates: 26% GR32191 33% placebo	$p = 0.02$
Serruys (23) (CARPORT)	697	R, DB, PC	GR32191B 80 mg/day; or placebo	Angio, clinical events	75	21% GR32191B 19% placebo Minimal luminal diameter: −0.31 mm GR3219B −0.31 mm placebo	NS NS
Bove (25) (M-HEART)	755	R, DB, PC	ASA 325 mg/day; or sulotroban 800 mg qid; or placebo	Angio	55	% stenosis at 6 mo.: 42.9% ASA 49.0% sulotroban 48.3% placebo	NS vs. placebo NS vs. placebo

						Minimal luminal diameter: −0.37 mm ASA −0.45 mm sulotroban −0.48 mm placebo	 NS vs. placebo NS vs. placebo
GIIb/IIIa receptor antagonists							
Topol (EPIC) (38)	2099	R, DB, PC	c7E3 iv bolus + 12h infusion ($n = 708$); or 7E3 bolus + placebo infusion ($n = 695$); or placebo bolus + placebo infusion ($n = 695$	Clinical events	—	Target vessel CABG/PTCA: placebo/placebo 22.3% c7E3 bolus/placebo 21.0% c7E3 bolus/c7E3 infusion 16.5%	$p = 0.007$ vs. placebo
IMPACT II (39)	4010	R, DB, PC	Integrel 135 g/kg bolus + 0.5 g/kg.min infusion; or Integralin 135 g/kg golus + 0.75 g/kg.min infusion; or placebo bolus + placebo infusion	Clinical events	—	Combined integrelin-treated 9.5% placebo 11.6%	$p = 0.046$
Ketanserin							
Klein (27)	43	R	ketanserin 0.1 mg/min ×24 h + ASA 300 mg/day + diltiazem 180 mg/day; or ASA 300 mg/day + diltiazem 180 mg/day	Angio	86	26% ketanserin + ASA 22% ASA	NS

Table 1 Continued

Study	Patients (n)	Study design	Therapy	Endpoint	Follow-up (%)	Results[a]	p
Serruys (28)	658	R, DB, PC	ketanserin 40 mg BID + ASA; or placebo + ASA	Angio, clinical events	90	Clinical endpoints: 28% ketanserin 32% placebo;	NS
						Minimal luminal diameter: −0.27 mm ketanserin −0.24 mm placebo	NS
Trapidil							
Okamoto (29)	97	R	trapidil 600 mg/day + nifedipine 40 mg/day; or ASA 300 mg/day + dipyridamole 150 mg/day +nifedipine 40 mg/day	Angio	74	19.4% trapidil 41.7% ASA/dip	$p < 0.05$
Nishikawa (30)	160	R	trapidil 200 mg tid + ASA; or dipyridamole 50 mg tid + ASA	Angio	86	20% trapidil 38% dip	—
Maresta (31) (STARC)	384	R, DB	trapidil 100 mg tid; or ASA 100 mg tid	Angio	66	24.2% trapidil vs. 39.7% ASA (patients);	$p < 0.01$
						23.3% trapidil vs. 36.9% ASA (lesions)	$p = 0.018$

[a]Restenosis rates are reported unless otherwise noted.
R = randomized; DB = double-blind; PC = placebo-controlled; ASA = aspirin; dip = dipyridamole; CCB = calcium channel blocker; nrd = nicorandil; tpd = ticlopidine; LD = low dose; HD = high dose; qd = once daily; bid = twice daily; tid = three times daily.

2. *Prostacyclin (PGI_2)*

Aspirin is known to inhibit platelet function by inhibiting cyclooxygenase and, at higher doses, it can also inhibit prostacyclin production. Short-term prostacyclin infusions at the time of PTCA have been evaluated in two restenosis trials. Prostacyclin (PGI_2) infusions before and at 4 ng/kg/min for 36 h (19) or 5–8 ng/kg/min for 48 h (20) following successful PTCA did not affect restenosis rates at 6 months compared to placebo infusions. Concomitant therapy in these studies was with aspirin (19) or with a combination of aspirin/dipyridamole (20). No effect on angioplasty-induced platelet activation was seen in the study of prostacyclin infusion at 4 ng/kg/min compared to placebo (19). Platelet function was not evaluated in the latter study. Nausea, flushing, hypotension, and bradycardia were side effects of prostacyclin infusions in these studies and limited the doses of prostacyclin that could be administered in the latter study (20).

3. *Thromboxane A_2 Inhibition*

Thromboxane A_2 is released by platelets which are activated during angioplasty. Thromboxane A_2 increases platelet aggregation and has a mitogenic effect on smooth muscle cells. A thromboxane A_2 synthase inhibitor and two thromboxane A_2 receptor antagonists have been evaluated in clinical trials of restenosis prevention. In a randomized, double-blind, placebo-controlled trial, inhibition of thromboxane A_2 with the thromboxane A_2 synthetase inhibitor CV-4151 (21) had no significant effect on restenosis rates at 3–6 months after coronary angioplasty. An assessment of platelet function was not performed in this study. Similarly, neither of the thromboxane A_2 receptor antagonists [GR32191B (22,23) or sulotroban (24,25)] had a significant effect on restenosis compared to placebo in randomized, double-blind trials. Therapy with these agents was begun before angioplasty and was continued through follow-up. In the GRASP study of GR32191B (22), there was a significant ($p = 0.02$) reduction in clinical event rate in the active treatment groups (26%) compared to the placebo group (33%), primarily due to a reduction in the incidence of myocardial infarction and re-PTCA in the active treatment groups. However, there was no difference in CABG between treatment groups. In the Coronary Artery Restenosis Prevention on Repeated Thromboxane-Antagonism (CARPORT) study of GR32191B (23), however, there were no differences in clinical events, restenosis rates, or minimal luminal diameter between treatment groups. Platelet aggregation studies were performed in the CARPORT study at one of the centers, and there was a significant lowering of U-46619 (thromboxane A_2 agonist)–stimulated aggregation in the active treatment group after 3 months of therapy. In the Multi-Hospital Eastern Atlantic Restenosis Trial II (M-HEART-II), neither sulotroban nor aspirin was different from placebo with regard to percent stenosis or stenosis diameter at 6 month follow-up (25). Platelet function studies were not performed in M-HEART-II; however, in a separate pilot study of 14 patients undergoing PTCA and randomized to aspirin 500 mg/day ($n = 7$) or sulotroban 800 mg tid ($n = 7$), sulotroban was shown to inhibit U-46619 stimulated aggregation. After 3 months of therapy, however, there was no difference in the degree of restenosis between the aspirin and sulotroban-treated groups in this pilot study (26).

4. GIIb/IIIa Antagonists

The final common pathway for platelet activation involves glycoprotein IIb/IIIa integrin. GIIb/IIIa antagonists are currently undergoing clinical evaluation for the prevention of restenosis following successful PTCA. One of these antagonists is c7E3, a chimeric 7E3 antibody Fab named abciximab or ReoPro®, which binds to glycoprotein IIb/IIIa integrin. In the Evaluation of c7E3 for the Prevention of Ischemic Complications (EPIC) trial (38), 2099 patients who had unstable angina, recent or evolving myocardial infarction, or high-risk angiographic morphology were randomized into three groups: placebo bolus and placebo 12-h infusion, active c7E3 bolus at 0.25 mg/kg and placebo 12-h infusion, or active c7E3 bolus at the same dose followed immediately by c7E3 at 10 μg/kg/min for 12 h. The bolus was given at least 10 min prior to PTCA. Patients also received aspirin 325 mg/day. After 30 days of follow-up, there was a significant reduction in major ischemic events in the c7E3 bolus/c7E3 infusion group (8.3%) compared to the placebo bolus/placebo infusion group (12.8%) ($p = 0.008$). After 6 months, the need for target vessel revascularization (CABG/PTCA) in the c7E3 bolus/c7E3 infusion group was 16.5 vs. 22.3% in the placebo bolus/placebo infusion group ($p = 0.007$). The c7E3 bolus/placebo infusion group had an intermediate outcome that was not significantly better than that of the placebo bolus/placebo infusion group.

Angiographic follow-up was not reported in this study. This therapy has only been studied in high-risk angioplasty patients and carries a risk of bleeding complications. c7E3 is a relatively nonspecific GIIb/IIIa antagonist in that it binds to other integrins, including the vitronectin receptor. Therapy with GIIb/IIIa antagonists that are more specific for the GIIb/IIIa receptor may be more or less efficacious than c7E3. IMPACT-II, a 4010-patient, 82-center, placebo-controlled trial of Integrelin® (a specific GIIb/IIIa receptor antagonist) in coronary angioplasty recently reported preliminary data (39). All Integrelin®-treated patients received a bolus injection of 135 μg/kg. Thereafter, patients in one active treatment arm received infusions at the rate of 0.5 μg/kg.min and patients in the other active treatment arm received infusions at the rate of 0.75 μg/kg.min. The trial also included a placebo-treated group. The occurrence of a composite endpoint of death, myocardial infarction, and the need for urgent intervention within 30 days following PTCA was 9.5% in the Integrelin®-treated patients and 11.6% in the placebo-treated patients ($p = 0.046$) (39). Data at 6 months are equally negative.

5. *Ketanserin*

Ketanserin is a serotonin S2-receptor antagonist that inhibits the platelet activation and vasoconstriction induced by serotonin and also inhibits the mitogenic effect of serotonin on vascular smooth muscle cells. In a dose-finding study in patients, intravenous ketanserin 0.1 and 0.2 mg/min induced a strong inhibition of ADP- and adrenaline-induced platelet aggregation (27). At 0.2 mg/min, however, side effects such as dizziness, hypotension, and nausea were frequently observed. In a randomized study, ketanserin 0.1 mg/min infused for 24 h following coronary angioplasty in addition to aspirin 300 mg/day and diltiazem 180 mg/day had no effect on restenosis rate after 4–9 months compared to aspirin and diltiazem alone (27). In a randomized, placebo-controlled trial of 6 months of therapy with aspirin plus oral ketanserin 40 mg bid compared to aspirin plus placebo, there were no differences in clinical events or minimal luminal diameter between treatment groups (28).

6. *Trapidil*

Some promising results have been reported with trapidil, a phosphodiesterase inhibitor and platelet-derived growth factor (PDGF) antagonist, which could potentially inhibit intimal proliferation after PTCA. Trapidil has been evaluated in three randomized, controlled studies of 6 months of therapy comparing trapidil to aspirin or to aspirin/dipyridamole. In a small study of 97 patients comparing trapidil 600 mg/day to aspirin 300 mg/day plus dipyridamole 150 mg/day, restenosis was present in 19.4% of patients in the trapidil group compared to 41.7% of the aspirin/dipyridamole group, which was a statistically significant result ($p < 0.05$). Trapidil was started one week prior to angioplasty and continued for 4–6 months. Of note, nifedipine 40 mg/day was also given to all patients in this study (29). In a small randomized trial of trapidil 200 mg tid vs. dipyridamole 50 mg tid, there was a trend toward a reduction in restenosis rate after 4 months. All patients received aspirin therapy in this trial (30). In the Studio Trapidil versus Aspirin nella Restenosi Coronarica (STARC) trial, 384 patients were randomized to either trapidil 100 mg tid or aspirin 100 mg tid starting at least 3 days prior to PTCA and continuing for 6 months thereafter. Restenosis occurred in 24.2% of the trapidil group and 39.7% of the aspirin group ($p < 0.01$). Clinical events at follow-up were similar in the two groups except that recurrent angina was significantly more frequent in the aspirin group (31).

B. Anticoagulant Therapies (Table 2)

1. Warfarin

Warfarin therapy has been evaluated in two randomized clinical trials. One trial compared warfarin to aspirin 325 mg/day (32), and the other compared warfarin and verapamil to verapamil alone (33). Therapeutic anticoagulation with warfarin did not prevent restenosis in either study compared to the alternate treatment; however, warfarin therapy was not started prior to angioplasty in either trial. In the trial conducted by Thornton et al. (32), patients with at least a 6-month history of angina demonstrated a significantly different response to treatment in that 44% of warfarin-treated patients had restenosis compared to 21% of aspirin-treated patients ($p < 0.05$).

2. Heparin and Low Molecular Weight Heparins

Heparin and low molecular weight heparins have also been evaluated in trials of restenosis prevention. Ellis et al. (34) compared intravenous heparin for 18–24 h post-PTCA to intravenous dextrose and found no significant difference in restenosis rates at 6 months post-PTCA. Aspirin 325 mg once daily up to four times daily was a concomitant therapy in both groups, and approximately 50% of patients in each group were also prescribed dipyridamole. Uncontrolled pilot studies of two low molecular weight heparins, reviparin (n = 39) (35) and fraxiparin (n = 20) (36), have been reported with restenosis rates at 3 months of 17–25% for reviparin and 30% for fraxiparin. In a large randomized, double-blind, placebo-controlled study of enoxaparin, a third low molecular weight heparin, 40 mg sc qd for one month, there was no difference in restenosis rates between active drug and placebo treatment groups at 6 months of follow-up (37).

3. Thrombin Inhibitors

Direct-acting thrombin inhibitors, such as hirudin and its analogs, have several theoretical advantages over heparin in the management of coronary angioplasty. They do not require a cofactor such as antithrombin III, are active against clot-bound thrombin, and have no known natural inhibitors (126). In the Hirulog Angioplasty study, the thrombin inhibitor, bivalirudin, in conjunction with aspirin was compared to heparin and aspirin (126). Both bivalirudin and heparin were each given as a bolus followed by sustaining infusions of up to approximately 24 h. There was no difference in the primary endpoint, defined as many of a number of acute complications during hospitalizations (e.g., death, myocardial infarction, abrupt closure of the dilated vessel, etc.) between the two treatment groups. At 6 months follow-up, the cumulative incidence of death, myocardial infarction or a need for repeated revascularization was similar in the two treatment groups as well. However, there are significantly lower rates of bleeding complications with bivalirudin than with heparin during the acute phase of coronary angioplasty.

Table 2 Anticoagulant Therapies

Study	Patients (*n*)	Study design	Therapy	Endpoint	Follow-up (%)	Results[a]	*p*
Warfarin							
Thornton (32)	248	R	ASA 325 mg/day; or warfarin	Angio, ETT	92	27% ASA 36% warfarin	NS
Urban (33)	110	R	warfarin + verapamil; or verapamil	Angio, ETT	77	29% warfarin vs. 37% control (patients);	NS
						25% warfarin vs. 33% control (lesions)	NS
Heparin and low molecular weight heparins							
Ellis (34)	416	R, PC	heparin × 18–24 h + aspirin; or dextrose × 18–24 h + aspirin	Angio	60	41.2% heparin 36.7% dextrose	NS
Faxon (37)	459	R, DB, PC	enoxaparin 40 mg sc qd × 1 month; or placebo	Angio	—	51% enoxaparin 52% placebo	NS
Thrombin inhibitors							
BITTL (126)	4098	R, DB	BIVALIRUDIN 1.0 mg/kg bolus +2.5 mg/kg × 4 h +0.2 mg/kg × 14–20 h +ASA OR heparin 175 U/kg bolus + 15 U/kg/h ×18–24 h + ASA	Clinical events	95	21% Bivalirudin +ASA vs. 21.3% heparin + ASA; in unstable angina patients, 17.8% and 18.4%, respectively	NS

[a]Restenosis rates are reported unless otherwise noted.

R = randomized; DB = double-blind; PC = placebo-controlled: ASA = aspirin; CCB = calcium channel blocker; sc = subcutaneous administration.

C. Lipid Lowering Therapies (Table 3)

1. *HMG-CoA Reductase Inhibitors*

On balance, lipid reduction with HMG-CoA reductase inhibitors has been unsuccessful in significantly decreasing restenosis rates following successful PTCA. In a randomized study, Sahni et al. (40) compared lovastatin 20–40 mg/day plus "conventional therapy" with aspirin 650 mg/day, dipyridamole 75 mg tid, and a calcium channel blocker to "conventional therapy" alone. The serum cholesterol level in the lovastatin group decreased from 212 to 175 mg/dl ($p < 0.001$), whereas in the control group it only decreased from 207 to 196 mg/dl ($p < 0.015$). In the lovastatin group 12% of patients had restenosis compared with 44% of patients in the control group ($p < 0.001$). In the lovastatin group 12.5% of vessels restenosed compared with 38.2% in the control group ($p < 0.001$). This study has been criticized since it was unblinded and there was only a 47% angiographic follow-up. In a larger, randomized, double-blind, placebo-controlled study, Weintraub et al. (41) found no difference in the restenosis of the index coronary lesion in the placebo group (46%) compared to the lovastatin group (44%) ($p = 0.50$) despite a 42% reduction in the serum level of LDL-cholesterol in the lovastatin group. There were no significant differences in minimal luminal diameter or other measures of restenosis after 6 months of treatment, and there were no differences between the two groups with respect to clinical events. The dose of lovastatin was 40 mg bid, and there was 91% angiographic follow-up at 6 months in this latter study. Results of a randomized, unblinded study of pravastatin 5–10 mg bid compared to no lipid-lowering therapy were also disappointing. Despite a decrease in the serum cholesterol from 215.7 to 181.2 mg/dl ($p < 0.001$) in the pravastatin group, there were no differences in angina, need for repeat PTCA, or angiographic restenosis between groups. Both groups of patients received aspirin 80 mg/day, dipyridamole 150 mg/day, and either diltiazem or nifedipine during the follow-up period (42). A large, multicenter, multinational, randomized, double-blind, placebo-controlled study (the Fluvastatin Angioplasty Restenosis or FLARE Trial) is currently ongoing and will evaluate the ability of fluvastatin 40 mg bid to reduce restenosis after successful single-lesion PTCA (43).

2. *Probucol*

Probucol, a lipid-lowering drug with antioxidant activity, has also been evaluated in a clinical trial of restenosis prevention. In a small trial, patients were randomly assigned to receive probucol 750–1000 mg qd or dipyridamole 150 mg qd, which was initiated 7 days prior to PTCA and continued for 3–6 months following PTCA. Patients also received

Table 3 Lipid-Lowering Therapies

Study	Patients (n)	Study design	Therapy	Endpoint	Follow-up (%)	Results[a]	p
HMG-CoA reductase inhibitors							
Sahni (40)	157	R	lovastatin 20–40 mg/day + ASA 650 mg/day + dipyridamole 75 mg tid + CCB; or ASA 650 mg/day + dipyridamole 75 mg tid + CCB	Angio	47%	12% lovastatin 44.4% control	$p < 0.001$
Weintraub (41)	354	R, DB, PC	lovastatin 40 mg bid; or placebo	Angio	91	% stenosis: 44% lovastatin 46% placebo	NS
Onaka (42)	66	R	pravastatin 5–10 mg bid + ASA 81 mg/day + dipyridamole 150 mg/day + CCB; or ASA 81 mg/day + dipyridamole 150 mg/day + CCB	Angio, symptoms	100	% stenosis; 53.4% pravastatin 61.9% untreated	NS
Probucol							
Setsuda (44)	67	R	750–1000 mg probucol + nifedipine 40 mg/day + ASA 300 mg/day; or dipyridamole 150 mg/day + nifedipine 40 mg/day + ASA 300 mg/day	Angio	76	19.4% probucol 41.7% dip	$p < 0.05$

Table 3 Continued

Study	Patients (*n*)	Study design	Therapy	Endpoint	Follow-up (%)	Results[a]	*p*
Fish oils							
Bairati (46)	205	R, DB, PC	2.7 g EPA/1.8 g DHA; or placebo	Angio	58	4 definitions (fish oil vs. placebo):	
						31% vs. 48%	<0.05
						31% vs. 42%	NS
						36% vs. 53%	<0.05
						22% vs. 44%	<0.03
Reis (47)	204	R, DB, PC	6g/day n-3 fatty acids + ASA 325 mg/day + dipyridamole 50 mg qid + CCB; or placebo + ASA 325 mg/day + dipyridamole 50 mg qid + CCB	Angio, clinical events, ETT,	37% angio; 100% clinical	34% fish oil 23% placebo	NS
Grigg (48)	108	R, DB, PC	1.8 g EPA/1.2 g DHA + ASA 150 mg/day + verapamil 80 mg tid; or placebo + ASA 150 mg/day + verapamil 80 mg tid	Angio	93	Patients: 34% fish oil 33% placebo	NS
						Lesions: 29% fish oil 31% placebo	NS
Franzen (49)	204	R, DB, PC	3.15 g n-3 fatty acids + aspirin 250 mg/day; or placebo + aspirin 250 mg/day	Angio	86	lesions: 31.2% fish oil 33.7% placebo	NS

Milner (50)	194	R	4.5 g n-3 fatty acid + ASA/CCB; or ASA/CCB	Angio, clinical events	29% angio; 100% clinical	Angio: 18% fish oil 27% control	NS
						Clinical: 19% fish oil 36% control	$p = 0.008$
Dehmer (51)	82	R	3.2 g EPA +ASA 325 mg/day +75 mg dipyridamole tid; or ASA 325 mg/day +dipyridamole 75 mg tid	Angio	100	Patients: 19% fish oil 46% control	$p = 0.007$
						Lesions: 16% fish oil 36% control	$p = 0.026$
Kaul (52)	107	R	1.8 g EPA/1.2 g DHA + ASA 150 mg/day + CCB; or ASA 150 mg/day +CCB	Angio, clinical events, ETT,	100	32% fish oil 27% control	NS
Nye (53)	108	R, PC	2.16 g EPA + ASA 300 mg/day + dipyridamole 75 mg tid; or placebo + ASA 300 mg/day + dipyridamole 75 mg tid	Angio, clinical events	92	17% ASA/dip 11% EPA 30% placebo	EPA vs. placebo, $p < 0.05$; EPA vs. ASA/dip, NS

[a]Restenosis rates are reported unless otherwise noted.
R = randomized; DB = double-blind; PC = placebo-controlled; ASA = aspirin; dip = dipyridamole; CCB = calcium channel blocker; qd = once daily; bid = twice daily; tid = three times daily; qid = four times daily; EPA = eicosapentaenoic acid; DHA = docosahexaenoic acid.

nifedipine 40 mg and aspirin 0.3 g daily. The restenosis rate was significantly lower in the probucol-treated group compared to the dipyridamole-treated group (19.4 vs. 41.7%, respectively, $p < 0.05$). There was no significant difference between groups in pre-PTCA serum cholesterol, however, at follow-up the serum cholesterol was significantly lower in the probucol-treated group than in the dipyridamole-treated group. In the subgroup with pre-PTCA serum cholesterol <200 mg/dl, there was no significant difference in the restenosis rate between probucol- and dipyridamole-treated patients; however, in the subgroup of patients with pre-PTCA serum cholesterol ≥ 200 mg/dl, the restenosis rate was significantly lower in the probucol-treated patients than in the dipyridamole-treated patients (44).

3. *LDL-Apheresis*

An interesting approach to lipid lowering in the prevention of restenosis following successful PTCA has been reported by Yamaguchi and coworkers (45). These investigators found that LDL-apheresis (LDL-apheresis Angioplasty Restenosis Trial or L-ART) was effective in preventing restenosis after 5 months of follow-up when combined with pravastatin 10 mg/day and niceritrol (nicotinic acid) 1500 mg/day. Fifty-four patients received LDL-apheresis 2 days prior to PTCA and 5 days post-PTCA and a subgroup of 29 of these 54 patients also received therapy with pravastatin and niceritrol for 5 months. A control group of 137 patients did not undergo LDL-apheresis treatment and were followed during the same period. All patients received apsirin, dipyridamole, and diltiazem as standard therapy. Thirty-three percent of all patients treated by LDL-apheresis experienced restenosis, while 38% of the 137 patients in the nonapheresis group experienced restenosis with no statistical significance between the two groups. There was also no difference in the restenosis rates between those patients who received lipid-lowering medications in addition to LDL-apheresis compared to those patients receiving LDL-apheresis alone. When restenosis rates were analyzed in relation to the reduction in plasma Lp(a), patients whose plasma Lp(a) levels were reduced by more than 50% showed a lower restenosis rate than those whose plasma Lp(a) levels were reduced by less than 50% (21.2 vs. 52.4%, $p = 0.0179$).

4. *Fish Oils*

Fish oils contain omega-3 fatty acids, which have been shown to decrease LDL-cholesterol, increase HDL-cholesterol and increase bleeding times. Variations in the study designs of the clinical trials of fish oils in the prevention of restenosis have made interpretation of the results very difficult. Four randomized, double-blind, placebo-controlled studies have evaluated n-3 fatty acids (combinations of eicosapentaenoic acid and docosahexaenoic acid) in the prevention of restenosis following PTCA (46–49). One of these four studies showed a significant reduction in the restenosis rate in the n-3 fatty acid group at 6 months (46), whereas the other three studies showed no significant effect of n-3 fatty acids compared to placebo (olive oil) therapy in reducing restenosis rates. The study, which demonstrated a beneficial effect of fish oils, utilized a dose of 4.5 g/day of n-3 fatty acids started 3 weeks before PTCA and continued for 6 months after PTCA. Four definitions of restenosis were used in this study, and a statistically significant result was obtained for three out of four of these definitions (46). A randomized, double-blind, placebo-controlled study utilizing a higher dose of 6 g n-3 fatty acids/day started 5 days before PTCA did not show a significant beneficial effect of fish oils on restenosis rates (47). Four randomized, unblinded studies have yielded variable results. Milner et al. (50) reported a significant reduction in restenosis rates with 4.5 g n-3 fatty acids/day started after PTCA in addition to "conventional therapy" with aspirin and calcium channel blockers compared to "conventional therapy" alone. This study was seriously flawed, however, since the endpoints were subjective (symptoms and exercise testing), randomization occurred after PTCA, and the study was unblinded. Indeed, when the authors reported on the "hard endpoints" of restenosis proven by angiography, there was no significant beneficial effect of n-3 fatty acids in addition to conventional therapy compared to conventional therapy alone. Dehmer et al. (51) compared 3 g n-3 fatty acids/day in addition to aspirin 300 mg/day and dipyridamole 75 mg tid to aspirin/dipyridamole alone and found a significant reduction in restenosis rates for patients (46 vs. 19%, respectively, $p = 0.007$) and lesions (36 vs. 16%, respectively, $p = 0.026$) in the n-3 fatty acid–treated patients compared to the control group. Kaul et al. (52) found no significant effect of n-3 fatty acids 3.0 g/day in addition to aspirin and calcium channel blockers compared to aspirin and calcium channel blockers alone. Nye et al. (53) compared eicosapentaenoic acid (EPA) 2.16 g/day vs. aspirin 300 mg/day and dipyridamole 75 mg tid vs. placebo (olive oil) and found a significant reduction in restenosis in the EPA-treated group compared to placebo, but could find no significant effect of EPA compared to aspirin/dipyridamole.

Therapy with fish oils is inconvenient, requiring the patient to swallow multiple capsules three times daily, and is associated with a significant incidence of gastrointestinal side effects (bad taste, regurgitation) (47). At the present time, dietary supplementation with fish oils has not been approved for the prevention of restenosis following PTCA.

D. Antiproliferative Therapies (Table 4)

1. ACE Inhibitors

Angiotensin-converting enzyme (ACE) inhibitors have recently received attention for their antiproliferative effects in animal models of vascular injury (55,56). It is believed that the most likely mechanism for this effect of ACE inhibitors is the inhibition of the mitogenic activity of angiotensin II. Enalapril 10 mg/day plus “conventional therapy” with aspirin 150 mg/day and a calcium channel blocker (nifedipine or diltiazem) was compared to “conventional therapy” alone in a small randomized trial (57). No significant differences were seen in restenosis rate or clinical events between treatment groups. In a large, randomized, double-blind, placebo-controlled trial of fosinopril 40 mg/day (58), there were no significant differences in restenosis rate, minimal luminal diameter, or clinical events between treatment groups. Both groups in this study were treated with aspirin. Cilazapril has been extensively evaluated in two large clinical trials of restenosis prevention. In the Multicenter European Research Trial with Cilazapril after Angioplasty to Prevent Transluminal Coronary Obstruction and Restenosis (MERCATOR) study (59), the effects of cilazapril 2.5 mg following successful PTCA and 5 mg bid for 6 months were compared to placebo in a randomized, double-blind clinical trial. All patients received aspirin for 6 months. There were no differences between cilazapril and placebo-treated groups with respect to minimal luminal diameter or clinical events. In the American version (MARCATOR), which was also randomized and double-blind (60), patients received cilazapril 1 or 2.5 mg following successful PTCA and then 1, 5, or 10 mg bid for 6 months or placebo. All patients in this trial received aspirin for 6 months. There was no significant difference in minimal luminal diameter between placebo-treated patients and patients treated with any dose of cilazapril.

It is interesting to note that the angiotensin II, AT-1 receptor antagonist losartan has been shown to prevent intimal proliferation in rat models (61–63). Angiotensin II receptor antagonists may be more efficacious in treating restenosis following PTCA since these drugs act at the tissue receptor level; however, the ability of animal models to predict efficacy in vascular injury in humans is suspect.

2. *Colchicine*

Colchicine, an antimitotic agent, has shown promise in preventing smooth muscle cell proliferation in animal models. Two clinical trials have evaluated colchicine for the prevention of restenosis following successful PTCA. In a randomized, double-blind trial of one month of therapy with colchicine 1 mg/day or placebo, there were no differences in clinical endpoints of restenosis or exercise thallium studies between colchicine- and placebo-treated patients after 6 months of follow-up. Colchicine therapy was initiated prior to PTCA (64). In another trial, patients were randomized in a 2:1 fashion to colchicine 0.6 mg bid or placebo for 6 months of therapy following coronary angioplasty. Therapy was initiated between 12 h before

Table 4 Antiproliferative Therapies

Study	Patients (n)	Study design	Therapy	Endpoint	Follow-up (%)	Results[a]	p
ACE inhibitors							
Kaul (57)	95	R	enalapril 10 mg/day + ASA 150 mg/day + CCB; or ASA 150 mg/day +CCB	Angio, clinical events, ETT	36% angio; 100% clinical	34% enalapril 31% control	NS
Desmet (58)	509	R, DB, PC	fosinopril 40 mg/day + ASA; or placebo + ASA	Angio, clinical events	60	Patients: 45.7% fosinopril 40.7% placebo	NS
						Minimal luminal diameter: −0.59 mm fosinopril −0.57 mm control	NS
MERCATOR (59)	735	R, DB, PC	cilazapril 5 mg bid + ASA; or placebo + ASA	Angio, clinical events	81	Minimal luminal diameter: −0.27 mm cilazapril −0.29 mm control	NS
Faxon for MARCATOR (60)	1436	R, DB, PC	Cilazapril 1, 5 or 10 mg bid + ASA; or placebo + ASA	Angio, clinical events	75	MLD difference: −0.35 mm placebo	
						−0.37 mm 1 mg bid	NS vs. placebo
						−0.45 mm 5 mg bid	NS vs. placebo
						−0.412 mm 10 mg bid	NS vs. placebo
Colchicine							
Grines (CART) (64)	253	R, DB, PC	colchicine 1 mg/day or placebo × 1 month	Clinical events, thallium exercise	79	48% colchicine 41% placebo	NS
O'Keefe (65)	197	R	colchicine 0.6 mg bid (n=130) or placebo (n=67)	Angio	74	41% colchicine 45% placebo	NS

[a]Restenosis rates are reported unless otherwise noted.

R = randomized; DB = double-blind; PC = placebo-controlled; ASA = aspirin; dip = dipyridamole; CCB = calcium channel blocker; qd = once daily; bid = twice daily; tid = three times daily; qid = four times daily.

and 24 h after angioplasty. There were no significant differences in percent lumen diameter narrowing or in restenosis rates between colchicine- and placebo-treated patients after 6 months of follow-up (65).

E. Anti-Inflammatory Therapies (Table 5)

1. Corticosteroids

Corticosteroids are potent inhibitors of monocyte and macrophage number and function and may stabilize lysosomal membranes, thereby limiting cellular injury. Two randomized clinical trials evaluated corticosteroid therapy given at the time of PTCA to prevent restenosis after 6 months of follow-up. The M-HEART investigators (66) randomized patients to either pulse methylprednisolone 1 g intravenously or placebo given in a double-blind fashion at 2–24 h prior to PTCA. All patients in this study were treated with aspirin 325 mg/day. In a second trial, Stone et al. (67) randomized patients to placebo or 125 mg methylprednisolone intramuscular the night before and morning of PTCA and then 60 mg orally once daily for one week. In the latter trial, patients who were studied were undergoing their second, third, or fourth dilation of the same coronary segment and were at increased risk of restenosis. In addition, these patients were treated with aspirin, dipyridamole, and a calcium channel blocker for at least 2 months after PTCA. In neither trial was there a significant effect of steroids on lesion restenosis rates or on clinical events compared to placebo. There was a trend toward reduction in clinical events in the latter trial (24% steroid-treated vs. 39% placebo-treated), which did not reach statistical significance ($p = 0.56$).

2. Ebselen

Ebselen is a selenium-containing heterocyclic compound exhibiting anti–inflammatory and antioxidant activities as shown by the prevention of inflammatory cell activation and lipid peroxidation, which may have a preventive effect on restenosis after PTCA. In a small randomized, placebo-controlled trial, 79 patients received either ebselen 200 mg orally bid ($n = 29$) or placebo ($n = 50$) starting 3 days before PTCA and continuing for 3 months following PTCA. The lesion restenosis rate was 38.2% in the placebo group and 18.6% in the ebselen group ($p < 0.05$). A statistically significant beneficial effect of ebselen vs. placebo therapy was also observed for quantitative luminal diameter (68).

F. Inhibition of Coronary Vasospasm

Coronary artery spasm and elastic recoil of the dilated coronary artery lesion may contribute to restenosis. Calcium channel blockers are given as

Table 5 Anti–Inflammatory Therapies

Study	Patients (n)	Study design	Therapy	Endpoint	Follow-up (%)	Results[a]	p
Corticosteroids							
Pepine (66)	722	R, DB, PC	1.0 g methylprednisolone iv 2-24 h prior +ASA 325 mg/day; or placebo +ASA 325 mg/day	Angio, clinical events	73.5%	Lesions: 40% methylprednisolone 39% placebo	NS
Stone (67)	102	R	125 mg methylprednisolone IM × 2 prior and then 60 mg qd × 1 week + ASA 325 mg tid + dipyridamole 75 mg tid + CCB; or no steroids +ASA 325 mg tid + dipyridamole 75 mg tid + CCB;	Angio, clinical events	53%	Patients: 42% steroids 48% control Lesions: 36% steroids 40% control	NS NS
Ebselen							
Hirayama (68)	79	R, PC	ebselen 200 mg bid for 3 months (n=29); or placebo (n=50)	Angio	—	18.6% ebselen 38.2% placebo	$p < 0.05$

[a]Restenosis rates are reported unless otherwise noted.

R = randomized; DB = double-blind; PC = placebo-controlled; ASA = aspirin; CCB = calcium channel blocker; iv = intravenous; IM = intramuscular injection; qd = once daily; bid = twice daily; tid = three times daily; qid = four times daily.

part of the PTCA procedure in an effort to reduce coronary artery spasm (Table 6) and are also included in the "conventional" therapies of many restenosis trials. Two clinical trials of restenosis prevention have evaluated diltiazem. A prospective randomized trial compared diltiazem 90 mg tid to control therapy for 3 months after PTCA. Active and control patients received aspirin 650 mg/day and dipyridamole 75 mg tid orally. There were no differences in restenosis rates or degree of restenosis between treatment groups after 5–10 months (69). A second randomized, double-blind trial evaluated a "high" dose of diltiazem 240–360 mg/day to placebo. All patients received aspirin and dipyridamole. After one year, there were no differences in restenosis rates or clinical events between treatment groups (70). Nifedipine was evaluated in a randomized, double-blind study of restenosis prevention. Patients were treated with nifedipine 10 mg qid or placebo for 6 months following angioplasty. There were no differences in restenosis rates or restenosis diameter between groups (71). A placebo-controlled, double-blind trial evaluated patients treated with 330 mg aspirin and 75 mg dipyridamole bid who were randomized to either verapamil 240 mg bid or placebo. At 6 months of follow-up, there was a trend toward reduction of restenosis rate in the verapamil group compared to placebo, which did not reach statistical significance (48.3 vs. 62.7%, $p = 0.059$). When noncompliant patients were eliminated from the analysis, the restenosis rate was 47.4% in the verapamil group and 63.9% in the placebo group ($p = 0.046$) in patients who had follow-up angiograms performed (72). Despite their widespread use, the results of clinical trials of restenosis prevention with calcium channel blockers have been disappointing.

G. Other Pharmacological Therapies (Table 7)

1. Angiopeptin

Angiopeptin is a cyclic octapeptide analog of somatostatin that has been shown to limit myointimal thickening in animal models following balloon injury. Parenterally administered angiopeptin therapy was evaluated in a randomized, double-blind, placebo-controlled trial of restenosis prevention (73). Patients received a continuous subcutaneous infusion of placebo or angiopeptin 6–24 h before PTCA and for 4 days after PTCA in addition to a bolus dose at the time of PTCA. Patients were also treated with aspirin 150 mg/day. There were no differences in minimal lumen diameter or in restenosis rates between treatment groups at 6 months. There was a trend toward reduction in clinical events at 12 months in patients treated with angiopeptin compared to placebo-treated patients (28.4 vs. 36.4%, respectively, $p = 0.046$) (75).

Table 6 Inhibition of Coronary Vasospasm

Study	Patients (n)	Study design	Therapy	Endpoint	Follow-up (%)	Results[a]	p
Calcium channel blockers							
Cocros (69)	92	R	diltiazem 90 mg tid × 3 months + ASA 650 mg qd + dipyridamole 75 mg tid; or ASA 650 mg qd + dipyridamole 75 mg tid	Angio	100%	15% diltiazem 22% control	NS
O'Keefe (70)	201	R, DB, PC	diltiazem 240–360 mg/day +ASA/dip; or placebo + ASA/dip	Angio, clinical events	60%	36% diltiazem 32% placebo	NS
Whitworth (71)	241	R, DB, PC	nifedipine 10 mg tid + ASA 325 mg/day; or placebo +ASA 325 mg/day	Angio	82%	28% nifedipine 29.5% placebo	NS
Hoberg (72)	196	R, DB, PC	verapamil 240 mg bid + ASA 330 mg qd+ dipyridamole 75 mg bid; or placebo + ASA 330 mg qd + dipyridamole 75 mg bid	Angio	88%	48.3% verapamil 62.7% placebo excluding noncompliant Patients: 47.4% verapamil 63.9% placebo	$p = 0.059$ $p = 0.046$

[a]Restenosis rates are reported unless otherwise noted.

R = randomized; DB = double-blind; PC = placebo-controlled; ASA = aspirin; dip = dipyridamole; CCB = calcium channel blocker; qd = once daily; bid = twice daily; tid = three times daily; qid = four times daily.

2. *Carvedilol*

Carvedilol is a novel, multiple-action cardiovascular agent with combined alpha/beta-blocker activity and a variety of other pharmacological properties. Carvedilol has antiproliferative activity in vascular smooth muscle cell culture and in animal models of vascular injury. Carvedilol also possesses antioxidant activity (74–76). Carvedilol was evaluated in a randomized, double-blind placebo controlled trial in restenosis prevention after PTCA. Patients received carvedilol 12.5 mg or matching placebo on the evening before PTCA and then 25 mg bid or placebo for 6 months starting on the morning before PTCA. There were no significant differences in restenosis rates or in clinical events after 6 months of follow-up (77).

V. PAUSE FOR REFLECTION

The failure of virtually every clinical study utilizing pharmacological agents to show consistent and clinically accepted benefit in the prevention of restenosis is disappointing. Indeed, many more questions have been raised by these failures than have been answered. In the most rigorously designed clinical protocols, criticisms have still been voiced that drug concentrations were not high enough to inhibit the events that cause restenosis or that patients were dosed for an inadequate duration either prior to or following angioplasty. With few exceptions most studies were conducted in a way such that the effect of a specific single agent was evaluated, rather than a combination of agents with different targets. In part this approach has been utilized by pharmaceutical companies who need to evaluate their agent versus placebo or "standard" therapy. While this approach has its regulatory merits, it is extraordinarily naive when the complexity of the process of vascular remodeling and restenosis injury is considered. Given the interdependencies of so many of the factors identified to date and the redundancy of the processes to ensure healing in the human body, in general, and in the coronary vascular bed, in particular, the concept of a single "magic bullet" can no longer be justified as the goal of an intervention to prevent clinically relevant restenosis.

The failed results of such pharmacological agents to prevent restenosis in humans is also an indictment of the animal models utilized to evaluate such potential agents. Clearly no single model or even combination of models appears to have predictive value for any agent's effect in humans. The carotid artery models, the nonatherosclerotic coronary artery models, and the peripheral vascular models, while elegant, have not provided adequate insight into the mechanisms associated with restenosis in humans. If the mechanism of restenosis injury and vascular remodeling is inherently different in the human diseased coronary, the animal models may have led

Table 7 Other Therapies

Study	Patients (n)	Study design	Therapy	Endpoint	Follow-up (%)	Results[a]	p
Angiopeptin							
Emanuelson(73)	553	R, DB, PC	3 mg/24 h sc pre-PTCA + 1.5 mg bolus sc at PTCA + 6 mg/24 h sc ×4 days post-PTCA +ASA 150 mg/day; or placebo +ASA 150 mg/day	Angio, clinical events	76% angio; 100% clinical	Patients: 36% angiopeptin 37% placebo	NS
						Minimal luminal diameter: −0.31 mm angiopeptin −0.30 mm placebo	NS
Carvedilol							
Desmet (77)	203	R, DB, PC	carvedilol 25 mg bid; or placebo	Angio, clinical events	71	44% carvedilol 34% placebo	NS
						Minimal luminal diameter: −0.53 mm carvedilol −0.30 mm placebo	$p = 0.01$

[a]Restenosis rates are reported unless otherwise noted.

R = randomized; DB = double-blind; PC = placebo-controlled; ASA = aspiring; dip = dipyridamole; CCB = calcium channel blocker; qd = once daily; bid = twice daily; tid = three times daily; qid = four times daily.

to conclusions and theories that are not at all applicable to humans. The costs of conducting clinical trials are becoming prohibitive such that much greater scrutiny will be given to any result in animals before there is enthusiasm for using the agent in humans in the future.

Since trials are expensive to conduct, where possible, a surrogate marker representative of the pharmacology of the investigational drug has been utilized for the purpose of dose selection. In considering the GPIIb/IIIa inhibitors, for example, inhibition of platelet aggregation was the surrogate. ReoPro® amd Integrelin® are the two GPIIb/IIIa inhibitors for which trial results have been reported. In addition to differences in trial design, target population, and specificity of receptor inhibition between the two agents, there was a difference in the amount of platelet aggregation inhibited by the doses tested in the trials. The dose of ReoPro® was selected based upon >90% inhibition of platelet aggregation, while the Integrelin® dose achieved lower degrees of platelet aggregation. The one-month data suggest that ReoPro® is a more effective agent, as has been previously discussed. Similarly treatment with the c7E3 bolus and infusion resulted in less need for target vessel revascularization at 6 months (16.5 vs. 22.3%), while data with Integrelin were negative in effect on restenosis.

The greatest impact of the plethora of negative data from clinical trials to date has been on the basic assumptions underpinning the accepted theories of restenosis injury. Until recently the prevailing hypothesis has been that the pathogenesis of restenosis is the development of neointimal hyperplasia at the site of the local vessel injury. The obstructive neointima is considered largely the result of uncontrolled medial smooth muscle cell proliferation at the arterial injury site (80). The lesion is fibroproliferative with cellular elements and abundant extracellular matrix; notably lipid deposition is not present. The three sequential stages are to include activation of platelets and thrombin (Phase IA), release of biologically active mediators [e.g., thromboxane, serotonin, platelet-derived growth factor, epidermal growth factor, transforming growth factor-beta (TGF-β), etc.] (Phase IB), medial smooth muscle cell replication (Phase IIa), media smooth muscle cell migration (Phase IIb), and intimal smooth muscle cell proliferation (Phase IIIa), with extracellular matrix modulation and vascular remodeling (Phase IIIb) (80). It is upon this theory and its sequence of events that pharmacological interventions have been based and have generally failed.

Thus, alternative theories have emerged (81,82). Less emphasis is being placed on smooth muscle cell proliferation and more attention on the role of the matrix and matrix metalloproteinases and their role in shaping the matrix. As pointed out by Schwartz et al. (81), the cellular components constitute only approximately 11% of neointimal volume; the rest is extracellular matrix. A leading alternative theory suggests that the fibrin matrix that results from endothelial damage from angioplasty is colonized by neointimal cells; that is, the fibrin matrix is laid down first, and into this matrix smooth muscle cells migrate, but they do not contribute significantly to the volume of restenotic lesion. If emerging data continue to support this theory, there will be major alterations in the approaches that have been considered to prevent restenosis.

VI. FUTURE CONSIDERATIONS

The angioplasty procedure is fairly violent with respect to the damage caused to the artery. As angiographers strive to create the largest luminal diameter during the procedure, greater damage will be done to the artery. The artery undergoes a reparative process, and every patient who undergoes angioplasty will have some degree of "restenosis." The goal of any therapeutic intervention should not be to stop the reparative process, but to attenuate the extent to which the reparative process results in a clinically relevant decrease in luminal diameter to cause ischemia. To date the risk of interference with the arterial repair process has been conjectural, primarily because no agent has worked. However, as advances allow more accurate and complete inhibition of coronary arterial healing, the risks of such intervention may become apparent. In the CAVEAT study (83), a trend toward an increased incidence of late sudden death after directional atherectomy may be explained by medial weakening as a result of partial resection and rupture of the vessel. There are no data to support this; nonetheless, it is important that such potential for negative outcomes be evaluated as much as positive outcomes in both animal experiments and clinical trials.

A. Local Delivery: Catheter-Related Delivery Systems

Because of concerns that systemic administration of drugs to prevent restenosis prevented the use of doses high enough to achieve local effect at the angioplasty site (59,60), a good deal of interest has been directed at the development of local delivery systems and technologies. The proof of concept for this approach has been demonstrated in a number of animal studies where polymers or reservoirs have been implanted on the exterior of the vessel wall (84–86). In effect the agent used diffused from the adventitia to the media and neointima. These techniques are not feasible in clinical medicine but did support further evaluation of local delivery from the lumen. Although direct application of an agent to the angioplasty site seems straightforward, it has become apparent that it is not. Very detailed reviews of the area have recently been published (87,88).

Local delivery balloon catheters appear to be the primary initiative, with three general types currently being evaluated. First, the Wolinsky perforated-balloon catheter (USCI Division of C.R. Bard, Inc.) has a number of 25-μm laser-drilled holes into a noncompliant balloon. As the balloon is inflated, the test drug flows out of holes (89). However, significant vascular trauma due to the jet stream of the test agent has been observed (90), in addition to inconsistent drug delivery due to blockage of the holes.

A second approach has been the microporous balloon (Cordis Corporation), which is characterized by a membrane surrounding the balloon with thousands of pores from which the test agent can exude. Several other catheters (Cardiovascular Dynamics, Sci Med Life Systems, Inc.) contain balloons, other than the one used for the angioplasty, that allow direct delivery at low flow rates to avert vascular trauma. The Dispatch® delivery catheter (Sci Med Life Systems, Inc.) functions as a temporary stent for periods up to 1 h, thus allowing a prolonged opportunity for drug delivery without impeding coronary blood flow.

The third approach has been to coat the angioplasty balloon with a layer of hydrophilic polyacrylic acid polymer (Hydrogel®, Boston Scientific Corporation) (91). The test agent becomes embedded into the vessel wall as the balloon is inflated. This technique circumvents to some extent the problem that may be inherent in the test agent to prevent prolonged residence time at the site of injury. Regardless of the technique utilized, however, the solubility of the test agent, its molecular size, its charge characteristics, and the presence of binding/receptor sites within the wall of the vessel will determine the duration of the local availability of the agent.

B. Biodegradable and Coated Stents

Metallic intracoronary stents have become widely accepted in clinical practice, and a number of studies have demonstrated their good tolerability and clinical outcome (92–94). It seems only natural then to consider placement of stents that are coated with a test agent to prevent clotting and restenosis. Since the need for a stent may be short-lived, biodegradable stents embedded with test agents are being considered and appear promising (95). Since the stent tends to be discontinuous and webbed in its appearance, the application of the test agent may be inconsistently applied over the surface of the lesion unless the test agent is very potent and diffuses well onto the vascular surface. The test agent will need to be stable in the vascular milieu for some prolonged period of time. Furthermore, the stent needs to be biocompatible to avoid creating an inflammatory response (96). To circumvent this problem, investigators from the Mayo Clinic have reported the use of a fibrin-coated tantalum coil stent (97). This stent is intended to be inert and act as a synthetic mural thrombus. In theory, thrombosis and smooth muscle cell prolilferation will be limited. While animal studies look encouraging, it will be interesting to see if it is equally effective in humans.

C. Facilitated Delivery

To enhance arterial delivery after local application, other techniques are being considered. Electroporation is a technique to create transient pores on all plasmalemma using pulsed electrical fields. The purpose of this approach would be to load a variety of different size molecules at high concentration directly into the cytoplasm (98). Another technique has been via iontophoresis, a process by which a charged test agent is transported across an electrical gradient established by an electrode catheter placed within the coronary artery (99). Early experience with iontophoresis in the dermatological application of drugs had resulted in direct damage to the skin, although recent experience is more encouraging (100).

Using technology developed for transdermal delivery of drugs, some investigators have utilized biodegradable mircospheres embedded with the test agent. The test agent diffuses through the pores and as the microspheres degrade (101,102). This approach enhances the test agent residence time at the angioplasty site. One report was able to document the presence of a fluorescent marker at the site for 4 weeks after application of the microspheres; in the absence of the microspheres the fluorescent marker disappeared after 72 h (103).

Yet another approach has recently been reported in the *Proceedings of the National Academy of Science* (104). Investigators utilized a nonionized, highly hydrated material (a hydrogel) to develop a resorbable, conformal barrier upon arterial surfaces in situ. This barrier is designed to block contact of blood with the vessel wall and thus block platelet deposition and thrombosis upon subendothelial tissues. This barrier virtually eliminated thrombosis in injured arteries in two animal models. The hydrogel could also be used as a vehicle containing other substances to prevent thrombosis and restenosis.

D. Miscellaneous Intraluminal Approaches

While the concept of local delivery seems to have focused on the delivery of a pharmacological agent, local applications of nonpharmacological agents have recently been proposed. Fischell et al. (105) have investigated the use of a 32P-impregnated titanium "stent" wire, which emits beta-particles to inhibit vascular smooth muscle cell and endothelial cell proliferation. While the studies were conducted in vitro, application to animal models is expected.

Another approach to inhibit smooth muscle cell growth has been to utilize the angioplasty catheter to provide ultraviolet light in order to inhibit smooth muscle cell growth (Restenosis Resistant Angioplasty™ Ultraviolet Light System; Angiomedics and SCIMED Life Systems, Inc.). The approach was reported by the company in a press release, and very little is known about this technology at this time.

E. Gene Therapy

Of all the interventions for restenosis that have been considered, the most intriguing and probably the most difficult to accomplish is gene therapy. The ability to genetically modify the response of the damaged coronary artery could be one of the first applications of gene therapy in humans. Some of the problems that have plagued application of gene therapy to the treatment of chronic diseases such as cystic fibrosis are not as great an issue in the rather acute disease state of vascular damage due to angioplasty. The techniques that have been recently considered include the use of naked DNA, liposomes, and retroviral and adenoviral vectors.

In the late 1980s, the application of gene therapy to vascular injury was to seed the vasculature with cells that had been transfected with a desired gene (106,107). These cells expressed and secreted the designated gene product. It was very well demonstrated by several investigators that vascular endothelial or smooth muscle cells transduced in vitro colonized the various layers of the arterial wall following reintroduction into the vasculature through balloons or stents. In theory these cells could be engineered to produce substances to block the various phases of arterial wall repair following angioplasty. Since heterologous sources of cells would need to be used, concerns about immunogenicity, longevity, and contamination have to be considered when applying this technology (80).

Technologies designed to deliver the genetic material directly to the target tissue without utilizing cellular vectors are being aggressively explored. The mechanisms by which this transfer of genetic material could be transferred include (1) in vivo gene transfer by infusion of naked DNA or antisense oligonucleotides (108,109), (2) use of cationic liposomes containing the DNA (108,110), (3) transport by hybrid liposomes containing viral coat particles as those from the hemagglutinating virus of Japan (111), or (4) via viral vectors using retro- or adenoviruses (110,112,113).

All of these approaches hold much promise, but much of the enthusiasm for these approaches has been promulgated by the publication of the successful experiments; the number of failures is unknown since data of this sort are generally not published. Aside from the potential problems of gene therapy (i.e., safety concerns, specifically extent and regulation of gene expression, etc.), there is the whole issue of which genes should be delivered to the arterial cells at the site of the angioplasty. In recent years the target, in keeping with the restenosis hypothesis, has been smooth muscle cells in order to prevent their proliferation. However, as the prevailing theory of restenosis injury is reexamined, a number of other targets have emerged including those involved in platelet adherence and aggregation, thrombus formation, penetration of inflammatory cells and production of their mediators, elaboration of a whole series of other mediators of tissue remodeling (i.e., TGF-β, basic fibroblast growth factor, etc.) and matrix production, and vascular remodeling. Will inhibition of any one of these targets be adequate, or will the delivered genetic "soup" need to contain a variety of genetic messages to cause a significant inhibition of restenosis?

Antisense technology may have less of the technological hurdles and potential safety problems than viral vector therapy; however, two recent reviews of the field raise considerable concern about both the specificity and consistency of directed antisense therapy in animals (114,115). Moreover the technology may not be as specific as originally conceived, since antisense oligodeoxynucleotides may cause degradation of both targeted and nontargeted mRNA (116).

Restenosis injury is a prime target for the experimental application of gene therapy. The application of this technology to this disease state is rational and promising, but many problems need to be addressed and solved for it to have clinical application in humans. An important issue that is usually never discussed in the published literature is the need to keep the cost of this type of therapy reasonable, particularly if results of clinical trials are not overwhelmingly positive. The full potential for this therapy will not be realized until there is firm understanding of the molecular mechanisms responsible for the development of restenosis in humans.

F. Pharmacological Intervention

Virtually any drug that appears to have direct or indirect antiproliferative properties in vitro or in animal models is being considered for potential use in restenosis injury including SCHAI-1 (Sheffield Medical Technologies), an agent being tested in Kaposi's sarcoma, hydroxycarbazole compounds (SmithKline Beecham/Boehringer Ingelheim), which may inhibit smooth muscle migration and proliferation, and Taxol (Bristol-Myers Squibb). Studies in rats have shown that Taxol has the ability to induce stable and nonfunctional chains of microtubules at doses 100 times lower than those used in cancer chemotherapy (117). A press release from Japan's Kissei Pharmaceuticals indicates that tranilast, which is currently marketed as an antiallergy agent in Japan, has shown significant benefit in preventing restenosis (14.7%) when compared to the control group (46.5%) in blood vessels following myocardial infarction (118). Details of this study are unknown, and further information is needed to interpret the implications of this study.

Despite the negative result obtained with lovastatin, both investigators in Japan and the United States continue to pursue lipid lowering as a means to reduce stenosis (45,119). Using low-denisty lipoprotein (LDL) apheresis on a dextran sulfate cellulose column, Daida et al. (119) reduced both plasma Lp(a) and LDL cholesterol levels. The rational for this approach comes from the proposal that Lp(a) may play a role in causing restenosis through its suppression of fibrolytic activity. In this study restenosis rates were lower when Lp(a) was reduced by greater than 50% of baseline. However, the study was small ($n = 66$ patients). Similar investigations are currently being conducted in both the United States and Europe. Larger trials will need to be undertaken to understand the impact of this approach.

The impact that ReoPro®, the GPIIb/IIIa inhibitor, appears to have on restenosis injury has caused cautious optimism about the impact that other cell adhesion molecules may have in this arena. A recent report from Austria demonstrated elevations in sELAM-1, sL-selectin, and IL-8 levels following PTCA with a positive correlation noted between these parameters and the number of dilations (120). Following angioplasty, the endothelium is activated to express the adhesion molecules ICAM-1, E-selectin, P-selectin, and VCAM-1. Macrophages and fibroblasts migrate into the injury site by means of this enhancement of integrins (121). Future therapies that inhibit the action of the integrins, perhaps in concert with a vitronectin-inhibiting GPIIb/IIIa inhibitor, may attenuate the restenosis process early in its inception.

Taking a cue from cancer chemotherapy tactics and experimental transplant strategies, investigators have considered the use of a recombinant chimeric toxin to prevent restenosis. In brief, a gene encoding a ligand is fused to a mutant toxin gene, such as the *Pseudomonas* exotoxin. The chimeric toxin expressed by this fusion gene specifically targets those cells with cell surface receptors recognizing the ligand. Once enveloped into the cell, the cytotoxic effect is delivered, and cell death ensues (122). This technology has been applied to specific ligands (cytokine interleukin-2, epidermal growth factor, and basic fibroblast growth factor) to result in reduced smooth muscle cell proliferation (123–125). From a clinical perspective this approach is more worrisome than other approaches primarily because the events result in cellular death. If the technique is not exceedingly specific, the vessel could be at risk for aneurysm development. Moreover, cellular death could result in worsening inflammatory response and thus negate the potential benefit of such an approach.

VII. CONCLUSION

While there is considerable speculation about future interventions, the evidence to date for successful intervention in the prevention of restenosis is truly damning: more than 56 clinical trials have been conducted in an effort to evaluate therapies that, at the time, seemed to be very good candidates to prevent restenosis injury. All results have been negative. The sole exception may be ReoPro®, but the data from the clinical trials were inferential, based upon clinical outcomes, rather than on direct demonstration of reduced restenosis angiographically. The uptake of ReoPro® by cardiologists in the United States has been very slow, probably for a number of reasons (cost, risk/benefit ratio, etc.). Yet therapies that have not been shown to be of any benefit in clinical trials continue to be prescribed. Aspirin, calcium channel blockers, and dipyridamole, for example, continue to be used in "standard" therapy. An effective agent or intervention to prevent restenosis remains a great unmet need in clinical medicine.

REFERENCES

1. Hermans WRM, Rensing BJ, Strauss BH, Serruys PW. Prevention of restenosis after percutaneous transluminal coronary angioplasty: the search for a "magic bullet." Am Heart J 1991; 122:171–187.
2. Franklin SM, Faxon DP. Pharmacologic prevention of restenosis after coronary angioplasty: review of the randomized clinical trials. Coronary Artery Dis 1993; 4:232–242.
3. Pepine CJ. Restenosis after angioplasty. Proc Annu Meet Med Sect Am Counc Life Insur 1991; 77–84.
4. Califf RM, Fortin DF, Frid DJ, Harlan WR, Ohman EM, Bengston JR, Nelson CL, Tcheng JE, Mark DB, Stack RS. Restenosis after coronary angioplasty: an overview. J Am Coll Cardiol 1991; 17:2B–13B.
5. Blackshear JL, O'Callaghan WG, Califf RM. Medical approaches to prevention of restenosis after coronary angioplasty. J Am Coll Cardiol 1987; 9:834–848.
6. Rensing BJ, Hermans WRM, Vos J, Tijssen JGP, Rutch W, Danchin N, Heyndrickx GR, Mast G, Wijns W, Serruys PW. Luminal narrowing after percutaneous transluminal coronary angioplasty. A study of clinical, procedural, and lesional factors related to long-term angiographic outcome. Circulation 1993; 88:975–985.
7. Holmes DR, Vlietstra RE, Smith HC, Vetrovec GW, Kent KM, Cowley MJ, Faxon DP, Greuntzig AR, Kelsey SF, Detre KM, Van Raden J, Mock MB. Restenosis after percutaneous transluminal coronary angioplasty (PTCA): a report from the PTCA registry of the National Heart, Lung, and Blood Institute. Am J Cardiol 1984; 53:77C–81C.
8. Serruys PW, Luijten HE, Beatt KJ, Geuskens R, De Feyter PJ, Van Den Brand M, Reiber JHC, Ten Katen HJ, Van ES GA, Hugenholtz PG. Incidence of restenosis after successful coronary angioplasty: a time-related phenomenon. Circulation 1988; 77:361–371.

9. Kalbfleisch SJ, McGillem MJ, Pinto IMF, Kavanaugh KM, DeBoe SF, Mancini J. Comparison of automated quantitative coronary angiography with caliper measurements of percent diameter stenosis. Am J Cardiol 1990; 65:1181–1184.
10. Finci L, Meier B, Steffenino G, Rutishauser W. Aspirin versus placebo after coronary angioplasty for prevention of restenosis (abstract). Eur Heart J 1988; 9:156.
11. Taylor RR, Gibbons FA, Cope GD, Cumpston GN, Mews GC, Luke P. Effects of low-dose aspirin on restenosis after coronary angioplasty. Am J Cardiol 1991; 68:874–878.
12. Schwartz L, Bourassa MG, Lesperance J, Aldridge HE, Kazim F, Salvatori VA, Henderson M, Bonan R, David PR. Aspirin and dipyridamole in the prevention of restenosis after percutaneous transluminal coronary angioplasty. N Engl J Med 1988; 318:1714–1719.
13. Chesebro JH, Webster MWI, Reeder GS, Mock MB, Grill DE, Bailey KR, Steichen S, Fuster V. Coronary angioplasty: antiplatelet therapy reduces acute complications but not restenosis (abstract). Circulation 1989; 80(suppl II): II–64.
14. Mufson L, Black A, Roubin G, Wilenz J, Mead S, MacFarland K, Weintraub W, Douglas JS, King SB. A randomized trial of aspirin in PTCA: Effect of high vs low dose aspirin on major complications and restenosis (abstract). J Am Coll Cardiol 1988; 11:236A.
15. Dykmans J, Thonnes W, Ozbek C, Muller M, Bach R, Schwerdt H, Sen S, Schieffer H, Bette L. High vs low dosage of acetylic salicylic acid for prevention of restenosis after successful PTCA. Preliminary results of a randomized trial (abstract). Eur Heart J 1988; 9:58.
16. Schanzenbacher P, Grimmer M, Maisch B, Koschsiek K. Effect of high dose and low dose aspirin on restenosis after primary successful angioplasty (abstract). Circulation 1989; 80:II–99.
17. White CW, Knudson M, Schmidt D, Chisholm RJ, Vandormael M, Morton B, Roy L, Khaja F, Reitman M. Neither ticlopidine nor aspirin-dipyridamole prevents restenosis post PTCA: results from a randomized placebo-controlled multicenter trial (abstract). Circulation 1987; 77:IV–213.
18. Kitazume H, Kubo I, Iwama T, Ageishi Y, Suzuki A. Combined use of aspirin, ticlopidine and nicorandil prevented restenosis after coronary angioplasty (abstract). Circulation 1988; 78:II–633.
19. Gershlick AH, Spriggins D, Davies SW, Syndercombe-Court YD, Timmins J, Timmis AD, Rothman MT, Layton C, Balcon R. Failure of epoprostenol (prostacyclin, PGI_2) to inhibit platelet aggregation and to prevent restenosis after coronary angioplasty: results of a randomized placebo controlled trial. Br Heart J 1994; 71:7–15.
20. Knudtson ML, Flintoft VF, Roth DL, Hansen JL, Duff HJ. Effect of short-term prostacyclin administration on restenosis after percutaneous transluminal coronary angioplasty. J Am Coll Cardiol 1990; 15:691-697.
21. Hattori R, Kodama K, Takatsu F, Yui Y, Kawai C. Randomized trial of a

selective inhibitor of thromboxane A2 synthase (E)-7-(3-pyridyl)-6-heptenoic acid (CV-4151), for prevention of restenosis after coronary angioplasty. Jpn Circ J 1991; 55:324–329.
22. Feldman RL, Bengston JR, Pryor DB, Zimmerman MB. The GRASP study: use of a thromboxane A2 receptor blocker to reduce advese clinical events after coronary angioplasty (abstract). J Am Coll Cardiol 1992; 19:259A.
23. Serruys PW, Rutsch W, Heyndrickx GR, Danchin N, Mast G, Wijns W, Rensing BJ, Vos J, Stibbe J for the Coronary Artery Restenosis Prevention on Repeated Thromboxane-Antagonism study group (CARPORT). Prevention of restenosis after percutaneous transluminal coronary angioplasty with thromboxane A_2-receptor blockade: a randomized, double-blind, placebo-controlled trial. Circulation 1991; 84:1568–1580.
24. Savage MP, Goldberg S, Macdonald RG, Bass TA, Margolis JR, Whitworth HB, Taussig AS, Vetrovec G, Cowley M, Bove AA, Kleaveland P, Hirshfeld JW, Hill JA, Gilmore P, Pepine CJ. Multi-Hospital Eastern Atlantic Restenosis Trial II: A placebo-controlled trial of thromboxane blockade in the prevention of restenosis following coronary angioplasty. Am Heart J 1991; 122:1239–1244.
25. Bove A, Savage M, Deutsch E, Macdonald R, Bass T, Vetrovec G, Whitworth H, Cowley M, Goldberg S, Margolis J, Hill J, Hirshfeld J, Granett J, Pepine C for the M-HEART investigators (abstract). J Am Coll Cardiol 1992; 19:259A.
26. Reiss H, Holfing B, von Arnim T, Hiller E. Thromboxane receptor blockade versus cyclooxigenase inhibition: Antiplatelet effects in patients. Thromb Res 1986; 42:235–245.
27. Klein W, Eber B, Dusleag J, Rotman B, Koltringer P, Luha O, Vanhoutte PM. Ketanserin prevents early restenosis following percutaneous transluminal coronary angioplasty. Clin Physiol Biochem 1990; 8(suppl 3):101–107.
28. Serruys PW, Klein W, Tijssen JPG, Rutsch W, Heyndrickx GR, Emanuelson H, Ball SG, Decoster O, Schroeder E, Liberman H, Eichhorn E, Willerson JT, Anderson HV, Khaja F, Alexander RW, Baim D, Melkert R, van Oene JC, Van Gool R. Evaluation of ketanserin in the prevention of restenosis after percutaneous coronary angioplasty. A multicenter randomized double-blind placebo-controlled trial. Circulation 1993; 88:1588–1601.
29. Okamoto S, Inden M, Setsuda M, Konishi T, Nakano T. Effects of trapidil (triazolopyrimidine), a platelet-derived growth factor antagonist, in preventing restenosis after percutaneous transluminal angioplasty. Am Heart J 1992; 123:1439–1444.
30. Nishikawa H, Ono N, Motoyasu M, Aoki T, Shimizu Y, Fukui A, Kakuta Y, Nakano T. Preventive effects of trapidil (PDGF antagonist) on restenosis after PTCA (abstract). Circulation 1992; 86:I–53.
31. Maresta A, Balducelli M, Cantini L, Casari A, Chioin R, Fabbri M, Fontanelli A, Monici PPA, Repetto S, De Servi S, et al. Trapidil (triazolopyrimidine), a platelet-derived growth factor antagonist, reduces restenosis after percutaneous transluminal coronary angioplasty. Results of the randomized, double-blind STARC study. Studio Trapidil versus Asirin nella Restenosi Coronarica. Circulation 1994; 90:2710–2715.

32. Thornton MA, Gruentzig AR, Hollman J, King SB, Douglas JS. Coumadin and aspirin in prevention of recurrence after transluminal coronary angioplasty: a randomized study. Circulation 1984; 69:721–727.
33. Urban P, Buller N, Fox K, Shapiro L, Bayliss J, Rickards A. Lack of effect of warfarin on the restenosis rate or on clinical outcome after balloon coronary angioplasty. Br Heart J 1988; 60:485–488.
34. Ellis SG, Roubin GS, Wilentz J, Douglas JS, King SB. Effect of 18- to 24-hour heparin administration for prevention of restenosis after uncomplicated coronary angioplasty. Am Heart J 1989; 117:777–782.
35. Schmid KM, Preisack M, Voelker W, Sujatta M, Karsch KR. First clinical experience with low molecular weight heparin LU 47311 (Reviparin) for prevention of restenosis after percutaneous transluminal coronary angioplasty. Semin Thromb Hemost 1993; 19(suppl 1):155–159.
36. Amann FW, Neuenschwander C, Meyer BJ. Fraxiparin for prevention of restenosis after percutaneous coronary angioplasty. Semin Thromb Hemost 1993; 19(suppl 1):160–163.
37. Faxon D, Spiro T, Minor S, Douglas J, Cote G, Dorosti K, Gottlieb R, Califf R, Topol E, Gordon J. Enoxaprin, a low molecular weight heparin, in the prevention of restenosis after angioplasty: results of a double blind randomized trial (abstract). J Am Coll Cardiol 1992; 19:158A.
38. Topol EJ, Califf RM, Weisman HF, Ellis SG, Tcheng JE, Worley S, Ivanhoe R, George BS, Fintel D, Weston M, Sigmon K, Anderson KM, Lee KL, Willerson JT on behalf of the EPIC investigators. Randomised trial of coronary intervention with antibody against platelet IIb/IIIa integrin for reduction of clinical restenosis: results at six months. Lancet 1994; 343:881–886.
39. Cor Therapeutics announces preliminary results of phase III clinical trial of Integrelin. Hoover NewsAlert Article. Dow Jones News Service, June 14, 1995, 7:47 am.
40. Sahni R, Maniet AR, Voci G, Banka VS. Prevention of restenosis by lovastatin after successful coronary angioplasty. Am Heart J 1991; 121:1600–1608.
41. Weintraub WS, Boccuzzi SJ, Klein JL, Kosinski AS, King SB, Ivanhoe R. Cedarholm JC, Stillabower ME, Talley JD, Demaio SJ, O'Neill WW, Frazier JE, Cohen-Bernstein CL, Robbins DC, Brown CL, Alexander RW for the Lovastatin Restenosis Trial Group. Lack of effect of lovastatin on restenosis after coronary angioplasty. N Engl J Med 1994; 331:1331–1337.
42. Onaka H, Hirota Y, Kita Y, Tsuji R, Ishii K, Ishimura T, Kawamura K. The effect of pravastatin on prevention of restenosis after successful percutaneous transluminal coronary angioplasty. Jpn Circ J 1994; 58:100–106.
43. Foley DP, Bonnier H, Jackson G, Macaya C, Shepherd J, Vrolix M, Serruys PW. Prevention of restenosis after coronary balloon angioplasty: FLARE Trial. Am J Cardiol 1994; 73:50D–61D.
44. Setsuda M, Inden M, Hiraoka N, Okamoto S, Tanaka H, Okinaka T, Nishimura Y, Okano H, Kouji T, Konishi T, Nakano T. Probucol therapy in the prevention of restenosis after successful percutaneous transluminal coronary angioplasty. Clin Ther 1993; 15:374–382.
45. Yamaguchi H, Lee YJ, Daida H, Yokoi H, Miyano H, Kanoh T, Ishiwata S,

Kato K, Nishikawa H, Takatsu F, Kutsumi Y, Mokuno H, Yamada N, Noma A. Effectiveness of LDL-apheresis in preventing restenosis after percutaneous transluminal coronary angioplasty (PTCA): LDL apheresis angioplasty restenosis trial (L-ART). Chem Phys Lip 1994; 67/68:399–403.
46. Bairati I, Roy L, Meyer F. Double-blind, randomized, controlled trial of fish oil supplements in prevention of recurrence of stenosis after coronary angioplasty. Circulation 1992; 85:950–956.
47. Reis GJ, Sipperly ME, McCabe CH, Sacks FM, Boucher TM, Silverman DI, Baim DS, Grossman W, Pasternak RC. Randomized trial of fish oil for prevention of restenosis after coronary angioplasty. Lancet 1989; 2:177–181.
48. Grigg LE, Kay TWH, Valentine PA, Larkins R, Flower DJ, Manolas EG, O'Dea K, Sinclair AJ, Hopper JL, Hunt D. Determinants of restenosis and lack of effect of dietary supplementation with eicosapentaenoic acid on the incidence of coronary artery restenosis after angioplasty. J Am Coll Cardiol 1989; 13:665–672.
49. Franzen D, Schannwell M, Oette K, Hopp HW. A prospective, randomized, and double-blind trial on the effect of fish oil on the incidence of restenosis following PTCA. Cathet Cardiovasc Diagn 1993; 28:301–310.
50. Milner MR, Gallino RA, Lefffingwell A, Pichard AD, Brooks-Robinson S, Rosenberg J, Little T, Lindsay J. Usefulness of fish oil supplements in preventing clinical evidence of restenosis after percutaneous transluminal coronary angioplasty. Am J Cardiol 1989; 64:294–299.
51. Dehmer GJ, Popma JJ, Van Den Berg EK, Eichhorn EJ, Prewitt JB, Campbell WB, Jennings L, Willerson JT, Schmitz JM. Reduction in the rate of early restenosis after coronary angioplasty by a diet supplemented with n-3 fatty acids. N Engl J Med 1988; 319:733–740.
52. Kaul U, Sanghvi S, Bahl VK, Dev V, Wasir HS. Fish oil supplements for prevention of restenosis after coronary angioplasty. Int J Cardiol 1992; 35:87–93.
53. Nye ER, Ablett MB, Robertson MC, Ilsley CD, Sutherland WHF. Effect of eicosapentaenoic acid on restenosis rate, clinical course and blood lipids in patients after percutaneous transluminal angioplasty. Aust NZJ Med 1990; 20:549–552.
54. Powell JS, Clozel JP, Muller RKM, Kuhn H, Hefti F, Hosang M, Baumgartner HR. Inhibitors of angiotensin-converting enzyme prevent myointimal proliferation after vascular injury. Science 1989; 245:186–188.
55. Powell JS, Muller RKM, Rouge M, Kuhn H, Hefti F, Baumgartner HR. The proliferative response to vascular injury is suppressed by angiotensin-converting enzyme inhibition. J Cardiovasc Pharmacol 1990; 16(suppl 1):S42–S49.
56. Powell JS, Muller RKM, Baumgartner HR. Suppression of the vascular response to injury: The role of angiotensin-converting enzyme inhibitors. J Am Coll Cardiol 1991; 17:137B–142B.
57. Kaul U, Chandra S, Bahl VK, Sharma S, Wasir HS. Enalapril for prevention of restenosis after coronary angioplasty. Indian Heart J 1993; 45:469–473.
58. Desmet W, Vrolix M, De Scheerder I, Van Lierde J, Willems JL, Piessens J.

Angiotensin-converting enzyme inhibition with fosinopril sodium in the prevention of restenosis after coronary angioplasty. Circulation 1994; 89:385–392.
59. MERCATOR study group. Does the new angiotensin converting enzyme inhibitor cilazapril prevent restenosis after percutaneous transluminal coronary angioplasty? Results of the MERCATOR study: a multicenter, randomized, double-blind placebo-controlled trial. Circulation 1992; 86:100–110.
60. Faxon DP on behalf of the MARCATOR study group. Effect of high dose angiotensin-converting enzyme inhibition on restenosis: Final results of the MARCATOR study, a multicenter, double-blind, placebo-controlled trial of cilazapril. J Am Coll Cardiol 1995; 25:362–369.
61. Kaufman RF, Bean JS, Zimmerman KM, Brown RF, Steinberg MI. Losartan, a nonpeptide angiotensin II (ang II) receptor antagonist, inhibits neointima formation following balloon injury to rat carotid arteries. Life Sci 1991; 49:223–228.
62. Prescott MF, Webb RL, Reidy MA. Angiotensin-converting enzyme inhibitor versus angiotensin II, AT1 receptor antagonist. Effects on smooth muscle cell migration and proliferation after balloon catheter injury. Am J Pathol 1991; 139:1291–1296.
63. Azuma H, Niimi Y, Hamasaki H. Prevention of intimal thickening after endothelial removal by a nonpeptide angiotensin II receptor antagonist, losartan. Br J Pharmacol 1992; 106:665–671.
64. Grines CL, Rizik D, Levine A, Schreiber T, Gangadharan V, Ramos R, Choski N, Gangadharan C, Timmis GC. Colchicine angioplasty restenosis trial (CART) (abstract). Circulation 1991; 84:II–365.
65. O'Keefe JH, McCallister BD, Bateman TM, Kuhnlein DL, Ligon RW, Hartzler GO. Ineffectiveness of colchicine for the prevention of restenosis after coronary angioplasty. J Am Coll Cardiol 1992; 19:1597–1600.
66. Pepine CJ, Hirshfeld JW, Macdonald RG, Henderson MA, Bass TA, Goldberg S, Savage MP, Vetrovec G, Cowley M, Taussig AS, Whitworth HB, Margolis JR, Hill JA, bove AA, Jugo R. A controlled trial of corticosteroids to prevent restenosis after coronary angioplasty. Circulation 1990; 81:1753–1761.
67. Stone GW, Rutherford BD, McConahy DR, Johnson WL, Giorgi LV, Ligon RW, Hartzler GO. A randomized trial of corticosteroids for the prevention of restenosis in 102 patients undergoing repeat coronary angioplasty. Cathet Cardiovasc Diagn 1989; 18:227–231.
68. Hirayama A, Nanto S, Ohara T, Nishida K, Okuyama, Kodama K. Preventive effect on restenosis after PTCA by ebselen: a newly synthesized anti-inflammatory agent (abstract). J Am Coll Cardiol 1992; 19:259A.
69. Corcos T, David PR, Guiteras P, Renkin J, Dangoisse V, Rapold HG, Bourassa MG. Failure of diltiazem to prevent restenosis after percutaneous coronary angioplasty. Am Heart J 1985; 109:926–931.
70. O'Keefe JH, Giorgi LV, Hartzler GO, Good TH, Ligon RW, Webb DL, McCallister BD. Effects of diltiazem on complications and restenosis after coronary angioplasty. Am J Cardiol 1991; 67:373–376.
71. Whitworth HB, Roubin GS, Hollman J, Meier B, Leimgruber PP, Douglas JS,

King SB, Gruentzig AR. Effect of nifedipine on recurrent stenosis after percutaneous transluminal coronary angioplasty. J Am Coll Cardiol 1986; 8:1271–1276.
72. Hoberg E, Dietz R, Frees U, Katus HA, Rauch B, Schomig A, Schuler G, Schwartz F, Tillmanns H, Niebauer J, Kubler W. Verapamil treatment after coronary angioplasty in patients at high risk of recurrent stenosis. Br Heart J 1994; 71:254–260.
73. Emanuelsson H, Beatt KJ, Bagger JP, Balcon R, Heikkila J, Piessens J, Schaeffer M, Suryapranata H, Foegh M. Long-term effects of angiopeptin treatment in coronary angioplasty. reduction of clinical events but not angiographic restenosis. Circulation 1995; 91:1689–1696.
74. Yue TL, Cheng HY, Lysko PG, McKenna PJ, Feuerstein R, Gu JL, Lysko KA, Davis LL, Feuerstein G. Carvedilol, a new vasodilator and beta adrenoceptor antagonist, is an antioxidant and free radical scavenger. J Pharmacol Exp Ther 1992; 263:92–98.
75. Ohlstein EH, Douglas SA, Sung CP, Yue TL, Louden C, Arleth A, Poste G, Ruffolo RR, Feuerstein GZ. Carvedilol, a cardiovascular drug, prevents vascular smooth muscle cell proliferation, migration, and neointimal formation following vascular injury. Proc Natl Acad Sci USA 1993; 90:6189–6193.
76. Sung CP, Arleth AJ, Ohlstein EH. Carvedilol inhibits vascular smooth muscle cell proliferation. J Cardiovasc Pharmacol 1993; 21:221–227.
77. Desmet W, De Scheerder I, Emaneulsson H, Hjalmarsson A, Piessens J. Carvedilol in the prevention of restenosis after coronary angioplasty. Circulation in press.
78. Epic Investigators. Use of a monoclonal antibody directed against the platelet glycoprotein IIb/IIIa receptor in high-risk coronary angioplasty. N Engl J Med 1994; 330:956–61.
79. Jang Y, Lincoff M, Plow EF, Topol EJ. Cell adhesion molecules in coronary artery disease. J Am Coll Cardiol 1994; 7:1591–601.
80. Lee PC, Gibbons GH, Dzau VJ. Cellular and molecular mechanisms of coronary artery restenosis. Coron Artery Dis 1993; 4:254–259.
81. Schwartz RS, Holmes DR, Topol EJ. The restenosis paradigm revisited: An alternative proposal for cellular mechanisms. J Am Coll Cardiol 1992; 20:1284–93.
82. Casscells W, Engler D, Willerson JT. Mechanisms of restenosis. Tex Heart Inst J 1994; 21:68–77.
83. Topol EJ, Leya F, Pinkerton CA, Whitlow PL, Hofling B, Semonton CA, Masden RR, Serruys PW, Leon MB, Williams DO, King SBI, Mark DB, Isner JM, Holmes DRJ, Ellis SG, Lee KL, Keeler G, Berdan LG, Hinohara T, Califf RM, on behalf of the CAVEAT Study Group. A comparison of coronary angioplasty with directional atherectomy in patients with coronary artery disease. N Engl J Med 1993; 329:221–227.
84. Edelman ER, Adams DH, Karnovsky MJ. Effect of controlled adventitial heparin delivery on smooth muscle cell proliferation following endothelial injury. Proc Natl Acad Sci USA 1990; 87:3773–3777.
85. Simons M, Edeman ER, DeKeyser JL, Langer R, Rosenberg RD. Antisense

c-myb oligonucleotides inhibit intimal arterial smooth muscle cell accumulation in vivo. Nature 1992; 359:67–70.
86. Villa AE, Guzman LA, Chen W, Golomb G, Levy RJ, Topol EJ. Local delivery of dexamethasone for prevention of neointimal proliferation in a rat model of balloon angioplasty. J Clin Invest 1994; 93:1243–1249.
87. Lincoff AM, Topol EJ, Ellis SG. Local drug delivery for the prevention of restenosis: Fact, fancy, future. Circulation 1994; 4:2070–84.
88. Sigwart U. Coronary stents for the prevention of restenosis. Restenosis Summit VII, Cleveland, Ohio, May 18–19, 1995.
89. Wolinsky H, Thung SN. Use of a perforated balloon catheter to deliver concentrated heparin into the wall of the normal canine artery. J Am Coll Cardiol 1990; 15:475–481.
90. Lambert CR, Leone JE, Rowland SM. Local drug delivery catheters: functional comparison of porous and microporous designs. Coronary Artery Dis 1993; 4:469–475.
91. Azrin MA, Mitchel JF, Bow LM, Alberghini TV, Peck R, Fram DB, Waters D, McKay RG. Effect of local delivery of heparin on platelet disposition during in vivo balloon angioplasty using hydrogel-coated balloons (abstract). Circulation 1993; 88(suppl I):I–310.
92. Carrozza JP, Kuntz RE, Levine MJ, Pomerantz RM, Fishman RF, Mansour M, Gibson CM, Senerchia CC, Diver DJ, Safian RD, Baim DS. Angiographic and clinical outcome of intracoronary stenting: immediate and long-term results from a large single-center experience. J Am Coll Cardiol 1992; 20:328–337.
93. Kimura T, Nosaka H, Yokoi H, Iwabuchi M, Nobuyoshi M. Serial angiographic follow-up after Palmaz-Schatz stent implantation: comparison with conventional balloon angioplasty. J Am Coll Cardiol 1993; 21:1557–1563.
94. Emanuelsson H, van der Giessen WJ, Serruys P, on behalf of the Benestent Group. Benestent II: Back to the future. J Int Cardiol 1994; 7:587–592.
95. Tanguay JF, Zndar JP, Phillips HR, Stack RS. Current status of biodegradable stents. Cardiol Clin 1994; 12:699–713.
96. Lincoff Am, van der Giessen WJ, Schwartz RS, van Beusekom HMM, Serruys PW, Holmes DR, Ellis SG, Topol EJ: Biodegradable and biostable polymers may both cause vigorous inflammatory responses when implanted in the porcine coronary artery (abstract). J Am Coll Cardiol 1993; 21:179A.
97. Holmes DR, Edwards WD, Camrud AR, Jorgenson MA, Schwartz RS. Differential arterial response to stents in a porcine coronary model: Exogenous fibrin vs polyurethane vs polyethylene terephthalate (abstract). J Am Coll Cardiol 1993; 21:179A.
98. Chronos NAF, Robinson KA, Schieffer E, Crawford N, Dev K, Hofmann G, Brown JE, King SB. Enhanced uptake of propidium iodide marker into nuclei of SMC in pig aorta in vitro, and pig carotid artery in vivo, by direct vessel wall electroporation. Restenosis Summit VII, Cleveland, Ohio, May 18–19, 1995.
99. Fernández-Ortiz A, Meyer BJ, Mailhac A, Falk E, Badimon L, Fallon JT, Fuster V, Chesebro JH, Badimon JJ. A new approach for local intravascular drug delivery. Iontrophoretic balloon. Circulation 1994; 89:1518–1522.

100. Costello CT, Jeske AH. Iontophoresis: applications in transdermal medication delivery. Phys Ther 1995; 75:554–563.
101. Dev V, Zeng H, Forrester J, Eigler N, Hickey AJ, Fishbein MC, Litvack F. Biodegradable microspheres for sustained drug delivery to the arterial wall (abstract). Circulation 1993; 88(suppl I):I–311.
102. Farb A, Carlson GC, Virmani R. In vivo local delivery and persistence of small and large particles following balloon angioplasty of atherosclerotic arteries: histologic confirmation (abstract). Circulation 1993; 88(suppl I):I–310.
103. Dev V, Zeng H, Forrester JS, Eigler N, Tian Y, Hickey AJ, Fishbein MC, Kupfer J, Livack F. Microspheres for drug delivery to the arterial wall: a study of kinetics, toxicity, and effects of coroticosteroid loaded microspheres (abstract). J Am Coll Cardiol 1994; 23:19A.
104. Hill-West JL, Chowdhury SM, Slepian MJ, Hubbell JA. Inhibition of thrombosis and intimal thickening by in situ photopolymerization of thin hydrogel barriers. Proc Natl Acad Sci USA 1994; 91:5967–5971.
105. Fischell TA, Kharma BK, Fischell DR, Loges PG, Coffey CW, Duggan DM, Naftelan AJ. Low-dose, beta-particle emission from 'stent' wire results in complete localized inhibition of smooth muscle cell proliferation. Circulation 1994; 90:2956–63.
106. Dichek DA, Neville RF, Zwiebel JA, Freeman SM, Leon MB, Anderson WF. Seeding of intravascular stents with genetically engineered endothelial cells. Circulation 1989; 80:1347–1353.
107. Plautz G, Nabel E, Nabel J. Introduction of vascular smooth muscle cells expressing recombinant genes in vivo. Circulation 1991; 83:578–583.
108. Chapman G, Lim CS, Gammon RS, Culp SC, Desper JS, Bauman RP, Swain J, Stack R. Gene transfer into coronary arteries of intact animals with a percutaneous balloon catheter. Circ Res 1992; 71:27–33.
109. Shi Y, Hutchinson HG, Hall DJ, Zalewski A. Downregulation of C-myc expression by antisense oligonucleotides inhibits proliferation of human smooth muscle cells. Circulation 1993; 88:1190–1195.
110. Mazur W, Ali NM, Grinstead WC, Schulz DG, Raizner AE, French BA. Lipofectin-mediated versus adenovirus-mediated gene transfer in vitro and in vivo: comparison of canine and porcine model systems. Coronary Artery Dis 1994; 5:779–786.
111. Morishita R, Gibbons GH, Kaneda Y, Ogihara T, Dzau VJ. Novel in vitro gene transfer method for study of local modulators in vascular smooth muscle cells. Hypertension 1993; 21:894–899.
112. French BA, Mazur W, Ali NM, Geske RS, Finnigan JP, Rodgers GP, Roberts R, Raizner AE. Percutaneous transluminal in vivo gene transfer by recombinant adenovirus in normal porcine coronary arteries, atherosclerotic arteries, and two models of coronary restenosis. Circulation 1994; 90:2402–2413.
113. Kahn ML, Lee SW, Dichek D. Optimization of retroviral vector-mediated gene transfer into endothelial cells in vitro. Circ Res 1992; 71:1508–1517.
114. Epstein SE, Speir E, Finkel T. Do antisense approaches to the problem of restenosis make sense? Circulation 1993; 88:1351–1353.

115. Villa AE, Guzman LA, Poptu EJ, Labhasetwar V, D'Souza S, Farrell CL, Plow EF, Levy RJ, DiCorleto PE, Topol EJ. Effects of antisense C-myb oligonucleotides on vascular smooth muscle cell proliferation and response to vessel wall injury, Circ Res 1995; 76:505–513.
116. Woolf TM, Melton DA, Jennings CGB. Specificity of antisense nucleotides in vivo. Proc Natl Acad Sci USA 1992; 89:7305–7309.
117. Sollott SJ, Cheng L, Pauly RR, Jenkins G-M, Monticone RE, Kuzuya M, Froehlich JP, Crow MT, Lakotta EC, Rowinsky EK, Kinsella JL. Taxol inhibits neointimal smooth muscle cell accumulation after angioplasty in the rat. J Clin Invest 1995; 95:1869–1876.
118. Comline biotechnology wire via First. Tranilast appears effective against vascular restenosis. Pharm Jpn 1/16/95.
119. Daida H, Lee YJ, Yokoi H, Kanoh T, Ishiwata S, Kato K, Nishikawa H, Takatsu F, Kato H, Kutsumi Y, Yamada N, Noma A, Yamaguchi H, and the Low-Density Lipoprotein Apheresis Angioplasty Restenosis Trial (L-ART) Group. Prevention of restenosis after percutaneous transluminal coronary angioplasty by reducing lipoprotein (a) levels with low-density lipoprotein apheresis. Am J Cardiol 1994; 73:1037–1040.
120. Kurz RW, Graf B, Gremmel F, Wurnig C, Stockenhuber F. Increased serum concentrations of adhesion molecules after coronary angioplasty. Clin Sci 1994; 87:627–633.
121. Heino J, MaQsaque J. Transforming growth factor-B switches the pattern of integrins expressed in MG63 human osteosarcoma cells and causes a selective loss of cell adhesion to laminin. J Biol Chem 1989; 264:21800–11.
122. Epstein SE, Speir E, Unger EF, Guzman RJ, Finkel T. The basis of molecular strategies for treating coronary restenosis after angioplasty. J Am Coll Cardiol 1994; 23:1278–88.
123. Casscells W, Lappi DA, Olwin B, et al. Elimination of smooth muscle cells in experimental restenosis: targeting of fibroblast growth factor receptors. Proc Natl Acad Sci USA 1991; 89:7159–63.
124. Miller DD, Paige SB, Tio FO, et al. Lymphocyte/monocyte interleukin-2 receptor targeted fusion toxin therapy with DAB486-IL2 prevents proliferative post-angioplasty restenosis (abstract). Circulation 1991; 84(suppl II):11–70.
125. Pickering JG, Bacha P, Jekanowski J, Weir L, Nichols JC, Isner JM. Prevention of smooth muscle cell proliferation and outgrowth from human atherosclerotic plaque by a recombinant fusion protein (abstract). Circulation 1992; 86:226.
126. Bittl JA, Strony J, Brinker JA, Ahmed WH, Meckel CR, Chaitman BR, Maraganore J, Deutsch E, Adelman B for the Hirulog Angioplasty Study Investigators. Treatment with bivalirudin (Hirulog) as compared with heparin during coronary angioplasty for unstable or postinfarction angina. N Engl J Med 1995; 333:764–769.

19

Coronary Stenting: Past, Present, and Future

Arvinder S. Kurbaan and U. Sigwart
Royal Brompton Hospital and National Heart and Lung Institute, London, England

Coronary stenting has been advocated as the most significant advance in interventional cardiology since the advent of balloon angioplasty by Andreas Gruentzig 18 years ago (1). Even prior to the publication of two large multicenter trials (2,3) supporting the additional benefit of stenting in reducing restenosis, interventional cardiologists were rapidly applying the technique. Recently, there has been rapid development in the types of stents available and adjuvant treatment such as anticoagulation and antiplatelet regimens (4) and local drug delivery systems (5). The complication rate has been reduced by improved stent-implantation techniques and better management of the local puncture site (6). This is in turn leading to an improved cost-benefit ratio (7), contributing to an increase in both the absolute and relative number of intracoronary procedures with stents.

The original concept of vascular stenting has been attributed to Alexis Carrel. In 1912, Carrel advocated the use of glass canine tubes to maintain the patency of the lumen under various conditons (8). His recommendation was not followed until Charles Dotter in 1968 implanted simple metal spirals in animal arteries (9). Dotter found that the metal elements remained free from thrombus, became firmly embedded in the arterial wall, and were coated with neoendothelium. In the 1970s Senning suggested a similar concept. His work led to the development of a large-diameter spiral prosthesis made from surgical steel alloys. This double helix device, consisting of two spring-type spirals made out of stainless steel metal bands connected by individually spaced bridges, was assessed in large vessels and, interestingly, was found to be free from thrombotic occlusion in 52 implants (10). Placement of this device in the vena cava and jugular and iliac veins was well tolerated in dogs despite this challenging experimental model with low blood flow. However, the device appeared unsuitable for smaller vessels because of its relatively large metal surface area. The reduction of the foreign body surface area has been a central tenet in subsequent stent design. Gianturco and coworkers produced a zig-zag design composed of straight metal strands that form a spring-type cylindrical zig-zag pattern when released from the delivery catheter (11). For technical reasons only short stents of this type are possible. Palmaz and coworkers developed a balloon-expandable slotted tube stent made of malleable surgical steel (12), which after extensive testing in animals was introduced into clinical practice (13). The first stent used in human peripheral and coronary arteries was the self-expanding Wallstent (14), which was developed in Lausanne (Switzerland). This elastic woven wire mesh tube consists of elastic metal braids of about 80 μm thickness. The elastic wire mesh tube is geometrically stable, has a very large expansion ratio, remains flexible when compressed into a small diameter, and conforms to structures of a different diameter. It also maintains a residual expansion force once implanted in a vessel sightly smaller than its unconstrained diameter. This expansion force makes any dislocation unlikely and continues to expand the artery over time.

A dedicated delivery device was developed prior to carrying out the first animal experiments. This consisted of a 5F co-axial catheter on which a compressed stent is held by a constraining membrane. The stent is deployed in blood vessels by retraction of the outer layer of the doubled-over membrane. To minimize friction between the two layers of the plastic membrane, the space between the inner and outer membrane layer is filled with fluid, preferably contrast medium, to make it visible under a pressure of 3–4 atm. When the membrane is retracted, the stent gradually opens up and is deployed from distally to proximally.

Some of the initial enthusiasm for the concept of stenting and the Wallstent evaporated when the somewhat ambiguous results of a multicenter registry were published in 1991 (15). The restenosis rate in this observation was only 13% despite a heterogeneous patient group with complicated pathology, a large percentage of whom had been treated for documented restenosis or graft lesions. The thrombosis rate, however, was prohibitively high. The reasons for this high thrombosis rate have never been fully elucidated. They may have been due to the initial learning curve of stenting of several investigators who had not agreed upon a uniform strategy.

I. CLASSIFICATION OF STENTS

Classification may be made according to a number of criteria including material, mode of delivery, length of stay in the body, absence or presence of active ingredients. The following is an attempt to describe the currently used stents, their advantages, disadvantages and potential applications in clinical practice. With the current pace of developments in coronary stenting any classification is likely to be imperfect. It is also important to note that there is only a limited amount of information directly comparing various stents in particular clinical situations.

II. PERMANENT STENTS

All permanent stents which have been used in clinical practice thus far are made of metal alloys. Spring-type metals are used in self-expanding stents and plastically deformable alloys for balloon expandable stents.

A. Self-Expanding Stents

In early 1986 clinical stenting was initiated with the Wallstent (Medinvent; Fig. 1) (16). Animal experiments with this stent in the mid-1980s demonstrated the reliability of the delivery instrument. It was also shown that the stent was biocompatible, not causing excessive thrombosis despite the lack of anticoagulation therapy. Within a few weeks the stent was generally embedded into the arterial wall and covered by a thin shiny layer of neointima. The thickness of this intimal layer normally measured between 150 and 350 μm. The top layer of the new tissue was composed of a monolayer of cells similar to the natural intima. It is uncertain whether

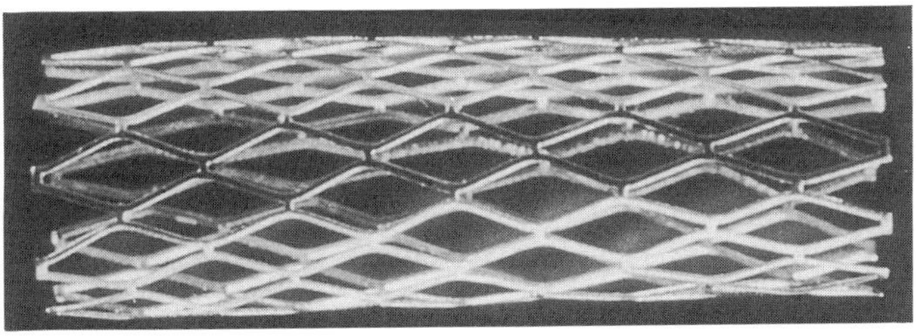

Figure 1 Wallstent (Medinvent).

this top layer is as functionally competent as the natural endothelium or not. Some observations point towards the latter: in particular, the phenomena of leakage with red cells trapped in the subintimal layers may indicate a lesser performance index of this type of cell. In vessels larger than 3 mm in diameter, complications with self-expanding mesh stents are rare. If vessels of less than 3 mm diameter are stented with this device, the chances of thrombosis and/or intrastent restenosis become significant (17,18). On the other hand, the self-expanding mesh stent has a number of important advantages. It is flexible on the delivery device, and after implantation it maintains a limited radial expansion force (provided the nominal size of the stent is chosen to be slightly larger than the actual size of the artery). The stent is geometrically stable and, if the vessel is large enough, provides excellent flow characteristics. Its elasticity enables it to be extended to cover long lesions, and it has an excellent expansion ratio allowing 1.5-mm delivery devices to carry 6.5-mm stents. The latter is of importance when dealing with large degenerate bypass grafts, which can frequently be stented with this device without even predilating the graft, an important feature reducing the risk of distal emolization of material (19). A modified version of the stent, which among other minor changes shortens less on expansion, is currently gradually being reintroduced into clinical practice.

B. Balloon-Expandable Stents

1. Flexible Stents

The Gianturco-Roubin stent (Cook; Fig. 2) (20) was the first to receive FDA approval for clinical use in bail-out situations at the time of angioplasty and the first to be implanted in human coronary arteries in North America (21). Clinical evaluation with the stent was conducted systematically. In the initial phase only candidates for bypass surgery received a stent

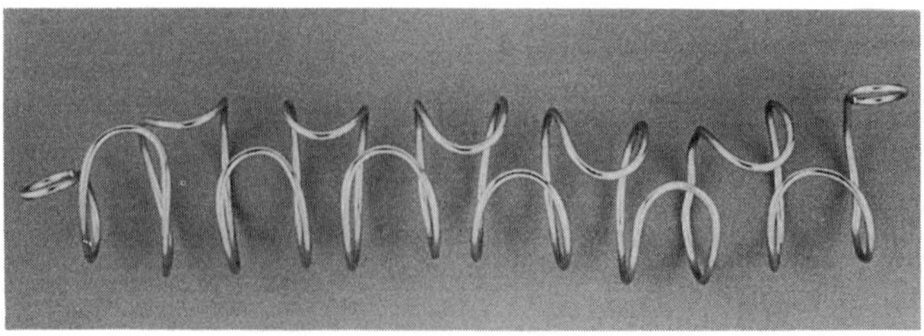

Figure 2 Gianturco-Roubin stent (Cook).

as a bridge to surgery. After this positive initial experience, a second phase was planned with patients having a stent implanted as a definitive treatment after abrupt postangioplasty closure. The advantages of this device would lie in its flexibility and the lack of shortening during expansion. Its disadvantages are the delivery balloon, some recoil, and relatively large spacing of the wires. The wires are also fairly thick, with a diameter of 150 μm. The large spacing and wire profile may explain why restenosis after use of this stent is probably more frequent (22). Unlike most balloon-expandable stents, it comes in two lengths: 12 and 20 mm. The 20-mm version may be long enough for most dissections, but for very short lesions a 12-mm stent is sufficient. A newer version of the stent will soon become available.

The Wiktor stent (Medtronic; Fig. 3) is made of tantalum, which is highly radiopaque (23). Tantalum was thought to have more favorable characteristics than stainless steel when reacting with blood. Extensive experiments have failed to substantiate this hypothesis. Tantalum is somewhat more brittle than stainless steel. The wire spacing of this stent is large and dictated by the shape of the compressed, unexpanded coil. The wire diameter is similar to that of the Gianturco-Roubin stent. The overall length is 17 mm, and the stent is considerably shorter than the delivery balloon. In a multicenter study using this stent in patients with restenosis, some recoil of the stented segment was observed. In this study the restenosis rate was about 30% and the subacute occlusion rate was 10% (24). Recent observations seem to indicate a lower restenosis rate. Its hemodynamic characteristics may be similar to those of the Gianturco-Roubin stent. Angiographic analysis of the stented segment is complicated by the high density of the tantalum wires. Newer developments include a delivery system with a lower profile.

The Multilink stent (ACS; Fig. 4) was developed with the aim of creating a balloon-expandable metallic stent with good structural support, low

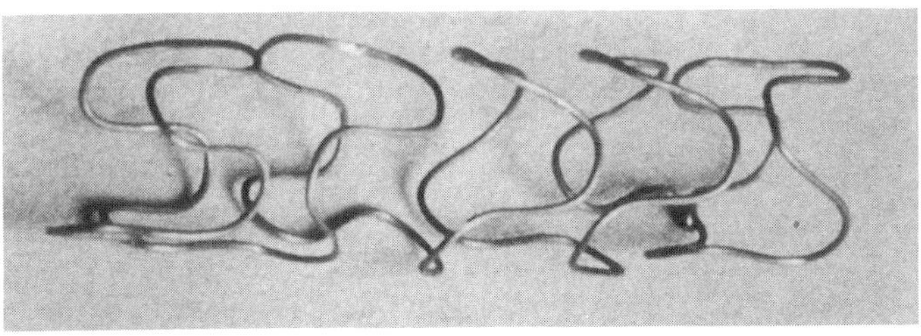

Figure 3 Wiktor stent (Medtronic).

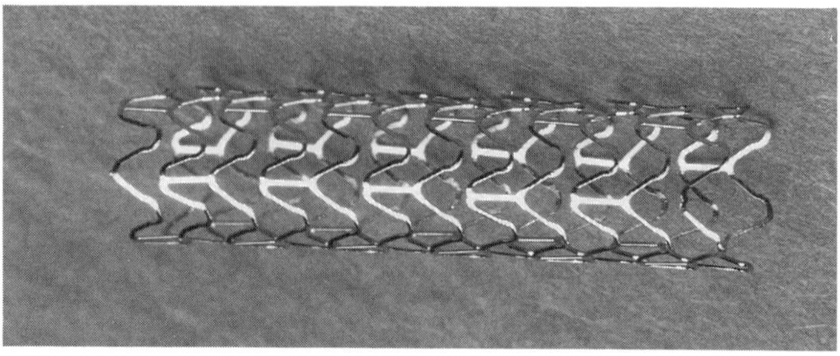

Figure 4 Multilink stent (ACS).

strut thickness, flexibility, and easy safe delivery (25). In contrast to the flexible balloon-expandable stents described above, this stent is not made with wires but is made from a stainless steel tube (like the Palmaz-Schatz stent). The strut thickness is approximately 50 μm, and the stent is composed of individual corrugated rings interconnected by a number of bridges. This geometry makes the stent very flexible. The gaps are smaller than in other stents, resulting in a smoother surface and reducing the amount of turbulence. Smaller gaps also produce a uniform support, which is able to seal small flaps and dissections. The collapse pressure of the Multilink stent is slightly lower than that of the Palmaz-Schatz stent but significantly higher than those of the self-expanding mesh stent, the Gianturco-Roubin stent, and Wiktor stent. The structure of the stent allows easy side branch access and even dilatation of bifurcations. By refining the mesh, the metal-to-air ratio of the stent surface has been reduced by 35% compared to the Palmaz-Schatz stent. The stent was tested in a purpose-built pulse duplicator, which, in addition to the pulsatile action causing repetitive radial distension, also simulates the bending of the coronary arteries during systole and diastole. Stents were tested to 380 million cycles, corresponding to 10 years of actual life.

The Multilink stent is mounted on a stretchable elastic sleeve, which covers the delivery balloon in order to protect the balloon, guarantee even expansion, and prevent the stent from dislodging from the delivery balloon. The stent itself is covered by another sleeve (5F), which, like the Palmaz-Schatz or the self-expanding mesh stent sleeve, protects the stent during its passage through the guiding equipment and through the target vessel. This delivery system is equipped with a manipulator allowing a retraction operation to be performed with one hand.

The Multilink stent comes in various lengths and diameters. In order to control the amount of stress and avoid cracks during expansion, the expansion ratio must be kept within certain limits. For this reason different stents are being used for different arterial sizes. The mounted stent comes in differing lengths, and it does not shorten significantly during expansion.

Animal experiments with the Multilink stent have demonstrated easy and precise delivery without any failures. There were no acute or subacute closures, and all stents were endothelialized after 1–6 months. Human experience is limited to suboptimal results postangioplasty. There were no subacute thrombotic occlusions, and the restenosis rate appeared to be approximately 10%.

The Cordis stent is a tantalum stent with some similarities to the Wiktor stent. The main difference is its smaller gap size, aiming to reduce restenosis. At present it is being clinically evaluated.

The Strecker stent (Boston Scientific; Fig. 5) is made of knitted tantalum wire, which forms a network similar to chicken wire fences. This stent has the advantage of being flexible with relatively small pore size. On the other hand, the tantalum wires present cross points similar to the self-expanding stent but without the advantage of continuous radial force. The Strecker stent probably has the lowest collapse pressure and the largest recoil of all the balloon-expandable stents described here (26). By virtue of the wire crossings, there is an increased risk of thrombosis (27), which has been seen in experimental and clinical studies (28,29). Like the Wallstent it may be suited for large, old, degenerate, and friable vein grafts, for the thrombosis risk in small vessels is high, as is the restenosis rate. The stent has been tried mainly in bail-out situations (30).

A newer version of the AVE microstent (Fig. 6) has recently been introduced into clinical practice (31). This short stent is deployed using a simple balloon-expandable technique. The design consists of 0.2-mm stainless struts with partial radiopacity and a zig-zag structure. Once expanded, its surface area is 8.4% with a 3.5-mm diameter. It is composed of 4-mm welded and unconnected segments providing a range of lengths from 4 to

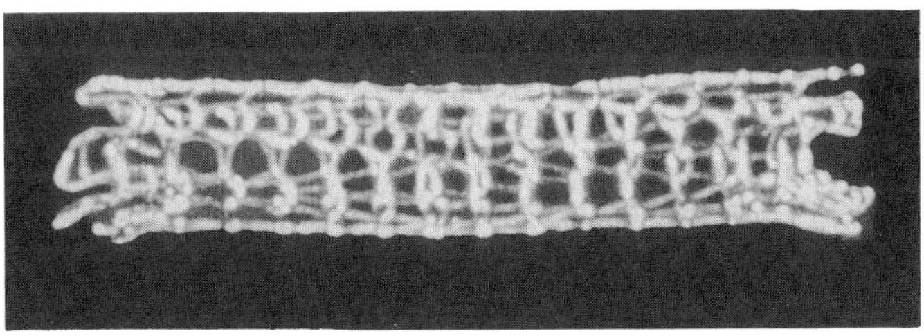

Figure 5 Strecker stent (Boston Scientific).

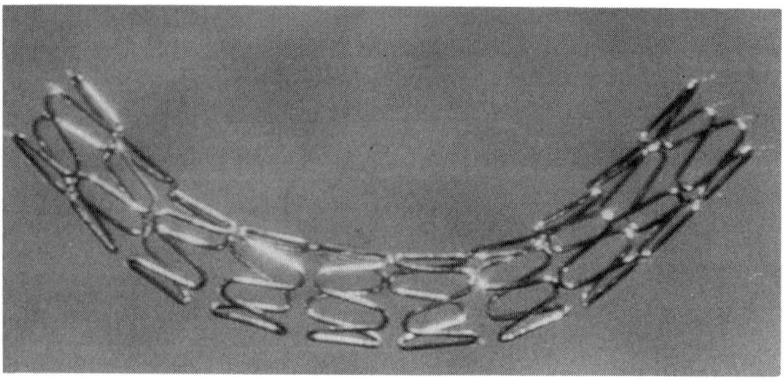

Figure 6 AVE stent (AVE).

16 mm. In a recent study it was successfully deployed in 20 patients who developed acute or threatened closure after angioplasty. Further clinical reports are needed before its full role can be defined.

2. *Articulated Balloon-Expandable Stents*

The Palmaz-Schatz stent (Johnson and Johnson; Fig. 7) is the prototype of the articulated slotted tube stent (32–37). The stent has relatively wide open pores, the surface of which depends on the degree of expansion (32). It also shortens with expansion, although not as much as the self-expanding stent (33). The shortening makes implantation in larger vessels, e.g., 6 mm, somewhat problematic because the original length of 15 mm may be reduced to only 11 mm. Some investigators have pointed out that the use of multiple stents in normal-size coronary arteries is associated with a high risk of restenosis (38,39), others, however, cannot confirm this observation. The stent is available in several lengths: the shortest, unarticulated, is 8 mm long in the unexpanded state; the longest, consisting of three elements connected by a new spiral articulation, is 21 mm long. This recent modification addresses the problem of inadequate coverage of long lesions, which previously could only be overcome by placing two stents in tandem on one long balloon; this helped to avoid a gap of undefined length between two independently implanted stents as well as the potential overlap (40).

The stent delivery device manufactured by Johnson and Johnson provides a protective sheath, which can be withdrawn once the stent is positioned in the stenosis or slightly distal to the stenosis. Radiopaque markers on the sheath help to indicate whether or not the sheath has been sufficiently retracted prior to stent expansion. The balloon used with this device is unsuitable for high-presure expansion. If such expansion is required, a different balloon should be used after the initial deployment. Some operators, particularly in Europe, prefer hand crimping of the stent to a balloon

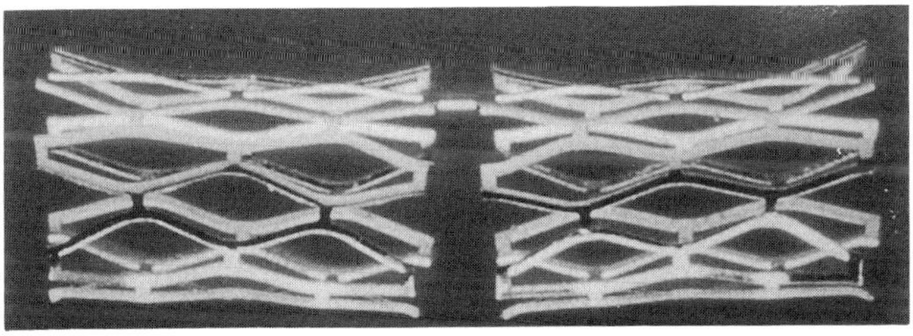

Figure 7 Palmaz-Schatz stent (Johnson & Johnson).

of their choice and to work without sheath protection, accepting the small risk of stent embolization. It is helpful to pressurize the balloon to 0.2–0.3 atm after crimping. This method slightly expands the distal and proximal free portions of the balloon without expanding the stent. In our experience, this technique helps prevent embolization of stents. The gap between the two articulated segments is of concern. Angioscopic, long-term angiographic, and intravascular ultrasound observations have confirmed the suspicion that restenosis is likely to develop in this gap (41,42). A new version of a more elaborate articulation designed to eliminate the gap while maintaining the feature of flexibility is now being evaluated. The articulation produces some torsion of the individual segments during expansion.

III. TEMPORARY STENTS

Permanently implanted metallic stents are a source of continuing injury, stimulating intimal neoplasia. Temporary stenting supports the vessel wall for a short period, sealing dissection flaps and limiting recoil. The short deployment period may overcome some of the limitations of permanent stents. These stents may be either removable or biodegradable. The latter may find a place in the treatment of restenosis.

A. Catheter-Mounted Temporary Stents

1. Perfusion Balloons

All perfusion balloons conceptually work like catheter-mounted temporary stents (43). Side branches leaving the target lesion must inevitably remain occluded during the balloon inflation. In cases where large side branches leave the target area, this may result in ischemic symptoms and, if the balloon is used for more than 1 or 2 h, in myocardial necrosis. Perfusion balloons also display unfavorable hemodynamic characteristics; they typically produce pressure gradients and reduce the flow to the distal arterial segments. Even under optimal circumstances only 40–60 ml of blood per minute are expected to reach the distal artery (44). Thus, other concepts have been developed allowing side branch perfusion and lesser obstruction to flow.

2. Flow Support Catheter (Advanced Cardiac Systems)

This wire basket–type stent expands by passive shortening of its long axis (45). This shortening is achieved by a graded mechanism at the proximal end of the catheter. Delivery catheters are either co-axial or monorail with a shaft size of 3F. Clinical experience with temporary stents is limited to some 50 cases worldwide. Excellent perfusion of distal segments can be obtained with this device, but the long-term results are not satisfactory in the majority of cases. Meticulous anticoagulation must be maintained during temporary stenting. In most clinical investigations 30 min of temporary stenting was followed by another 30 min if the result was not satisfactory. In a multicenter open, nonrandomized observational study, 37 patients were subjected to temporary stenting. At the end of the procedure, which lasted 30–60 min, only one quarter of the cases were considered satisfactory and did not require any further treatment. About 40% of the cases were improved, and the rest were unchanged or worse (45). At present this device has an uncertain future.

B. Retrievable Temporary Stents

1. The HARTS Device (Advanced Coronary Technologies)

The HARTS (Heat Activated Recoverable Tissue Support) device is a nickel-titanium alloy (nitinol) with thermoelastic shape memory (46,47). It exists in either the martensite or the austenite crystal phase. The stent is inserted in the deformable martensite fraction (Martensite I). The mechanical expansion of the alloy induces a change in the crystalline structure (Martensite II). Removal is facilitated by inserting a recovery catheter coaxially through the stent over the guide wire. Three to five ml of lactated Ringers solution at or near the transition temperature is infused and the stent undergoes thermoelastic phase change, returning to its memorized shape, collapsing on the recovery catheter in the austenite crystal phase. Animal studies indicate successful deployment and removal within the first week. After 6 weeks, fibrous overgrowth prevents removal (48). The stent is currently undergoing further evaluation.

2. The Instent

The Instent is a self-expandable nitinol stent that uses the thermoelastic properties of the alloy for expansion and deployment at body temperatures (49). It consists of a coil with two terminal balls. In the expanded austenite phase, the alloy is stiffer and provides greater radial strength. It can be removed by a dedicated retrieval device. The wire loop of this device catches the stent by clockwise rotation, is locked, and then pulled into the catheter. In a caninie model, stents were successfully inserted and removed within 24 h. Postremoval angiography confirmed patent arteries, and there was no macroscopic evidence of intimal tear or damage in excised arteries. The results of further evaluation are awaited.

3. *Biodegradable Stents*

Stents that remain in place only as long as needed, without having to be removed, are an appealing concept. Considerable research is being directed to the development of biodegradeble polymers. Bioerosive stents may be attractive if they are not accompanied by detrimental effects such as an increased inflammatory response. Polymer paving (50) involves creation of an artificial arterial wall tapestry capable of controlling and modulating the healing process after angioplasty. How this new lining may be materialized is still unclear; as far as publications are concerned, no significant progress can be observed over the last years.

4. *Biodegradable Mesh Stents*

Biodegradable mesh stents have been investigated at the Mayo Clinic in Rochester, Minnesota (51), at Duke University Medical Center in Durham, North Carolina (52), and at the Thorax Center in Rotterdam in the Netherlands (53). All three groups have been working with self-expanding mesh stents, geometrically similar to the Wallstent (16). The Thorax Center stent is composed of individual strands of 150 μm thickness woven into the dual counterhelical stent, which has been tested in pig coronary arteries. No results from rapidly biodegradable stents of this design are available. The Duke stent uses a self-expanding structure again similar to the Wallstent (52). It is made from eight strands of a highly specialized polymer that includes poly-L-lactic acid (PLLA). The Mayo stent can be elongated to assume a long profile for loading into deployment apparatus. In dogs, five deployed stents remained patent in coronaries without significant inflammatory response. Endothelialization of the stent had occurred by 2 weeks. All dogs had received heparin at the time of implantation followed by aspirin alone.

These results, reported from the Mayo Clinic, are somewhat in contrast to the pig coronary experience in Rotterdam using a very similar geometric model for a PET stent with a molecular weight of 30,000 (53). The strands were slightly thicker than those discussed previously, being 176 μm in diameter. The relatively bulky PET filaments were rapidly covered by endothelium in most places, but large areas without coverage were also observed. In the pig model the amount of intimal hyperplasia was acceptable. When truly bioabsorbable stents were used, there was an important degree of inflammatory reaction correlating with the rapidity of the bioerosion; in other words, slow biodegradation caused less intimal hyperplasia.

The prospects for biodegradable stents are unclear. First, in order to provide comparable structural support to metal stents they require relatively thicker elements, but these generate more turbulence (and consequently more thrombosis). Second, they seem to generate a greater inflammatory response and intimal hyperplasia compared to metal, which may limit their additional benefit. Third, thus far only self-expanding stents have been tested, which require loading of the stent onto the delivery device just before use. Other concepts using coiled sheet designs are under evaluation and may overcome some of the drawbacks of the present geometry.

5. *Collagen Tube Stent*

Some preliminary data are available on a collagen tube stent that expands upon hydration (55). This concept is limited by very simple mechanical problems: the stent has low radial strength and high wall compliance and may not be able to withstand elastic recoil. In many ways the concept resembles endoluminal paving.

IV. COATED STENTS

A number of approaches have been advocated to enable stents to become more compatible with blood and tissue. Bare metal, whether polished or not, strongly attracts thrombin and platelets as well as other blood constituents that promote thrombosis and may trigger the self-perpetuating process of smooth muscle cell proliferation leading to restenosis (20). Alteration of the surface chemistry, surface structure, and surface charge in order to minimize thrombosis has failed to reduce the thrombosis significantly (56). Polymer coating seems attractive since it combines the structural properties of metal along with the surface characteristics of polymers, which may be potentially beneficial. Polymers may not by themselves be ideally suited with respect to biocompatibility, but they can be impregnated with active substances that enhance tissue and blood compatibility. With the incorporation of specific thrombin inhibitors into a polymer matrix, total suppression of platelet adhesion and thrombosis may be possible. Binding of such agents onto friendly substances like phosphoryl choline appears to be a promising approach currently under investigation. Drugs like heparin, hirudin, other antithrombin components, or even antiproliferative agents can be incorporated comparatively easily in polymer matrices wrapped around the artery (57,58). Preliminary investigations have shown that such techniques may indeed reduce thrombosis as well as hyperplasia. Coating with biologically active cells that express substances like t-PA is feasible. Recently, a preliminary study showed that antiplatelet GPIIb/IIIa antibody passively bound to polymer-coated stents reduced platelet adhesion to the stents (106). The stent has also been used as a local delivery vehicle for radioactive implants. Palmaz-Schatz stents made radioactive in the cyclotron inhibit smooth muscle cell proliferation and neointimal hyperplasia in a rabbit model (107,108). It remains to be seen whether or not some of these substances are practical (or acceptable) for use in humans in the routine clinical setting.

The pace and direction of current research is likely to lead to the majority of stents becoming coated in the near future. At present we are awaiting the results of the large Benestent II trial, which compares heparin-coated (59) and noncoated Palmaz-Schatz stents.

V. LOCAL DRUG DELIVERY

Thrombosis and restenosis are localized events occurring at the site of angioplasty and stent insertion. The ability of agents, such as enoxaparin, to successfully inhibit neointimal proliferation in animal studies (60) but not in placebo-controlled human trials (61) may be due to the high systemic doses required to achieve a local effect. Doses in animal studies were 10–70 times higher than those used in human trials. Thus, specific targeting with concentrated therapeutic interventions and minimizing the systemic actions would appear logical. As discussed above, coated and biodegradable stents can be used for this purpose. Interest has also focused on specifically designed catheter delivery systems.

The simplest devices, such as the Dispatch catheter (SciMed) (62), rely upon prolonged contact with the wall, enabling the transfer of material transmurally. In an attempt to prolong the availability, the active agent has been incorporated into a hydrophilic gel [Hydrogel Balloon (Boston Scientific)] (63). Pressure-driven devices force the agent into the arterial wall, achieving a deeper penetration and a greater concentration. Again a number of systems exist, such as the Infusasleeve (LocalMed) (64), which has the advantage of being able to be placed over a standard angioplasty catheter. To ensure even greater transmural delivery, physical methods have been developed. The needle catheter (BMT Ltd) directly injects the agent into the arterial wall. It appears to cause minimal trauma, and adventitial deposition for up to 3 weeks has been shown (65). The iontophoretic balloon catheter (Cor Trak) utilizes electrical current to atraumatically transfer charged molecules into the wall (66).

At present there are a variety of devices at various stages of development, but none as yet has been shown to be effective in the clinical setting (67). This field does, however, offer promise for the future, particularly as newer antithrombotic and antiproliferative agents become available. Interest has also focused on the local transfer of genetic material such as antisense oligomers targeting the c-*myc* protooncogene to modulate smooth muscle proliferation (68).

VI. INDICATIONS FOR STENTING

In vessels with a diameter of 3 mm or greater, stenting can repair abrupt closure after angioplasty better than any other technique (69–73). The choice of stents in this situation depends on the operator experience and the vessel anatomy. For tortuous vessels a flexible stent has the greatest chance of being deployed correctly. Although in many instances it may be adequate to seal just the entry site, it appears to be important to cover the dissection site completely.

Bail-out stenting appears to have a higher recurrence rate than primary stenting (74). In most studies the restenosis rate after emergency stenting is approximately 30% (29,75–77). The reasons for this higher restenosis rate are unclear. It may be due in part to the differences in the local arterial enviroment postdissection. Furthermore, acute dissection is often managed by repeat balloon inflations, which increase the degree of trauma to the arterial wall, and among other actions, stimulate smooth muscle cell hyperplasia. It appears logical to insert stents rapidly once the dissection has been diagnosed. With this strategy the restenosis rate of a pilot study using the self-expanding mesh stent was 18% (78). There also seems to be a higher incidence of subacute thrombosis of stents compared to the primary indication. Figures of subacute thrombosis rates after bail-out stenting range between 5 and 30% (29,73–79). This means that, in the worst scenario, the major problems encountered after bail-out stenting, i.e., subacute thrombosis plus restenosis, amount to 60% of such cases. These unacceptable results show that delayed decision making, use of short stents, and implantation in arteries less than 3 mm in diameter may be the main reason for a poor outcome.

VII. STENTING FOR THE PREVENTION OF RESTENOSIS

Different stents may have a different potential to prevent restenosis. Desirable features for such stents are adequate radial strength to counteract recoil and contraction during the healing process, optimal gap size to avoid bulging of arterial wall segments not covered by the stent into the lumen, low strut thickness, and low thrombogenicity (56,80). Analyzing the different stent designs, it is not surprising to see relatively high restenosis rates with stents that are primarily designed to deal with postangioplasty dissections at the exprense of reduced structural support. The stent with the highest structural support is the self-expanding Wallstent (16). This stent may induce more thrombosis because of its wire crossings and the relatively large amount of metal. It also may stimulate smooth muscle growth by virtue of the persisting radial expansion force when excessively oversized. Stents like the Wiktor stent with comparatively low structural support or the Strecker stent with considerable recoil would not seem to be the ideal stent targeted to the reduction of restenosis. Clinical data tend to support this impression. Even in the most challenging clinical study, restenosis rates with the self-expanding Wallstent were only 13% (15), whereas the Wiktor stent experience and the Strecker stent experience yielded much higher restenosis rates (24,28,29). Data from Japan obtained in a nonrandomized study with the Palmaz-Schatz stent (81) report restenosis rates in primary indication with this stent similar to the Wallstent experience, whereas experience with the Wiktor stent reveals restenosis rates about twice as high (24). In a multicenter trial restenosis rates in selected indications with the Palmaz-Schatz stent were as low as 5.6% if the primary result after stenting was ideal, i.e., virtually no residual stenosis (82).

From these data it appears that the initial luminal gain after stenting determines the amount of restenosis. Even if smooth muscle cell proliferation is greater after stenting compared with balloon angioplasty (late loss), the vessel can accommodate significantly more tissue ingrowth before restenosis occurs (83). Two major trials have answered this question for the Palmaz-Schatz stent (STRESS trial in the United States and Benestent trial in Europe) (2,3). All patients in these trials were investigated by quantitative coronary angiography after 6 months. The initial results after stenting are significantly better when compared to balloon angioplasty, and this advantage is maintained, to a lesser degree, over the 6 month follow-up until repeat angiography is carried out. Furthermore, patients with stents have fewer clinical events and fewer repeat interventions, even over an extended period of observation of up to one year. Among 520 randomized patients, 259 had a stent implanted as a primary treatment. The baseline characteristics of both groups were similar. The mean luminal diameter of the target lesion in the stent group increased from 1.07 ± 0.31 to 2.51 ± 0.36 mm, whereas the balloon only postreatment diameter was 2.05 ± 0.32 mm. In-hospital complications (repeat PTCA, surgical revascularization, emergency stenting, myocardial infarction, cerebrovascular accidents) were more frequent in the balloon-only group (12% vs. 9%). On the other hand, stent patients stayed in the hospital longer [8.3 ± 5.8 days (6.4 ± 3.5 days if no complications were observed)]than balloon-only patients (2.9 ± 3.4 days). Local complications were more frequent in the stent group. Using the 50% dichotomous criterion balloon angioplasty had a restenosis rate of 33% compared to 20% restenosis in the stent group. The STRESS trial has yielded very similar results, with both the PTCA and the stent restenosis rates being slightly higher. Both studies suffered from an elevated local complication rate, largely due to too generous anticoagulation during the first 24 h (blood transfusion for local hematoma in 7%, pseudoaneurysm in 6%, hematoma or gastrointestinal bleeding in 3% in the Benestent group).

The importance of stent design in reducing restenosis (and thrombosis) extends beyond minimizing the surface area to reduce tissue and blood reaction while still providing adequate support. There is increasing evidence that arteries remodel themselves in response to long-term flow changes. The luminal diameter and wall mass is reshaped to maintain stable flow and wall tensile stress. Under low-flow conditions shear stress is reduced, resulting in a reduction of radius until wall shear stress is restored to baseline levels (84). There are corresponding proliferative changes in the vessel wall in response to the reduced tensile stress. Optimally inserted stents facilitate good blood flow, which should enable local levels of wall shear stress to reach baseline levels, limiting the stimulus for proliferation and subsequent restenosis (85). Furthermore, keeping the amount of metal and expansion constant but reducing the number of strut-strut intersections by one third reduced disruptions of the internal elastic lamina and the tunica media by nearly a half. There was a corresponding twofold reduction in neointimal hyperplasia and near elimination of thrombosis (86).

Restenosis of the site of stent insertion can be managed by conventional approaches. Standard balloon angioplasty appears to be effective in this scenario, with a 6-month restenosis rate of about one third. This is comparable to that seen after balloon angioplasty of the native coronary stenoses (87).

VIII. STENTING OF BYPASS GRAFTS

The pathology of bypass venous grafts requires particular attention in regard to angioplasty techniques. It appears that virtually all saphenous veins used as aorto-coronary conduits for longer than one year develop atherosclerotic plaques. The changes affect not only the intima and media layers, but also the adventitia (88). Within 2 months after coronary artery bypass grafting, the predominant intimal change is proliferation of fibrous tissue. This may develop into an extremely hard, almost undilatable connective tissue stenosis. Late changes include lipid deposition, thrombus, and aneurysm formation. Degeneration, including sclerosis and calcification of valves within the saphenous vein, may also play an important clinical role (89). Other critical parameters associated with problems after bypass surgery are the proximal and distal surgical anastomotic sites. Luminal narrowing has been observed at the distal coronary anastomosis as well as the proximal aortic site. These stenoses are mainly secondary to problems with surgical techniques rather than being due to underlying degenerative changes. This complex pathology requires a specific approach to angioplasty techniques. Balloon angioplasty carries a high risk of producing embolization in old grafts (90). Restenosis after graft angioplasty, particularly the proximal and midportions, can be expected in 60% or more of treated patients (91). Removal techniques (directional atherectomy, rotational atherectomy, extraction atherectomy) fail to yield significantly lower restenosis rates compared to balloon angioplasty—hence the great interest in stents in this pathology.

It is difficult to give general recommendations for the choice of stents in graft lesions. Stents with smaller gaps are likely to achieve better results in friable grafts simply because they prevent embolization of atheromatous material more reliably than stents with large gaps. In fibrotic graft lesions stents should exert sufficient radial force to counteract the significant recoil. The individual choice of the appropriate stent should be made according to these criteria.

The self-expanding mesh stent has a good track record in vein grafts. In our experience with this stent, restenosis or occlusion in coronary artery bypass grafts more than 3 mm in diameter occurred in only 11% of all cases (92). These encouraging results, however, have not been seen by all investigators. The Palmaz-Schatz stent has been used extensively in graft lesions and, in primary indication, has yielded a 14% restenosis rate in a multicenter trial (93).

Particular problems arise from ostial lesions, the results of which are not always acceptable after balloon angioplasty. Stents in this situation have a high success rate and a low complication rate (94). If the ostial lesion is short, a single element of a Palmaz-Schatz stent or a very short self-expanding stent may be enough to cover the entire diseased area (95). Short stents in this situation have the advantage of allowing extremely precise positioning while avoiding the protrusion into the aorta. As with native coronary arteries, stents are at present the only means of effectively reducing the initial complication rate and the restenosis rate after bypass graft angioplasty.

IX. THE PROBLEM OF STENT THROMBOSIS

After insertion of intracoronary stents, spasm, infection, and inflammatory responses are rare. Thrombosis, however, is not uncommon, particularly if stents are not firmly embedded into the arterial wall by high-pressure inflations with slightly (10–20%) oversized balloons. If this strategy is employed and an "ideal" result is obtained (judged by high-resolution angiography and/or intravascular ultrasound imaging), long-term anticoagulation can probably be dispensed with (96). This could be even more important for the prevention of hyperplasia, as thrombus may provide the matrix for subsequent smooth muscle cell proliferation and ultimately restenosis (97). All patients after stent placements receive antiplatelet agents such as aspirin. Heparin is given during the implantation procedure, and most clinicians still follow with overlapping oral anticoagulation with coumadins for several weeks or months. Anticoagulation is associated with hemorrhagic complications and involves significant financial costs. The evidence to support the routine use of such regimens is equivocal. Certainly there appears to be little role for coumadins in preventing restenosis. In view of this, attention has focused on antiplatelet agents. Early results from French multicenter studies (such as the TASTE registry) suggest that intensive antiplatelet therapy with aspirin or ticlopidine, a newer antiplatelet agent, is an effective alternative to classical anticoagulation and may permit early patient discharge (5,99). Individual clinical scenarios such as intimal dissection may require different approaches, perhaps reflecting the differing local arterial enviroments. In the absence of large prospective trials, the roles of anticoagulation, antiplatelet agents, thrombolytics, and other adjuncts are still unclear.

From clinical experience, early sheath removal is the best way of fighting the problem of local hemorrhagic complications. During the first 24 h, thrombosis of the stent itself is rare, and therefore this early period should be exploited to deal with the local problems. Collagen plugs may have been proposed for stent patients (100), but their value is still unclear (101). Prolonged pressure controlled local compression using an inflatable compression device such as the FemoStop may be the best way of dealing with the problem of puncture site bleeding (6). Most groups report a dramatic drop in bleeding complications after having adopted such a regimen. Another approach to reduce puncture site problems is stent insertion using the radial artery approach. Unfortunately, this may prove to be possible only in highly selected cases (102). Despite the improvements in puncture site management, stent occlusion, primarily between the fourth and eighth days after implantation, may become a problem if the stent is not optimally expanded. The subacute occlusion rate may be between 2 and 10% depending on the stent employed, the indication, and the vessel size. Prothrombin factors 1 and 2 (F1,2) as well as factor X have been implicated in playing a major role in the etiology of these subacute occlusions. Heparin may be unable to counteract stent thrombosis for a number of reasons. Activated platelets release platelet-specific heparin-binding proteins, like platelet factor IV, and therefore neutralize heparin. Also, clotbound thrombin may not be bound by heparin and may continue to activate platelets (103). Low molecular weight heparin injected subcutaneously by the patient himself may be used to cover this period after discharge from the hospital. The future will determine whether replacement of heparin by low molecular weight heparin or other agents given systemically or locally will improve the clinical results, including restenosis.

X. CONCLUSION

Stents hold the greatest promise of all the available newer angioplasty techniques. They predictably reverse postangioplasty occlusions, improve primary postangioplasty results, and reduce restenosis rates after angioplasty. Subacute thrombosis after stenting may be the result of incomplete stent expansion and suboptimal primary results. Aggressive systemic anticoagulation with heparin and warfarin reduces the thrombosis rate in these circumstances at the expense of more frequent local complications. However, it fails to eliminate it, possibly due to the failure to react with specific elements of the clotting cascade. Improved puncture site management has markedly reduced local complications. According to the results of randomized controlled studies, stents do reduce the incidence of restenosis after angioplasty. Newer agents such as low molecular weight heparin given systemically or locally and genetic material transferred locally may be beneficial. Stent designs currently being developed reflect the greater understanding of the role of geometry in influencing fluid dynamics and the arterial wall. This should further reduce the thrombosis and restenosis rates, enhancing the role of stenting in the management of coronary artery disease.

REFERENCES

1. Gruentzig A. Transluminal dilatation of coronary artery stenosis. Lancet 1978; 1:263.
2. Serruys PW, de Jaegere P, Kiemeneiji C, Macaya H, RutschW, Heyndrickx G, Emanuelsson G, Marco J, Legrand V, Maren P, Belardi J, Sigwart U, et al. A comparison of balloon expandable stent implantation with balloon angioplasty in patients with coronary artery disease. (The Benestent study). N Engl J Med 1994; 331:489–495.

3. Fischman DL, Leon MB, Baim DS, Schatz RA, Savage MP, Penn I, Detre K, Veltri L, Ricci DR, Nobuyoshi M, et al. A randomized comparison of coronary stent placement and balloon angioplasty in the treatment of coronary artery disease. (The trial). N Engl J Med 1994; 331:496–501.
4. Hoefling B, Huehns TY. Intravascular local drug delivery after angioplasty. Eur Heart J 1995; 16:437–440.
5. Morice, et al. Intracoronary stenting without coumadin: one month results of a French multicentre study. Cath Cardiovasc Diag 1995; 35:1–17.
6. Sridhar K, Porter D, Gupta B, et al. Reduction in peripheral vascular complications after coronary artery stenting by the use of a pneumatic vascular compression device. Circulation 1994; 90:1621.
7. Wong SC, Popma JJ, Chuang YC, Mintz GS, et al. Economic impact of reduced anticoagulation after saphenous vein graft stent placement. J Am Coll Cardiol 1995; 25:80A.
8. Carrel A. Results of the permanent intubation of the thoracic aorta. Surg Gyn Obstet 1912; 16:245–248.
9. Dotter CT. Transluminally placed coil spring arterial tube grafts: long term patency in canine popliteal artery. Invest Rad 1969; 4:329–332.
10. Maas D, Zollikofer CL, Largiader F, Senning A. Radiological follow-up of transluminally inserted vascular endoprostheses: an experimental study using expanding spirals. Radiology 1984; 152:639–663.
11. Gianturco C, Wright KC, Wallace S, Charnsangavej C, Carrasco CH. Percutaneous endovascular stents: an experimental evalutaion. Radiology 1982; 156:69–72.
12. Palmaz JC, Windeler SAM, Garcia FM, Tio FO, Sibbitt RR, Reuter SR. Atherosclerotic rabbit aortas: expandable intraluminal grafting. Radiology 1986; 160:723–726.
13. Palmaz JC. Balloon expandable intravascular stent. Am J Radiol 1988; 150:1263–1269.
14. Sigwart U, Puel J, Mirkovitch V, Joffre F, Kappengberger L. Intravascular stents to prevent occlusion and restenosis after transluminal angioplasty. N Engl J Med 1987; 316:701–706.
15. Serruys PW, Strauss BH, Beatt KJ, Bertrand M, Puel J, Rickards AF, Meier B, Goy JJ, Vogt P, Kappenberger L, Sigwart U. Angiographic follow-up after placement of a self-expanding coronary artery stent. N Engl J Med 1991; 324:13–17.
16. Sigwart U. The self-expanding stent. In: Topol E, ed. Textbook of Interventional Cardiology. Philadelphia: W.B. Saunders, 1990:605–622.
17. Sigwart U, Imbert C, Essinger A, Fischer A, et al. Analysis of complications associated with coronary artery stenting. Circulation 1987; 76(suppl. IV):
18. Stewart JT, Sigwart U, Rickards AF, Goy JJ, et al. Self-expanding coronary stents: Late results from Lausanne and London. Eur Heart J Suppl 1991; 12:166.
19. Urban P, Sigwart U, Golf S, Kaufman U, Sadeghi H, et al. Intravascular stenting for stenosis of aortacoronary venous bypass grafts. J Am Coll Cardiol 1989; 13:1085–1091.

20. Roubin GS, Robinson KA, King SB, Gianturco C, Black AJ, Brown JE, et al. Early and late results of intracoronary arterial stenting after coronary angioplasty in dogs. Circulation 1987; 76:891–897.
21. Roubin GS, King SB, Douglas JS Jr, Lembo NJ, Robinson, KA. Intracoronary stenting during percutaneous transluminal coronary angioplasty. Circulation 1990; 81:92–100.
22. Hirshfeld JW, Schwartz JS, Jugo R. Restenosis after coronary angioplasty: a multivariate statistical model to relate lesion and procedure variables to restenosis. J Am Coll Cardiol 1991; 18(3):647–656.
23. White CJ, Ramee SR, Banks AK, Mesa JE, Chokshi S, Isner JM. A new balloon-expandable tantalum coil stent: angiographic patency and histologic findings in an atherogenic swine model. J Am Coll Cardiol 1992; 19:870–876.
24. de Jaegere PP, Serruys PW, Bertrand M, Wiegand V, Kober, et al. Wiktor stent implantation in patients with restenosis following balloon angioplasty of a native coronary artery. Am J Cardiol 1992; 69:598–602.
25. Sigwart U, Khosravi F, Virmani R, Buller N, Haber R, Simonton C, Kowlachuk G. Bronco: Ein neuer, balloon-expandierbarer, flexibler Stent. Z Kardiol 1993; 71:219.
26. Reifart N, Langer A, Stoerger H, Schwarz F. Strecker stent as a bail-out device following percutaneous transluminal coronary angioplasty. J Intervent Cardiol 1992; 5:79–83.
27. Barth KH. Does experimental evidence favor any of the balloon-expandable stents? Angiology 1992; 43:265.
28. Beytien C, Terres W, Kupper W, Hamm C. In vitro model to test the thrombogenicity of coronary stents. Eur Heart J 1992; 13:266.
29. Geschwind H, Nakamura F, Kvasnicka J, Dubois-Rande JL, Elbadaoui G. Coronary Strecker stent. Does it look promising? Angiology 1992; 43:272–273.
30. Reifart N, Preusler W, Schwarz F, Stoerger H. Strecker stents: Are they the answer? Angiology 1992; 43:279.
31. Ozaki Y, Keane D, Ruygrok P, de Feyter P, Stertzer S, Serruys PW. Acute clinical and angiographic results with the new AVE micro coronary stent in bail out management. Am J Cardiol 1995; 76:112–116.
32. Schatz RA, Palmaz JC, Tio FO, Garcia F, Garcia O, Reuter SR. Balloon-expandable intracoronary stents in the adult dog. Circulation 1987; 76:450–457.
33. van der Gessen WJ, Slager CJ, van Beusekom HM, Schenau DS, et al. Development of a polymer endovascular prosthesis and its implantation in porcine arteries. J Intervent Cardiol 1992; 5:175–185.
34. Schatz RA. A view of vascular stents. Circulation 1989; 79:445–457.
35. Schatz RA. An introduction to intravascular stents. Cardiol Clin 1988; 6:357–372.
36. Schatz RA, Baim DS, Leon M, Ellis G, et al. Clinical experience with the Palmaz-Schatz coronary stent. Circulation 1991; 83:148–161.
37. Schatz RA, Tierstein PS, Hirschfeld JW, Cabin HS, et al. Report of the initial experience with the Palmaz-Schatz coronary stent following elective angio-

plasty. In: Sigwart U, Frank GI, eds. Coronary Stents. Berlin: Springer-Verlag, 1992:45–55.
38. Fajadet J, Marco J, Cassagneau B, Laurent JP, Robert G. Multiple intracoronary balloon expandable stent: early experience. Eur Heart J 1990; 11:370.
39. Fajadet J. Marco J, Cassagneau B, Robert G, van Dormael M. Coronary stenting with the Palmaz-Schatz stent: the Clinique Pasteur Interventional Cardiology Unit Experience. In: Sigwart U, Frank GI, eds. Coronary Stents. Berlin: Springer-Verlag, 1992:57–77.
40. Nordrehaug JE, Priestley K, Rickards AF, Buller N, Sigwart U. Simultaneous implantation of two Palmaz-Schatz stents mounted on a long angioplasty balloon. J Intervent Cardiol.
41. Zeiher AM, Holnloser S, Fassbender S, Wollschlaeger H, Just H. Intracoronary ultrasound morphology following interventional therapy in coronary heart disease. Eur Heart J 1992; 13:308.
42. George G, Erbel R, Ge T, Grber T, Haude M, Meyer J. Intravascular ultrasound after stent implantation: Can stent recoil or compression occur? Eur Heart J 1992; 13:308.
43. Hinohara T, Simpson JB, Phillips HR, Behar VS, et al. Transluminal catheter reperfusion: a new technique to reestablish blood flow after coronary occlusion during percutaneous transluminal coronary angioplasty. Am J Cardiol 1986; 57:684–686.
44. Stack RS, Quigley PJ, Collins G, Phillips HR. Perfusion balloon catheter. Am J Cardiol 1988; 61:77G–80G.
45. Whitlow P, Gaspard P, Kent K, Baim DS, et al. Improvement of coronary dissection with a removal flow support catheter. J Am Coll Cardiol 1992; 19:217.
46. Shetky LM. Shape memory alloys. Sci Am 1979; 241:74–83.
47. Mehran JK, Neal LE, Robert L, Hess JP, et al. Implantation and recovery of balloon delivered removable stents. J Am Coll Cardiol 1992; 19:218a.
48. Khorsandi MJ, Eigler NL, Lambert T, et al. Temporary stenting with heat activated recoverable temporary stent: implantantation up to six weeks. Circulation 1992; 86:I–800A.
49. Beyar R, Henry M. Removable self expanding nitinol coil stent: initial report on in vitro canine and human results. J Am Coll Cardiol 1993; 21:439A.
50. Slepian MJ, Schindler A. Polymer endoluminal paving/sealing: a bioabsorbable alternative to intracoronary stenting. Circulation 1988; 78(suppl II):409.
51. Schwartz RS, Murphy JG, Edwards WD, Holmes DR. Bioabsorbable, drug-eluting, intracoronary stents: design and future applications. In: Sigwart U, Frank GI, eds. Coronary Stents. Berlin: Springer-Verlag, 1992:135–154.
52. Gammon RS, Chapman GD, Bauman RP, Stack RS. Bioabsorbable endovascular stent prostheses. In: Sigwart U, Frank GI, eds. Coronary Stents. Berlin: Springer-Verlag, 1992:155–167.
53. Van der Giessen WJ, Slager CJ, van Beusekom H,van Ingen, Schenau DS, et al. Development of a polymer endovascular prosthesis and its implantation in porcine arteries. J Intervent Cardiol 1992; 5:175–185.

54. Beyar R, Shofti R, Grendier E, Henry M, Globerman O, Beyar M. Self expandable Nitinol stent for cardiovascular applications: canine and human experience. Cath Cardiovasc Diag 1994;
55. Bier JD, Zalesky P, Li S-T, Sasken H, Williams DO. A new bioabsorbable intravascular stent: in vitro assessment of hemodynamic and morphometric characteristics. J Intervent Cardiol 1992; 5:187–194.
56. Sigwart U. Coronary stents: Will they survive? In:Sigwart U, Frank GI, eds. Coronary Stents. Berlin: Springer-Verlag, 1992:169–177.
57. Edelman ER, Adams DH, Karnovsky MJ. Effects of controlled adventitial heparin delivery on smooth muscle cell proliferation following endothelial injury. Proc Natl Acad Sci 1991; 87:3773–3777.
58. Rogers C, Edelman ER. Controlled release of heparin reduces neointimal hyperplasia in stents rabbit arteries: ramifications for local therapy. J Intervent Cardiol 1992; 5:195–202.
59. Van der Giessen WJ, Hardhammar PA,van Beusekom HMM, et al. Reduction of thrombotic occlusion of heparin coated vs. non heparin coated Palmaz-Schatz stents in normal coronary arteries in pigs. Eur Heart J 1993; 14:352A.
60. Currier JW, Pow TK, Haudenschild CC, Minihan AC, Faxon DP. Low molecular weight heparin (Enoxaprin) reduces restenosis after iliac angioplasty in the hypercholesterolaemic rabbit. J Am Coll Cardiol 1991; 17:118B–125B.
61. Faxon D, Spiro T, Minor S, Douglas J, Cote G, Dovosti K, Gottlieb R, Califf R, Topol E, Gordon J. Enoxaprin, a low molecular weight heparin in the prevention of restenosis after agioplasty: results of a double blind randomised trial, double blind placebo controlled trial. J Am Coll Cardiol 1992; 19:258A.
62. McKay RG, Fram DB, Hirst JA, et al. Treatment of intracoronary thrombus with local urokinase infusion using a new site specific drug delivery system: the dispatch catheter. Cath Cardiovasc Diag 1994; 33:181–188.
63. Fram DB, Aretz T, Azrin MA, et al. Localised intra mural drug delivery during balloon angioplasty using hydrogel coated ballons and pressure augmented diffusion. J Am Coll Cardiol 1994; 23:1570–1577.
64. Kaplan AV, Kermode J, Grant, et al. Intramural delivery of marker agent in ex vivo and in vivo models using a novel drug delivery sleeve. J Am Coll Cardiol 1994; 23:189A.
65. Gonschior P, Goetz AE, Heuhns TY, Hoefling B. A new catheter for prolonged local drug application. Coronary Artery Dis 1995; 6:329–334.
66. Fernandez-Ortiz A, Meyer BJ, Mailhac A, et al. A new approach for local intravascular drug delivery. Circulation 1994; 89:1518–1522.
67. Lincoff AM, Topol EJ, Ellis SG. Local drug delivery for the prevention of restenosis. Fact, fancy, and future. Circulation 1994; 90(4):2070–2084.
68. Roque F, Belardi J, Rodriguez L, et al. Safety trial of intracoronary admission of c-myc antisense in patients undergoing percutaneous transluminal coronary angioplasty. Eur Heart J 1995; 16:2479A.
69. Sigwart U, Urban P, Golf S, Kaufmann U, Imbert, et al. Emergency stenting for acute occlusion after coronary balloon angioplasty. Circulation 1988; 72:1121–1127.

70. Strauss BH, Serruys PW, Bertrand ME, Puel J, Meier B, et al. Quantitative angiographic follow-up of the coronary Wallstent in native vessels and bypass grafts: the evolving European experience from March 1986 to March 1990. Am J Cardiol 1992; 69:475–481.
71. Roubin GS, Cannon AD, Agrawal SK, Macander PJ, et al. Intracoronary stenting for acute and threatened closure complicating percutaneous transluminal coronary angioplasty. Circulation 1992; 85:916–927.
72. Goy JJ, Vogt R, Stauffer JC, Sigwart U, Kappenberger L. Stenting versus prolonged inflation to manage acute occlusion of the right coronary artery following PTCA: a long term follow-up. Z Kardiol 1992; 81:109.
73. Satler LF, Leon MB, Kent KM, Pichard AD. Strategies for acute occlusion after coronary angioplasty (editorial comment). J Am Coll Cardiol 1992; 19:936–938.
74. Serruys PW, Strauss BH, van Beusekom H, van der Giessen WJ. Stenting of coronary arteries: Has a modern Pandora's box been opened? J Am Coll Cardiol 1991; 17:143B–154B.
75. Roubin GS, Pinkerton CA. Gianturco-Roubin stent: development and investigation. In: Sigwart U, Frank GI, eds. Coronary Stents. Berlin: Springer-Verlag, 1992:79–99.
76. Haude M, Erbel R, Straub U, Dietz U, Schatz R, Meyer J. Results of intracoronary stents for management of coronary dissection after balloon angioplasty. J Am Coll Cardiol 1991; 67:691–696.
77. Fajadet J, Marco J, Cassagneau B, Robert G, Vandormael M. Coronary stenting with the Palmaz-Schatz stent: the Clinique Pasteur Interventional Cardiology Unit Experience. In: Sigwart U, Frank GI, eds. Coronary Stents. Berlin: Springer-Verlag, 1992:57–77.
78. Urban P, Sigwart U. The self-expanding mesh stent. In: Sigwart U, Frank GI, eds. Coronary Stents. Berlin: Springer-Verlag, 1992:21–44.
79. Schatz RA, Goldberg S, Leon M. Coronary stenting following suboptimal coronary angioplasty results (abstract). Circulation 1990; 82(suppl. III):540.
80. Tominga R, Kambic HE, Emoto H, Harasaki H, Sutton CS, Hollman J. Effects of design geometry of intravascular endoprostheses on stenosis rate in normal rabbits. Am Heart J 1992; 123:21–28.
81. Kimura T, Nosaka H, Nibuyoshi M. Serial angiographic follow up after Palmaz-Schatz stent implantation retrospective comparison with conventional balloon angioplasty. J Am Coll Cardiol 1992; 19:197.
82. Ellis SG, Savage M, Fischman D, Baim DS, Leon M, Goldberg S, Hirshfeld JW, Cleman MW, et al. Restenosis after placement of Palmaz-Schatz stent in native coronar arteries; initial results of a multicenter experience. Circulation 1992; 86:1836–1844.
83. Kuntz RE, Gibson M, Nobuyoshi M, Baim DS. Generalised model of restenosis after conventional balloon angioplasty, stenting and directional atherectomy. J Am Coll Cardiol 1993; 21:15–25.
84. Zarins CK, Zatina MA, Giddens DP, Ku DN, Glagov S. Shear stress regulation of artery diameter in experimental atherogenesis. J Vasc Surg 1987; 105:393–400.

85. Glagov S. Intimal hyperplasia, vascular remodelling and the restenosis problem. Circulation 1994; 89:2888–2891.
86. Rogers C, Edelman ER. Endovascular stent design dictates experimental restenosis and thrombosis. Circulation 1995; 91:2995–3001.
87. Debbas N, Eeckhout E, Stauffer JC, et al. Traitement par angioplastie au ballonnet de restenosis servenues sur prosthesis endocoronaires. Arch Mal Coeur 1995; 88:987–991.
88. Kalan JM, Roberts CW. Morphologic findings in saphenous veins used as coronary arterial bypass conduits for longer than 1 year: necropsy analysis of 53 patients 123 saphenous veins and 1865 5mm segments of veins. Progr Cardiol 1990; 119:1164–1184.
89. Mills NL. Saphenous vein graft valves "the bad guys." Ann Thorac Surg 1989; 48:613–614.
90. Bourassa MG, Campeau I, Lesperance J. Changes in grafts and in coronary arteries after coronary bypass surgery. In: Waters DD, Bourassa MG, eds. Care of the Patient with Previous Coronary Bypass Surgery. Davis, 1991:83–100.
91. Kussmaul WG. Percutaneous angioplasty of coronary bypass grafts: an emerging consensus. Cathet Cardiovasc Diagn 1988; 15:1–4.
92. Stewart JT, William MG, Goy JJ, Buller N, Rickards AF, Sigwart U. Self-expanding stents for diseased saphenous vein coronary artery bypass grafts. J Am Coll Cardiol 1992; 19:49.
93. Leon MB, Ellis SG, Pichard AD, Baim DS, Heuser RR, Schatz RA. Stents may be the preferred treatment for focal aortacoronary vein graft disease. Circulation 1991; 84(suppl. 4):II–249.
94. Nordrehaug JE, Chronos N, Denne L, Rickards AF, Buller N, Sigwart U. Self expanding stents for the management of aorto-ostial stenoses in saphenous vein bypass grafts. Br Heart J 1994; 72:285–287.
95. Nordrehaug JE, Priestly K, Chronos N, Buller N, Sigwart U. Usefulness of implanting half Palmaz-Schatz stents in short aorto-ostial lesions. Cathet Cardiovasc Diagn 1993; 29:141–143.
96. Hall P. Colombo A, Nakamura S, Maiello L, Blenigo S, Ferraro M, Martini G. A prospective study of the Gianturco-Roubin coronary stent implantation without subsequent anticoagulation. Ciculation 1994; 90(4):662A.
97. Schwartz RS, Holmes, D Jr, Topol EJ. The restenosis paradigm revisited: an alternative proposal for cellular mechanism. J Am Coll Cardiol 1992; 20:1284–1293.
98. Blengino S, Maiello L, Hall P, Nakamura S, Martini G, Colombo A. Randomised trial of coronary stent implantation without anti-coagulation: aspirin v ticlopidine. Ciculation 1994; 90(4):665A.
99. Lablanche JM, Bonnet JL, Grollier G, Danchin N, Bedossa M, Van Belle E, Bauters C, Bertrand ME. Ticlopidine Aspirin Stents Evaluation (TASTE): a French multicentre study. Eur Heart J 1995; 16:1408A.
100. Ernst J, Kloos R, Schrader R, Kaltenbach M, Sigwart U, Sanborn TA. Immediate sealing of arterial puncture site after catheterisation and PTCA using a vascular haemostatic device with collagen: an international registery. Circulation 1991; 84(suppl. 2):69.

101. Gibbs JSR, Slade AKB, Blake J, Nordrehaug JE, et al. Femoral arterial hemostasis using a collagen plug after coronary artery stent implantation. J Intervent Card 1992; 5:85–88.
102. Kiemeneiji F, Laarman GJ. Percutaneous transradial artery approach for coronary Palmaz-Schatz stent implantation. Am Heart J 1994; 128(1):167–174.
103. Harker LA, Kelly AB, Hanson SR. Experimental arterial thrombosis in nonhuman primates. Circulation 1991; 83(suppl. 4):41–55.
104. Aggraval RK, Ireland DC, Ezekowitz MD, de Bono DP, Gershlick AH. Antiplatelet glycoprotein IIb/IIIa antibody adsorbed onto polymer coated stents reduces platelet deposition and abolishes cyclical flow variation. Eur Heart J 1995; 16:1406A.
105. Hehrlein C, Gollan C, Dünges K, Metz J, Riessen R, Fehnsenfeld P, von Hodenberg E, Kübler W. Low dose radioactive endovascular stents prevent smooth muscle cell proliferation and neointimal hyperplasia in rabbits. Circulation 1995; 92:1570–1575.
106. Waksman R, Robinson KA, Crocker IR, Gravanis MB, Palmer SJ, Wang C, Cipolla GD, King III SB. Intracoronary radiation before stent implantation inhibits neointima formation in stented porcine coronary arteries. Circulation 1995; 92:1383–1386.

20

Gene Therapy for Restenosis: Status, Issues, and Future Directions

Giora Z. Feuerstein and Robert R. Ruffolo, Jr.
SmithKline Beecham Pharmaceuticals, King of Prussia, Pennsylvania

I. INTRODUCTION

The blood vessel response to injury introduced by PTCA, stents, or artherectomies induces a broad array of transcriptional changes marked by immediate, early, and late gene expression and their products. As reviewed in previous chapters (see Chaps. 2 and 4), numerous growth factors, cytokines, transcription factors, and signal transduction processes as well as cell cycle–associated genes are activated following the injury to the blood vessel wall. Attempts to modulate the expression of specific genes considered essential in the process of restenosis are driven in part by the persistent failure so far of numerous pharmacological interventions to prevent restenosis. The refractory nature of "neointima formation" to treatment by drugs has led many investigators to explore the utility of recombinant genes, introduced directly into vascular cells, for inhibition of cell proliferation—one of the most prominent cellular events in neointima formation. This new field of gene therapy (1), which at the present time can only be viewed as an early experimental endeavor, adds exciting new possibilities for the discovery of new drugs. In this chapter, attempts will be made to analyze the conceptual framework that underpins "gene therapy" for restenosis, the various technical strategies utilized to achieve effective gene transfer, the experimental successes and limitations of this approach, as well as hurdles that must be overcome in order to make gene therapy a clinical reality.

II. METHODOLOGY OF GENE TRANSFER

A. DNA Transfer

Direct administration of cDNA into cells has proven to be a feasible strategy to enable new gene expression in somatic cells. Direct DNA transfer has the obvious advantage of avoiding exposure to viral nucleotides (DNA and RNA), which, as indicated below, is an inherent problem when using viral vectors for gene transfer. However, the rate of transfetion (or efficiency of uptake) with "naked DNA" is very low (<1%), and for vascular targets, systemic injections are impractical. Targeted DNA transfer can be enhanced by local administration of the DNA in a carrier medium (e.g., hydrogel coating) that is applied on the vessel wall directly. In fact, the first approved human protocol for vascular gene transfer is based on direct transfer of DNA encoding vascular endothelial growth factor (VEGF). An important additional advantage of the "direct DNA" transfer strategy is that the "transgene" (the gene that is transferred) is not incorporated into the cell's genomic DNA, thus avoiding the possibility of insertional mutations. Obviously, the limitation of this approach is that the expression of the transgene is transient, as the nonprotected DNA is eventually destroyed or the transgene product is diluted out by cell proliferation.

B. Liposome-Mediated Gene Transfer

Liposomes have been used extensively to aid in DNA transfer. Liposomes are a mixture of cationic and neutral lipids that form micellar structures in an aqueous environment. Liposome components are capable of complexing with DNA and fusing with cell membranes, thereby delivering the liposome-associated DNA into the cell. Liposomes have been used for recombinant gene transfer in vascular cells in vitro and in vivo. In a pioneer study, Nabel et al. (2) demonstrated the expression of a reporter gene, lacZ, in endothelial cells and smooth muscle cells of Yucatan minipigs treated with a lipofectin reagent complexed with the lacZ gene. Although the efficiency of gene transfer in this experiment (as judged by the percentage of endothelial cells and smooth muscle cells expressing lacZ) was below 1%, the same investigators were able to show that phenotypic consequences could be elicited by the DNA-liposome gene-transfer method (3). Most notably, liposomes complexed with the recombinant fibroblast growth factor (FGF) gene or the recombinant platelet-derived growth factor (PDGF-B) gene (4) were able to cause intimal hyperplasia and angiogenesis (3–5) in pig arteries. Successful expression of reporter genes with comparable low efficacy has also been reported by other groups (6,7).

These studies clearly demonstrate the usefulness of liposomes to make possible gene transfer to vascular tissue and, in particular, to endothelial and smooth muscle cells. While the efficiency of gene transfer by this method is extremely low, the functinal outcomes as demonstrated in several of these studies, such as the FGF gene-transfer study (5), are remarkable as reflected by the robust phenotypic modification of the vessel histology and the ultimate appearance of neointima that shares significant resemblence to the neointima formed after PTCA. These studies, while proving the potential utility of liposome vehicles for effective gene transfer, are still quite remote from being utilized as therapeutic vehicles.

III. VIRAL VECTORS FOR GENE TRANSFER

A. Retroviruses

The utility of viruses for gene transfer has been primarily motivated by the need to improve the efficiency of the gene-transfer process. The superior efficiency of viral vectors has been clearly demonstrated in direct comparisons with "naked" DNA and liposome-DNA complexes (2,8). The most significant limitation in using retroviruses for gene transfer is that the retrovirus integrates into the genome of the transfected cells and, therefore, may carry the liability of insertional mutagenesis (i.e., disruption of a host gene at the site of the transferred gene). Insertional mutagenesis may result in either "silencing" or "activation" of host genes that could persist as long as the infection with the viral vector is active. For successful retroviral-mediated gene transfer, cell replication appears to be important (9). This prerequisite minimizes the succes rate of gene transfer into somatic vascular cells that are known to replicate at a very low rate (especially smooth muscle and endothelium). Retroviruses have found widespread use in in vitro transfection studies for gene transfer to smooth muscle cells (10–12) and endothelial cells (13–15) that actively undergo cellular replication. Such cells have been then "seeded" onto the arterial wall, where successful cell viability and gene expression could be maintained for extended periods (months). The practical wide scale utility of ex vivo cell transfection and in vivo implantation are at present a remote possibility in vascular therapy.

B. Adenoviruses

Replication-deficient adenoviruses have been engineered, and these currently represent the most advanced and promising technology for transient, high-efficiency, and versatile gene transfer (16,17). These engineered adenoviruses provide the following advantages for gene transfer:

1. Adenoviruses are capable of infecting a wide variety of cells, either replicating or nonreplicating.
2. A high rate of gene transfer can be demonstrated by diverse routes of administration (intravenous, intraarterial, intramuscular, inhalational) (17–19).
3. Engineered adenoviruses are capable of accommodating relatively large cDNA inserts (approximately 10 kb).
4. Very high titer stocks of these viruses can be produced (10^{11} PFU/ml) (20), which are 4–5 orders of magnitude higher than those used in retroviral vectors.
5. Adenoviruses do not integrate into the host genome and are not considered oncogenic or associated with chronic infections (20).

Wild-type adenoviruses are double-stranded, linear DNA viruses known to cause mild flulike symptoms (20). The adenovirus genome is approximately 34 kb in size. The replication-defective adenoviruses engineered for gene therapy have a deletion of the E1 region of their genome. Because the E1 region encodes two early transcriptional regulatory proteins (E1A and E1B) that induce late viral genes important in the viral lytic cycle, these engineered adenoviruses do not replicate. Some adenoviruses also carry deletions of the E3 region (a non–replication-essential region) that provide further "space" in the viral genome for large promoter cDNA insertions. E1-deleted adenoviruses are grown in "permissive" cell lines that express the E1 protein. Such cells are then transfected with a linearized plasmid containing part of the adenovirus genome, a promoter-cDNA cassette, and the remaining part of the wild-type adenovirus genome. A recombinant replication-defective adenovirus is generated through an intracellular homologous recombination event between the plasmid and the adenovirus DNA. After plaque purification, high titer viral stocks are produced by infection of "permissive" cells in vitro. Successful gene transfer using replication deficient adenoviruses has been demonstrated in myocardium, coronary arteries, and large peripheral blood vessels. For example, infusion of 10^9 PFU of AdRSVβGal containing the lacZ marker gene into neonatal mice resulted in lacZ expression in many organs, including the heart, where approximately 0.2% of the myocytes were actively expressing the lacZ gene (21). Most interesting was the observation that the expression of the lacZ gene persisted more than one year without evidence of incorporation of the adenovirus genome into the mouse chromosome.

In a sheep model, 10^9–10^{10} PFU of AdRSVβ*Gal containing the lacZ gene or Ad* α1AT (human α_1-antitrypsin cDNA driven by the Ad2 major late promoter) were infused (over 15 min) into the lumens of occluded carotid arteries or internal jugular vein segments; the expression of the α_1-AT genes was observed for 2 weeks. The expression of both genes was highly efficient, but was restricted to the endothelial layer (22).

The efficiency and stability of recombinant gene expression in the heart and coronary arteries after percutaneous, transluminal administration of replication-defective adenoviruses into the coronary arteries was also demonstrated by Barr et al. (17). In these studies, 10^9–10^{10} PFU of AdCMV-lacZ (lacZ gene controlled by cytomegalovirus promoter/enhancer) were infused directly into the coronary arteries of adult rabbits. LacZ gene expression and viral DNA (monitored by PCR) were followed for 2 months. At 5 days after the infection, 60–80% of the cardiac myocytes demonstrated β-galactosidase staining throughout the heart, and the levels were 50- to 100-fold higher compared to injection of "naked" DNA (23). Interestingly, high levels of lacZ expression were also observed throughout the vascular tree and in particular in the terminal capillaries. The overall efficiency of this method was also 50- to 100-fold greater than that observed with liposome-mediated gene transfer into vascular tissue (2,6).

Although the efficiency of gene transfer to the heart after intracoronary administration of the adenovirus construct was impressively high, the period of gene expression was relatively short; after 2 weeks, the expression levels were markedly reduced, and no evidence of lacZ gene expression was observed at 1 month. It is also important to note that while the recombinant viral inoculation was local (intracoronary), PCR for adenovirus DNA revealed widespread presence in lung, liver, brain, kidney, and other organs.

In summary, replication-defective adenovirus vectors represent a highly efficient strategy for gene transfer into many cell types of the cardiovascular system. However, key issues that remain to be resolved include (1) the transient nature of gene expression, especially in adult humans; (2) immune response directed against the infected cells; (3) safety issues resulting from widespread adenovirus infection of most, if not all, organs; and (4) the potential (although rare) for recombination between the recombinant virus and any wild-type adenovirus that might be present in the host cells.

These concerns, while subject to significant research, cannot overshadow the promise of potential usefulness of the recombinant adenovirus technology for treatment of some cardiovascular diseases and in particular restenosis following PTCA. However, significant efforts over many years will be required to resolve these issues.

IV. GENES AND OLIGONUCLEOTIDE TREATMENT FOR RESTENOSIS

A. Transgenes

The ability to deliver specific genes to vascular cells in vitro and in vivo, using any of the technologies described above, has stimulated many investigations aimed at utilizing these technologies for specific gene therapy in vascular diseases. In particular, restenosis has been targeted as one of the primary cardiovascular diseases for recombinant DNA–based therapeutics, since early studies using primarily antisense DNA transfer technology have been encouraging. In particular, experiments in animal models have demonstrated the feasibility to express specific genes and their products in vivo and to modulate the phenomenon of vascular remodeling (cell proliferation, migration, activation).

1. Dominant Negative Transgenes

Genes associated with vascular smooth muscle cell replication have been extensively studied, and most notable among these are growth factors, cell-cycle promoters, and transcription factors. As noted above, PDGF and FGF have been implicated in neointima formation due to their growth-promoting actions on vascular smooth muscle cells. As both PDGF and FGF gene transfer to blood vessels have been shown to produce neointima-like growth (4,5), these growth factor genes could become potential targets for gene-transfer therapy with the aim of interrupting the production and/or signal transduction elements that mediate the PDGF and FGF pro-proliferative effects. Such a strategy could include a dominant-negative *ras*-gene, a common component of the PDGF, FGF, and EGF signal-transduction pathways in smooth muscle cells (25,26).

Another strategy to inhibit the robust proliferative response of smooth muscle cells would exploit essential cell-cycle elements that are critical for cell replication. Candidate genes include Rb (retinoblastoma gene family), the cyclins and cyclin-dependent kinases (CDKs), as well as phosphatases and the CDK inhibitory gene, p53. A most promising strategy is that of a recombinant gene that produces a dominant-negative mutant protein (e.g., a nonphosphorylatable variant), which interrupts the cell-cycle progression by overwhelming the cell with a protein variant that does not allow progression of cell cycle. An example of this possibility is the capacity to block smooth muscle cell-cycle progression by insertion of an Rb-mutant gene (encoding a nonphosphorylatable Rb variant) whose expression in vivo suppresses neointima formation.

2. *Suppressor Transgenes*

A different strategy for inhibiting restenosis involves a suppression of vascular smooth muscle proliferation utilizing genes that provide products that inhibit smooth muscle cell growth. This strategy may have the advantage of utilizing diffusable factors that may affect cells that have not been directly transfected (intentionally or nonintentionally) by the transgene. The number of candidate genes that could deliver such soluble factors is rather diverse, and careful selection of the most appropriate genes is clearly an issue. A recent example of successful inhibition of restenosis (in animals) using this strategy involved nitric oxide synthase transgene overexpression (27). Nitric oxide is a potent regulator of vascular smooth muscle cell activation (by suppression of smooth muscle cell responsiveness to mitogenic and contractile stimuli). Thus, the production of nitric oxide at the vessel injury site by even a small percentage of the cells could afford significant protection to all of the cells because of the highly diffusable nature of this molecule, thereby inhibiting neighboring cells even though transfection of the gene has not occurred. This particular example may be of special interest because nitric oxide is an inhibitor of smooth muscle cell activation by a variety of mitogens and is also a potent vasodilating factor (thereby providing for a larger lumen diameter) and a potent inhibitor of platelet aggregation (which will minimize the potential for thrombosis).

3. *Pro-Drug Gene Therapy*

A third strategy that has been successfully deployed to inhibit neointima formation by transgene utilizes genes that express enzymes capable of converting an inert drug to a highly cytotoxic chemical at a certain desired locale. Such a strategy is exemplified by transfer of the herpes simplex virus (HSV) gene, thymidine kinase (tk), into a site where inhibition of cell proliferation is desired. In several recent studies, an adenovirus encoding HSV-tk has been utilized to inhibit smooth muscle cell proliferation after balloon angioplasty of pig femoral vessels (28) or rat carotid arteries (29,30). In each study, successful expression of the tk gene allowed for treatment of the animals with ganciclovir (a nonactive pro-drug), which is phosphorylated locally in the cells that expressed tk, thereby converting the pro-drug ganciclovir to a nucleoside analog that is incorporated into the elongating DNA of the replicating cells, which ultimately results in termination of replication and cell-growth arrest. This strategy was effective in reducing neointima formation by approximately 50%, as shown in Figure 1. Other pro-drug transgene therapy may exploit bacterial cytosine deaminase, an enzyme that metabolizes 5-fluorocytosine (an antifungal agent) to 5-fluorouracil, a potent antiproliferative chemotherapeutic agent (31). The

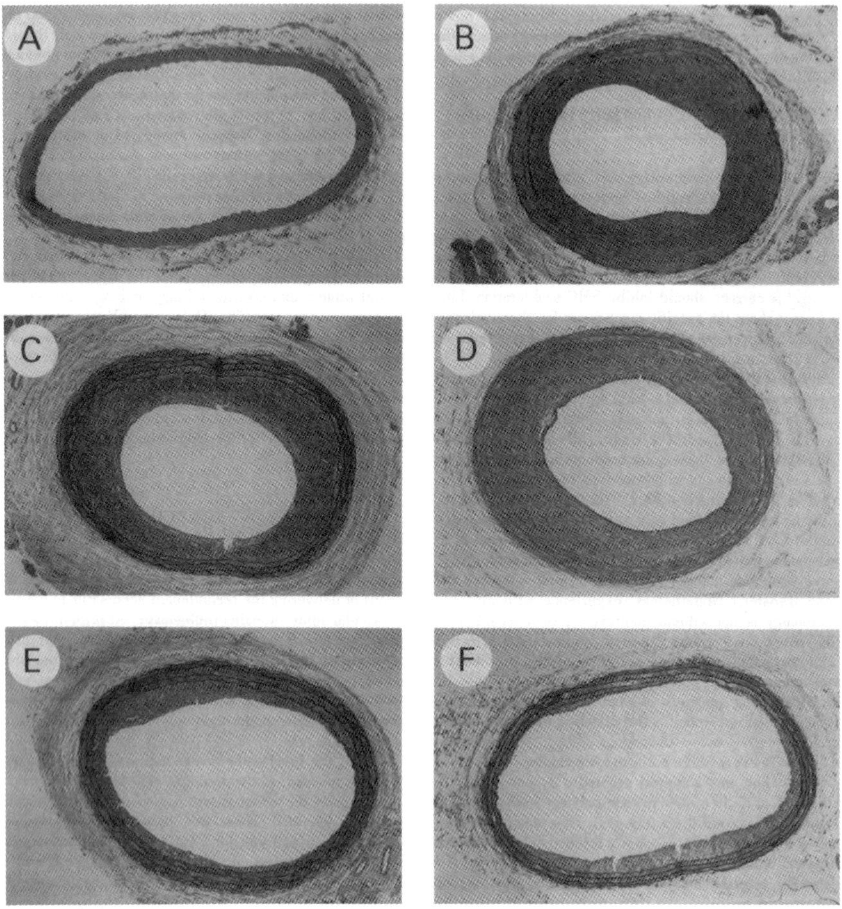

Figure 1 Examples of the therapeutic use of adenoviral gene transfer in an animal model of balloon injury. Rat carotid arteries were balloon-injured and subsequently exposed to either a control adenovirus (AdRSV.β/CAL) or the therapeutic virus (AdMLP.HSTK). Animals were then randomized to receive ganciclovir or saline injections. As described in the text, only HSV-tk expression along with ganciclovir treatment should result in inhibition of smooth muscle proliferation. The panels show (A) uninjured carotid artery; (B) arterial segment exposed to vehicle only; (C) arterial segment infected with 1×10^9 pfu of AdRSV.βgal with systemic ganciclovir treatment (30 mg/kg twice daily); (D) arterial segment infected with 1×10^9 pfu of AdMLP.HSTK without ganciclovir treatment; (E) arterial segment infected with 1×10^9 pfu of AdMLP.HSTK with systemic ganciclovir treatment (30 mg/kg twice daily); and (F) additional arterial segment infected with 1×10^9 pfu of AdMLP.HSTK and treated with systemic ganciclovir (30 mg/kg twice daily). (From Ref. 44.)

main advantage of a pro-drug gene-therapy approach is safety, inasmuch as the cytotoxic effects are confined to a specific locale, and the pro-drug agent can be delivered in a highly regulated manner including by systemic routes.

The strategies discussed above are not selective for blood vessel, as the adenovirus (nonreplicating) vehicle for the gene to be transferred has no particular selectivity for vascular cells. Therefore, local delivery at the blood vessel wall is likely to be required to minimize side effects and to maximize therapeutic efficacy. Indeed, local delivery systems are now being extensively explored with new experimental balloon catheters and stent technology.

B. Antisense Oligonucleotide Strategies for Treatment of Restenosis

Antisense nucleotides are short (15–30 bp) DNA molecules that correspond in sequence to the noncoding DNA strand or the antisense sequence of a target mRNA. Such oligonucleotides are capable of suppressing the expression of specific genes by (1) annealing to the complementary portion of the target mRNA, thereby preventing transport of the mRNA from the nucleus into the cytoplasm; (2) enhancing mRNA degradation by RNAase H; (3) interfering with translation (32); (4) interacting with double-stranded DNA; and (5) interaction with proteins. Antisense nucleotides possess features that make them attractive tools and potential drugs for regulation of cellular DNA transcription and mRNA translation processes. In particular, oligonucleotides can enter cells by simple diffusion across the cell membrane, and therefore have the potential to access all cell types in vivo. Furthermore, antisense oligonucleotides act in a non-replication-dependent manner (unlike retroviruses). In addition, antisense oligonucleotides carry no hazard of incorporation into the cell genome, thereby improving the safety profile. Most importantly, antisense oligonucleotides are synthetic molecules that can be synthesized in large quantities, are of high purity and relatively low cost. Finally, antisense nucleotides, unlike any form of viral vector, are not expected to serve as templates for foreign proteins that could be subject to immune response.

While antisense oligonucleotides have many significant advantages, they are not free of limitations. First, as in the case with "naked" DNA, they are not specific for any cell type and therefore must be delivered locally to minimize spread. Second, the efficiency of DNA delivery to the cells is low, requiring very high concentrations and longer "contact time" with the tissue. Although improved stability of antisense oligonucleotides by chemical modification has been progressing steadily, the uptake rate remains quite low. Third, the pharmacokinetics of even the most stable antisense oligonucleotides is still far from satisfactory and is still in the order of minutes (32).

Antisense oligonucleotides have been used rather extensively in experimental models of restenosis. Early studies using antisense oligonucleotides directed towards the proto-oncogene c-myb, a transcription-activation factor associated with vascular smooth muscle cell proliferation, resulted in significant suppression of neointima formation after PTCA when applied locally (using pluronic gel) to rat carotid artery adventitia (33,34). These studies demonstrated the suppression of c-myb mRNA, which is normally robustly expressed in smooth muscle cells at the injury site. Successful in vivo experiments using a variety of antisense oligonucleotides to inhibit neointima formation and restenosis have been reported. These include antisense oligonucleotides to c-myc (35–38), cdc 2 kinase (39–41), and PCNA (42,43). These gene products are all localized to the nucleus of the cell, where they play a critical role in regulating cell-cycle progression and cell replication. The results from those studies emphasize the potential of antisense oligonucleotide technology in regulating vascular pathologies associated with acute or chronic injuries. However, the key issues in transforming antisense oligonucleotide from basic research tools to drug therapy remain largely unresolved. The most important issues in the development hurdles are delivery of the antisense oligonucleotides and pharmacokinetics.

V. SUMMARY

The proliferation of knowledge concerning the pathophysiological mechanisms involved in neointima formation and vascular remodeling has revealed a number of exciting opportunities for nontraditional strategies to combat restenosis. The recognition of the role of new gene expression in the proliferation, migration, and activation of vascular smooth muscle cells subjected to acute injury by the various procedures (PTCA, stent, endarterectomy) has led to a number of novel approaches directed at inhibiting the variety of responses that comprise the vascular response to injury. Proof of concept has been achieved by using direct cDNA transfer or sophisticated vehicles to deliver transgenes in the form of viral carriers that produce high levels of transfection in vivo. Synthetic oligonucleotides (antisense) have also been deployed with no lesser efficacy than transgene therapy. However, regardless of the strategy adopted, the key issues remain formidable: efficacy in gene transfer to humans, safety, delivery, immune reactions, and long-term consequences.

These difficulties, however, are primarily technical in nature and may not deter the drive for clinical development of one or another form of gene/DNA therapy that provides patients with benefits that far surpass the risk.

In fact, experimental clinical trials with transgenes have commenced (e.g., VEGF transgene to provide angiogenesis in areas of insufficient circulation). It is likely that regulatory agencies will continue to grant approval for investigation of many such therapies (transgene, antisense oligonucleotide, "naked" cDNA) well beyond the turn of the century.

REFERENCES

1. Swain JL. Gene therapy: a new approach to the treatment of cardiovascular disease. Circulation 1989; 80:1495–1496.
2. Nabel E, Plautz G, Nabel GJ. Site-specific gene expression in vivo by direct gene transfer into the arterial wall. Science 1990; 249:1285–1288.
3. Nabel E, Plautz G, Nabel GJ. Transduction of a foreign histocompatibility gene into the arterial wall induces vasculitis. Proc Natl Acad Sci 1992; 89:5157–5161.
4. Nabel E, Yang Z, Lipay S, San H, Gordon D, Haudenschild CC, Nabel GJ. Recombinant platelet-derived growth factor B gene expression in porcine arteries induces intimal hyperplasia in vivo. J Clin Invest 1993; 91:1822–1829.
5. Nabel E, Yang Z, Plautz G, et al. Recombinant fibroblast growth factor-1 promotes intimal hyperplasia and angiogenesis in arteries in vivo. Nature 1993; 362:844–846.
6. Leclerc G, Gal D, Takeshita S, et al. Percutaneous arterial gene transfer in a rabbit model: efficiency in normal and balloon-dilated atherosclerotic arteries. J Clin Invest 1992; 90:936, 944.
7. Lim C, Chapman G, Gammon RS, et al. Direct in vivo gene transfer into the coronary and peripheral vasculature of the intact dog. Circulation 1991; 83:2007–2011.
8. Flugelman MY, Yaklitsch MT, Newman KD, Cassells W, Branthauer GL, Dichek DA. Low level in vivo gene transfer into the arterial wall through a perforated balloon catheter. Circulation 1992; 85:1110–1117.
9. Miller DG, Adam MA, Miller AD. Gene transfer by retrovirus vectors occurs only in cells that are actively replicating at the time of infection. Mol Cell Biol 1990; 10:4239–4242.
10. Plautz G, Nabel EG, Nabel GJ. Introduction of vascular smooth muscle cells expressing recombinant genes in vivo. Circulation 1991; 83:578–583.
11. Lynch CM, Clowes MM, Osborne WRA, Clowes AW, Miller AD. Long term expression of human adenosine deaminase in vascular smooth muscle cells in rats: a model for gene therapy. Proc Natl Acad Sci 192; 89:1138–1142.
12. Clowes MM, Lynch CM, Miller AD, Miller DG, Osborne WR, Clowes AW. Long term biological response of injured rat carotid artery seeded with smooth muscle cells expressing retrovirally introduced human genes. J Clin Invest 1994; 93:644–651.
13. Nabel EG, Plautz G, Boyce FM, Stanley JC, Nabel GJ. Recombinant gene expression in vivo within endothelial cells of the arterial wall. Science 1989; 244:1342–1344.

14. Wilson JM, Birinyi LK, Salomon RN, Libby P, Callows AD, Mulligan RC. Implantation of vascular grafts lined with genetically modified endothelial cells. Science 1989; 244:1344–1346.
15. Messina LM, Podrazik RM, Whitehill TA, Eshterae D, Brothers TE, Wilson JM, Burkel WE, Stanley JC. Adhesion and incorporation of lac2-transfected endothelial cells into the intact capillary wall in the rat. Proc Natl Acad Sci 1992; 80:12018–12022.
16. Yoshimura K, Rosenfeld M, Seth P, et al. Adenovirus-mediated augmentation of cell transfection with unmodified plasmid vectors. J Biol Chem 1993; 268:2300–2303.
17. Barr E, Caroll J, Tripathy SK, Kozarsky K, Wilson J, Leiden JM. Efficient cathet-mediated gene transfer into the heart using replication-defective adenovirus. Gene Ther 1994; 1:51–58.
18. Rosenfeld M, Siegfried L, Yoshimura M, et al. In vivo transfer of the human cystic fibrosis transmembrane conductance regulator gene to the airway epithelium. Cell 1992; 68:143–155.
19. Quantin B, Perricaudet L, Jajbakhsh S, et al. Adenovirus as an expression vector in muscle cells in vivo. Proc Natl Acad Sci 1992; 89:2581–2586.
20. Berkner K. Development of adenovirus vectors of the expression of heterologous genes. Biotechniques 1988; 6:616–629.
21. Stratford-Perricaudet L, Makeh I, Perricaudet M, et al. Widespread long term gene transfer to mouse skeletal muscle and heart. J Clin Invest 1992; 90:626–630.
22. Lemarchand P, Jones M, Yamada I, et al. In vivo gene transfer and expression in normal uninjured blood vessels using replication-deficient recombinant adenovirus vectors. Circ Res 1993; 72:1132–1138.
23. Lin H, Parmacek M, Morle G, et al. Expression of recombinant genes in myocardium in vivo after direct injection of DNA. Circulation 1990; 82:2217–2221.
24. Cai H, Szeberenyl J, Cooper G. Effect of dominant inhibitory Ha-ras mutation on mitogenic signal transduction in NIH 3T3 cells. Mol Cell Biol 1990; 10:5314–5323.
25. Irani K, Herzlinger S, Finkel T. Ras proteins regulate multiple mitogenic pathways in A10 vascular smooth muscle cells. Biochem Biophys Res Commun 1994; 202:1252–1258.
26. Chang MW, Barr E, Seltzer J, Jiang Y-Q, Nabel GJ, Nabel EG, Parmacek MS, Leiden JM. Cytostatic gene therapy for vascular proliferative disorders with a constitutively active form of the retinoblastoma gene product. Science 1995; 267:518–522.
27. Leyen von der HE, Gibbons GH, Morishita, Lewis NP, Zhang L, Nakajima M, Kaneda Y, Cooke JP, Dzau VJ. Gene therapy inhibiting neointimal vascular lesion: in vivo transfer of endothelial cell nitric oxide synthene gene. Proc Natl Acad Sci 1995; 92:1137–1141.
28. Ohno T, Gordon D, San H, Pompili VJ, Imperiale MJ, Nabel GJ, Nabel EG. Gene therapy for vascular smooth muscle cell proliferation after arterial injury. Science 1994; 265:781–784.

29. Guznau RJ, Hirschowitz EA, Brody SL, Crystal RG, Epstein SE, Finkel T. In vivo suppression of injury induced vascular smooth muscle cell accumulation using adenovirus mediated transfer of the herpes simplex virus thymidine kinase gene. Proc Natl Acad Sci 1994; 91:10732–10736.
30. Chang, MW, Ohno T, Gordon D, Lu MM, Nabel GJ, Nabel EG, Leiden JM. Adenovirus-mediated transfer of the herpes simplex virus thymidine kinase gene inhibits vascular smooth muscle cell proliferation and neointima formation following balloon angioplasty of the rat carotid artry. Mol Med 1995; 1:172–181.
31. Huber BE, Austin EA, Richards CA, Davis ST, Good SS. Metabolism of 5-fluorocytosine to 5-fluorouracil in human colorectal tumor cells transduced with the cytosine deaminase gene: significant antitumor effects when only a small percentage of tumor cells express cytosine deaminase. Proc Natl Acad Sci 1994; 91:8302–8306.
32. Leonetti J, Degols G, Clarone JP, et al. Cell delivery and mechanisms of action of antisense oligonucleotides. Prog Nuc Acid Res Mol Biol 1993; 44:143–166.
33. Simons M, Rosenberg R. Antisense nonmuscle myosin heavy chain and c-myb oligonucleotides suppress smooth muscle cell proliferation in vitro. Circ Res 1992; 70:835–843.
34. Simons M, Edelman E, Dekeyser J-L, et al. Antisense c-myb, oligonucleotides inhibit intimal arterial smooth muscle cell accumulation in vivo. Nature 1992; 359:67–70.
35. Biro S, Fu YM, Yu ZX, Epstein SE. Inhibitory effects of antisense oligodeoxynucleotides targeting c-myc mRNA on smooth muscle cell proliferation and migration. Proc Natl Acad Sci USA 1993; 90:654–658.
36. Shi Y, Hutchinson HG, Hall DJ, Zalewski A. Downregulation of c-myc expression by antisense oligonucleotides inhibits proliferation of human smooth muscle cells. Circulation 1993; 88:1190–1195.
37. Shi Y, Fard A, Galeo A, Hutchinson HG, Vermani P, Dodge GR, Hall DJ, Shaheen F, Zalewski A. Transcatheter delivery of c-myc antisense oligomers reduces neointimal formation in a procine model of coronary artery balloon injury. Circulation 1994; 90:944–951.
38. Bennett MR, Anglin S, McEwan JR, Jagoe R, Newby AC, Evan CI. Inhibition of vascular smooth muscle cell proliferation *in vitro* and *in vivo* by c-myc antisense oligodeoxynucleotides. J Clin Invest 1994; 93:820–828.
39. Morishita R, Gibbons GH, Ellison KE, Nakajima M, Zhang, L, Kaneda Y, Ogihara T, Dzau VJ. Single intraluminal delivery of antisense CDC2 kinase and PCNA oligonucleotides results in chronic inhibition of neointimal hyperplasia. Proc Natl Acad Sci USA 1993; 90:8474–8478.
40. Morishita R, Gibbons GH, Ellison KE, Nakajima M, von der Leyen H, Zhang L, Kaneda Y, Ogihara T, Dzau VJ. Intimal hyperplasia after vascular injury is inhibited by antisense cdk 2 kinase oligonucleotides. J Clin Invest 1994; 93:1458–1464.
41. Abe J, Zhou W, Taguchi J, Takuwa N, Miki K, Okazaki H, Kurokawa K, Kumada M, Takuwa Y. Suppression of neointimal smooth muscle cell accumu-

lation *in vivo* by antisense cdc2 and cdk2 oligonucleotides in rat carotid artery. Biochem Biophys Res Commun 1994; 198:161–24.
42. Speir E, Epstein SE. Inhibition of smooth muscle cell proliferation by an antisense oligodeoxynucleotide targeting the mRNA encoding PCNA. Circulation 1992; 86:538–547.
43. Simons M, Edelman ER, Rosenberg RD. Antisense proliferating cell nuclear antigen oligonucleotides inhibit intimal hyperplasia in a rat carotid artery injury model. J Clin Invest 1994; 93:2351–2356.
44. Finkel T, Epstein SE. Gene therapy for vascular disease. FASEB J 1995; 843–851.

Index

About the Editor

GIORA Z. FEUERSTEIN is Director of the Department of Cardiovascular Pharmacology at SmithKline Beecham Pharmaceuticals, King of Prussia, Pennsylvania. The author or coauthor of over 500 professional papers, he is a member of the American Heart Association and the American Society for Pharmacology and Experimental Therapeutics, among other organizations. Dr. Feuerstein received the M.Sc. degree (1970) in pharmacology from the Hebrew University of Jerusalem, Israel, and the M.D. degree (1973) from Hadassah Medical School, Jerusalem, Israel.